SEVENTH EDITION

Nursing Diagnosis Reference Manual

"Problem" (Nanda Nursing Diagnosis) (ex Spiritual distress)

as related to "cause" - What causes or

contributes to the development of the problem

(Spiritual distress related to death of husband)

as evidenced by - defining characteristics of the problem

Spiritual distress related to the death of husband as evidenced by tearfulness and subjective comment "Why did God allow this to happen?"

Never state a medical diagnosis

SEVENTH EDITION

Nursing Diagnosis Reference Manual

Sheila Sparks Ralph, RN, PhD, FAAN
Professor, Division of Nursing
Shenandoah University
Winchester, Virginia
Member NANDA-I Foundation
Philadelphia

Cynthia M. Taylor, RN, MS
Nurse Consultant
Coordinator, Parish Nurse Program
St. Michael's Church
Kailua Kona, Hawaii

 Wolters Kluwer | Lippincott Williams & Wilkins
Health
Philadelphia · Baltimore · New York · London
Buenos Aires · Hong Kong · Sydney · Tokyo

STAFF

Executive Publisher
Judith A. Schilling McCann, RN, MSN

Editorial Director
H. Nancy Holmes

Clinical Director
Joan M. Robinson, RN, MSN

Art Director
Elaine Kasmer

Editorial Project Manager
Jennifer L.D. Kowalak

Copy Editors
Kimberly Bilotta (supervisor),
Carol Brown, Heather Ditch,
Jeannine Fielding, Shana Harrington,
Liz Mooney, Dona Perkins,
Carolyn Petersen, Lisa Stockslager,
Dorothy P. Terry, Pamela Wingrod

Designers
Susan Hopkins Rodzewich (project
manager), Joseph John Clark

Digital Composition Services
Diane Paluba (manager),
Joyce Rossi Biletz, Donald G. Knauss,
Donna S. Morris

Associate Manufacturing Manager
Beth J. Welsh

Editorial Assistants
Karen J. Kirk, Jeri O'Shea,
Linda K. Ruhf

Indexer
Barbara E. Hodgson

Credits
NANDA-I nursing diagnoses, definitions, defining
characteristics or risk factors: © NANDA-
International (2007). *NANDA-I Nursing
Diagnoses: Definitions and Classification 2007-
2008.* Philadelphia: NANDA-I, 2007.
Suggested NOC labels: Moorhead, S., Johnson,
M., and Maas, M. *Nursing Outcomes Classification
(NOC),* 3rd ed. St. Louis: Mosby, 2004.
Suggested NIC labels: Dochterman, J.M., and
Bulechek, G.M.. *Nursing Interventions Classifica-
tion (NIC),* 4th ed. St. Louis: Mosby, 2004.

NDRM7E011107

Library of Congress Cataloging-in-Publication
Data

Ralph, Sheila Sparks.
  Sparks and Taylor's nursing diagnosis reference
manual / Sheila Sparks Ralph, Cynthia M. Taylor.—
7th ed.
    p. ; cm.
  Includes bibliographical references and index.
  1. Nursing diagnosis—Handbooks, manuals, etc.
I. Taylor, Cynthia M. II. Title. III. Title: Nursing
diagnosis reference manual.
  [DNLM: 1. Nursing Diagnosis—Handbooks. 2.
Patient Care Planning—Handbooks. WY 49 R163s
2008]
RT48.6.S66 2008
616.07′5—dc22
ISBN-13: 978-0-7817-7178-8 (alk. paper)
ISBN-10: 0-7817-7178-1 (alk. paper)   2007032753

Contents

Contributors

Blair Belkin, MSN, RN-C, CHPN
Shenandoah University
Winchester, Va.

Elizabeth Tayloe Courts, RN, MSN, CFNP
Assistant Professor
Shenandoah University
Winchester, Va.

Kathryn M. Ganske PhD, RN
Assistant Professor
Shenandoah University
Winchester, Va.

Eleanor L. Gooch, RN,C, MSN
Adjunct Faculty
Shenandoah University
Winchester, Va.

Pauline M. Green, RN, PhD
Professor
Howard University Division of Nursing
Washington, D.C.

Kathryn Van Dyke Hayes, RN, PhD,
  BC, CNE
Professor
Holy Family University
Philadelphia

Jennifer H. Matthews, APRN,BC, PhD
Associate Professor
Shenandoah University
Winchester, Va.

Helen H. Mautner, RN, MSN
Assistant Professor
Shenandoah University
Winchester, Va.

Marian Newton, PhD, MN, APRN, BC, PMHNP
Professor
Shenandoah University
Winchester, Va.

Nancy J. Pauling, RN, PhD
Associate Professor
Shenandoah University
Winchester, Va.

Laura V. Polk, RN, DNSc
Associate Professor
College of Southern Maryland
La Plata

Janice S. Smith RN, PhD
Assistant Professor
Shenandoah University
Winchester, Va.

Caroline Ann Teames, RN, BSN
Pediatric Nurse
Leesburg, Va.

Preface

For student nurses as well as expert clinicians, *Nursing Diagnosis Reference Manual*, Seventh Edition, offers clearly written, authoritative care plans to help meet patients' health care needs throughout the life span. For this new edition, we added care plans for the 15 newest diagnoses as well as a new section on Wellness. The book also includes the linkages between NANDA International (NANDA-I) and the Nursing Interventions Classification (NIC) and Nursing Outcomes Classification (NOC) labels. You'll find the care plans in this book invaluable in every health care setting you encounter throughout your career.

The nursing process is thoroughly integrated into the material on every page of this book. Providing care based on the nursing process offers benefits to both beginning and experienced nurses. The nursing process:
■ provides a framework for independent nursing action
■ promotes a consistent structure for professional practice
■ helps you focus more precisely on each patient's health care needs.

Nursing Diagnosis Reference Manual, Seventh Edition, provides the information you need to accurately apply the nursing process. It focuses on health problems that you can diagnose legally and treat independently. This manual incorporates all diagnoses approved by NANDA-I.

Nursing Diagnosis Reference Manual, Seventh Edition, begins with an explanation of each step of the nursing process—assessment, nursing diagnosis, outcome identification, planning, implementation, and evaluation. Included in this introductory section are clear guidelines for writing a clinically accurate diagnostic statement. This section also clarifies the distinction between a nursing diagnosis and a medical diagnosis.

After this section come the manual's eight major parts: adult health, adolescent health, child health, maternal-neonatal health, geriatric health, psychiatric and mental health, community-based health, and wellness. Together, these parts include comprehensive care plans for more than 300 nursing diagnostic statements. Each care plan has been written and reviewed by leading nursing clinicians, educators, and researchers. Each one can be used independently and is complete, thereby eliminating the need to search for material in different places.

Care plans

All care plans contain the following sections:
■ *Diagnostic statement.* Each diagnostic statement includes a NANDA-I-approved diagnosis and, in most cases, a related etiology. This edition of the

Nursing Diagnosis Reference Manual contains all the diagnoses approved by NANDA-I to date.

■ *Definition.* This section offers a brief explanation of the diagnosis.

■ *Assessment.* This section suggests parameters to use when collecting data to ensure an accurate diagnosis. Data may include health history, physical findings, psychosocial status, laboratory studies, patient statements, and other subjective and objective information.

■ *Defining characteristics.* This section lists clinical findings that confirm the diagnosis. For diagnoses expressing the possibility of a problem, such as "Risk for injury," this section is labeled *Risk factors.*

■ *Expected outcomes.* Here you'll find realistic goals for resolving or ameliorating the patient's health problem, written in measurable behavioral terms. You should select outcomes that are appropriate to the condition of your patient. Outcomes are arranged to flow logically from admission to discharge of the patient. Outcomes identified by NOC research have been added to correlate with the NANDA-I expected outcomes.

■ *Interventions and rationales.* This section provides specific activities you carry out to help attain expected outcomes. Each intervention contains a rationale, highlighted in italic type. Rationales receive typographic emphasis because they form the premise for every nursing action. You'll find it helpful to consider rationales before intervening. Understanding the why of your actions can help you see that carrying out repetitive or difficult interventions are essential elements of your nursing practice. More importantly, it can improve critical thinking and help you to avoid mistakes. Interventions from NIC research have been added to correlate with the interventions.

■ *Evaluations for expected outcomes.* Here you'll find evaluation criteria for the expected outcomes. These criteria will help you determine whether expected outcomes have been attained or provide support for revising outcomes or interventions to meet changing patient conditions.

■ *Documentation.* This section lists critical topics to include in your documentation—for example, patient perceptions, status, and response to treatment as well as nursing observations and interventions. Using the information provided in this section will enable you to write the careful, concise documentation required to meet professional nursing standards.

Appendices

The manual includes an appendix that lists nursing diagnoses commonly found in patients with specific medical diagnoses or medical issues as well as one that groups nursing diagnoses by Gordon's functional health patterns. You will also find appendices labeled NANDA-I taxonomy II domains, classes, and diagnoses; and NNN taxonomy of nursing practice: Placement of nursing diagnoses.

Acknowledgments

We would like to express our sincere appreciation to the nurses who contributed to the *Nursing Diagnosis Reference Manual*, Seventh Edition. Their expertise and commitment to quality patient care made this work possible. We are also grateful to Nancy Holmes, Jennifer Kowalak, and Jean Rodenberger from Lippincott Williams & Wilkins for their assistance and enthusiastic support of our work.

Finally, we dedicate this book to nursing students and clinicians who are striving to provide quality care in today's turbulent health care arena.

Sheila Sparks Ralph, RN, PhD, FAAN
Cynthia M. Taylor, RN, MS

SEVENTH EDITION

Nursing Diagnosis
Reference Manual

The nursing process

The cornerstone of clinical nursing, the nursing process is a systematic method for taking independent nursing action. Steps in the nursing process include:
- assessing the patient's problems
- forming a diagnostic statement
- identifying expected outcomes
- creating a plan to achieve expected outcomes and solve the patient's problems
- implementing the plan or assigning others to implement it
- evaluating the plan's effectiveness.

These phases of the nursing process — assessment, nursing diagnosis formation, outcome identification, care planning, implementation, and evaluation — are dynamic and flexible; they commonly overlap.

Becoming familiar with this process has many benefits. It will allow you to apply your knowledge and skills in an organized, goal-oriented manner. It will also enable you to communicate about professional topics with colleagues from all clinical specialties and practice settings. Using the nursing process is essential to documenting nursing's role in the provision of comprehensive, quality patient care.

The recognition of the nursing process is an important development in the struggle for greater professional autonomy. By clearly defining those problems a nurse may treat independently, the nursing process has helped to dispel the notion that nursing practice is based solely on carrying out physician's orders.

Nursing remains in a state of professional evolution. Nurse researchers and expert practitioners continue to develop a body of knowledge specific to the field. Nursing literature is gradually providing direction to students and seasoned practitioners for evidence-based practice. A strong foundation in the nursing process will enable you to better assimilate emerging concepts and to incorporate these concepts into your practice. (See *Nursing's approach to problem solving*.)

ASSESSMENT

The vital first phase in the nursing process — assessment — consists of the patient history, the physical examination, and pertinent diagnostic studies. The other nursing process phases — nursing diagnosis formation, outcome identification, care planning, implementation, and evaluation — depend on the quality of the assessment data for their effectiveness.

A properly recorded initial assessment provides:
- a way to communicate patient information to other caregivers
- a method of documenting initial baseline data
- the foundation on which to build an effective care plan.

Your initial patient assessment begins with the collection of data (patient history, physical examination findings, and diagnostic study data) and ends with a

Nursing's approach to problem solving

Dynamic and flexible, the phases of the nursing process resemble the steps that many other professions rely on to identify and correct problems. Here's how the nursing process phases correspond to the standard problem-solving method.

NURSING PROCESS	PROBLEM-SOLVING METHOD
Assessment ■ Collect and analyze subjective and objective data about the patient's health problem.	■ Recognize the problem. ■ Learn about the problem by obtaining facts.
Diagnosis ■ State the health problem.	■ State the nature of the problem.
Outcome identification ■ Identify expected outcomes.	■ Establish goals and a time frame for achieving them.
Planning ■ Write a care plan that includes the nursing interventions designed to achieve expected outcomes.	■ Think of and select ways to achieve goals and solve the problem.
Implementation ■ Put the care plan into action. ■ Document the actions taken and their results.	■ Act on ways to solve the problem.
Evaluation ■ Critically examine the results achieved. ■ Review and revise the care plan as needed.	■ Decide if the actions taken have effectively solved the problem.

statement of the patient's risk for, deficiency in, or readiness for enhancement of a nursing diagnosis.

Building a database

The information you collect in taking the patient's history, performing a physical examination, and analyzing test results serves as your assessment database. Your goal is to gather and record information that will be most helpful in assessing your patient. You can't realistically collect — or use — *all* the information that exists about the patient. To limit your database appropriately, ask yourself these questions:

■ What data do I want to collect?

■ How should I collect the data?

■ How should I organize the data to make care planning decisions?

Your answers will help you to be selective in collecting meaningful data during patient assessment.

The well-defined database for a patient may begin with admission signs and symptoms, chief complaint, or medical diagnosis. It may also center on the type of patient care given in a specific setting, such as the intensive care unit (ICU), the emergency department (ED), or an outpatient care center. For example, you wouldn't ask a trauma victim in the ED if she has a family history of breast cancer, nor would you perform a routine breast examination on her. You would, however, do these types of assessment during a comprehensive health checkup in an outpatient care setting.

If you work in a setting where patients with similar diagnoses are treated, choose your database from information pertinent to this specific patient population. Even when addressing patients with similar diagnoses, however, complete a thorough assessment to make sure unanticipated problems don't go unnoticed.

Subjective and objective data

The assessment data you collect and analyze fall into two important categories: subjective and objective. The patient's history, embodying a *personal perspective* of problems and strengths, provides *subjective data*. It's your most important assessment data source. Because it's also the most subjective source of patient information, it must be interpreted carefully.

In the *physical examination* of a patient — involving inspection, palpation, percussion, and auscultation — you collect one form of *objective data* about the patient's health status or about the pathologic processes that may be related to his illness or injury. In addition to adding to the patient's database, this information helps you interpret his history more accurately by providing a basis for comparison. Use it to validate and amplify the historical data. However, don't allow the physical examination to assume undue importance — formulate your nursing diagnosis by considering *all* the elements of your assessment, not just the examination.

Laboratory test results are another objective form of assessment data and the third essential element in developing your assessment. Laboratory values will help you to interpret — and usually, clarify — your history and physical examination findings. The advanced technology used in laboratory tests enables you to assess anatomic, physiologic, and chemical processes that can't be assessed subjectively or by physical examination alone. For example, if the patient complains of fatigue (history) and you observe conjunctival pallor (physical examination), check his hemoglobin level and hematocrit (laboratory data).

Both subjective (history) and objective (physical examination and laboratory test results) data are essential for comprehensive patient assessment. They validate each other and together provide more data than either can provide alone. By considering history, physical examination, and laboratory data in their appropriate relationships to one another, you'll be able to develop a nursing diagnosis on which to formulate an effective care plan.

Taking a complete health history

This portion of the assessment consists of the subjective data you collect from the patient. A complete health history provides the following information about a patient:

- biographical data, including ethnic, cultural, health-seeking and spiritual factors
- chief complaint (or concern)
- history of present illness (or current health status)
- health promotion behaviors, motivation
- past health history
- family medical history
- psychosocial history
- activities of daily living (ADLs)
- review of systems.

Follow this orderly format in taking the patient's history, but allow for modifications based on his chief complaint or concern. For example, the health history of a patient with a localized allergic reaction will be much shorter than that of a patient who complains vaguely of mental confusion and severe headaches.

If the patient has a chief complaint, use information from his health history to decide whether his problems stem from physiologic causes or psychophysiologic maladaptation and how your nursing interventions may help. The depth of such a history depends on the patient's cooperation and your skill in asking insightful questions.

A patient may request a complete physical checkup as part of a periodic (perhaps annual) health maintenance routine. Such a patient may not have a chief complaint; therefore, this patient's health history should be comprehensive, with detailed information about lifestyle, self-image, family and other interpersonal relationships, and degree of satisfaction with current health status.

Be sure to record health history data in an organized fashion so that the information will be meaningful to everyone involved in the patient's care. Some health care facilities provide patient questionnaires or computerized checklists. (See *Using an assessment checklist,* page xvi.) These forms make history-taking easier, but they aren't always available. Therefore, you must know how to take a comprehensive health history without them. This is easy to do if you develop an orderly and systematic method of interviewing. Ask the history questions in the same order every time. With experience, you'll know which types of questions to ask in specific patient situations.

Review of systems

When interviewing the patient, use this review of systems as a guide.

- *General:* overall state of health, ability to carry out ADLs, weight changes, fatigue, exercise tolerance, fever, night sweats, repeated infections
- *Skin:* changes in color, pigmentation, temperature, moisture, or hair distribution; eruptions; pruritus; scaling; bruising; bleeding; dryness; excessive oiliness; growths; moles; scars; rashes; scalp lesions; brittle, soft, or abnormally formed nails; cyanotic nail beds; pressure ulcers
- *Head:* trauma, lumps, alopecia, headaches

Using an assessment checklist

Use an assessment checklist such as this to ensure that you cover all key points during your health history interview. Although the format may vary from one facility to another, all assessment checklist guides include the same key elements.

❏ *Reason for hospitalization or chief complaint:* As patient sees it

❏ *Duration of this problem:* As patient recalls it (Has it affected his lifestyle?)

❏ *Other illnesses and previous experience with hospitalization(s):* Reason, date(s), results, impressions of previous hospitalizations, problems encountered, effect of this hospitalization on education, family, child care, employment, finances

❏ *Observation of patient's condition:* Level of consciousness, well-nourished, healthy, color, skin turgor, senses, headaches, cough, syncope, nausea, seizures, edema, lumps, bruises or bleeding, inflammation, integrity of skin, pressure areas, temperature, range of motion, unusual sensations, paralysis, odors, discharges, pain

❏ *Mental and emotional status:* Cooperative, understanding, anxious, language, expectations, feelings about illness, state of consciousness, mood, self-image, reaction to stress, rapport with interviewer and staff, compatibility with roommate

❏ *Review of systems:* Neurologic, EENT, pulmonary, cardiovascular, GI, genitourinary, skin, reproductive, musculoskeletal, and so forth

❏ *Allergies:* Food, drugs, other allergens, type of reaction

❏ *Medication:* Dosage, why taken, when taken, last dose, does he have it with him, any others taken occasionally, recently, why, use of over-the-counter drugs or cough preparations, use of alcohol or recreational drugs

❏ *Prostheses:* Pacemaker, intermittent positive-pressure breathing unit, tracheostomy tube, drainage tubes, feeding tube, catheter, ostomy appliance, breast form, hearing aid, glasses or contact lenses, dentures, false eye, prosthetic leg, cane, brace, walker, does the patient have the device with him, need anything

❏ *Hygiene patterns:* Dentures, gums, teeth, bath or shower, when taken

❏ *Rest and sleep patterns:* Usual times, aids, difficulties

❏ *Activity status:* Self-care, ambulatory, aids, daily exercise

❏ *Bladder and bowel patterns:* Continent, frequency, nocturia, characteristics of stools and urine, discharge, pain, ostomy, appliances, who cares for these, laxatives, medications

❏ *Meals and diet:* Feeds self, diet restrictions (therapeutic and cultural or preferential), frequency, snacks, allergies, dislikes, fad diets, usual dietary intake

❏ *Health practices:* Breast self-examination, physical examination, Papanicolaou test, testicular self-examination, digital rectal examination, smoking, electrocardiogram, annual chest X-ray, practices related to other conditions, such as glaucoma testing, urine testing, weight control

❏ *Lifestyle:* Parent, family, number of children, residence, occupation, recreation, diversion, interests, financial status, religion, sexuality, education, ethnic background, living environment

❏ *Typical day profile:* As patient describes it

❏ *Informant:* From whom did you obtain this information, patient, family, old records, ambulance driver

■ *Eyes:* nearsightedness, farsightedness, glaucoma, cataracts, blurred vision, double vision, tearing, burning, itching, photophobia, pain, inflammation, swelling, color blindness, injuries (also ask about use of glasses or contact lenses, date of last eye examination, and past surgery to correct vision problems)

■ *Ears:* deafness, tinnitus, vertigo, discharge, pain, tenderness behind the ears, mastoiditis, otitis or other ear infections, earaches, ear surgery

■ *Nose:* sinusitis, discharge, colds, or coryza more than four times per year; rhinitis; trauma; sneezing; loss of sense of smell; obstruction; breathing problems; epistaxis

■ *Mouth and throat:* changes in color or sores on tongue, dental caries, loss of teeth, toothaches, bleeding gums, lesions, loss of taste, hoarseness, sore throats (streptococcal), tonsillitis, voice changes, dysphagia, date of last dental checkup, use of dentures, bridges, or other dental appliances

■ *Neck:* pain, stiffness, swelling, limited movement, or injuries

■ *Breasts:* change in development or lactation pattern, trauma, lumps, pain, discharge from nipples, gynecomastia, changes in contour or in nipples, history of breast cancer (also ask if the patient knows how to perform breast self-examination)

■ *Cardiovascular:* palpitations, tachycardia, or other rhythm irregularities; pain in chest; dyspnea on exertion; orthopnea; cyanosis; edema; ascites; intermittent claudication; cold extremities; phlebitis; orthostatic hypotension; hypertension; rheumatic fever (also ask if an electrocardiogram has been performed recently)

■ *Respiratory:* dyspnea, shortness of breath, pain, wheezing, paroxysmal nocturnal dyspnea, orthopnea (number of pillows used), cough, sputum, hemoptysis, night sweats, emphysema, pleurisy, bronchitis, tuberculosis (contacts), pneumonia, asthma, upper respiratory tract infections (also ask about results of chest X-ray and tuberculin skin test)

■ *Gastrointestinal:* changes in appetite or weight, dysphagia, nausea, vomiting, heartburn, eructation, flatulence, abdominal pain, colic, hematemesis, jaundice (pain, fever, intensity, duration, color of urine), stools (color, frequency, consistency, odor, use of laxatives), hemorrhoids, rectal bleeding, changes in bowel habits

■ *Renal and genitourinary:* color of urine, polyuria, oliguria, nocturia (number of times per night), dysuria, frequency, urgency, problem with stream, dribbling, pyuria, retention, passage of calculi or gravel, sexually transmitted disease (discharge), infections, perineal rashes and irritations, incontinence (stress, functional, total, reflex, urge), protein or sugar ever found in urine

■ *Reproductive:* male—lesions, impotence, prostate problems (also ask about use of contraceptives and whether the patient knows how to perform a testicular self-examination); female—irregular bleeding, discharge, pruritus, pain on intercourse, protrusions, dysmenorrhea, vaginal infections (also ask about number of pregnancies; delivery dates; complications; abortions; onset, regularity, and amount of flow during menarche; last normal menses; use of contraceptives; date of menopause; last Papanicolaou test)

■ *Neurologic:* headaches, seizures, fainting spells, dizziness, tremors, twitches, aphasia, loss of sensation, weakness, paralysis, numbness, tingling, balance problems

■ *Psychiatric:* changes in mood, anxiety, depression, inability to concentrate, phobias, suicidal or homicidal thoughts, hallucinations, delusions

■ *Musculoskeletal:* muscle pain, swelling, redness, pain in joints, back problems, injuries (such as fractured bones, pulled tendons), gait problems, weakness, paralysis, deformities, range of motion, contractures

■ *Hematopoietic:* anemia (type, degree, treatment, response), bleeding, fatigue, bruising (also ask if patient is receiving anticoagulant therapy)

■ *Endocrine* and *metabolic:* polyuria, polydipsia, polyphagia, thyroid problem, heat or cold intolerance, excessive sweating, changes in hair distribution and amount, nervousness, swollen neck (goiter), moon face, buffalo hump

Ensuring a thorough history

When documenting the health history, be sure to record negative findings as well as positive ones; that is, note the absence of symptoms that other history data indicate might be present. For example, if a patient reports pain and burning in his abdomen, ask him if he has experienced nausea and vomiting or noticed blood in his stools. Record the presence or absence of these symptoms.

Remember that the information you record will be used by others who will be caring for the patient. It could even be used as a legal document in a liability case, a malpractice suit, or an insurance disability claim. With these considerations in mind, record history data thoroughly and precisely. Continue your questioning until you're satisfied that you've recorded sufficient detail. Don't be satisfied with inadequate answers, such as "a lot" or "a little"; such subjective terms must be explained within the patient's context to be meaningful. If taking notes seems to make the patient anxious, explain the importance of keeping a written record. To facilitate accurate recording of the patient's answers, familiarize yourself with standard history data abbreviations.

When you complete the patient's health history, it becomes part of the permanent written record. It will serve as a subjective database with which you and other health care professionals can monitor the patient's progress. Remember that history data must be specific and precise. Avoid generalities. Instead, provide pertinent, concise, detailed information that will help determine the direction and sequence of the physical examination — the next phase in your patient assessment.

Physical examination

After taking the patient's health history, the next step in the assessment process is the *physical examination.* During this assessment phase, you obtain objective data that usually confirm or rule out suspicions raised during the health history interview.

Use four basic techniques to perform a physical examination: *inspection, palpation, percussion,* and *auscultation* (IPPA). These skills require you to use your senses of sight, hearing, touch, and smell to formulate an accurate appraisal of the structures and functions of body systems. Using IPPA skills effectively lessens the chances that you'll overlook something important during the physical examination. In addition, each examination technique collects data that validate and amplify data collected through other IPPA techniques.

Accurate and complete physical assessments depend on two interrelated elements. One is the critical act of sensory perception, by which you receive and perceive external stimuli. The other element is the conceptual, or cognitive, process by which you relate these stimuli to your knowledge base. This two-step process gives meaning to your assessment data.

Develop a system for assessing patients that identifies their problem areas in priority order. By performing physical assessments systematically and efficiently instead of in a random or indiscriminate manner, you'll save time and identify priority problems quickly. First, choose an *examination method.* The most commonly used methods for completing a total systematic physical assessment are *head-to-toe* and *major body systems.*

The head-to-toe method is performed by systematically assessing the patient by —as the name suggests—beginning at the head and working toward the toes. Examine all parts of one body region before progressing to the next region to save time and to avoid tiring the patient or yourself. Proceed from left to right within each region so you can make symmetrical comparisons; that is, when examining the head, proceed from the left side of the head to the right side. After completing both sides of one body region, proceed to the next.

The major body systems method of examination involves systematically assessing the patient by examining each body system in priority order or in an established sequence.

Both the head-to-toe and the major-body-systems methods are systematic and provide a logical, organized framework for collecting physical assessment data. They also provide the same information; therefore, neither is more correct than the other. Choose the method (or a variation of it) that works well for you and is appropriate for your patient population. Follow this routine whenever you assess a patient, and try not to deviate from it.

To decide which method to use, first determine whether the patient's condition is life-threatening. Identifying the *priority* problems of a patient suffering from a life-threatening illness or injury—for example, severe trauma, a heart attack, or GI hemorrhage—is essential to preserve his life and function and prevent additional damage.

Next, identify the *patient population* to which the patient belongs, and take the common characteristics of that population into account in choosing an examination method. For example, elderly or debilitated patients tire easily; for these patients, you should select a method that requires minimal position changes. You may also defer parts of the examination to avoid tiring the patient.

Try to view the patient as an integrated whole rather than as a collection of parts, regardless of the examination method you use. Remember, the integrity of a body *region* may reflect adequate functioning of many body *systems,* both inside and outside the region in question. For example, the integrity of the chest region may provide important clues about the functioning of the cardiovascular and respiratory systems. Similarly, the integrity of a body *system* may reflect adequate functioning of many body *regions* and of the various systems within these regions.

You may want to plan your physical examination around the patient's *chief complaint* or *concern.* To do this, begin by examining the body system or region that corresponds to the chief complaint. This allows you to identify priority prob-

Documentation tips

Remember these rules about documenting your initial assessment:

■ Always document your findings as soon as possible after you take the health history and perform the physical examination.

■ Complete your documentation of your assessment away from the patient's bedside. Jot down only key points while you're with the patient.

■ If you're using an assessment form, answer every question. If a question doesn't apply to your patient, write "N/A" or "not applicable" in the space.

■ Focus your questions on areas that relate to the patient's chief complaint. Record information that has significance and will help you build a care plan.

■ If you delegate the job of filling out the first section of the form to another nurse or an ancillary nursing person, remember — you must review the information gathered and validate it if you aren't sure it's correct.

■ Always accept accountability for your assessment by signing your name to the areas you've completed.

■ Always directly quote the patient or family member who gave you the information if you fear that summarizing will lose some of its meaning.

■ Always write or print legibly, in ink.

■ Be concise, specific, and exact when you describe your physical findings.

■ Always go back to the patient's bedside to clarify or validate information that seems incomplete.

lems promptly and reassures the patient that you're paying attention to his chief complaint.

Physical examination findings are crucial to arriving at a nursing diagnosis and, ultimately, to developing a sound nursing care plan. Record your examination results thoroughly, accurately, and clearly. Although some examiners don't like to use a printed form to record physical assessment findings, preferring to work with a blank paper, others believe that standardized data collection forms can make recording physical examination results easier. These forms simplify comprehensive data collection and documentation by providing a concise format for outlining and recording pertinent information. They also remind you to include all essential assessment data.

When documenting, describe exactly what you've inspected, palpated, percussed, or auscultated. Don't use general terms, such as *normal, abnormal, good,* or *poor.* Instead, be specific. Include positive and negative findings. Try to document as soon as possible after completing your assessment. Remember that abbreviations aid conciseness. (See *Documentation tips.*)

NURSING DIAGNOSIS

According to NANDA International (NANDA-I), the nursing diagnosis is a "clinical judgment about individual, family, or community responses to actual or potential health problems or life processes. Nursing diagnoses provide the basis for selection of nursing interventions to achieve outcomes for which the nurse is accountable." The nursing diagnosis must be supported by clinical information obtained during patient assessment. (See *Nursing diagnoses and the nursing process,* page xxii.)

Each nursing diagnosis describes a patient problem that a nurse can legally manage. Becoming familiar with nursing diagnoses will enable you to better understand how nursing practice is distinct from medical practice. Although the identification of problems commonly overlaps in nursing and medicine, the approach to treatment clearly differs. Medicine focuses on curing disease; nursing focuses on holistic care that includes care and comfort. Nurses can independently diagnose and treat the patient's response to illness, certain health problems and risk for health problems, readiness to improve health behaviors, and the need to learn new health information. Nurses comfort, counsel, and care for patients and their families until they're physically, emotionally, and spiritually ready to provide self-care.

Developing your diagnosis

The nursing diagnosis expresses your professional judgment of the patient's clinical status, responses to treatment, and nursing care needs. You perform this step so that you can develop your care plan. In effect, the nursing diagnosis *defines* the practice of nursing. Translating the history, physical examination, and laboratory data about a patient into a nursing diagnosis involves organizing the data into clusters and interpreting what the clusters reveal about the patient's ability to meet basic needs. In addition to identifying the patient's needs in coping with the effects of illness, consider what assistance the patient requires to grow and develop to the fullest extent possible.

Your nursing diagnosis describes the cluster of signs and symptoms indicating an actual or potential health problem that you can identify — and that your care can resolve. Nursing diagnoses that indicate potential health problems can be identified by the words "risk for," which appear in the diagnostic label. There are also nursing diagnoses that focus on prevention of health problems and enhanced wellness.

Creating your nursing diagnosis is a logical extension of collecting assessment data. In your patient assessment, you asked each history question, performed each physical examination technique, and considered each laboratory test result because it provided evidence of how the patient could be helped by your care or because the data could affect nursing care.

To develop the nursing diagnosis, use the assessment data you've collected to develop a problem list. Less formal in structure than a fully developed nursing diagnosis, this list describes the patient's problems or needs. It's easy to generate such a list if you use a conceptual model or an accepted set of criterion norms. Examples of such norms include normal physical and psychological development and Gordon's functional health patterns.

You can identify the patient's problems and needs with simple phrases, such as *poor circulation, high fever,* or *poor hydration.* Next, prioritize the problems on the list and then develop the working nursing diagnosis.

Nursing diagnoses and the nursing process

When first described, the nursing process included only assessment, planning, implementation, and evaluation. However, during the past three decades, several important events have helped to establish diagnosis as a distinct part of the nursing process.

■ The American Nurses Association (ANA), in its 1973 publication *Standards of Nursing Practice,* mentioned nursing diagnosis as a separate and definable act performed by the registered nurse. In 1991, the ANA published its revised standards of clinical practice, which continued to list nursing diagnosis as a distinct step of the nursing process.

■ Individual states passed nurse practice acts that listed diagnosis as part of the nurse's legal responsibility.

■ In 1973, the North American Nursing Diagnosis Association, now NANDA International (NANDA-I), began a formal effort to classify nursing diagnoses. NANDA-I continues to meet biennially to review proposed new nursing diagnoses and examine applications of nursing diagnoses in clinical practice, education, and research. Their most recent meeting was held in April, 2006 in Philadelphia, Pennsylvania. NANDA-I also publishes *NANDA-I Nursing Diagnoses: Definitions and Classification 2007-2008,* a complete list of nursing diagnoses, definitions, and defining characteristics. Currently, members of NANDA-I are working in cooperation with the ANA and the International Council of Nurses to develop an International Classification of Nursing Practice.

■ The emergence of the computer-based patient record has underscored the need for a standardized nomenclature for nursing.

Writing a nursing diagnosis

Some nurses are confused about how to document a nursing diagnosis because they think the language is too complex. By remembering the following basic guidelines, however, you can ensure that your diagnostic statement is correct:

■ Use proper terminology that reflects the patient's *nursing* needs.

■ Make your statement concise so it's easily understood by other health care team members.

■ Use the most precise words possible.

■ Use a problem and cause format, stating the problem and its related cause.

Whenever possible, use the terminology recommended by NANDA-I.

NANDA-I diagnostic headings, when combined with suspected etiology, provide a clear picture of the patient's needs. Thus, for clarity in charting, start with one of the NANDA-I categories as a heading for the diagnostic statement. The category can reflect an actual or potential problem. Consider this sample diagnosis:

■ *Heading:* Impaired physical mobility

■ *Etiology:* Related to pain and discomfort following surgery

■ *Signs and symptoms:* "I can't walk without help." Patient hasn't ambulated since surgery on (give date and time). Range of motion limited to 10 degrees flexion in the right hip. Patient can't walk 3′ from the bed to the chair without the help of two nurses.

This format links the patient's problem to the etiology without stating a direct cause-and-effect relationship (which may be hard to prove). Remember to state only the patient's problems and the probable origin. Omit references to possible solutions. (Your solutions will derive from your nursing diagnosis, but they aren't part of it.)

Avoiding common errors

One major pitfall in developing a nursing diagnosis is writing one that nursing interventions can't treat. Errors can also occur when nurses take shortcuts in the nursing process, either by omitting or hurrying through assessment or by basing the diagnosis on inaccurate assessment data.

Keep in mind that a nursing diagnosis is a statement of a health problem that a nurse is licensed to treat — a problem for which you'll assume responsibility for therapeutic decisions and accountability for the outcomes. A nursing diagnosis is *not* a:
- diagnostic test ("schedule for cardiac angiography")
- piece of equipment ("set up intermittent suction apparatus")
- problem with equipment ("the patient has trouble using a commode")
- nurse's problem with a patient ("Mr. Jones is a difficult patient; he's rude and won't take his medication.")
- nursing goal ("encourage fluids up to 2,000 ml per day")
- nursing need ("I have to get through to the family that they must accept the fact that their father is dying.")
- medical diagnosis ("cervical cancer")
- treatment ("catheterize after each voiding for residual urine").

At first, these distinctions may not be clear. The following examples should help clarify what a nursing diagnosis is:
- Don't state a need instead of a problem.
- Incorrect: Fluid replacement related to fever
- Correct: Deficient fluid volume related to fever
- Don't reverse the two parts of the statement.
- Incorrect: Lack of understanding related to noncompliance with diabetic diet
- Correct: Noncompliance with diabetic diet related to lack of understanding
- Don't identify an untreatable condition instead of the problem it indicates (which can be treated).
- Incorrect: Inability to speak related to laryngectomy
- Correct: Social isolation related to inability to speak because of laryngectomy
- Don't write a legally inadvisable statement.
- Incorrect: Skin integrity impairment related to improper positioning
- Correct: Impaired skin integrity related to immobility
- Don't identify as unhealthful a response that would be appropriate, allowed for, or culturally acceptable.
- Incorrect: Anger related to terminal illness
- Correct: Ineffective therapeutic regimen management related to anger over terminal illness

■ Don't make a tautological statement (one in which both parts of the statement say the same thing).
– Incorrect: Pain related to alteration in comfort
– Correct: Acute pain related to postoperative abdominal distention and anxiety
■ Don't identify a nursing problem instead of a patient problem.
– Incorrect: Difficulty suctioning related to thick secretions
– Correct: Ineffective airway clearance related to thick tracheal secretions

How nursing and medical diagnoses differ

You assess your patient to obtain data in order to make a nursing diagnosis, just as the physician examines a patient to establish a medical diagnosis. Learn the differences between the two, and remember that sometimes they overlap. You perform a complete assessment to identify patient problems that your nursing interventions can help resolve; your nursing diagnoses state these problems. (Some may occur secondary to medical treatment.) If you plan your care of a patient around only the medical aspects of his illness, you'll probably overlook significant problems.

For example, suppose the patient's medical diagnosis is a fractured femur. In your assessment, take a careful history. Include questions to determine if the patient has adequate financial resources to cope with prolonged disability. To assess the patient's capacity to adjust to the physical restrictions caused by the disability, gather data about his previous lifestyle.

Suppose your physical examination of this patient — in addition to uncovering signs and symptoms pertaining to the medical diagnosis — reveals actual or potential skin breakdown secondary to immobility. Your nursing diagnoses, in that case, may include home maintenance management impairment, diversional activity deficit (related to prolonged immobility), and risk for skin integrity impairment.

The care plan you prepare for this patient should include the nursing interventions suggested by your nursing diagnoses as well as the nursing actions necessary to fulfill the patient's medical treatment plan. When integrated into a care plan, the nursing and medical diagnoses describe the complete nursing care the patient needs.

Examples

Study the examples here to better understand the difference between medical and nursing diagnoses.
■ Frank Smith, age 67, complains of "stubborn, old muscles." He has difficulty walking, as you can see by his shuffling gait. During the interview, Mr. Smith speaks in a monotone and seems very depressed. Physical examination shows a pill-rolling hand tremor. Laboratory tests reveal a decreased dopamine level.
– *Medical diagnosis:* Parkinson's disease
– *Nursing diagnoses:* Impaired physical mobility related to decreased muscle control; disturbed body image related to physical alterations; deficient knowledge related to lack of information about progressive nature of illness
■ For 5 consecutive days, Judy Wilson, age 26, has had sporadic abdominal cramps of increasing intensity. Most recently, the pain has been accompanied by

vomiting and a slight fever. Your examination reveals rebound tenderness and muscle guarding.

– *Medical diagnosis:* Appendicitis

– *Nursing diagnoses:* Acute pain related to biological agents; deficient fluid volume related to vomiting

■ During an extensive bout with respiratory tract infections, Tom Bradley, age 7, complains of throbbing ear pain. Tom's mother notes his hearing difficulty and his fear of the pain and possible hearing loss. On inspection, his tympanic membrane appears red and bulging.

– *Medical diagnosis:* Acute suppurative otitis media

– *Nursing diagnoses:* Acute pain related to swollen tympanic membrane; fear related to progressive hearing loss; disturbed sensory perception (auditory) related to obstructed middle ear.

OUTCOME IDENTIFICATION

During this phase of the nursing process, you identify expected outcomes for the patient. Expected outcomes are measurable, patient-focused goals that are derived from the patient's nursing diagnoses. These goals may be short- or long-term. Short-term goals include those of immediate concern that can be achieved quickly. Long-term goals take more time to achieve and usually involve prevention, patient teaching, and rehabilitation.

In many cases, you can identify expected outcomes by converting the nursing diagnosis into a positive statement. For instance, for the nursing diagnosis "impaired physical mobility related to a fracture of the right hip," the expected outcome might be "The patient will ambulate independently before discharge."

When writing the care plan, state expected outcomes in terms of the patient's behavior — for example, "the patient correctly demonstrates turning, coughing, and deep breathing." Also identify a target time or date by which the expected outcomes should be accomplished. The expected outcomes will serve as the basis for evaluating your nursing interventions.

Keep in mind that each expected outcome must be stated in measurable terms. If possible, consult with the patient and his family when establishing expected outcomes. As the patient progresses, expected outcomes should be increasingly directed toward planning for discharge and follow-up care.

Outcome statements should be tailored to your practice setting. For example, on the intensive care unit you may focus on maintaining hemodynamic stability, whereas on a rehabilitation unit you would focus on maximizing the patient's independence and preventing complications. (See *Understanding NOC*, page xxvi.)

Writing expected outcome statements

When writing expected outcomes in your care plan, always start with a specific action verb that focuses on the patient's behavior. By telling your reader how the patient should *look, walk, eat, drink, turn, cough, speak,* or *stand,* for example, you give a clear picture of how to evaluate progress.

Understanding NOC

The Nursing Outcomes Classification (NOC) is a standardized language of patient/client outcomes that was developed by a nursing research team at the University of Iowa. It contains 330 outcomes organized into 29 classes and seven domains. Each outcome has a definition, list of measurable indicators, and references. The outcomes are research-based, and studies are ongoing to evaluate their reliability, validity, and sensitivity. More information about NOC can be found at the Center for Nursing Classification and Clinical Effectiveness (*www.nursing.uiowa.edu/cnc*).

Avoid starting expected outcome statements with *allow, let, enable,* or similar verbs. Such words focus attention on your own and other health care team members' behavior—not on the patient's.

With many documentation formats, you won't need to include the phrase "The patient will..." with each expected outcome statement. You will, however, have to specify which person the goals refer to when family, friends, or others are directly concerned.

Make sure target dates are realistic. Be flexible enough to adjust the date if the patient needs more time to respond to your interventions.

PLANNING

The nursing care plan refers to a written plan of action designed to help you deliver quality patient care. It includes relevant nursing diagnoses, expected outcomes, and nursing interventions. Keep in mind that the care plan usually forms a permanent part of the patient's health record and will be used by other members of the nursing team. The care plan may be integrated into an interdisciplinary plan for the patient. In this instance, clear guidelines should outline the role of each member of the health care team in providing care.

Benefits of a care plan

To provide quality care for each patient, you must plan and direct that care. Writing a care plan lets you document the scientific method you have used throughout the nursing process. On the care plan, you summarize the patient's problems and needs (as nursing diagnoses) and identify appropriate nursing interventions and expected outcomes. A care plan that's well conceived and properly written helps decrease the risk of incomplete or incorrect care by:

■ *Giving direction.* A written care plan gives direction by showing colleagues the goals you have set for the patient and giving clear instructions for helping to achieve them. It also makes clear exactly what to document on the patient's progress notes. For instance, it lists what observations to make and how often, what nursing measures to take and how to implement them, and what to teach the patient and his family before discharge.

■ *Providing continuity of care.* A written care plan identifies the patient's needs to each caregiver and tells what must be done to meet those needs. With this information, nurses caring for the patient at different times can adjust their routines to meet the patient's care demands. A care plan also provides caregivers with specific instructions on patient care, eliminating the confusion that can exist. If the patient is discharged from your health care facility to another, your care plan can help ease this transition.

■ *Establishing communication between you and other nurses who will care for the patient, between you and health care team members in other departments, and between you and the patient.* By soliciting the patient's input as you develop the care plan, you build a rapport that lets the patient know you value his opinions and feelings. By reviewing the care plan with other health care team members, and with other nurses, you can regularly evaluate the patient's response or lack of response to the nursing care and medical regimen.

■ *Serving as a key for patient care assignments.* If you're a team leader, you may want to delegate some specific routines or duties described in each nursing intervention — not all of them need your professional attention.

Reviewing the planning stages

Formulating the care plan involves three stages:

■ *Assigning* priorities to the nursing diagnoses: Any time you develop more than one nursing diagnosis for the patient, you must assign priorities to them and begin your care plan with those having the highest priority. High-priority nursing diagnoses involve the patient's most urgent needs (such as emergency or immediate physical needs). Intermediate-priority diagnoses involve nonemergency needs, and low-priority diagnoses involve needs that don't directly relate to the patient's specific illness or prognosis.

■ *Selecting* appropriate nursing actions (interventions): Next, you'll select one or more nursing interventions to achieve each of the expected outcomes identified for the patient. For example, if one expected outcome statement reads "The patient will transfer to chair with assistance," the appropriate nursing interventions include placing the wheelchair facing the foot of the bed and assisting the patient to stand and pivot to the chair. If another expected outcome statement reads "The patient will express feelings related to recent injury," appropriate interventions might include spending time with the patient each shift, conveying an open and nonjudgmental attitude, and asking open-ended questions.

■ *Documenting* the nursing diagnoses, expected outcomes, nursing interventions, and evaluations on the care plan: Reviewing the second part of the nursing diagnosis statement (the part describing etiologic factors) may help guide your choice of nursing interventions. For example, for the nursing diagnosis "Risk for injury related to inadequate blood glucose levels," you would determine the best nursing interventions for maintaining an adequate blood glucose level. Typical interventions for this goal include observing the patient for evidence of hypoglycemia and providing an appropriate diet. Try to think creatively during this step in the nursing process. It's an opportunity to describe exactly what you and your patient would like to have happen and to establish the criteria against which you'll judge further nursing actions.

The planning phase culminates when you write the care plan and document the nursing diagnoses, expected outcomes, nursing interventions, and evaluations for expected outcomes. Write your care plan in concise, specific terms so that other health care team members can follow it. Keep in mind that because the patient's problems and needs will change, you'll have to review your care plan frequently and modify it when necessary.

Elements of the care plan

Care-planning formats vary from one health care facility to another. For example, you may write your care plan on a form supplied by the hospital or you can use software that's approved by your facility. Nearly all care-planning formats include space in which to document the nursing diagnoses, expected outcomes, and nursing interventions. In many health care facilities, you may also document assessment data and discharge planning on the care plan.

No matter which format you use, be sure to write the care plan in ink (and sign it), even though you may have to make revisions if your nursing interventions don't work. Remember — the patient's care plan becomes part of the permanent record and shouldn't be erased or destroyed. If you write it in pencil — so you can erase to revise — you make it seem unimportant. The information must remain intact, enabling you and other health care team members to readily refer to nursing interventions used in the past. (See *Guidelines for writing the care plan.*)

Be specific when writing your care plan. By discussing specific problems, expected outcomes, nursing interventions, and evaluations for expected outcomes, you leave no doubt as to what needs to be done by other health care team members. When listing nursing interventions, for example, be sure to include *when* the action should be implemented, *who* should be involved in each aspect of implementation, and the *frequency, quantity,* and *method* to be used. Specify dates and times when appropriate. List target dates for each expected outcome.

If your nursing interventions have resolved the problem on which you've based the nursing diagnosis, write "discontinued" next to the diagnostic statement on the care plan, and list the date you discontinued the interventions. If your nursing interventions haven't resolved the problem by the target date, reevaluate your plan and do one of the following:

■ Extend the target date and continue the intervention until the patient responds as expected.

■ Discontinue the intervention and select a new one that will achieve the expected outcome.

You'll need to update and modify a patient's care plan as problems (or their priorities) change and resolve, new assessment information becomes available, and you evaluate the patient's responses to nursing interventions.

IMPLEMENTATION

During this phase, you put your care plan into action. Implementation encompasses all nursing interventions directed toward solving the patient's nursing problems and meeting health care needs. While you coordinate implementation, you also seek help from other caregivers, the patient, and the patient's family. (See *Understanding* NIC, page xxx.)

Guidelines for writing the care plan

Keeping these tips in mind will help you write an accurate and useful care plan.

■ Write your patient's care plan in ink—it's part of the permanent record. Sign your name.

■ Be specific; don't use vague terms or generalities on the care plan.

■ Never use abbreviations that may be confused or misinterpreted. In general, it's better to use only established abbreviations and acronyms.

■ Take time to review all your assessment data *before* you select an approach for each problem. (*Note:* If you can't complete the initial assessment, immediately note "insufficient database" on your records.)

■ Write down a specific expected outcome for each problem you identify, and record a target date for its completion.

■ Avoid setting an initial goal that's too high to be achieved. For example, the outcome for a newly admitted patient with stroke stating, "Patient will ambulate with assistance," is an unrealistic initial goal because several patient outcomes will need to be achieved before this goal can be addressed.

■ Consider the following three phases of patient care when writing nursing interventions: What observations to make and how often, what nursing measures to do and how to do them, and what to teach the patient and family before discharge.

■ Make each nursing intervention specific.

■ Make sure nursing interventions match the resources and capabilities of the staff. Combine what's necessary to correct or modify the problem with what's reasonably possible in your setting.

■ Be creative when you write your patient's care plan; include a drawing or an innovative procedure if either will make your directions more specific.

■ Don't overlook any of the patient's problems or concerns. Include them on the care plan so they won't be forgotten.

■ Make sure your care plan is implemented correctly.

■ Evaluate the results of your care plan, and discontinue any nursing diagnoses that have been resolved. Select new approaches, if necessary, for problems that haven't been resolved.

Implementation requires some (or all) of the following interventions:

■ assessing and monitoring (for example, recording vital signs)

■ therapeutic interventions (for example, giving medications)

■ making the patient more comfortable and helping him with activities of daily living

■ supporting his respiratory and elimination functions

■ providing skin care

■ managing the environment (for example, controlling noise to ensure a good night's sleep)

■ providing food and fluids

■ giving emotional support

■ teaching and counseling

Understanding NIC

The Nursing Interventions Classification (NIC) is a standardized language of treatments that was developed by a nursing research team at the University of Iowa. It contains 514 interventions organized into 30 classes and seven domains. Each intervention has a definition, list of detailed activities, and references. The interventions are research-based and studies are ongoing to evaluate the effectiveness and cost of nursing treatments. More information about NIC can be found at the Center for Nursing Classification and Clinical Effectiveness (*www.nursing.uiowa.edu/cnc*).

■ referring the patient to appropriate agencies or services.

Incorporate these elements into the implementation stage:

■ *Reassessing.* Although it may be brief or narrowly focused, reassessment should confirm that the planned interventions remain appropriate.

■ *Reviewing and modifying the care plan.* Never static, an appropriate care plan changes with the patient's condition. As necessary, update the assessment, nursing diagnoses, implementation, and evaluation sections. (Entering the new data in a different color of ink alerts other staff members to the revisions.) Date the revisions.

■ *Seeking assistance.* Determine, for example, whether you need help from other staff members or additional information before you can intervene.

Documentation

Implementation isn't complete until you've documented each intervention, the time it occurred, the patient's response, and any other pertinent information. Make sure each entry relates to a nursing diagnosis. Remember that any action not documented may be overlooked during quality assurance monitoring or evaluation of care. Another good reason for thorough documentation: It offers a way for you to take rightful credit for your contribution in helping a patient achieve the highest possible level of wellness. After all, nurses use a unique and worthwhile combination of interpersonal, intellectual, and technical skills when providing care. (See *Nursing interventions: Three types.*)

EVALUATION

In this phase of the nursing process, you assess the effectiveness of the care plan by answering such questions as:

■ How has the patient progressed in terms of the plan's projected outcomes?

■ Does the patient have new needs?

■ Does the care plan need to be revised?

Evaluation also helps you determine whether the patient received high-quality care from the nursing staff and the health care facility. Your facility bases its own nursing quality assurance system on nursing evaluations.

Nursing interventions: Three types

Knowing the three types of nursing interventions will help you document implementation appropriately.

1. *Independent interventions.* These interventions fall within the purview of nursing practice and don't require a physician's direction or supervision. Most nursing actions required by the patient's care plan are independent interventions. Examples include patient teaching, health promotion, counseling, and helping the patient with activities of daily living.

2. *Dependent interventions.* Based on written or oral instructions from another professional — usually a physician — dependent interventions include administering medication, inserting indwelling urinary catheters, and obtaining specimens for laboratory tests.

3. *Interdependent interventions.* Performed in collaboration with other professionals, interdependent interventions include following a protocol and carrying out standing orders.

Steps in the evaluation process

Include the patient, family members, and other health care professionals in the evaluation. Then follow these steps:

■ *Select evaluation criteria.* The care plan's projected outcomes — the desired effects of nursing interventions — form the basis for evaluation.

■ *Compare the patient's response with the evaluation criteria.* Did the patient respond as expected? If not, the care plan may need revision.

■ *Analyze your findings.* If your plan wasn't effective, determine why. You may conclude, for example, that several nursing diagnoses were inaccurate.

■ *Modify the care plan.* Make revisions (for example, change inaccurate nursing diagnoses) and implement the new plan.

■ *Reevaluate.* Like all steps in the nursing process, evaluation is ongoing. Continue to assess, plan, implement, and evaluate for as long as you care for the patient.

Questions to answer

When evaluating and documenting the patient's care, collect information from all available sources — for example, the patient's medical record, family members, other caregivers, and the patient. Include your own observations.

During the evaluation process, ask yourself these questions:

■ Has the patient's condition improved, deteriorated, or remained the same?

■ Were the nursing diagnoses accurate?

■ Have the patient's nursing needs been met?

■ Did the patient meet the outcome criteria documented in the care plan?

■ Which nursing interventions should I revise or discontinue?

■ Why did the patient fail to meet some goals (if applicable)?

■ Should I reorder priorities? Revise expected outcomes?

Nursing diagnoses and critical pathways

In a growing number of health care settings—inpatient and outpatient, acute and long-term care—critical pathways are being used to guide the process of care for a patient. Critical pathways describe the course of a specific health-related condition. A critical pathway may be used along with or instead of a nursing care plan, depending on the standards set by the individual health care facility. These tools may also be referred to as clinical pathways, care maps, collaborative care plans, or multidisciplinary action plans. (See *Developing a critical pathway.*)

The concept of the critical pathway evolved out of the growth of managed care and the development of the case management model in the early 1990s. Pressure from managed care organizations to control costs led to the evolution of case management.

In case management, one professional—usually a nurse or a social worker—assumes responsibility for coordinating care so that patients move through the health care system in the shortest time and at the lowest cost possible.

Early on, case managers used the nursing process and based their plans on nursing diagnoses. Over time, however, it became evident that a multidisciplinary approach was needed to adequately monitor length of stay and reduce overall costs. This led to the development of the critical pathway concept.

In critical pathways, a time line is defined for each condition and for the achievement of expected outcomes. By reading the critical pathway, caregivers can determine on any given day where the patient should be in his progress toward optimal health.

The critical pathway provides a method for physicians and nurses to standardize and organize care for routine conditions. These pathways also make it easier for case managers to track data needed to:

■ streamline utilization of material resources and labor
■ ensure that patients receive quality care
■ improve the coordination of care
■ reduce the cost of providing care.

The most successful critical pathways have been developed for medical diagnoses with predictable outcomes, such as hip replacement, mastectomy, myocardial infarction, and cardiac catheterization. Critical pathways work best with high-volume, high-risk, high-cost conditions or procedures for which there are predictable outcomes.

Developing a critical pathway

The critical pathway is an interdisciplinary tool that requires the collaborative efforts of all disciplines involved in patient care. The interdisciplinary team must decide on a diagnosis, select a set of achievable outcomes, and agree on a plausible time line for achieving the desired outcomes. Note that when establishing standard practices for treatment of a given condition, it has usually proved difficult for physicians to achieve consensus.

Establishing a time line

Time intervals allocated on a critical pathway vary according to the patient's condition and its acuity. For a hip replacement, the time line extends over days; for a cardiac catheterization procedure, time intervals are expressed in hours. In the postanesthesia period, a critical pathway can be defined in minutes.

Average length of stay is an important concept in developing a critical pathway. If agency data indicate that the average length of stay for an inpatient who has had a modified radical mastectomy with reconstruction is 4 days, then the team begins planning around a 4-day stay.

Building the pathway

The interdisciplinary team must choose a framework for developing outcomes and interventions. Some agencies build pathways around nursing diagnoses. If interdisciplinary collaboration is strong, an agency may build pathways around general aspects of care; for example, pain, activity, nutrition, assessment, medications, psychosocial status, treatments, teaching, and discharge planning.

In an acute care setting, outcomes and interventions for each aspect of care are determined for each day of an expected length of stay. In long-term care and other community-based settings, progress may be measured in longer intervals.

CARE PLANNING FOR STUDENTS

Developing a care plan helps the nursing student improve problem-solving technique, learn the nursing process, and improve written and verbal communication and organizational skills. More important, it shows how to apply classroom and textbook knowledge to practice.

Because it aims to teach the care-planning process, the student care plan is longer than the standard plan used in most health care facilities. In a step-by step manner, it progresses from assessment to evaluation. However, some teaching institutions model the student care plan on the plan used by the affiliated health care institution, adding a space for the scientific rationale for each nursing intervention selected.

Writing out all of your planned actions enables you to review planned nursing activities with your clinical instructor. This is an opportunity to consider whether you have complete assessment data to support your diagnoses and interventions and if you've taken into consideration all the problems that a more experienced nurse is likely to identify.

THE IMPORTANCE OF NURSING DIAGNOSES

Using a critical pathway can be helpful, especially for nursing students and new graduates. You may be assigned to provide care to a particular patient for only 1 or 2 days. Seeing the entire pathway and examining the outcomes the patient is expected to achieve will help you obtain a broader clinical perspective on care.

Using a critical pathway as a guide for delivering care doesn't, however, negate the need to formulate and utilize nursing diagnoses. Nursing diagnoses continue to define the primary responsibility of nursing—to diagnose and treat human responses to actual or potential health problems. The full nursing care needs of any patient are unlikely to be documented on a critical pathway. When using a pathway, always keep in mind that the patient may require nursing intervention beyond what's specified in the critical pathway.

For example, a patient enters a hospital for a hip replacement and can't communicate verbally because of a recent stroke. The critical pathway wouldn't include measures to assist the patient to make his needs known. Therefore, you would develop a nursing care plan around the diagnosis "Impaired verbal communication related to decreased circulation to the brain."

Even if you practice in a clinical setting that relies on critical pathways to fill documentation requirements, the *Nursing Diagnosis Reference Manual,* Seventh Edition, will prove to be a valuable resource for identifying and treating each patient's unique nursing needs. Creating a care plan based on carefully selected nursing diagnoses and using it along with a critical pathway will enable you to provide your patients with high-quality collaborative care that includes a strong nursing component.

I Adult health

INTRODUCTION

This section includes approximately 200 alphabetically organized diagnostic labels and associated care plans that identify adult health problems responsive to independent nursing action. Many focus on meeting the patient's actual physiologic needs. For example, you'll find care plans that will assist you to plan the care of a patient with decreased cardiac output, help an injured patient maintain joint range of motion, and teach an immunosuppressed patient measures to prevent infection. In addition, you'll find plans for warding off potential health problems, such as risk for infection or injury.

Other care plans focus on the psychological and psychosocial problems of adulthood. For example, if a patient with a chronic illness experiences related emotional difficulties, such diagnostic labels as *hopelessness, ineffective role performance,* and *disturbed body image* may help pinpoint his needs. If a patient lacks adequate financial, social, or spiritual resources, appropriate care plans provide instructions for documenting such hardships and interventions for ameliorating them.

Still other care plans focus on more specialized patient problems. For example, you'll find plans for patients undergoing surgery.

In summary, the diagnostic labels and associated care plans covered in this section encompass the full range of nursing responsibilities. To make full use of this broad database, you'll need to perform a complete and careful nursing assessment. When appropriate, include questions about the patient's cultural background. Ask about self-concept, stressors, daily living habits, and coping mechanisms. Discuss the patient's health goals. How well does the patient understand his condition? Will family members or friends take an active role in his care? Your assessment should also include information derived from your own observations.

Use information gathered during assessment to select an accurate diagnostic statement and an appropriate care plan. That way, you can ensure your adult patient comprehensive, individualized, and consistent nursing care.

ACTIVITY INTOLERANCE
related to imbalance between oxygen supply and demand

Definition
Insufficient physiologic or psychological energy to endure or complete required or desired daily activities

Assessment
- History of circulatory disease, respiratory disease, or both
- Patient's perception of tolerance for activity
- Current medications, effectiveness
- Respiratory status, including pulse oximetry, pulmonary function studies, and respiratory rate, depth, and pattern at rest and with activity
- Cardiovascular status, including blood pressure, complete blood count, stress electrocardiogram (ECG) results, and heart rate and rhythm at rest and with activity
- Knowledge, including understanding of present condition, perception of need to maintain or restore an activity level consistent with capabilities, and physical, mental, and emotional readiness to learn

Defining characteristics
- Abnormal heart rate or blood pressure in response to activity
- Arrhythmia or ischemic changes on ECG
- Exertional discomfort or dyspnea
- Verbal report of fatigue or weakness

Expected outcomes
- Patient will state desire to increase activity level.
- Patient will state understanding of the need to increase activity level gradually.
- Patient will identify controllable factors that cause fatigue.
- Patient's blood pressure and pulse and respiratory rates will remain within prescribed limits during activity.
- Patient will state sense of satisfaction with each new level of activity attained.
- Patient will demonstrate skill in conserving energy while carrying out daily activities to tolerance level.
- Patient will explain illness and connect symptoms of activity intolerance with deficit in oxygen supply or use.

Suggested NOC outcomes
Activity Tolerance; Discharge Readiness; Endurance; Energy Conservation; Psychomotor Energy; Self-Care: Activities of Daily Living (ADL); Self-Care: Instrumental Activities of Daily Living (IADL)

Interventions and rationales
- Discuss with patient the need for activity. *Lack of activity causes physical deconditioning and may also have a negative impact on psychological well-being.*

■ Identify activities patient considers desirable and meaningful. *Engaging patient in activities that have personal meaning may motivate patient to continue developing tolerance.*

■ Encourage patient to help plan activity progression, being sure to include activities he considers essential. *Participation in planning may encourage patient compliance with the plan.*

■ Instruct and help patient to alternate periods of rest and activity. *Providing rest periods prevents fatigue and encourages patient to continue improving activity tolerance.*

■ Remove barriers that prevent patient from achieving goals that have been established *to minimize factors that may decrease patient's exercise tolerance.*

■ Monitor physiologic responses to increased activity (including respirations, pulse oximetry, heart rate and rhythm, and blood pressure). Document the time after each period of exercise. *Values should return to normal within five minutes or less.*

■ Teach patient how to conserve energy while performing ADLs—for example, sitting in a chair while dressing, wearing lightweight clothing that fastens with Velcro or a few large buttons, and wearing slip-on shoes. *These measures reduce cellular metabolism and oxygen demand.*

■ Teach patient exercises for increasing strength and endurance *to improve breathing and promote general physical reconditioning.*

■ Support and encourage activity to patient's level of tolerance *to help foster patient's independence.*

■ Before discharge, formulate a plan with patient and caregivers that will enable the patient either to continue functioning at maximum activity tolerance or to gradually increase tolerance. For example, teach patient and caregivers to monitor patient's pulse during activities, to recognize need for oxygen (if prescribed), and to use oxygen equipment properly. *Participation in discharge planning encourages patient satisfaction and compliance.*

Suggested NIC interventions

Body Mechanics Promotion; Energy Management; Environmental Management; Exercise Promotion; Exercise Therapy: Muscle Control; Mutual Goal Setting; Oxygen Therapy; Progressive Muscle Relaxation

Evaluations for expected outcomes

■ Patient states a desire to increase activity level.

■ Patient identifies a plan to increase activity level.

■ Patient lists factors that cause fatigue.

■ Patient's blood pressure and pulse and respiratory rates remain within normal parameters.

■ Patient expresses satisfaction with increase in activity level.

■ Patient is proficient in conserving energy while performing ADLs.

■ Patient demonstrates an understanding of relationship between signs and symptoms of activity intolerance and deficit in oxygen supply or use.

Documentation
- Patient's perception of need for activity
- Patient's priorities in performing selected activities
- Patient's description of physical effects of various activities
- Observations made while patient performs activities
- Skills demonstrated by patient in conserving energy during activity
- New activities patient was able to perform
- Evaluations for expected outcomes

Reference
Garcia-Aymerich, J., et al. "Regular Physical Activity Reduces Hospital Admission and Mortality in Chronic Obstructive Pulmonary Disease: A Population-based Cohort Study," *Thorax* 61(9):772-78, September 2006.

ACTIVITY INTOLERANCE
related to immobility

Definition
Insufficient physiologic or psychological energy to endure or complete required or desired daily activities

Assessment
- History of present illness
- Past experience with prolonged bed rest
- Neurologic status, including level of consciousness, orientation, motor status, and sensory status
- Respiratory status, including arterial blood gas analysis, breath sounds, and rate, depth, and pattern of respiration at rest and with activity
- Cardiovascular status, including blood pressure, skin color, hemoglobin level and hematocrit, and heart rate and rhythm at rest and with activity
- Musculoskeletal status, including range of motion (ROM) and muscle size, strength, and tone

Defining characteristics
- Abnormal heart rate or blood pressure in response to activity
- Arrhythmia or ischemic changes on electrocardiogram
- Exertional discomfort or dyspnea
- Verbal report of weakness or fatigue

Expected outcomes
- Patient will regain and maintain muscle mass and strength.
- Patient will maintain maximum joint ROM.
- Patient will perform isometric exercises.
- Patient will help perform self-care activities.
- Heart rate and rhythm and blood pressure will remain within expected range during periods of activity.

■ Patient will state understanding of and willingness to cooperate in maximizing activity level.

■ Patient will perform self-care activities to tolerance level.

Suggested NOC outcomes

Activity Tolerance; Endurance; Energy Conservation; Self-Care: Activities of Daily Living (ADL); Self-Care: Instrumental Activities of Daily Living (IADL)

Interventions and rationales

■ Perform active or passive ROM exercises to all extremities every 2 to 4 hours. *These exercises foster muscle strength and tone, maintain joint mobility, and prevent contractures.*

■ Turn and reposition patient at least every 2 hours. Establish a turning schedule for the dependent patient. Post schedule at bedside and monitor frequency. *Turning and repositioning prevents skin breakdown and atelectasis and improves lung expansion.*

■ Maintain proper body alignment at all times *to avoid contractures and to maintain optimal musculoskeletal balance and physiologic function.*

■ Encourage active exercise:

– Provide a trapeze or other assistive device whenever possible. *Such devices simplify moving and turning for many patients and help them to strengthen upper-body muscles.*

– Teach isometric exercises *to help patient maintain or increase muscle tone and joint mobility.*

– Have patient perform self-care activities. Begin slowly and increase daily, as tolerated. *Performing self-care activities helps patient regain independence and enhances self-esteem.*

■ Provide emotional support and encouragement *to improve patient's self-concept and motivate patient to perform ADLs.*

■ Involve patient in planning and decision making *to encourage greater compliance with activity plan.*

■ Monitor physiologic responses to increased activity level, including respirations, heart rate and rhythm, and blood pressure *to ensure they return to normal within 2 to 5 minutes after stopping exercise.*

■ Teach caregivers to assist patient with self-care activities in a way that maximizes patient's potential. *This enables caregivers to participate in patient's care and encourages them to support patient's independence.*

■ Make sure that a case manager or social worker has assessed patient's home and made the appropriate modifications to accommodate patient's level of mobility. *Making adjustments in the home allows patient a greater degree of independence in performing ADLs, thus better conserving energy.*

Suggested NIC interventions

Activity Therapy; Body Mechanics Promotion; Energy Management; Exercise Promotion: Strength Training; Exercise Therapy: Ambulation; Exercise Therapy: Balance; Exercise Therapy: Joint Mobility; Exercise Therapy: Muscle Control

Evaluations for expected outcomes

■ Patient regains and maintains pre-illness muscle mass and strength, as demonstrated by increased activity level.

■ Patient demonstrates maximum joint ROM.

■ Patient performs isometric exercise _____ times per day.

■ Patient assists caregiver in performing self-care activities.

■ Patient's blood pressure and pulse rate and rhythm remain within normal parameters.

■ Patient verbalizes understanding of need to maximize activity level.

■ Patient performs self-care activities at optimal level within restrictions imposed by illness.

Documentation

■ Patient's perceptions about the importance of maintaining optimal levels of activity within restrictions imposed by the illness

■ Activities performed by patient

■ Observations of physical findings in response to activity

■ Teaching activities performed with patient or caregivers

Reference

Shin, Y., et al. "A Tailored Program for the Promotion of Physical Exercise Among Korean Adults," *Applied Nursing Research* 19(2):88-94, May 2006.

Risk for
ACTIVITY INTOLERANCE

related to presence of circulatory or respiratory problems

Definition

At risk for experiencing insufficient physiologic or psychological energy to endure or complete required or desired activity

Assessment

■ History of present illness

■ Past experience with immobility or prescribed bed rest

■ Cardiovascular status, including blood pressure, heart rate and rhythm at rest and with activity, complete blood count, skin temperature and color, edema, and chest pain or discomfort

■ Respiratory status, including arterial blood gas analysis, auscultation of breath sounds, pain or discomfort associated with respiration, and rate, rhythm, depth, and pattern of respirations at rest and with activity

■ Neurologic status, including level of consciousness, orientation, and mental, sensory, and motor status

■ Musculoskeletal status, including range of motion (ROM), muscle size, strength, and tone, and functional mobility as follows:

0 = completely independent

1 = requires use of equipment or device
2 = requires help, supervision, or teaching from another person
3 = requires help from another person and equipment or device
4 = dependent; doesn't participate in activity

Risk factors

- Circulatory or respiratory problems
- History of previous intolerance
- Inexperience with a particular activity
- Deconditioned status

Expected outcomes

- Patient will maintain muscle strength and joint ROM.
- Patient will carry out isometric exercise regimen.
- Patient will communicate understanding of rationale for maintaining activity level.
- Patient will avoid risk factors that may lead to activity intolerance.
- Patient will perform self-care activities to tolerance level.
- Patient's blood pressure, pulse, and respiratory rate will remain within prescribed range during periods of activity (specify).

Suggested NOC outcomes

Activity Tolerance; Endurance; Energy Conservation; Self-Care: Activities of Daily Living (ADL); Self-Care: Instrumental Activities of Daily Living (IADL)

Interventions and rationales

- Position patient to maintain proper body alignment. Use assistive devices as needed *to maintain joint function and prevent musculoskeletal deformities.*
- Turn and position the patient at least every 2 hours. Establish turning schedule for dependent patient. Post at bedside and monitor frequency. *Turning helps prevent skin breakdown by relieving pressure.*
- Assess patient's level of functioning using the functional mobility scale *to determine patient's capabilities.*
- Communicate patient's level of functioning to all staff. *Communication among staff members ensures continuity of care and enables patient to preserve identified level of independence.*
- Unless contraindicated, perform ROM exercises every 2 to 4 hours. Progress from passive to active, according to patient tolerance. *ROM exercises prevent joint contractures and muscular atrophy.*
- Encourage active movement by helping patient use trapeze or other assistive devices *to improve muscle tone and enhance self-esteem.*
- Teach patient how to perform isometric exercises *to maintain and improve muscle tone and joint mobility.*
- Assist patient in carrying out self-care activities. Increase patient's participation in self-care, as tolerated, *to foster independence and improve mobility.*

■ Encourage patient to become involved in planning care and making decisions related to treatment. *Participation in planning enhances patient compliance.*

■ Teach patient, family member, or other caregiver methods to maximize patient's participation in self-care. *Informed caregivers can encourage patient to become more independent.*

■ Assess patient's physiologic response to increased activity (blood pressure, respirations, heart rate, and rhythm). *Monitoring vital signs helps to assess tolerance for increased exertion and activity.*

■ Teach patient symptoms of overexertion, such as dizziness, chest pain, and dyspnea *to help patient take responsibility for monitoring his own activity level.*

■ Explain rationale for maintaining or improving activity level. Discuss factors that increase risk of activity intolerance. *Education helps patient avoid activity intolerance.*

■ Encourage patient to carry out ADLs. Provide emotional support, and offer positive feedback when patient displays initiative. *Offering emotional support enhances patient's self-esteem and motivation.*

Suggested NIC interventions

Energy Management; Exercise Promotion: Strength Training; Exercise Therapy: Joint Mobility; Hope Instillation; Self-Care Assistance; Teaching: Prescribed Activity/Exercise

Evaluations for expected outcomes

■ Functional mobility scale indicates that muscle strength and joint ROM remain stable.

■ Patient demonstrates isometric exercises.

■ Patient explains rationale for maintaining activity level.

■ Patient states at least five risk factors for activity intolerance.

■ Patient performs self-care activities in preparation for discharge.

■ Patient doesn't exhibit evidence of cardiovascular or respiratory complications during or after activity.

Documentation

■ Patient's expressions of motivation to maintain maximum activity level within restrictions imposed by illness

■ Activities performed by patient

■ Teaching instructions provided to patient and family member or other caregivers

■ Patient's physiologic response to increased activity

■ Evaluations for expected outcomes

References

Killey, B., and Watt, E. "The Effect of Extra Walking on the Mobility, Independence, and Exercise Self-efficacy of Elderly Patients: A Pilot Study," *Contemporary Nurse* 22(1):120-33, July 2006.

Tucker, D., et al. "Walking for Wellness: A Collaborative Program to Maintain Mobility in Hospitalized Older Adults," *Geriatric Nursing* 25(4):242-45, July-August 2004.

Ineffective
AIRWAY CLEARANCE
related to retained secretions

Definition
Inability to clear secretions or obstructions from the respiratory tract to maintain a clear airway

Assessment
- History of present illness
- Patient's perception of ability to clear airway
- Knowledge of physical condition
- Neurologic status, including level of consciousness, orientation, and sensory and motor status
- Respiratory status, including symmetry of chest expansion; use of accessory muscles; cough (productive or nonproductive); respiratory rate, depth, and pattern; sputum characteristics (color, consistency, amount, odor, and changes from patient's norm); palpation for fremitus; percussion of lung fields; auscultation for breath sounds; pulse oximetry; chest X-ray; arterial blood gas (ABG) values; and hemoglobin level and hematocrit
- Pulmonary function studies
- Psychosocial status, including interest, motivation, and knowledge

Defining characteristics
- Adventitious breath sounds, such as crackles, rhonchi, and wheezes
- Changes in respiratory rate and rhythm
- Cyanosis
- Diminished breath sounds
- Difficulty vocalizing
- Dyspnea
- Ineffective or absent cough
- Orthopnea
- Restlessness
- Sputum production
- Wide-eyed

Expected outcomes
- Airway will remain patent.
- Adventitious breath sounds (crackles, rhonchi, wheezes, or stridor) will be absent.
- Chest X-ray will show no abnormality.
- Oxygen level will be in normal range.
- Patient will breathe deeply and cough to remove secretions.
- Patient will expectorate sputum.
- Patient will demonstrate controlled coughing techniques.
- Ventilation will be adequate.

■ Patient will demonstrate skill in conserving energy while attempting to clear airway.

■ Patient will state understanding of changes needed to diminish oxygen demands.

Suggested NOC outcomes

Anxiety Level; Aspiration Prevention; Respiratory Status: Airway Patency; Respiratory Status: Ventilation

Interventions and rationales

■ Assess respiratory status at least every 4 hours or according to established standards. *Obstruction in the airway leads to atelectasis, pneumonia, or respiratory failure.*

■ Turn patient every 2 hours. Always position for maximal aeration of lung fields and mobilization of secretions. *This prevents pooling and stasis of respiratory secretions.*

■ Mobilize patient to full capabilities *to facilitate chest expansion and ventilation.*

■ Avoid placing patient in supine position for extended periods. Encourage lateral, sitting, prone, and upright positions as much as possible *to enhance lung expansion and ventilation.*

■ When helping patient cough and deep-breathe, use whatever position best ensures cooperation and minimizes energy expenditure, such as high Fowler's position or sitting on side of bed. *Such positions promote chest expansion and ventilation of basilar lung fields.*

■ Suction, as ordered, to stimulate cough and clear airways. Be alert for progression of airway compromise. *These steps prevent respiratory distress.*

■ Perform postural drainage, percussion, and vibration to facilitate secretion movement. Monitor sputum, noting amount, odor, and consistency. *Sputum amount and consistency may indicate hydration status and effectiveness of therapy. Foul-smelling sputum may indicate respiratory infection.*

■ Teach patient an easily performed cough technique *to clear airway without fatigue.*

■ Provide adequate humidification *to loosen secretions.*

■ Encourage adequate water intake (3 to 4 qt [3 to 4 L/day]) *to ensure optimal hydration and loosening of secretions, unless contraindicated.*

■ Encourage sputum expectoration *to remove pathogens and prevent spread of infection.* Provide tissues and paper bags for hygienic disposal.

■ Give expectorants, bronchodilators, and other drugs, as ordered, and monitor effectiveness. *These measures enhance clearance of secretions from airways.*

■ Provide bronchodilator treatments before chest physiotherapy *to optimize results of the treatment.*

■ Administer oxygen, as ordered, t*o promote oxygenation of cells throughout the body.*

■ Monitor ABG values and hemoglobin levels *to assess oxygenation and ventilatory status.* Report deviations from baseline levels; oxygen saturation should be higher than 90%.

■ If conservative measures fail to maintain partial pressure of arterial oxygen (PaO_2) within an acceptable range, prepare for endotracheal intubation, as ordered, *to maintain artificial airway and optimize PaO_2 level.*

■ Assess patient's learning needs, and provide appropriate information *to help prevent recurrence of obstruction and promote change in daily activities to reduce oxygen demands.*

Suggested NIC interventions

Airway Management; Aspiration Precautions; Cough Enhancement; Infection Protection; Oxygen Therapy; Positioning; Respiratory Monitoring; Ventilation Assistance

Evaluations for expected outcomes

■ Patient's airway remains clear and allows for adequate ventilation.
■ Auscultation of patient's lung fields doesn't reveal adventitious breath sounds (crackles, rhonchi, wheezes, or stridor).
■ Patient's chest X-ray is normal.
■ Patient's oxygen level remains within normal range.
■ Patient coughs and deep breathes to expectorate secretions.
■ Patient expectorates sputum.
■ Patient performs controlled coughing techniques.
■ Patient doesn't experience dyspnea or change in respiratory pattern.
■ Patient performs energy conservation techniques.
■ Patient demonstrates understanding of changes needed to diminish oxygen demands.

Documentation

■ Patient's perceptions of ability to cough
■ Observations of physical findings
■ Effectiveness of medications
■ Patient's attempts to clear airway
■ Maneuvers performed to clear airway
■ Evaluations for expected outcomes

Reference

Cigna, J.A., and Turner-Cigna, L.M. "Rehabilitation for the Home Care Patient with COPD," *Home Healthcare Nurse* 23(9):578-84, September 2005.

Latex
ALLERGY RESPONSE
related to absent immune system response

Definition

An allergic response to natural latex rubber products

Assessment

■ Age and gender
■ Weight
■ Occupation
■ Health history, including past episodes of latex allergy; food, pollen, or drug allergy; multiple surgical history; spina bifida; and asthma
■ Current health status, including temperature, blood pressure, respiratory status, and other vital signs
■ Integumentary status, including color, elasticity, hygiene, lesions, moisture, sensation, texture, and turgor
■ Reports of contact with latex products, including when, where, and what
■ Laboratory studies, including arterial blood gas levels, complete blood count, immunoglobulin E level, radioallergosorbent test, and scratch test

Defining characteristics

■ Immediate reactions (less than 1 hour) to latex proteins (can be life-threatening)
■ Contact urticaria progressing to generalized symptoms
■ Edema of the lips, tongue, uvula, and/or throat
■ Shortness of breath or tightness in the chest, wheezing, and bronchospasm leading to respiratory arrest
■ Hypotension, syncope, and cardiac arrest
■ Orofacial characteristics: edema of sclera or eyelids, erythema or itching of the eyes, tearing of the eyes, nasal congestion, rhinorrhea, facial erythema, facial itching, and oral itching
■ Abdominal pain or nausea
■ Flushing
■ General discomfort, generalized edema, and complaints of increasing body warmth
■ Restlessness

Expected outcomes

■ Patient's vital signs, respiratory status, and laboratory values will return to normal.
■ Patient's skin will be clear, moist, and free from erythema, edema, itching, urticaria, and breakdown.
■ Patient will express awareness of allergic response to latex-containing products.
■ Patient will state intention to avoid contact with latex-containing products.

Suggested NOC outcomes

Comfort Level; Immune Hypersensitivity Response; Knowledge: Infection Control; Tissue Integrity: Skin & Mucous Membranes

Interventions and rationales

■ If patient exhibits compromised respiratory status, implement treatment immediately and document the findings. *Airway maintenance is a primary health consideration and must be attended to immediately.*

■ Conduct a nursing assessment and document the results *to allow for development of an individualized care plan.*

■ Monitor respiratory status and document the findings *to detect changes in status and respond appropriately.* Accurate documentation is necessary to maintain continuity of care among staff.

■ Administer prescribed drugs and treatments in a timely fashion. *Wheezing and shortness of breath can quickly deteriorate to respiratory distress and failure. Skin with urticaria and itching is uncomfortable and unsightly, so patients appreciate timely treatment.*

■ Become familiar with the potential adverse effects of administered drugs. Bronchodilators, antihistamines, and corticosteroids may cause systemic adverse effects; *becoming familiar with these effects and ways to respond to them may help prevent serious reactions.*

■ When latex allergy is confirmed, document on the patient record and label the record clearly *to prevent future contact with the allergen.*

■ Remove all latex products from the immediate proximity of patient and the staff treating patient. *If latex products are nearby, they may be inadvertently used by the staff or patient, increasing risk for contact and allergic reaction.*

■ Educate patient and family about allergic reaction to latex products *to prevent future contact and allergic reactions.*

■ Give patient and family a list of household items containing latex, and emphasize the importance of avoiding these. Tell them about nonlatex product substitutes. *Prevention is the foundation of treatment of latex allergy.*

■ Educate patient and family members about the importance of quickly seeking medical treatment for allergic reaction *to foster timely intervention.*

■ Emphasize the need to inform all health care providers — including emergency medical service — about patient's latex sensitivity. Stress the importance of wearing a medical identification bracelet that specifies latex sensitivity *to prevent future contact and allergic reactions.*

■ Provide documentation of latex allergy for patient to take to his employer. With patient's permission, communicate with the employee health department and discuss patient's need to avoid contact with latex products *to help prevent patient's further contact with latex products and avoid latex allergy reaction.*

Suggested NIC interventions

Allergy Management; Anaphylaxis Management; Environmental Risk Protection; Latex Precautions; Risk Identification; Teaching: Individual

Evaluations for expected outcomes

■ Patient's vital signs, respiratory status, and laboratory values return to normal levels.

■ Patient's skin is clear, moist, and free from erythema, edema, itching, urticaria, and breakdown.

■ Patient expresses awareness of allergic response to latex-containing products.

■ Patient expresses intention to avoid contact with latex-containing products.

Documentation

■ Results of nursing assessment

- Diagnosis of latex allergy
- Treatment of allergic reaction, including drugs administered
- Respiratory status throughout episode of allergic reaction
- Integumentary status throughout episode of allergic reaction
- Evidence of refrain from latex product use during patient's care and of removal of latex products from immediate patient area; explanation of latex product substitutes
- Evidence of patient and family education regarding latex allergy and avoidance of latex products
- Evaluations for expected outcomes

Reference
Reines, H.D., and Seifert, P.C. "Patient Safety: Latex Allergy," *Surgical Clinics of North America* 85(6):1329-40, December 2005.

Risk for latex
ALLERGY RESPONSE

Definition
At risk for allergic response to natural latex rubber products

Assessment
- Age, gender, weight
- Occupation
- Current health status, including vital signs, respiratory status, and integumentary status
- Health history, including drug, food, or pollen allergies; surgical history; chronic disease such as spina bifida; and previous local or systemic allergic reactions
- Laboratory studies, such as immunoglobulin E level, complete blood count, radioallergosorbent test, and scratch tests

Risk factors
- Diagnosis of spina bifida
- Frequent medical or occupational exposure to latex
- History of atopy
- History of food allergies, such as allergy to bananas, kiwi, avocados, chestnuts, or pineapples
- Professions with daily exposure to latex
- Conditions associated with continuous or intermittent catheterizations
- History of reaction to latex
- Allergy to poinsettia plants
- History of allergies and asthma

Expected outcomes

- Patient's vital signs, especially respirations, will remain within normal limits.
- Patient's skin will remain free from erythema, edema, urticaria, and breakdown.
- Patient's nasal passages and laryngeal area will remain clear and free from edema and secretions.
- Patient and family members will express understanding of risk of latex allergy.
- Patient and family members will state intention to take precautions to avoid contact with latex products.

Suggested NOC outcomes

Allergy Response: Localized; Immune Hypersensitivity Response; Knowledge: Health Behavior; Risk Control; Risk Detection

Interventions and rationales

- Conduct a nursing assessment and document the results *to allow for development of an individualized care plan.*
- Remove all latex-containing products from patient's room *to reduce risk of allergic reaction.*
- Use only nonlatex products when caring for patient *to reduce risk of latex allergy reaction in patient.*
- Make sure all personnel are aware of the risk of latex allergy and refrain from using latex products during diagnostic procedures. *Communication with other health care personnel allows for continuity of care and reduces the risk of latex allergy reaction.*
- Educate patient and family about the risk of latex allergy *to prevent allergic reaction due to contact with latex products.*
- Explain that although some reactions to latex are relatively minor (such as sneezing and runny nose), others are life-threatening. *This will foster awareness of serious nature of risk.*
- Educate patient and family regarding the symptoms of allergic reaction and the need for quick treatment if symptoms appear. *Rapid response to allergic reaction may help prevent complications, such as skin infection (with local reaction) and respiratory failure (with systemic reaction).*
- Give patient and family a list of household items containing latex and emphasize the importance of avoiding these. Tell them about nonlatex product substitutes. *Prevention is the foundation of treatment of latex allergy.*
- Emphasize the need to inform all health care providers — including emergency medical service — about patient's latex sensitivity. Stress the importance of wearing a medical identification bracelet that specifies latex sensitivity *to prevent future contact and allergic reactions.*
- Provide emotional support to help patient cope with stress. *Fear of latex exposure can cause a high level of stress in a latex-sensitive patient. Some patients are afraid to seek medical help for fear of latex exposure.*

Suggested NIC interventions

Allergy Management; Environmental Management; Health System Guidance; Latex Precautions; Risk Identification; Teaching: Individual

Evaluations for expected outcomes

■ Patient's vital signs, especially respirations, remain within patient's normal limits.
■ Patient's skin remains free from erythema, edema, urticaria, and breakdown.
■ Patient's nasal passages and laryngeal area remain clear and free from edema and secretions.
■ Patient and family members express understanding of risk of latex allergy.
■ Patient and family members state intention to take precautions to avoid contact with latex products.

Documentation

■ Results of nursing assessment
■ Presence of risk factors
■ Communication of risk factors to health care personnel involved in care or diagnostic studies of patient
■ Teaching provided to patient and family members about risk factors and symptoms of allergic reactions
■ Patient's and family members' statements indicating understanding of risk factors and symptoms of allergic reactions
■ Evaluations for expected outcomes

Reference

Crippa, M., et al. "Prevention of Latex Allergy Among Health Care Workers and in the General Population: Latex Protein Content in Devices Commonly Used in Hospitals and General Practice," *International Archives of Occupational and Environmental Health* 79(7):550-57, August 2006.

ANXIETY

related to situational crisis

Definition

Vague uneasy feeling of discomfort or dread accompanied by an autonomic response (the source commonly non-specific or unknown to the individual); a feeling of apprehension caused by anticipation of danger — an alerting signal that warns of impending danger and enables the individual to take measures to deal with threat

Assessment

■ Current health status
■ Patient's perception of problem, onset of problem, recent stressors, life changes, and other precipitants

■ Mental status, including orientation to time, place, and person; insight regarding current situation; judgment; abstract thinking; general information; mood; affect; recent and remote memory; thought processes; and thought content
■ Coping and problem-solving ability
■ Ability to perform activities of daily living
■ Sleep habits
■ Dietary and nutritional status
■ Available support systems, including family members, friends, clergy, and health care agencies

Defining characteristics
Behavioral
■ Diminished productivity
■ Scanning and vigilance
■ Poor eye contact
■ Restlessness
■ Extraneous movement
■ Expressed concerns due to change in life events
■ Insomnia
■ Fidgeting

Affective
■ Regretful
■ Irritable
■ Anguished
■ Fearful
■ Jittery
■ Uncertain
■ Wary
■ Distressed

Physiologic
■ Quivering voice
■ Shakiness
■ Increased respiration
■ Urinary urgency
■ Dilated pupils
■ Increased reflexes
■ Abdominal pain
■ Dry mouth
■ Weakness
■ Decreased pulse

Cognitive
■ Blocking of thoughts
■ Confusion
■ Preoccupation
■ Forgetfulness

■ Impaired attention
■ Rumination

Expected outcomes

■ Patient will identify factors that elicit anxious behaviors.
■ Patient will discuss activities that tend to decrease anxious behaviors.
■ Patient will practice progressive relaxation techniques a specified number of times per day.
■ Patient will cope with current medical situation without demonstrating severe signs of anxiety.

Suggested NOC outcomes

Anxiety Level; Coping; Grief Resolution; Hyperactivity Level; Impulse Self-Control; Psychosocial Adjustment: Life Change; Social Interaction Skills; Stress Level; Symptom Control

Interventions and rationales

■ Spend 10 minutes with patient twice per shift. Convey a willingness to listen. Offer understanding and empathy; for example, "I know you're frightened. I'll stay with you." *Specific amount of uninterrupted, non-care-related time spent with anxious patient builds trust and reduces tension. Active listening helps patient ventilate feelings.*
■ Give patient clear, concise explanations of anything that's about to occur. Avoid information overload; an anxious patient can't assimilate many details. *Anxiety may impair patient's cognitive abilities.*
■ Listen attentively; allow patient to express feelings verbally. *This may allow patient to identify anxious behaviors and discover source of anxiety.*
■ Make no demands on patient. *Anxious patient may respond to excessive demands with hostility and abuse.*
■ Identify and reduce as many environmental stressors (including people) as possible. *Anxiety commonly results from lack of trust in the environment.*
■ Have patient state what kinds of activities promote feelings of comfort, and encourage patient to perform them. *This gives patient a sense of control.*
■ Remain with patient during severe anxiety. *Anxiety is usually related to fear of being left alone.*
■ Include patient in decisions related to care, when feasible. *Anxious patient may mistrust own abilities; involvement in decision making may reduce anxious behaviors.*
■ Support family members in coping with patient's anxious behavior. *Involving family members in process of reassurance and explanation allays patient's anxiety as well as their own.*
■ Allow extra visiting periods with family if this seems to allay patient's anxiety. *This allows anxious patient and family to support each other according to their abilities and at their own pace.*
■ Teach patient relaxation techniques to be performed at least every 4 hours, such as guided imagery, progressive muscle relaxation, and meditation. *These measures restore psychological and physical equilibrium by decreasing autonomic response to anxiety.*

■ Offer relaxing types of music to patient for quiet listening periods. *Listening to relaxing music may have a calming effect on patient.*

■ Refer patient to community or professional mental health resources to provide ongoing mental health assistance. *Encouraging the use of community resources reinforces the notion that anxiety reduction is a long-term process.*

Suggested NIC interventions

Anger Control Assistance; Anticipatory Guidance; Anxiety Reduction; Behavior Modification: Social Skills; Calming Technique; Coping Enhancement; Simple Guided Imagery; Support Group

Evaluations for expected outcomes

■ Patient describes at least two situations that increase anxious behaviors.

■ Patient states at least two ways to eliminate or minimize anxious behaviors.

■ Patient demonstrates progressive relaxation exercises and practices them a specified number of times per day.

■ Patient reports being able to cope with current situation without experiencing severe anxiety.

Documentation

■ Patient's statement of anxiety and feelings of relief

■ Statements about observable signs of patient's anxiety

■ Interventions to reduce patient's anxiety

■ Effectiveness of nursing interventions that can be observed

■ Evaluations for expected outcomes

References

Buffum, M.D., et al. "A Music Intervention to Reduce Anxiety Before Vascular Angiography Procedures," *Journal of Vascular Nursing* 24(3):68-73, September 2006.

Richardson, C., et al. "Psychological Approaches for the Nursing Management of Chronic Pain: Part 2," *Journal of Clinical Nursing* 15(9):1196-202, September 2006.

Death
ANXIETY
related to terminal illness

Definition
Apprehension, worry, or fear related to death or dying

Assessment
■ Age

■ History of present illness

■ Mental status, including level of consciousness, orientation, cognition, memory, and insight

■ Self-care status, including ability to carry out activities of daily living

■ Sleep pattern, including hours of sleep, energy level before and after sleep, rest and relaxation patterns, and difficulty falling asleep

■ Pain assessment, including location, quality, intensity on a scale of 1 to 10, temporal factors, sources of provocation, and relief

■ Psychological status, including reaction to illness and dying, and expressions of fear, anger, hope, and anxiety

■ Spiritual status, including that which gives purpose or meaning in life, religious affiliation, current perception of faith, religious practices, changes in religious beliefs or practices brought on by illness, and evidence of unmet spiritual needs (meaning and purpose, love and relatedness, forgiveness)

■ Family status, including marital status, family roles, family communications, family's ability to meet patient's physical and emotional needs, extent to which religion defines family's value system, and changes patient's illness and impending death will make in family functioning

Defining characteristics

■ Worry about the impact of one's death on significant others

■ Powerlessness over issues related to dying

■ Fear of loss of physical and mental abilities when dying

■ Anticipated pain related to dying

■ Concerns about overworking the caregiver as terminal illness incapacitates self

■ Concern about meeting one's creator or feeling doubtful about the existence of a god or higher being

■ Total loss of control over aspects of one's own death

■ Negative death images or unpleasant thoughts about any event related to death or dying

■ Fear of delayed demise

■ Fear of premature death because it prevents accomplishment of important life goals

■ Worry about being the cause of other's grief or suffering

■ Fear of leaving family alone after death

■ Fear of developing a terminal illness

■ Denial of one's own mortality or impending death

Expected outcomes

■ Patient will identify need for time with others and need for time alone.

■ Patient will identify comfort measures that enhance feelings of well-being.

■ Patient will communicate important thoughts and feelings to family members.

■ Patient will obtain the level of spiritual support he requests.

■ Patient will use available support systems to cope with dying.

■ Patient will express feelings of comfort and peacefulness.

■ Patient will experience dying with dignity, sensitivity, and love.

Suggested NOC outcomes

Acceptance: Health Status; Anxiety Level; Depression Level; Dignified Life Closure; Fear Self-Control; Hope

Interventions and rationales

■ Assess how much help patient wants. *Patient may need a higher degree of independence than caregiver wants to allow.*

■ Offer to spend time either reading to patient or sitting quietly beside him. *Typically, patient approaching death desires the presence of another but isn't interested in conversing.*

■ If patient is confused, provide reassurance by telling him who's in the room. *This information may help to reduce anxiety.*

■ Provide comfort measures — bathing, massage, regulation of environmental temperature, mouth care, administration of ice chips or wet washcloth — according to patient's preferences. *Some patients may prefer not to be bothered unless they specifically request comfort measures.*

■ Help family members identify, discuss, and resolve issues related to patient's dying. *Patient needs the support of family members. Family members may need help removing emotional blocks that prevent them from providing full support to patient.*

■ Demonstrate to patient your willingness to discuss spiritual aspects of death and dying *to foster open discussion.* Keep conversation focused on patient's spiritual values and the role they play in coping with dying *to ensure that your interaction with patient remains therapeutic.*

■ Refer patient to a priest, minister, rabbi, or spiritual counselor, according to his preference, *to show respect for patient's beliefs and provide expert spiritual care.*

■ Ask patient or family members if there's a prayer or words of spiritual comfort that are especially meaningful to him. If patient seems comfortable with your request, recite this special prayer with him. *Doing so will demonstrate support for patient's spiritual needs and convey caring and acceptance.*

■ Help patient cope by listening actively to him and by communicating acceptance of his thoughts and feelings. *Dying patients need the opportunity to express their feelings.*

■ Provide simple physical gestures of support such as holding hands with patient. Encourage family members to do the same. Verify with patient that your actions aren't intrusive. *As patients begin to let go, they sometimes want to experience less touching.*

■ Reassure patient that he won't be left alone; however, respect patient's requests to be alone. *For some patients, asking to be alone is part of the process of letting go.*

Suggested NIC interventions

Active Listening; Anticipatory Guidance; Family Involvement Promotion; Pain Management; Spiritual Support; Touch

Evaluations for expected outcomes

■ Patient expresses satisfaction with private time and time spent with others.

■ Patient uses those comfort measures that enhance individual well-being and reduce physical symptoms associated with anxiety.

- Patient engages in conversation and activities with family, caregivers, and other support people.
- Patient expresses satisfaction with spiritual support that is offered.
- Patient makes appropriate use of available support systems to cope with the dying process.
- Patient exhibits sense of comfort and overall peace.
- Patient dies in a dignified manner in an environment of sensitivity and love.

Documentation
- Behavioral manifestations of anxiety
- Patient's expressions of feelings related to death and dying
- Patient's requests for visitors or expression of desire for solitude
- Conferences with family members
- Patient's requests for comfort measures and their effectiveness
- Referrals to clergy, spiritual advisors, or others
- Patient's response to nursing interventions
- Evaluations for expected outcomes

Reference
Duggleby, W., and Berry, P. "Transitions and Shifting Goals of Care for Palliative Patients and Their Families," *Clinical Journal of Oncology Nursing* 9(4):425-28, August 2005.

Risk for
ASPIRATION
related to presence of endotracheal or tracheostomy tube

Definition
At risk for entry of GI secretions, oropharyngeal secretions, solids, or fluids into tracheobronchial passages

Assessment
- Neurologic status, including level of consciousness (LOC), orientation, and mental status
- GI status, including gag and swallow reflexes, inspection of abdomen, abdominal girth, auscultation of bowel sounds, palpation for masses and tenderness, percussion of abdomen, and medications
- Nutritional status, including continuous and intermittent tube feeding
- Respiratory status, including skin color, rate and depth of respiration, cough (productive or nonproductive), auscultation of breath sounds, palpation for fremitus, sputum characteristics (color, consistency, amount, and odor), arterial blood gas values, and chest X-ray
- Vital signs
- Laboratory studies, such as white blood cell (WBC) count and sputum culture

Risk factors

- Increased intragastric pressure
- Tube feedings
- Situations hindering elevation of the upper body
- Reduced LOC
- Presence of endotracheal or tracheostomy tube
- Medication administration
- Wired jaws
- Increased gastric residual
- Incompetent lower esophageal sphincter
- Impaired swallowing
- Depressed gag reflexes
- Decreased GI motility

Expected outcomes

- Patient will tolerate ____ ml of tube feeding.
- Patient's temperature and WBC count will remain normal.
- No pathogens will appear in cultures.
- Respiratory secretions will be clear and odorless.
- Auscultation will reveal no adventitious breath sounds.
- Auscultation will reveal normal bowel sounds.
- Patient and caregiver will discuss measures to prevent aspiration.

Suggested NOC outcomes

Aspiration Prevention; Mechanical Ventilation Response: Adult; Respiratory Status: Airway Patency; Respiratory Status: Ventilation; Risk Control; Swallowing Status

Interventions and rationales

- Assess respiratory status at least every 4 hours *for signs of possible aspiration (increased respiratory rate, cough, sputum production, or diminished breath sounds).*
- Monitor and record neurologic status *to detect altered LOC, which could affect intake of food or saliva.*
- Monitor and record vital signs *to detect signs of aspiration or impaired gas exchange due to aspiration.*
- Suction as needed *to keep airway clear.*
- Assess patient for gag and swallow reflexes. *Decreased gag or swallow reflex may cause aspiration.*
- Encourage patient to cough and expectorate sputum *to mobilize secretions.* Provide tissues and paper bags for hygienic sputum disposal *to prevent spreading infection.*
- Auscultate for bowel sounds every shift and report changes. *Delayed gastric emptying and elevated intragastric pressure may promote regurgitation of stomach contents.*

■ If patient is receiving tube feedings:

– Assess cuff inflation for patient with artificial airway and adjust appropriately *to protect lower airways from oropharyngeal secretions.*

– Add food coloring to tube feeding if patient has altered state of consciousness, diminished gag reflex, or history of aspiration *to help monitor gastric secretions for aspiration.*

– Begin regimen with a small, diluted amount, as tolerated and ordered, *to allow adjustment to formula osmolality and avoid nausea, vomiting, and diarrhea.*

– Elevate head of bed during and after feedings unless contraindicated *to prevent aspiration.*

– Check for residual tube feeding every shift and record amount. If more than 50 ml remains, withhold feeding *to prevent vomiting and aspiration.* Report findings to physician.

– Place tube properly before feeding or giving medication *to protect airway.*

– Stop feeding immediately if you suspect aspiration; then apply suction, as needed, and turn patient on side *to avoid further aspiration.*

■ Assess need for antiemetic drug *to reduce nausea and vomiting.* Administer, if ordered, and monitor for effectiveness.

■ Review test results *to identify signs of infection;* report abnormalities.

■ Explain treatment to patient and caregivers *to encourage compliance.*

Suggested NIC interventions

Airway Suctioning; Artificial Airway Management; Aspiration Precautions; Enteral Tube Feeding; Positioning; Vomiting Management

Evaluations for expected outcomes

■ Patient tolerates _____ ml of tube feeding.

■ Patient's temperature and WBC count remain within normal parameters.

■ No pathogens appear in patient's cultures.

■ Patient's respiratory secretions remain clear and odorless.

■ Auscultation of lungs reveals no adventitious breath sounds.

■ Auscultation of abdomen reveals normal bowel sounds.

■ Patient and caregiver discuss measures necessary to prevent aspiration.

Documentation

■ Verification of tube placement

■ Tolerance of tube feedings

■ Residuals of tube feedings

■ Vomiting or aspiration

■ Breath sounds

■ Patient's indication of situations that may lead to aspiration

■ Observations of physical findings

■ Interventions performed to prevent aspiration

■ Evaluations for expected outcomes

Reference

Williams, T.A., and Leslie, G.D. "A Review of the Nursing Care of Enteral Feeding Tubes in Critically Ill Adults: Part II," *Intensive & Critical Care Nursing* 21(1):5-15, February 2005.

AUTONOMIC DYSREFLEXIA

Definition

Life-threatening, uninhibited sympathetic response of nervous system to noxious stimulus after spinal cord injury at T7 or above

Assessment

■ History of spinal cord trauma, including level of injury or lesion, and previous episodes of dysreflexia

■ Patient's description of symptoms, including headache, nasal congestion, blurred vision, chest pain, diaphoresis and flushing above level of lesion, chilling, paresthesia, cutis anserina ("goose flesh") above level of lesion, metallic taste, and nausea

■ Neurologic status, including level of consciousness, orientation, pupillary response, sensory status, and motor status

■ Cardiovascular status, including blood pressure, heart rate and rhythm, and skin temperature and color

■ Genitourinary status, including urine output, palpation of bladder, signs of urinary tract infection (UTI), and examination of urinary assistive devices such as catheter

■ GI status, including nausea and vomiting, usual bowel elimination pattern, last bowel movement, inspection of abdomen, auscultation of bowel sounds, palpation for masses, and percussion for areas of dullness

■ Environmental conditions, including changes in temperature (for example, cold draft) and objects putting pressure on skin

Defining characteristics

■ Paroxysmal hypertension (sudden periodic elevated blood pressure, systolic over 140 mm Hg and diastolic over 90 mm Hg); bradycardia or tachycardia (pulse under 60 or over 100 beats/minute); diaphoresis above injury; red splotches (vasodilation) on skin above injury; pallor below injury; or diffuse headache not confined to any nerve distribution area

■ Bladder distention

■ Bowel distention

■ Lack of caregiver and patient knowledge

■ Chilling, conjunctival congestion, Horner's syndrome (contracted pupils, partial ptosis, enophthalmos, loss of sweating on affected side of face [sometimes]), paresthesia, pilomotor reflex, blurred vision, chest pain, metallic taste, or nasal congestion

Expected outcomes

■ Cause of dysreflexia will be identified and corrected.
■ Patient will experience cardiovascular stability as evidenced by _____ systolic range, _____ diastolic range, and _____ heart rate range.
■ Patient will avoid bladder distention and UTI.
■ Patient will have no fecal impaction.
■ Patient's environment will have no noxious stimuli.
■ Patient will state relief from symptoms of dysreflexia.
■ Patient will have few if any complications.
■ Patient's bladder elimination pattern will remain normal.
■ Patient's bowel elimination pattern will remain normal.
■ Patient, family members, or caregiver will demonstrate knowledge and understanding of dysreflexia and will describe care measures.
■ Patient will experience few or no dysreflexic episodes.

Suggested NOC outcomes

Knowledge: Disease Process; Neurologic Status; Neurologic Status: Autonomic; Sensory Function Status; Vital Signs Status

Interventions and rationales

■ Assess for signs of dysreflexia (especially severe hypertension) *to detect condition so that prompt treatment may be initiated.*
■ Place patient in sitting position or elevate head of bed *to aid venous drainage from brain, lower intracranial pressure, and temporarily reduce blood pressure.*
■ Ascertain and correct probable cause of dysreflexia:
– Check for bladder distention and patency of catheter. If necessary, irrigate catheter with small amount of solution, or insert a new catheter immediately. *A blocked urinary catheter can trigger dysreflexia.*
– Check for fecal mass in rectum. Apply dibucaine ointment (Nupercainal) or another product, as ordered, to anus and 1" (2.5 cm) into rectum 10 to 15 minutes before removing impaction. *Failure to use ointment may aggravate autonomic response.*
– Check environment for cold drafts and objects putting pressure on patient's skin, *which could act as dysreflexia stimuli.*
– Send urine for culture if no other cause becomes apparent *to detect possible UTI.*
■ If hypertension persists despite other measures, administer ganglionic blocking agent, vasodilator, or other medication as ordered. *Drugs may be required if hypertension persists or if noxious stimuli can't be removed.*
■ Take vital signs frequently *to monitor effectiveness of prescribed medications.*
■ Instruct patient, family members, or caregiver about dysreflexia, including its causes, signs and symptoms, and care measures *to prepare them to handle possible emergencies related to condition.*
■ Implement and maintain bowel and bladder elimination programs *to avoid stimuli that could trigger dysreflexia.*

Suggested NIC interventions

Airway Management; Bowel Management; Dysreflexia Management; Fluid Management; Neurologic Monitoring; Surveillance; Temperature Management; Vital Signs Monitoring

Evaluations for expected outcomes

■ Cause of dysreflexia is identified and corrected.
■ Patient experiences cardiovascular stability as evidenced by ___ systolic range, _____ diastolic range, and ___ heart rate range.
■ Palpation doesn't reveal a distended bladder or signs of UTI.
■ Patient's bowel elimination program is successfully implemented and maintained. Fecal impaction is absent.
■ Patient's environment remains free from noxious stimuli.
■ Patient expresses relief from signs and symptoms of dysreflexia.
■ Patient doesn't experience complications of dysreflexia, including contractures, venous stasis, thrombus formation, skin breakdown, and hypostatic pneumonia.
■ Patient's bladder elimination program is successfully implemented and maintained, urinary catheter is patent and without kinking or blockage, and urine output remains within specified volume.
■ Patient's bowel elimination pattern remains normal.
■ Patient, family member, or caregiver expresses understanding of causes, signs and symptoms, and treatment of autonomic dysreflexia and demonstrates measures to implement if dysreflexia occurs.
■ Because of successful maintenance of bladder and bowel elimination programs, preventive skin care measures, and patient and family teaching, patient experiences few or no dysreflexic episodes.

Documentation

■ Objective assessment of dysreflexic episode
■ Patient's description of dysreflexic episode
■ Interventions to identify and eliminate causes of dysreflexia and patient's response to these
■ Instructions given to patient, family, and caregiver
■ Patient's expressions of understanding and demonstrated ability to prevent or manage dysreflexic episode
■ Implementation, alteration, or continuation of bladder and bowel programs
■ Evaluations for expected outcomes

Reference

Karlsson, A.K. "Autonomic Dysfunction in Spinal Cord Injury: Clinical Presentation of Symptoms and Signs," *Progress in Brain Research* 152:1-8, 2006.

Risk for
AUTONOMIC DYSREFLEXIA

Definition
At risk for life-threatening, uninhibited sympathetic response of nervous system to noxious stimulus after spinal cord injury at T7 or above

Assessment
- History of spinal cord trauma or spinal cord tumor, including level of injury or lesion; previous episodes of dysreflexia
- Neurologic status, including level of consciousness, orientation, pupillary response, sensory status, and motor status
- Cardiovascular status, including blood pressure, heart rate and rhythm, and skin temperature and color
- Genitourinary status, including urine output, palpation of bladder, signs of urinary tract infection (UTI), and urinary assistive devices such as catheter
- GI status, including nausea and vomiting, usual bowel pattern, bowel habits, last bowel movement, inspection of abdomen, auscultation of bowel sounds, palpation for masses and tenderness, and percussion for areas of tympany and dullness
- Environmental conditions, including changes in temperature (for example, cold drafts) and objects putting pressure on skin

Risk factors
An injury or lesion at T6 or above and at least one of the following noxious stimuli:
- Painful stimuli below level of injury
- Bladder distention
- Detrusor sphincter dyssynergia
- Bladder spasm
- Instrumentation or surgery
- Epididymitis
- Urethritis
- Urinary tract infection
- Calculi
- Cystitis
- Catheterization
- Constipation or fecal impaction
- Digital stimulation
- Suppositories
- Hemorrhoids
- Difficult passage of stool
- Enemas
- Gastric ulcers
- Esophageal reflux

- Gallstones
- Menstruation
- Sexual intercourse
- Pregnancy
- Ovarian cyst
- Ejaculation
- Pressures over boney prominences
- Fractures
- Wounds
- Temperature fluctuations
- Positioning
- Constrictive clothing
- Drug reactions
- Pulmonary emboli
- Deep vein thrombosis

Expected outcomes

- Risk factors for dysreflexia will be identified and reduced.
- Patient will avoid bladder distention.
- Patient won't experience UTI.
- Patient will maintain normal urinary and bowel elimination patterns.
- Patient will be free from fecal impaction.
- Patient's environment will be free from noxious stimuli that may cause dysreflexia.
- Patient, family member, or caregiver will express understanding of causes of dysreflexia.
- Patient, family member, or caregiver will demonstrate understanding of measures to prevent dysreflexia.

Suggested NOC outcomes

Neurologic Status: Autonomic; Symptom Severity; Vital Signs Status

Interventions and rationales

- Assess for risk factors of dysreflexia, such as constipation, fecal impaction, distended bladder, and presence of noxious stimuli. *Identifying risk factors can prevent or minimize dysreflexic episodes.*
- Monitor and record intake and output accurately *to ensure adequate fluid replacement, thereby helping to prevent constipation.*
- Check for bladder distention and patency of catheter. *A blocked catheter can trigger dysreflexia.*
- Check for abdominal distention and assess bowel sounds. Monitor and record characteristics and frequency of stools. *Fecal impaction may lead to dysreflexia.*
- Encourage fluid intake of 2½ qt (2.5 L) daily, unless contraindicated. *Adequate fluid intake helps maintain patency of catheter and aids bowel elimination.*
- Administer laxative, enema, or suppositories, as prescribed, *to promote elimination of solids and gases from GI tract.* Monitor effectiveness.

■ Consult with dietitian about increasing fiber and bulk in diet to maximum prescribed by physician *to improve intestinal muscle tone and promote comfortable elimination.*

■ Implement and maintain bowel and bladder programs *to avoid stimuli that could trigger dysreflexia.*

■ Monitor vital signs frequently *to ensure effectiveness of preventive measures.* Severe hypertension may indicate dysreflexia.

■ Instruct patient, family member, or caregiver about risk factors, signs and symptoms, and care measures for dysreflexia *to help prevent a possible dysreflexic episode and help him respond appropriately should dysreflexia occur.*

Suggested NIC interventions
Dysreflexia Management; Neurologic Monitoring; Vital Signs Monitoring

Evaluations for expected outcomes
■ Risk factors for dysreflexia are identified and reduced.

■ Patient avoids bladder distention.

■ Patient doesn't experience UTI.

■ Patient maintains normal urinary and bowel elimination patterns.

■ Patient remains free from fecal impaction.

■ Patient's environment is free from noxious stimuli that may cause dysreflexia.

■ Patient, family member, or caregiver expresses understanding of causes of dysreflexia.

■ Patient, family member, or caregiver demonstrates understanding of measures to prevent dysreflexia.

Documentation
■ Presence of risk factors for dysreflexia

■ Interventions to minimize risk of dysreflexia and patient's response

■ Patient's, family members', or caregiver's expressions of concern about risk of dysreflexia

■ Instructions given to patient, family member, or caregiver regarding prevention of dysreflexic episodes

■ Implementation or alteration of bowel and bladder program

■ Evaluations for expected outcomes

Reference
Joseph, A.C., and Albo, M. "Urodynamics: The Incidence of Urinary Tract Infection and Autonomic Dysreflexia in a Challenging Population," *Urologic Nursing* 24(5):390-93, October 2004.

Risk-prone health
BEHAVIOR

related to disability or health status change requiring change in lifestyle

Definition
Inability to modify lifestyle/behavior in a manner consistent with changed health status

Assessment
■ Nature and impact of medical diagnosis
■ Behavioral responses, including verbal or nonverbal, engagement or disengagement, interest or apathy, acceptance or denial, and independence or dependence
■ Knowledge of health condition
■ Past experiences with family, friends, and media
■ Psychosocial factors, such as age, gender, ethnic and cultural background, religious preference and beliefs, values, occupation, family support, and coping style
■ Nutritional status, including modifications in diet and weight changes

Defining characteristics
■ Demonstration of nonacceptance of health status change
■ Failure to achieve optimal sense of control
■ Failure to take action to prevent further health problems
■ Denial of health status change

Expected outcomes
■ Patient will identify inability to cope and will adjust adequately.
■ Patient will express understanding of the illness or disease.
■ Patient will participate in health care regimen and will plan care activities.
■ Patient will demonstrate ability to manage health problem.
■ Patient will show ability to accept and adapt to a new health status and integrate learning.
■ Patient will demonstrate new coping strategies.

Suggested NOC outcomes
Acceptance: Health Status; Adaptation to Physical Disability; Coping; Health Seeking Behavior; Participation in Health Care Decisions; Psychosocial Adjustment: Life Change; Social Support; Treatment Behavior: Illness or Injury

Interventions and rationales
■ Encourage patient to express feelings in a safe, nonthreatening environment. *This allows patient to gain insight into and rationally define fears, goals, and potential problems.*
■ Allow patient to grieve. Grieving is a normal and essential aspect with any kind of negative change in health status. *After working through denial and isolation, anger, bargaining, and depression, patient will progress toward acceptance.*

■ Provide reassurance that patient's feelings, under these circumstances, are normal. *By realizing that it's acceptable to grieve, the patient will be ready to look for positive ways of coping.*

■ Begin teaching patient and caregivers the skills needed to adequately manage care *to encourage compliance and adjustment to optimum wellness.*

■ Spend 15 minutes per shift listening to patient's feelings. *This helps reassure patient you're interested and care.*

■ Help patient identify areas where it's possible to maintain control. *This avoids feelings of powerlessness and lets patient feel part of a team effort.*

■ Encourage patient to plan for care activities, such as time of treatment, personal hygiene, and rest periods. *Doing this offers patient an opportunity to control facets of care and increases feelings of self-determination.*

■ Arrange for others who have suffered similar health problems to speak with patient and family. *This exposes patient to suitable role models and may allow a trusting, supportive relationship to develop.*

■ Discuss health problems and implications with family members *to enable them to participate in patient's care and to foster a trusting relationship.*

■ Obtain a consultation with a mental health specialist if patient develops severe depression or other psychiatric problems. *Although trauma or illness commonly causes some depression, consultation with a mental health professional may help minimize it.*

Suggested NIC interventions

Anxiety Reduction; Behavior Modification; Coping Enhancement; Counseling; Decision-Making Support; Emotional Support; Mutual Goal Setting; Role Enhancement; Simple Relaxation Therapy; Support System Enhancement

Evaluations for expected outcomes

■ Patient recognizes necessity of learning to live with impairment.

■ Patient understands that grieving is a normal response to impairment.

■ Patient meets learning objectives before discharge.

■ Patient identifies and contacts sources of continued psychological support if needed.

■ Patient identifies two areas in which he can maintain control despite altered health status.

■ Patient meets with individual who has similar health problem and reports results of meeting.

Documentation

■ Patient's nonverbal behaviors

■ Patient's verbal expressions of denial, anger, or guilt because of the illness or disease process

■ Patient's ability or inability to participate in care

■ Evaluations for expected outcomes

Reference

Telford, K., et al. "Acceptance and Denial: Implications for People Adapting to Chronic Illness: Literature Review," *Journal of Advanced Nursing* 55(4):457-64, August 2006.

Disturbed
BODY IMAGE
related to biophysical changes

Definition
Confusion in mental picture of one's physical self

Assessment
- Physiologic changes
- Behavioral changes
- Patient's and family's perception of patient's present health problem
- Patient's usual pattern of coping with stress
- Marital status
- Patient's role in family
- Patient's past experiences with health problems
- Sleep pattern
- Appetite
- Hobbies and interests
- Occupational history
- Ethnic background and cultural perceptions

Defining characteristics
- Actual change in structure or function
- Verbalization of feelings and perceptions that reflect an altered view of one's body in appearance, structure, or function
- Behaviors of avoiding, monitoring, or acknowledging one's body
- Hiding or overexposing body part (intentional or unintentional)
- Missing body part
- Nonverbal or verbal response to actual or perceived change in structure or function
- Not looking at or touching body part
- Trauma to nonfunctioning part
- Preoccupation with change or loss
- Personalization of part or loss by name
- Depersonalization of part or loss by impersonal pronouns
- Extension of body boundary to incorporate environmental objects
- Negative feelings about body
- Verbalization of change in lifestyle
- Focus on past strength, function, or appearance
- Fear of rejection by others

■ Emphasis on remaining strengths
■ Heightened achievement

Expected outcomes
■ Patient will acknowledge change in body image.
■ Patient will participate in decision making about his care (specify).
■ Patient will communicate feelings about change in body image.
■ Patient will express positive feelings about self.
■ Patient will talk with someone who has experienced the same problem.
■ Patient will demonstrate ability to practice two new coping behaviors.

Suggested NOC outcomes

Adaptation to Physical Disability; Body Image; Coping; Grief Resolution; Psychosocial Adjustment: Life Change; Self-Esteem

Interventions and rationales
■ While assisting with self-care measures, involve patient in discussions that will provide further insights into patient's coping patterns and self-esteem. *Patient's usual coping patterns and self-perception provide baseline data for assessing potential threat of current situation.*
■ Accept patient's perception of self. *The nurse's acceptance validates patient's self-perception and provides reassurance that he can successfully overcome crisis.*
■ Assess patient's readiness for decision making; then involve him in making choices and decisions related to care. *This gives patient sense of control over environment.*
■ Encourage patient to participate actively in performing care. *This gives patient sense of independence and increases self-esteem.*
■ Give patient opportunities to voice feelings. *This helps patient ventilate doubts and resolve concerns.*
■ Provide positive reinforcement to patient's efforts to adapt *to increase probability that healthy adaptation will continue.*
■ Arrange for patient to interact with others who have similar problems. *A support group allows patient to share mutual support and caring with others who can fully understand.*
■ Refer patient to a mental health professional for further counseling. *Referral to psychiatric liaison nurse is indicated when patient is adapting poorly to situation.*
■ Teach patient coping strategies (specify) *to help overcome maladaptive coping behaviors.*
■ Have patient provide feedback about coping behaviors that seem to work. Reinforce the practice of these behaviors. *This allows you to evaluate patient's adaptive abilities.* Positive feedback reinforces adaptability and encourages similar behaviors in future.

Suggested NIC interventions

Active Listening; Anticipatory Guidance; Body Image Enhancement; Coping Enhancement; Counseling; Grief Work Facilitation; Presence; Self-Care Assistance; Spiritual Support; Support System Enhancement

Evaluations for expected outcomes
- Patient acknowledges change in body image.
- Patient takes an active role in planning aspects of care (specify).
- Patient expresses emotions associated with change in body image.
- Patient expresses at least one positive feeling about self daily.
- Patient participates in discussions with support group composed of individuals with a similar change in body image (specify).
- Patient uses at least two healthy coping skills to deal with change in body image.

Documentation
- Words patient uses to describe self, prostheses, adaptive equipment, and limitations
- Body parts that patient focuses on or ignores
- Observations related to change in structure or function of body part
- Observed responses of patient to change in body part, such as touching or not touching
- Health education or counseling provided to help patient cope with altered body image
- Patient's response to nursing interventions
- Evaluations for expected outcomes

Reference
Alfano, C.M., and Rowland, J.H. "Recovery Issues in Cancer Survivorship: A New Challenge for Supportive Care," *Cancer Journal* 12(5):432-43, September-October 2006.

BOWEL INCONTINENCE
related to impaired cognition

Definition
Change in normal bowel habits characterized by involuntary passage of stool

Assessment
- History of neurologic or psychiatric disorder
- Fluid and electrolyte status, including intake and output, skin turgor, urine specific gravity, and mucous membranes
- GI status, including usual bowel elimination habits, change in bowel habits, stool characteristics (color, amount, size, and consistency), pain or discomfort, inspection of abdomen, auscultation of bowel sounds, palpation for masses and tenderness, percussion for tympany and dullness, and laxative and enema use
- Characteristics of incontinence, including frequency, time of day, before or after meals, relationship to activity, and behavior pattern (restlessness)
- Neurologic status, including orientation, level of consciousness, memory, and cognitive ability

Defining characteristics

- Constant dribbling of soft stool
- Fecal odor
- Fecal staining of clothing or bedding
- Feeling of rectal fullness
- Ignoring of urge to defecate
- Inability to delay defecation
- Inability to feel rectal fullness or urge to defecate
- Red perianal skin
- Urgency

Expected outcomes

- Patient will experience bowel movement every ___ day(s) when placed on commode or toilet at ___ a.m./p.m.
- Patient's skin will remain clean and intact.
- Patient will improve control of incontinent episodes.
- Caregiver will state understanding of bowel routine.
- Caregiver will demonstrate skill in placing patient on commode.
- Caregiver will demonstrate skill in use of suppository if indicated.
- Caregiver will understand and explain relationship of food and fluid regulation to promotion of continence.
- Patient will maintain self-respect and dignity through participation and acceptance within group.

Suggested NOC outcomes

Bowel Continence; Bowel Elimination; Cognition; Self-Care: Toileting; Tissue Integrity: Skin & Mucous Membranes

Interventions and rationales

- Establish a regular pattern for bowel care; for example, after breakfast every other day, place patient on commode chair 1 hour after inserting suppository, and allow patient to remain upright for 30 minutes for maximum response; then clean anal area. *Procedure encourages adaptation and routine physiologic function.*
- Monitor and record incontinent episodes; keep baseline record for 3 to 7 days *to track effectiveness of toileting routine.*
- Discuss bowel care routine with family or caregiver *to foster compliance.*
- Demonstrate bowel care routine to family or caregiver *to reduce anxiety from lack of knowledge or involvement in care.*
- Arrange for return demonstration of bowel care routine *to help establish therapeutic relationship with patient and family or caregiver.*
- Establish a date when family or caregiver will carry out bowel care routine with supportive assistance; *this will ensure that patient receives dependable care.*
- Instruct family or caregiver on need to regulate foods and fluids that cause diarrhea or constipation *to encourage helpful nutritional habits.*
- Maintain diet log *to identify irritating foods,* and then eliminate them from patient's diet.
- Clean and dry perianal area after each incontinent episode *to prevent infection and promote comfort.*

■ Maintain patient's dignity by using protective padding under clothing, by removing patient from group activity after incontinent episode, and by cleaning and returning patient to group without undue attention. *These measures prevent odor, skin breakdown, and embarrassment and promote patient's positive self-image.*

Suggested NIC interventions
Bowel Incontinence Care; Bowel Management; Perineal Care; Skin Surveillance

Evaluations for expected outcomes
■ Patient has one soft bowel movement every _____ day(s).
■ Patient's skin remains clean, dry, and intact.
■ Patients' episodes of incontinence decrease by 50%.
■ Caregiver can explain bowel routine.
■ Caregiver successfully demonstrates placing patient on commode.
■ Caregiver successfully demonstrates insertion of suppositories.
■ Caregiver explains relationship between food and fluid intake and regulation of continence and plans appropriate diet for patient.
■ Patient expresses positive self-image.

Documentation
■ Patient's level of awareness, response to incontinent episodes, and acceptance of bowel care routine
■ Family's or caregiver's response to incontinence and to establishment and implementation of a bowel care routine
■ Observation of effects of bowel care routine, episodes of incontinence, stool characteristics, and condition of skin
■ Family's or caregiver's skill in carrying out bowel care routine and modifying diet
■ Evaluations for expected outcomes

Reference
Dowd, T., and Dowd, E.T. "A Cognitive Therapy Approach to Promote Continence," *Journal of Wound, Ostomy, and Continence Nursing* 33(1):63-68, January-February 2006.

BOWEL INCONTINENCE
related to lower motor nerve damage

Definition
Change in normal bowel habits characterized by involuntary passage of stool

Assessment
■ History of neuromuscular disorder

■ GI status, including usual bowel elimination pattern, history of bowel disorder, laxative or enema use, incontinence characteristics (frequency, awareness of need to defecate, and precipitating factors), presence or absence of anal sphincter reflex, and bowel sounds
■ Fluid and electrolyte status, including intake and output, urine specific gravity, skin turgor, and mucous membranes
■ Nutritional status, including usual dietary pattern, appetite, tolerance or intolerance for foods, current (and normal) weight
■ Activity status, including type of exercise, frequency, and duration

Defining characteristics
■ Constant dribbling of soft stool
■ Fecal odor
■ Fecal staining of clothing or bedding
■ Feeling of rectal fullness
■ Ignoring of urge to defecate
■ Inability to delay defecation
■ Inability to feel rectal fullness or urge to defecate
■ Red perianal skin
■ Urgency

Expected outcomes
■ Patient will establish and maintain a regular pattern of bowel care.
■ Patient will state understanding of bowel care routine.
■ Patient or caregiver will demonstrate skill in carrying out bowel care routine with help from nurse.
■ Patient or caregiver will demonstrate increasing skill in performing bowel care routine independently.
■ Patient will participate in social activities.

Suggested NOC outcomes
Bowel Continence; Bowel Elimination; Self Care: Hygiene; Self-Care: Toileting; Tissue Integrity: Skin & Mucous Membranes

Interventions and rationales
■ For upper motor neuron lesion (anal reflex intact):
– Establish regular pattern for bowel care; for example, after breakfast every other day, maintain patient in upright position after inserting suppository, and allow a half hour for suppository to melt and maximum reflex response to occur. *Regular pattern encourages adaptation and routine physiologic function.*
– Discuss bowel care routine with patient and family *to promote feelings of safety, adequacy, and comfort.*
– Demonstrate bowel care to patient and caregivers *to reduce anxiety from lack of knowledge or involvement in care.*
– Observe return demonstration of bowel care routine by patient and caregivers *to check skills and establish a therapeutic relationship.*
– Establish a date when patient or caregivers will carry out bowel routine independently, with supportive assistance, *to reassure patient of dependable care.*

– Instruct patient and family on need to regulate foods and fluids that cause diarrhea or constipation *to encourage good nutritional habits.*

– Maintain dietary intake diary *to identify irritating foods;* instruct patient to avoid foods that are spicy, rich, or produce gas *to prevent painful flatulence.*

– Obtain order allowing modified bowel preparations for tests and procedures *to avoid interrupting routine and to encourage regular bowel function.*

– Encourage patient to use protective padding under clothing, changing it as necessary *to prevent odor, skin breakdown, or embarrassment and to promote positive self-image.*

■ For lower motor neuron lesion (flaccid sphincter):

– Establish regular pattern for bowel care; for example, after breakfast every other day, turn patient on left side, put waterproof pads under buttocks, administer prescribed enema, and allow him to remain in place 2 to 5 minutes. Then perform digital removal of stool, clean perianal area, and remove soiled pads. *These procedures encourage regular physiologic function, stimulate peristalsis, minimize infection, and promote comfort and elimination.*

– Follow rest of interventions for upper motor neuron lesion.

Suggested NIC interventions

Bowel Incontinence Care; Bowel Training; Emotional Support; Fluid Management; Self-Care Assistance: Toileting; Skin Surveillance; Teaching: Toilet Training

Evaluations for expected outcomes

■ Patient establishes and maintains regular pattern of bowel care.

■ Patient states understanding of bowel care routine.

■ Patient or caregiver demonstrates competence in performing bowel care routine with assistance from nurse.

■ Patient or caregiver carries out bowel routine independently.

■ Patient attends social events without experiencing bowel incontinence.

Documentation

■ Patient's feelings about problem and bowel routine

■ Bowel care routine and administration of suppositories and enemas

■ Description of incontinent episodes, including known precipitating factors, time of day, and other relevant details

■ Patient's and caregivers' skills in bowel care

■ Evaluations for expected outcomes

Reference

Akhtar, A.J., and Padda, M. "Fecal Incontinence in Older Patients," *Journal of the American Medical Directors Association* 6(1):54-60, January-February 2005.

Ineffective
BREATHING PATTERN
related to pain

Definition
Inspiration or expiration that doesn't provide adequate ventilation

Assessment
■ History of medical or surgical problem that causes ineffective breathing
■ Respiratory status, including rate and depth of respiration, symmetry of chest expansion, use of accessory muscles, presence of cough, anterior-posterior chest diameter, palpation for fremitus, percussion of lung fields, auscultation of breath sounds, and arterial blood gas (ABG) levels
■ Cardiovascular status, including heart rate and rhythm and blood pressure
■ Neurologic status, including level of consciousness and sensory and motor status
■ Psychosocial status, including willingness to cooperate with treatment, coping mechanisms, and current understanding of physical condition

Defining characteristics
■ Accessory muscle use
■ Altered chest excursion
■ Altered respiratory rate or depth or both
■ Assumption of three-point position
■ Decreased inspiratory or expiratory pressure
■ Decreased minute ventilation
■ Decreased vital capacity
■ Dyspnea
■ Increased anterior-posterior diameter
■ Nasal flaring
■ Orthopnea
■ Prolonged expiration phase
■ Pursed-lip breathing
■ Shortness of breath

Expected outcomes
■ Patient's respiratory rate will stay within 5 breaths of baseline.
■ ABG levels will remain normal.
■ Patient will achieve comfort without depressing respirations.
■ Patient will demonstrate correct use of incentive spirometer.
■ Auscultation will reveal no adventitious breath sounds.
■ Patient will state importance of taking deep breaths periodically.
■ Patient will practice relaxation techniques ___ times per day.
■ Patient will report ability to breathe comfortably.

Suggested NOC outcomes

Respiratory Status: Airway Patency; Respiratory Status: Ventilation; Vital Signs

Interventions and rationales

■ Assess and record respiratory status at least every 4 hours *to detect early signs of compromise.* Also assess ABG levels, according to facility policy, *to monitor oxygenation and ventilation status.*

■ Assess for pain every 3 hours. Pain reduces respiratory effort and ventilation.

■ Give pain medication, as ordered, *to allow maximal chest expansion.* Record effectiveness, and monitor respiratory depression induced by opioid analgesic *to guide further therapy.*

■ Assist patient to a comfortable position that also allows for maximal chest expansion; for example, use Fowler's position or have patient lean on overbed table with pillow *to enhance chest expansion.*

■ Assist patient in using incentive spirometer or other device, as ordered, *to ensure proper use and help prevent atelectasis.*

■ Teach patient how to splint chest while coughing. Keep extra pillow for patient's use. *Splinting reduces pain during coughing.*

■ Perform chest physiotherapy *to aid mobilization and secretion removal* if ordered. Percussion, vibration, and postural drainage enhance airway clearance and respiratory effort.

■ Provide rest periods between breathing enhancement measures *to avoid fatigue.*

■ Encourage patient to use incentive spirometer independently. Praise patient's efforts *to encourage compliance.*

■ Provide oxygen, as ordered, *to help relieve respiratory distress caused by hypoxemia.*

■ Teach relaxation techniques, such as guided imagery, progressive muscle relaxation, breathing exercises, and meditation, *to reduce pain and anxiety and enhance patient's sense of self-control.*

■ Change patient's position frequently *to maximize comfort.*

■ Encourage patient to discuss fears *to help reduce anxiety.*

Suggested NIC interventions

Airway Management; Airway Suctioning; Cough Enhancement; Oxygen Therapy; Pain Management; Progressive Muscle Relaxation; Respiratory Monitoring

Evaluations for expected outcomes

■ Patient's respiratory rate remains within set limits (specify).

■ Patient's ABG levels remain within set limits (specify).

■ Patient doesn't express feelings of pain, either verbally or through behavior.

■ Patient uses incentive spirometer or other respiratory device unassisted every 2 hours or as ordered.

■ Patient's breath sounds remain clear.

■ Patient explains why periodic deep breathing is important to maintaining respiratory status.

■ Patient practices relaxation techniques ___ times daily.
■ Patient reports breathing comfortably, either verbally or through behavior.

Documentation
■ Patient's reports of pain
■ Patient's perception of need to take deep breaths and cough
■ Patient's expression of the effectiveness of pain medication
■ Observations of physical findings
■ Effectiveness of medications
■ Descriptions of patient's efforts to take deep breaths and cough
■ Interventions performed to enhance patient's ability to breathe effectively
■ Evaluations for expected outcomes

Reference
Smetana, G.W. "Preoperative Pulmonary Evaluation: Identifying and Reducing Risks for Pulmonary Complications," *Cleveland Clinic Journal of Medicine* 73(Suppl 1):S36-S41, March 2006.

Ineffective
BREATHING PATTERN
related to respiratory muscle fatigue

Definition
Inspiration or expiration that doesn't provide adequate ventilation

Assessment
■ History of respiratory disorder
■ Respiratory status, including rate and depth of respiration, symmetry of chest expansion, use of accessory muscles, presence of cough, anterior-posterior chest diameter, palpation for fremitus, percussion of lung fields, auscultation of breath sounds, and pulmonary function studies
■ Cardiovascular status, including heart rate and rhythm, blood pressure, and skin color, temperature, and turgor
■ Neurologic and mental status, including level of consciousness and emotional level
■ Knowledge, including current understanding of physical condition and physical, mental, and emotional readiness to learn

Defining characteristics
■ Accessory muscle use
■ Altered chest excursion
■ Altered respiratory rate or depth or both
■ Assumption of three-point position
■ Decreased inspiratory or expiratory pressure
■ Decreased minute ventilation

- Decreased vital capacity
- Decreased tidal volume (adult tidal volume 500 ml at rest)
- Dyspnea
- Increased anterior-posterior diameter
- Nasal flaring
- Orthopnea
- Prolonged expiration phase
- Pursed-lip breathing
- Shortness of breath

Expected outcomes

- Patient's respiratory rate will stay within 5 breaths/minute of baseline.
- Arterial blood gas (ABG) levels will return to baseline.
- Patient will report feeling comfortable when breathing.
- Patient will report feeling rested each day.
- Patient will demonstrate diaphragmatic pursed-lip breathing.
- Patient will achieve maximum lung expansion with adequate ventilation.
- Patient will demonstrate skill in conserving energy while carrying out activities of daily living (ADLs).

Suggested NOC outcomes

Mechanical Ventilation Response: Adult; Respiratory Status: Airway Patency; Respiratory Status: Gas Exchange; Respiratory Status: Ventilation; Vital Signs

Interventions and rationales

- Assess and record respiratory rate and depth at least every 4 hours *to detect early signs of respiratory compromise.* Also assess ABG levels, according to facility policy, *to monitor oxygenation and ventilation status.*
- Auscultate breath sounds at least every 4 hours *to detect decreased or adventitious breath sounds;* report changes.
- Assist patient to a comfortable position, such as by supporting upper extremities with pillows, providing overbed table with a pillow to lean on, and elevating head of bed. *These measures promote comfort, chest expansion, and ventilation of basilar lung fields.*
- Help patient with ADLs, as needed, *to conserve energy and avoid overexertion and fatigue.*
- Administer oxygen as ordered. *Supplemental oxygen helps reduce hypoxemia and relieve respiratory distress.*
- Suction airway as needed. *Retained secretions alter the ventilatory response, thus reducing oxygen, leading to hypoxemia.*
- Schedule necessary activities to provide periods of rest. *This prevents fatigue and reduces oxygen demands.*
- Teach patient about:
- pursed-lip breathing
- abdominal breathing
- performing relaxation techniques

– taking prescribed medications (ensuring accuracy of dose and frequency and monitoring adverse effects)

– scheduling activities to avoid fatigue and provide for rest periods.

These measures allow patient to participate in maintaining health status and improve ventilation.

■ Refer patient for evaluation of exercise potential and development of individualized exercise program. *Exercise promotes conditioning of respiratory muscles and patient's sense of well-being.*

Suggested NIC interventions

Acid-Base Monitoring; Airway Management; Airway Suctioning; Anxiety Reduction; Exercise Promotion; Oxygen Therapy; Progressive Muscle Relaxation; Respiratory Monitoring; Ventilation Assistance

Evaluations for expected outcomes

■ Patient's respiratory rate remains within established limits.

■ Patient's ABG levels return to and remain within established limits.

■ Patient indicates, either verbally or through behavior, feeling comfortable when breathing.

■ Patient reports feeling rested each day.

■ Patient performs diaphragmatic pursed-lip breathing.

■ Patient demonstrates maximum lung expansion with adequate ventilation.

■ When patient carries out ADLs, breathing pattern remains normal.

Documentation

■ Patient's expressions of comfort in breathing, emotional state, understanding of medical diagnosis, and readiness to learn

■ Physical findings from pulmonary assessment

■ Interventions carried out and patient's responses to them

■ Evaluations for expected outcomes

Reference

Booker, R. "Chronic Obstructive Pulmonary Disease: Non-pharmacological Approaches," *British Journal of Nursing* 14(1):14-18, January 2005.

Decreased
CARDIAC OUTPUT
related to altered contractility

Definition

Inadequate blood pumped by the heart to meet metabolic needs.

Assessment

■ Mental status, including orientation and level of consciousness (LOC)

■ Cardiovascular status, including history of valvular disorder, capillary heart disease, or myopathy; skin color, temperature, turgor, and capillary refill time; jugular vein distention; hepatojugular reflux; heart rate and rhythm; heart sounds; blood pressure; peripheral pulses; electrocardiogram (ECG); exercise ECG; echocardiogram; and phonocardiogram

■ Respiratory status, including respiratory rate and depth, breath sounds, chest X-ray, and arterial blood gas values

■ Renal status, including weight, intake and output, and urine specific gravity

Defining characteristics
■ Altered heart rate and rhythm
■ Arrhythmias, palpitations, ECG changes
■ Abnormal chest X-ray and cardiac enzymes

Altered preload
■ Jugular vein distention, fatigue, edema, murmurs, increased/decreased central venous pressure, increased/decreased pulmonary wedge pressure, weight gain

Altered afterload
■ Cold, clammy skin; shortness of breath; oliguria; prolonged capillary refill; decreased peripheral pulses; variations in blood pressure; increased/decreased systemic vascular resistance; increased/decreased pulmonary vascular resistance; skin color changes

Altered contractility
■ Crackles, cough, orthopnea/paroxysmal nocturnal dyspnea, cardiac output (less than 4 L/minute), cardiac index (less than 2.5 L/minute), decreased ejection fraction, stroke volume index, audible S_3 or S_4 sounds

Behavioral/emotional
■ Anxiety, restlessness

Expected outcomes
■ Patient's pulse will be greater than _____ but not greater than _____.
■ Patient's blood pressure will be greater than _____ but not greater than _____.
■ Patient will exhibit no arrhythmias.
■ Skin will remain warm and dry.
■ Patient will exhibit no pedal edema.
■ Patient will perform activity within limits of prescribed heart rate.
■ Patient will express sense of physical comfort after activity.
■ Patient will maintain adequate cardiac output.
■ Patient will perform stress-reduction techniques every 4 hours while awake.
■ Patient will verbalize understanding of reportable signs and symptoms.
■ Patient will understand diet, medication regimen, and prescribed activity level.

Suggested NOC outcomes

Cardiac Pump Effectiveness; Circulation Status; Tissue Perfusion: Abdominal Organs; Tissue Perfusion: Peripheral; Vital Signs

Interventions and rationales

■ Monitor and record LOC, heart rate and rhythm, and blood pressure at least every 4 hours, or more often if necessary, *to detect cerebral hypoxia possibly resulting from decreased cardiac output.*

■ Auscultate for heart and breath sounds at least every 4 hours. Report abnormal sounds as soon as they develop. *Extra heart sounds may indicate early cardiac decompensation; adventitious breath sounds may indicate pulmonary congestion and diminished cardiac output.*

■ Measure and record intake and output accurately. *Decreased urine output without lowered fluid intake might indicate decreased renal perfusion, possibly from decreased cardiac output.*

■ Promptly treat life-threatening arrhythmias, as ordered, *to avoid crisis.*

■ Weigh patient daily before breakfast *to detect fluid retention.*

■ Inspect for pedal or sacral edema t*o detect venous stasis and reduced cardiac output.*

■ Provide skin care every 4 hours *to enhance skin perfusion and venous flow.*

■ Gradually increase patient's activities within limits of prescribed heart rate *to allow heart to adjust to increased oxygen demand.* Monitor pulse rate before and after activity *to compare rates and gauge tolerance.*

■ Plan patient's activities to avoid fatigue and increased myocardial workload.

■ Maintain dietary restrictions, as ordered, *to reduce risk of cardiac disease.*

■ Teach patient stress-reduction techniques *to reduce patient's anxiety and provide a sense of control.*

■ Explain all procedures and tests *to enhance understanding and reduce anxiety.*

■ Teach patient and family about chest pain and other reportable symptoms, prescribed diet, medications (name, dosage, frequency, and therapeutic and adverse effects), prescribed activity level, simple methods for lifting and bending, and stress-reduction techniques. *These measures involve patient and family in care.*

■ Administer oxygen, as prescribed, *to increase supply to myocardium.*

Suggested NIC interventions

Cardiac Precautions; Circulatory Precautions; Fluid Management; Hemodynamic Regulation; Vital Signs Monitoring

Evaluations for expected outcomes

■ Patient's pulse rate remains within set limits.

■ Patient's blood pressure remains within set limits.

■ Patient doesn't exhibit arrhythmias during monitoring or physical examination.

■ Patient's skin remains warm and dry to touch.

■ Inspection and palpation don't reveal pedal edema.

■ Patient carries out activities of daily living without heart rate exceeding or dropping below set limits.

■ Patient doesn't indicate, either verbally or through behavior, chest pain, dyspnea, fatigue, or other forms of discomfort after activity.

■ Patient performs stress-reduction techniques every 4 hours.

■ Patient describes signs and symptoms of decreased cardiac output, such as dizziness, syncope, clammy skin, fatigue, and dyspnea.

■ Patient understands importance of following prescribed diet, taking medications as ordered, and maintaining activity level.

Documentation

■ Patient's needs and perception of problem

■ Observations of physical findings

■ Patient's response to activity

■ Development of skills related to diet, medication, activity, and stress management

■ Evaluations for expected outcomes

References

Kodiath, K., et al. "Improving Quality of Life in Patients with Heart Failure: An Innovative Behavioral Intervention," *Journal of Cardiovascular Nursing* 20(1): 43-48, January-February 2005.

Masse, L., and Antonacci, M. "Low Cardiac Output Syndrome: Identification and Management," *Critical Care Nursing Clinics of North America* 17(4):375-83, December 2005.

Decreased
CARDIAC OUTPUT

related to reduced stroke volume as a result of electrophysiologic problems

Definition

Inadequate blood pumped by the heart to meet metabolic needs

Assessment

■ History of cardiac disorder

■ Mental status, including orientation and level of consciousness

■ Cardiovascular status, including history of arrhythmias and syncope, jugular vein distention, hepatojugular reflux, heart rate and rhythm, heart sounds, blood pressure, peripheral pulses, electrocardiogram (ECG), exercise ECG, echocardiogram, serum digoxin levels, and skin color, temperature, turgor, and capillary refill time

■ Respiratory status, including respiratory rate and depth, breath sounds, chest X-ray, and arterial blood gas values

■ Renal status, including weight, intake and output, urine specific gravity, and serum electrolytes

Defining characteristics

- Altered heart rate and rhythm
- Arrhythmias, palpitations, ECG changes

Altered preload

- Jugular vein distention, fatigue, edema, murmurs, increased/decreased central venous pressure, increased/decreased pulmonary wedge pressure, weight gain

Altered afterload

- Cold, clammy skin; shortness of breath; oliguria; prolonged capillary refill; decreased peripheral pulses; variations in blood pressure; increased/decreased systemic vascular resistance; increased/decreased pulmonary vascular resistance; skin color changes

Altered contractility

- Crackles, cough, orthopnea/paroxysmal nocturnal dyspnea, cardiac output (less than 4 L/minute), cardiac index (less than 2.5 L/minute), decreased ejection fraction, stroke volume index, audible S_3 or S_4 sounds

Behavioral/emotional

- Anxiety, restlessness

Expected outcomes

- Patient's pulse will be greater than _____ but not greater than _____.
- Patient's blood pressure will be greater than _____ but not greater than _____.
- Patient's skin will remain warm and dry.
- Patient will experience few or no dyspneic episodes.
- Patient will show no signs of dizziness or syncope.
- Patient will experience no chest pain.
- Patient will practice stress-reduction techniques every 2 hours.
- Patient's cardiac output will remain adequate.
- Patient will have no arrhythmias.
- Patient will verbalize knowledge of reportable signs and symptoms.
- Patient will understand diet, medication regimen, and prescribed activity level.

Suggested NOC outcomes

Cardiac Disease Self-Management; Cardiac Pump Effectiveness; Circulation Status; Tissue Perfusion: Abdominal Organs; Tissue Perfusion: Cardiac; Tissue Perfusion: Peripheral; Tissue Perfusion: Pulmonary; Vital Signs

Interventions and rationales

- Monitor patient at least every 4 hours for irregularities in cardiac rate or rhythm, dyspnea, fatigue, crackles in lungs, jugular venous distension, or chest pain. *Any or all of these may indicate impending cardiac failure or other complications.* Report them immediately.

■ Assess skin temperature every 4 hours. *Cool, clammy skin may indicate decreased cardiac output.*

■ Assess respiratory status at least every 4 hours. Report complaints of dyspnea or restlessness. *Adventitious breath sounds or dyspnea may indicate fluid buildup in lungs and pulmonary capillary bed (as in heart failure).*

■ Administer oxygen, as ordered, *to increase supply to myocardium.*

■ Report complaints of dizziness or syncope promptly; *these may indicate cerebral hypoxia resulting from a cardiac rhythm disturbance.*

■ Tell patient to report chest pain right away *because it may signal myocardial hypoxia or injury.*

■ Plan patient's care to avoid overexertion, *which increases myocardial oxygen demand.*

■ Change patient's position frequently *to promote comfort and avoid tachycardia and other sympathetic responses.*

■ Teach patient how to perform stress-reduction techniques, such as deep breathing and meditation, *to allay anxiety, avoid cardiac complications, and promote cardiac healing.*

■ Remind patient to practice stress-reduction techniques every 2 hours while awake *to help internalize learned techniques.*

■ Give antiarrhythmic drugs as prescribed *to reduce or eliminate arrhythmias.* Monitor for adverse effects.

■ Instruct patient to avoid straining during bowel movements, *which may cause stimulation of the vagus nerve resulting in bradycardia and decreased cardiac output.*

■ Administer stool softeners, as prescribed, *to reduce straining during bowel elimination.*

■ Teach patient about reportable symptoms (chest pain, palpitations, weakness, dizziness, and syncope), prescribed diet, medications (name, dosage, frequency, and therapeutic and adverse effects), and activity level. *These measures let patient and caregivers participate in patient's care and help patient make informed decisions about health status.*

Suggested NIC interventions

Cardiac Care; Energy Management; Fluid Monitoring; Hemodynamic Regulation; Laboratory Data Interpretation; Shock Prevention; Vital Signs Monitoring

Evaluations for expected outcomes

■ Patient's pulse rate remains within set limits.

■ Patient's blood pressure remains within set limits.

■ Patient's skin remains warm and dry.

■ Patient experiences fewer dyspneic episodes.

■ Patient doesn't experience dizziness or syncope.

■ Patient doesn't experience chest pain.

■ Patient practices stress-reduction techniques every 2 hours.

■ Patient's cardiac output remains adequate.

■ No arrhythmias are noted during monitoring or physical examination of patient.

■ Patient lists signs and symptoms of decreased cardiac output (dizziness, syncope, cool or clammy skin, fatigue, and dyspnea).
■ Patient expresses understanding of importance of following prescribed diet, taking medications, and maintaining activity level.

Documentation
■ Patient's symptoms
■ Observation of physical findings
■ Incidents of chest pain, including location, character, duration, and treatment
■ Patient's tolerance for activity
■ Interventions to control or monitor symptoms and patient's response
■ Patient teaching
■ Evaluations for expected outcomes

Reference
McCabe, P.T. "Spheres of Clinical Nurse Specialist Practice Influence Evidence-based Care for Patients with Atrial Fibrillation," *Clinical Nurse Specialist* 19(6):308-17, November-December 2005.

CAREGIVER ROLE STRAIN
related to increasing care needs/dependency

Definition
Difficulty in performing family caregiver's role

Assessment
■ Caregiver's physical and mental status, including chronic health problems, self-care abilities, mobility limitations, and level of cognitive function
■ Care recipient's physical and mental status, including illness, self-care limitations, mobility limitations, and level of cognitive function
■ Support systems, including financial resources, family members and friends, community services, health-related services such as geriatric day care, and home health aides
■ Home environment, including layout, structural barriers, need for equipment or assistive devices, and availability of transportation
■ Cultural, ethnic, and religious background
■ Perceived and actual obligations of caregiver
■ Caregiver's personal strengths, including coping and problem-solving abilities and participation in diversional activities or hobbies

Defining characteristics
Caregiving activities
■ Difficulty performing/completing required tasks
■ Preoccupation with care routine

■ Apprehension about care receiver's health and the caregivers' ability to provide care; the fate of the care receiver if the caregiver becomes ill or dies; or the possible institutionalization of care receiver

Caregiver health status
■ Physical
– GI upset
– Weight change
– Rash
– Hypertension
– Cardiovascular disease
– Diabetes
– Fatigue
– Headaches
■ Emotional
– Impaired individual coping
– Depression
– Disturbed sleep
– Anger
– Stress
– Somatization
– Increased nervousness and emotional lability
– Impatience
– Frustration
■ Socioeconomic
– Withdrawal from social life
– Changes in leisure activities
– Low work productivity
– Refusal of career advancement

Caregiver-care receiver relationship
■ Grief or uncertainty regarding changed relationship with care receiver
■ Difficulty with watching care receiver experience the illness

Expected outcomes
■ Caregiver will describe current stressors.
■ Caregiver will identify stressors that can and can't be controlled.
■ Caregiver will identify formal and informal sources of support.
■ Caregiver will show evidence of using support systems.
■ Caregiver will report increased ability to cope with stress.

Suggested NOC outcomes

Caregiver Emotional Health; Caregiver Lifestyle Disruption; Caregiver Stressors; Caregiver Well-Being; Caregiving Endurance Potential; Family Support During Treatment; Role Performance

Interventions and rationales

■ Help caregiver to identify current stressors *to evaluate the causes of role strain.*

■ Using a nonjudgmental approach, help caregiver evaluate which stressors are controllable and which aren't *to begin to develop strategies to reduce stress.*

■ Encourage caregiver to discuss coping skills used to overcome similar stressful situations in the past *to build confidence for managing the current situation.*

■ Encourage caregiver to participate in a support group. Provide information on organizations such as Alzheimer's Association, Children of Aging Parents, or the referral service of the community acquired immunodeficiency syndrome task force *to foster mutual support and provide an opportunity for caregiver to discuss personal feelings with empathetic listeners.*

■ Help caregiver identify informal sources of support, such as family members, friends, church groups, and community volunteers, *to provide resources for obtaining an occasional or regularly scheduled respite.*

■ Help caregiver identify available formal support services, such as home health agencies, municipal or county social services, hospital social workers, physicians, clinics, and day-care centers, *to enhance coping by providing a reliable structure for support.*

■ If caregiver seems overly anxious or distraught, gently point out facts about care recipient's mental and physical condition. *Many times, especially when care recipient is a family member, caregiver's perspective is clouded by a long history of emotional involvement. Your input may help caregiver view the situation more objectively.* If you believe that excessive emotional involvement is hindering caregiver's ability to function, consider recommending Codependents Anonymous, a support group for people whose preoccupation with a relationship leads to chronic suffering and diminished effectiveness, *to provide support.*

■ Suggest ways for caregiver to use time more efficiently. For example, caregiver may save time by filling out insurance forms while visiting and chatting with care recipient. *Better time management may help caregiver reduce stress.*

Suggested NIC interventions

Active Listening; Caregiver Support; Coping Enhancement; Counseling; Normalization Promotion; Role Enhancement; Support Group

Evaluations for expected outcomes

■ Caregiver identifies and develops a realistic appraisal of each stressful situation.
■ Caregiver describes emotional response to each stressful situation.
■ Caregiver identifies sources of support.
■ Caregiver uses available support systems.
■ Caregiver uses appropriate coping skills for each stressful situation.

Documentation

■ Stressors (perceived and actual) identified by caregiver
■ Observations of caregiver's response to stressful situations
■ Referrals provided
■ Caregiver's use of informal and formal support systems
■ Coping strategies identified by caregiver and nurse

■ Evidence of improvement in caregiver's ability to cope

■ Evaluations for expected outcomes

Reference

Schumacher, K., et al. "Family Caregivers: Caring for Older Adults, Working with Their Families," *AJN* 106(8):40-49, August 2006.

Risk for
CAREGIVER ROLE STRAIN
related to complexity of caregiving activities

Definition

Difficulty in performing family caregiver's role

Assessment

■ Caregiver's physical and mental status, including chronic health problems, self-care abilities, mobility limitations, and level of cognitive function

■ Care recipient's physical and mental status, including illness, self-care limitations, mobility limitations, and level of cognitive function

■ Support systems, including financial resources, family members and friends, community services, and health-related services, such as geriatric day care and home health aides

■ Home environment, including layout, structural barriers, need for equipment or assistive devices, and availability of transportation

■ Cultural, ethnic, and religious background

■ Perceived and actual obligations of caregiver

■ Caregiver's personal strengths, including usual coping and problem-solving abilities and participation in diversional activities or hobbies

Risk factors

■ Not developmentally ready for caregiver role (for example, young adult who must unexpectedly care for a middle-age parent)

■ Evidence of drug or alcohol addiction in caregiver or care recipient, health impairment of caregiver, severity or unpredictable course of illness, or instability of care recipient's health

■ Evidence of codependency; deviant, bizarre behavior of care recipient; dysfunctional family coping patterns that existed before the caregiving situation

■ Situational factors, such as close relationship between caregiver and care recipient; discharge of family member with significant home care needs; inadequate environment or facilities for providing care; isolation, inexperience, or overwork of caregiver; lack of recreation for caregiver; presence of abuse or violence; simultaneous occurrence of other events that cause stress for family (significant personal loss, natural disaster, economic hardship, or major life events)

Expected outcomes

■ Caregiver will identify current stressors.

■ Caregiver will identify appropriate coping strategies and will state plans to incorporate strategies into daily routine.

■ Caregiver will state intention to contact formal and informal sources of support.

■ Caregiver will state intention to incorporate recreational activities into daily routine.

■ Caregiver will report satisfaction with ability to cope with stress caused by caregiving responsibilities.

Suggested NOC outcomes

Caregiver Emotional Health; Caregiver Home Care Readiness; Caregiver Lifestyle Disruption; Caregiver-Patient Relationship; Caregiver Physical Health; Caregiver Stressors; Caregiving Endurance Potential; Rest

Interventions and rationales

■ Help caregiver identify current stressors. Ask whether stress is likely to increase or decrease in the future *to evaluate the risk of caregiver role strain.*

■ Encourage caregiver to discuss coping skills used to overcome similar stressful situations in the past *to bolster caregiver's confidence in ability to manage current situation and explore ways to apply coping strategies before caregiver becomes overwhelmed.*

■ Help caregiver identify informal sources of support, such as family members, friends, church groups, and community volunteers, *to plan for an occasional or regularly scheduled respite.*

■ Help caregiver identify available formal support services, such as home health agencies, municipal or county social services, hospital social workers, physicians, clinics, and day-care centers, *to help lessen risk of strain on caregiver.*

■ Encourage caregiver to discuss hobbies or diversional activities. *Incorporating enjoyable activities into the daily or weekly schedule will discipline caregiver to take needed breaks from caregiving responsibilities and thereby diminish stress.*

■ Encourage caregiver to participate in a support group. Provide information on organizations such as Alzheimer's Association, Children of Aging Parents, or the referral service of the community task force for acquired immunodeficiency syndrome *to foster mutual support and provide an outlet for expressing feelings before frustration becomes overwhelming.*

■ If caregiver seems overly anxious or distraught, gently point out facts about care recipient's mental and physical condition. *Many times, especially when care recipient is a family member, caregiver's perspective is clouded by a long history of emotional involvement. Your input may help caregiver view the situation more objectively.* If you believe that excessive emotional involvement is hindering caregiver's ability to function, consider recommending Codependents Anonymous, a support group for people whose preoccupation with a relationship leads to chronic suffering and diminished effectiveness, *to provide support.*

■ Suggest ways for caregiver to use time efficiently; for example, caregiver may save time by filling out insurance forms while visiting and chatting with care recipient. *Better time management may help caregiver reduce stress.*

Suggested NIC interventions

Caregiver Support; Coping Enhancement; Exercise Promotion; Home Maintenance Assistance; Referral; Respite Care; Role Enhancement; Support Group

Evaluations for expected outcomes

■ Caregiver identifies and develops a realistic appraisal of each stressful situation.
■ Caregiver describes coping strategies used in stressful situations.
■ Caregiver uses available support systems.
■ Caregiver incorporates recreational activities into daily routine.
■ Caregiver reports satisfaction in coping with stress.

Documentation

■ Current stressors identified by caregiver
■ Risk factors (developmental, pathophysiologic, psychological, and situational) for caregiver role strain identified by nurse
■ Caregiver's statements indicating intention to take action to minimize stress, such as seeking help from support services, participating in a caregiver support group, and scheduling time for recreational activities
■ Coping strategies identified by caregiver and nurse
■ Observations of caregiver's response to stressful situations
■ Referrals provided
■ Evaluations for expected outcomes

Reference

Perren, S., et al. "Caregivers' Adaptation to Change: The Impact of Increasing Impairment of Persons Suffering from Dementia on Their Caregivers' Subjective Well-being," *Aging and Mental Health* 10(5):539-48, September 2006.

Impaired verbal
COMMUNICATION

related to decreased circulation to brain

Definition

Decreased, delayed, or absent ability to receive, process, transmit, and use a system of symbols

Assessment

■ Neurologic status, including level of consciousness, orientation, cognition, memory (recent and remote), insight, and judgment
■ Speech characteristics, including pattern (garbled, incomprehensible, difficulty forming words), language and vocabulary, level of comprehension and expression, and ability to use other forms of communication (such as eye blinks, gestures, pictures, and nods)
■ Motor ability

■ Circulatory status, including a history of cardiac and circulatory problems, pulse, blood pressure, arteriogram, EEG, and computed tomography scan
■ Respiratory status, including dyspnea and use of accessory muscles

Defining characteristics
■ Disorientation
■ Difficulty comprehending and maintaining usual communication pattern
■ Difficulty expressing thoughts verbally (aphasia, dysphasia, apraxia, dyslexia)
■ Difficulty forming words or sentences (aphonia, dyslalia, dysarthria)
■ Difficulty using or inability to use facial expressions or body language
■ Dyspnea
■ Impaired articulation
■ Inability or lack of desire to speak
■ Inability to speak dominant language
■ Inappropriate verbalizations
■ Lack of eye contact or poor selective attention
■ Stuttering or slurring
■ Visual deficit (partial or total)

Expected outcomes
■ Patient's needs will be met by staff members.
■ Patient and family members will express satisfaction with level of communication ability.
■ Patient will maintain orientation.
■ Patient will maintain effective level of communication.
■ Patient will answer direct questions correctly.

Suggested NOC outcomes
Cognition; Communication; Communication: Expressive; Communication: Receptive; Information Processing; Sensory Function Status

Interventions and rationales
■ Observe patient closely for cues to his needs and desires, such as gestures, pointing to objects, looking at items, and pantomime *to enhance understanding.* Don't continually respond to gestures if the potential exists to improve speech *to avoid discouraging improvement.*
■ Monitor and record changes in patient's speech pattern or level of orientation. *Changes may indicate improvement or deterioration of condition.*
■ Speak slowly and distinctly in a normal tone when addressing patient, and stand where patient can see and hear you. *These actions promote comprehension.*
■ Reorient patient to reality.
– Call patient by name.
– Tell patient your name.
– Give patient background information (place, date, and time).
– Use television or radio to augment orientation.
– Use large calendars and reality orientation boards.
These measures develop orientation skills through repetition and recognition of familiar objects.

■ Use short, simple phrases and yes-or-no questions when patient is very frustrated *to reduce frustration.*

■ Encourage attempts at communication and provide positive reinforcement *to aid comprehension.*

■ Allow ample time for a response. Don't answer questions yourself if patient has the ability to respond. *This improves patient's self-concept and reduces frustration.*

■ Repeat or rephrase questions, if necessary, *to improve communication.* Don't pretend to understand if you don't *to avoid misunderstanding.*

■ Remove distractions from the environment during attempts at communication. *Reduced distractions improve comprehension.* Use communication boards (including alphabet and some common words and pictures), if appropriate, *to aid comprehension.*

■ Review diagnostic test results *to determine improvement or deterioration of the disease process.* Adjust the care plan accordingly.

Suggested NIC interventions

Active Listening; Anxiety Reduction; Communication Enhancement: Hearing Deficit; Communication Enhancement: Speech Deficit; Energy Management; Learning Facilitation; Touch

Evaluations for expected outcomes

■ Patient's needs are met by staff members.

■ Patient and family members communicate at satisfactory level.

■ Patient demonstrates orientation by consistently communicating thoughts to his family and staff.

■ Patient communicates effectively____ times every 8 hours (specify).

■ Patient correctly answers ____ direct questions (specify).

Documentation

■ Patient's current level of communication, orientation, and satisfaction with communication efforts

■ Observations of speech deficits, expressiveness and receptiveness, and ability to communicate

■ Interventions carried out to promote effective communication

■ Patient's response to nursing interventions

■ Evaluations for expected outcomes

Reference

Philpin, S.M., et al. "Giving People a Voice: Reflections on Conducting Interviews with Participants Experiencing Communication Impairment," *Journal of Advanced Nursing* 50(3):299-306, May 2005.

Impaired verbal
COMMUNICATION
related to physical barriers

Definition
Decreased, delayed, or absent ability to receive, process, transmit, and use a system of symbols

Assessment
■ History of respiratory, neurologic, or musculoskeletal disorder or surgery
■ Respiratory status, including dyspnea, use of accessory muscles, and respiratory pattern
■ Neurologic status, including mental status (level of consciousness, orientation, cognition, memory, insight, and judgment) and speech (pattern, signing, and such communication aids as artificial larynx, computer-assisted speech device, pen and pencil, slate, picture board, and alphabet board)
■ Musculoskeletal status, including range of motion and manual dexterity

Defining characteristics
■ Disorientation
■ Difficulty comprehending and maintaining usual communication pattern
■ Difficulty expressing thoughts verbally (aphasia, dysphasia, apraxia, dyslexia)
■ Difficulty forming words or sentences (aphonia, dyslalia, dysarthria)
■ Difficulty using or inability to use facial expressions or body language
■ Dyspnea
■ Impaired articulation
■ Inability or lack of desire to speak
■ Inability to speak dominant language
■ Inappropriate verbalizations
■ Lack of eye contact or poor selective attention
■ Stuttering or slurring
■ Visual deficit (partial or total)

Expected outcomes
■ Patient will communicate needs and desires without undue frustration.
■ Patient will use alternate means of communication.
■ Patient will demonstrate correct use of adaptive equipment.
■ Patient will express plans to use appropriate resources to maximize communication skills.

Suggested NOC outcomes
Client Satisfaction: Communication; Communication; Communication: Expressive; Communication: Receptive

Interventions and rationales

■ Maintain a consistent daily schedule of activities as much as possible. Observe patient closely for cues to needs and desires, such as gestures, pointing to or looking at objects, and pantomime, *to enhance understanding.*

■ Obtain communication aids for patient's use, such as an alphabet board, slate, pen, paper, and picture board, *to provide alternative communication methods.*

■ Use short, simple phrases and yes-or-no questions *to reduce frustration and anxiety.*

■ Encourage communication attempts; allow time to select or write words or pictures *to reduce pressure and improve interaction with others.*

■ Allow ample time for a response; don't answer questions for patient *to reduce frustration.*

■ Consult with a speech therapist to suggest such communication aids as an artificial larynx. Assist with its use. *Appropriate early referral encourages the use of communication aids.*

■ Demonstrate communication techniques, such as gestures, sign language, and eye blinking, to patient and family members *to develop alternative communication skills.*

■ Assist patient in energy-conserving techniques *to allow maximum breath for speech or use of communication aids.*

■ Use a tracheostomy plug *to facilitate speech,* if tolerated by patient.

■ Provide patient with emergency call system (bell or call light), and respond to all calls immediately and in person. Place a sign over the intercom to alert all staff members of the need to respond quickly. *Prompt responses reduce patient's fear and anxiety.*

■ Encourage attendance at a laryngectomy club or other appropriate support groups *to provide additional support.*

Suggested NIC interventions

Active Listening; Anxiety Reduction; Communication Enhancement: Speech Deficit; Energy Management; Environmental Management; Learning Facilitation; Referral

Evaluations for expected outcomes

■ Patient consistently communicates needs without frustration.

■ Patient successfully uses alternate means of communication (specify).

■ Patient uses adaptive equipment _____ times daily to improve communication (specify).

■ Patient identifies and contacts appropriate support resources, such as speech therapist and laryngectomy club.

Documentation

■ Patient's feelings about inability to communicate

■ Observations of patient's attempts to communicate, response to and ability to use alternate communication means, and level of frustration or fatigue

■ Patient's response to nursing interventions

■ Patient's preferences in daily care activities, such as when to shave or bathe and what kind of razor to use
■ Evaluations for expected outcomes

Reference
Happ, M.B., et al. "Patient Communication Following Head and Neck Cancer Surgery: A Pilot Study Using Electronic Speech-generating Devices," *Oncology Nursing Forum* 32(6):1179-87, November 2005.

Decisional
CONFLICT
related to health care options

Definition
State of uncertainty about health-related course of action when choice involves risk, potential loss, or challenge to personal life values

Assessment
■ Age and gender
■ Perception of health care options
■ Developmental state
■ Marital status
■ Family system (nuclear, extended role, and sibling position)
■ Sociocultural factors, including educational level, occupation, socioeconomic status, ethnic group, sexual preference, and religious beliefs
■ Level of functioning (cognitive, emotional, and behavioral)
■ Coping mechanisms
■ Past experience with decision making
■ Available support system

Defining characteristics
■ Delayed decision making
■ Focusing on self
■ Lack of experience or interference with decision making
■ Physical signs of distress or tension
■ Questioning personal values and beliefs while attempting to make a decision
■ Vacillation between alternative choices
■ Verbal statements describing undesired consequences of alternative actions being considered
■ Verbal expression of distress and uncertainty about making choices

Expected outcomes
■ Patient will state feelings about current situation.
■ Patient will discuss benefits and drawbacks of treatment options.
■ Patient will make minor decisions related to daily activities.

■ Patient will accept assistance from family, friends, clergy, and other people.

■ Patient will practice progressive muscle relaxation to decrease tension created by decisional conflict.

■ Patient will report feeling comfortable about ability to make an appropriate, rational choice.

Suggested NOC outcomes

Decision-Making; Information Processing; Participation in Health Care Decisions

Interventions and rationales

■ Listen to patient's concerns about making a decision. Use a nonjudgmental approach and encourage expression of feelings *to demonstrate acceptance of patient and respect for his culture, beliefs, and value system.*

■ Help patient identify available options and their possible consequences *to encourage rational decision making.*

■ Help patient make decisions about daily activities *to enhance his feelings of autonomy.*

■ Encourage visits with family, friends, and clergy; provide privacy during visits *to foster emotional support.*

■ Teach progressive muscle-relaxation techniques *to decrease physical and psychological signs of tension.*

■ Help patient identify decision-making areas that require assistance from others, and provide appropriate referrals. *Providing referrals will ensure ongoing support. Putting patient in touch with appropriate community resources will help promote feeling that others are genuinely interested in his well-being.*

Suggested NIC interventions

Active Listening; Assertiveness Training; Decision-Making Support; Learning Facilitation; Mutual Goal Setting

Evaluations for expected outcomes

■ Patient expresses anxiety, tension, and other feelings related to difficult medical treatment decisions.

■ Patient describes benefits and drawbacks of treatment options.

■ Patient makes minor decisions related to daily activities.

■ Patient accepts assistance from family, friends, clergy, and other people.

■ Patient practices progressive muscle relaxation to decrease tension created by decisional conflict.

■ Patient reports feeling at ease with ability to choose treatment option that's appropriate for him.

Documentation

■ Patient's statements that provide insight into conflict regarding treatment options

■ Cognitive, emotional, and behavioral functioning

■ Interventions to assist patient with resolving decisional conflict

■ Patient's response to nursing interventions
■ Evaluations for expected outcomes

Reference
Popejoy, L. "Health-related Decision-making by Older Adults and Their Families: How Clinicians Can Help," *Journal of Gerontological Nursing* 31(9):12-18, September 2005.

Acute
CONFUSION
related to dementia

Definition
Abrupt onset of changes in attention span, cognition, psychomotor activity, level of consciousness (LOC), or sleep-wake cycle

Assessment
■ Age, gender, level of education, occupation, and recent immigration status
■ Health history, including use of medications, recent surgery, allergies, history of alcoholism, drug abuse, and depression
■ Neurologic status, including LOC; orientation; thought and speech; mood; affect; memory; visual and spatial ability; judgment and insight; psychomotor activity; perceptions; delusions, illusions, and hallucinations; pain level; recent behavioral changes; and history of transient ischemic attacks, head injury, early dementia, acquired immunodeficiency syndrome, or schizophrenia
■ Cardiovascular status, including vital signs, skin color, auscultation of carotid artery and heart sounds, and history of coronary artery disease or hypertension
■ Respiratory status, including rate, depth, and pattern of respirations; auscultation for breath sounds; smoking history; shortness of breath; and history of chronic obstructive pulmonary disease, cancer, or tuberculosis
■ Sensory status, including results of vision and hearing examination, use of corrective lenses or hearing aid, and history of eye or ear disorders
■ Nutritional status, including typical daily food intake and weight loss
■ Sleep status, including recent change in sleep pattern or environment (recent hospitalization)

Defining characteristics
■ Fluctuations in LOC, psychomotor activity, cognition, and sleep-wake cycle
■ Hallucinations
■ Impaired perceptive ability
■ Increased agitation or restlessness
■ Misperceptions
■ Lack of motivation to initiate and follow through with goal-directed behavior

Expected outcomes

■ Patient will experience no injury.

■ Patient's neurologic status will remain stable.

■ Family members will report an improved ability to cope with the patient's confused state.

■ Patient will start to participate in activities of daily living (ADLs).

■ Patient will report feeling increasingly calm.

■ Patient and family members will state the causes of acute confusion.

■ Patient and family members will express an understanding of the importance of informing other health care providers about episodes of acute confusion.

Suggested NOC outcomes

Anxiety Level; Cognition; Cognitive Orientation; Distorted Thought Self-Control; Information Processing; Neurological Status: Consciousness; Safe Home Environment; Sleep

Interventions and rationales

■ Assess patient's LOC and changes in behavior *to provide baseline for comparison with ongoing assessment findings.*

■ Have a staff member stay at patient's bedside, if necessary, *to protect patient from harm.*

■ Enlist the aid of family member *to help calm patient.*

■ Limit noise and environmental stimulation *to prevent patient from becoming more confused.*

■ Monitor neurologic status on a regular basis to *detect any improvement or decline in patient's neurologic function.*

■ Use appropriate safety measures *to protect patient from injury.* Avoid physical restraints *to prevent agitating patient.*

■ Address patient by name and tell him your name *to foster his awareness of self and environment.*

■ Give patient short, simple explanations each time you perform a procedure or task *to decrease confusion.*

■ Schedule nursing care to provide quiet times for patient *to help avoid sensory overload.*

■ Mention time, place, and date frequently throughout day. Have a clock and a calendar where patient can easily see them. Refer to these aids when orienting him *to foster awareness of self and environment.*

■ Keep patient's possessions in the same place as much as possible. *A consistent, stable environment reduces confusion and frustration and aids completion of ADLs.*

■ Ask family members to bring labeled family photos and other favorite articles *to create a more secure environment for patient.*

■ Plan patient's routine, and be as consistent as possible in following it. *A consistent routine aids task completion and reduces confusion.*

■ Speak slowly and clearly and allow patient ample time to respond *to reduce his frustration and promote task completion.*

■ Encourage patient to perform ADLs, dividing tasks into small, critical units. Be patient and specific in providing instructions. Allow time for patient to perform each task. *These measures enhance his self-esteem as well as help prevent complications related to inactivity.*

■ Encourage family members to share stories and discuss familiar people and events with patient. *Sharing stories and familiar subjects promotes a sense of continuity, aids memory, and creates a sense of security and comfort.* Note that even if patient's short-term memory is impaired, his remote memory still may be intact.

■ Support family members' attempts to interact with patient *to provide positive reinforcement.*

■ Allow time before and after visits for family members to express feelings. *Listening to family members in an open and nonjudgmental manner helps them cope with patient's illness. Listening to their opinions may also help you assess and monitor patient's condition.*

■ Reassure patient and family that confusion will be temporary *to help relieve their anxiety.* Always include patient in discussions.

■ Confer with physician about diagnostic test results, patient's progress in behavior, and patient's LOC. *A collaborative approach to treatment helps ensure high-quality care and continuity of care.*

■ Discuss episodes of acute confusion with patient and family members *to make sure they understand the cause of confusion.*

■ Review measures family members can take at home to help patient if he begins to exhibit signs of confusion. Tell them to give patient short explanations of activities; remind him of time, place, and date frequently; speak slowly and clearly and allow patient time to respond; and provide patient with a consistent routine. *Teaching empowers patient and family members to take greater responsibility for their health care needs.*

■ Stress to patient and family that, in the future, they should inform health care providers about episodes of acute confusion *to help ensure continuity of care.*

Suggested NIC interventions

Behavior Management: Overactivity/Inattention; Cognitive Stimulation; Delirium Management; Fall Prevention; Hallucination Management; Medication Management; Reality Orientation; Sleep Enhancement

Evaluations for expected outcomes

■ Patient doesn't experience injury during episodes of acute confusion.

■ Patient exhibits a mental status within his normal range.

■ Family members report an increased ability to cope with patient's confused state.

■ Patient performs ADLs to the extent possible.

■ Patient reports feelings of increased calm.

■ Patient and family members express an understanding of the causes of acute confusion.

■ Patient and family members express an understanding of the importance of telling all health care providers about episodes of acute confusion.

Documentation

- Description of episodes of acute confusion
- Factors that precipitate and ameliorate periods of acute confusion
- Teaching sessions and referrals
- Evaluations for expected outcomes

Reference

Buettner, L., and Fitzsimmons, S. "Mixed Behaviors in Dementia: The Need for a Paradigm Shift," *Journal of Gerontological Nursing* 32(7):15-22, July 2006.

Chronic
CONFUSION

Definition

An irreversible, long-standing, or progressive deterioration of intellect and personality characterized by decreased ability to interpret environmental stimuli; decreased capacity for thought; and disturbances of memory, orientation, and behavior

Assessment

- Age and gender
- Neurologic status, including level of consciousness (LOC), orientation, thought and speech, mood, affect, memory, visual and spatial ability, judgment and insight, psychomotor activity, and perceptions; recent behavior changes; lethargy, restlessness, short- or long-term memory loss, and sleep disturbance; and history of multiple infarctions, transient ischemic attacks, Parkinson's disease, cerebral infarctions, seizures, and alcohol or drug abuse
- Self-care status, including ability to perform instrumental or routine activities of daily living (ADLs)
- Family status, including marital status, economic status, living arrangements, presence of caregiver and relationship to patient, and caregiver's perception of patient's abilities

Defining characteristics

- Altered interpretation and response to stimuli
- Altered personality
- Clinical evidence of organic impairment
- Impaired short-term and long-term memory
- Impaired socialization
- No change in LOC
- Progressive or long-standing cognitive impairment

Expected outcomes

- Patient will remain free of injury caused by confusion.
- Patient will exhibit no signs of depression.

■ Patient will maintain weight.

■ Family members will discuss their ability to provide care for the patient.

■ Patient will be provided with a structured environment to ensure maximum functioning.

■ Family members or caregiver will describe strategies to help patient cope with chronic confusion.

■ Patient will participate in selected activities to fullest extent possible.

■ Family members will maintain safety of patient's home environment.

■ The family will receive information on the various options available for long term care of the patient.

■ If necessary, patient and family members will prepare for relocation to long-term care facility.

■ Patient will receive adequate emotional support to help him cope with stress of moving to a new environment.

■ Staff at patient's new residence will receive clear instructions regarding measures to help patient cope with chronic confusion.

Suggested NOC outcomes

Client Satisfaction: Safety; Cognition; Cognitive Orientation; Concentration; Decision Making; Distorted Thought Self-Control; Identity; Information Processing; Memory

Interventions and rationales

■ Assess patient's cognitive abilities and changes in behavior *to provide baseline data for comparison with ongoing assessment findings.*

■ Encourage family members to watch you perform mental status assessments *to give them a more accurate view of patient's abilities.*

■ Evaluate patient's ability to care for himself, including his ability to function alone and drive a car. *Safety is a primary concern.*

■ Assess patient for depression *to determine need for treatment.*

■ Weigh patient, document your findings, and include instructions for regular weighing as part of care plan *to monitor patient's nutritional status.*

■ Ask family members about their ability to provide care for patient *to assess their need for assistance.* Project an attentive, nonjudgmental attitude when listening to them *to help ensure that you receive accurate information.*

■ Take steps to provide a stable physical environment and consistent daily routine for patient. *Stability and consistency enhance functioning.*

■ Teach family members or caregiver strategies to help patient cope with his condition:

– Place an identification bracelet on patient *to promote safety.*

– Touch patient *to convey acceptance.*

– Avoid unfamiliar situations when possible *to help ensure a consistent environment.*

– Provide structured rest periods *to prevent fatigue and reduce stress.*

– Avoid asking questions patient can't answer—for example, questions that test his orientation to time, place, person, or situation—*to avoid frustrating him.*

– Provide finger foods if patient won't sit and eat *to ensure adequate nutrition.*

– Select activities based on patient's interests and abilities and praise him for participating in activities *to enhance his sense of self-worth.*

– Use television and radio carefully *to avoid sensory overload, which may exacerbate confusion.*

– Limit choices patient has to make *to provide structure and avoid confusion.*

– Label familiar photos with names of individuals pictured *to provide a sense of security.*

– Use symbols, rather than written signs, to identify patient's room, bathroom, and other facilities *to help patient identify surroundings.*

– Place patient's name in large block letters on clothing and other belongings *to help patient recognize his belongings and prevent them from becoming lost.*

■ If possible, make a home visit *to assess safety of patient's living environment.*

■ Assist family members in contacting appropriate community services. If necessary, act as an advocate for patient within health care system *to help secure services needed for ongoing care.*

■ Provide family members with information concerning long-term health care facilities. If necessary, assist family members in moving patient to a nursing home or other long-term care setting. *A patient with chronic confusion may require ongoing skilled nursing care.*

■ If patient is to be moved to a long-term care facility, explain the decision to him in as simple and gentle terms as possible *to facilitate comprehension.* Allow patient to express his feelings regarding the move *to facilitate grieving over loss of independence.* Provide psychological support to patient and family members *to alleviate stress they may experience during relocation.*

■ Communicate all aspects of the discharge plan to staff members at patient's new residence, including measures to ensure a stable environment and consistent routine; need to monitor patient's ongoing ability to perform ADLs; measures to ensure adequate nutrition; and interventions to provide emotional support to patient and family members. *Documenting a discharge plan and communicating it to caregivers helps ensure continuity of care. Interventions should ensure patient's dignity and rights.*

Suggested NIC interventions

Anxiety Reduction; Area Restriction; Calming Technique; Cognitive Stimulation; Dementia Management; Emotional Support; Energy Management; Family Involvement Promotion; Medication Management; Reality Orientation; Sleep Enhancement

Evaluations for expected outcomes

■ Patient experiences no injury because of chronic confusion.

■ Patient exhibits no sign of depression.

■ Patient eats enough to maintain weight.

■ Family members discuss openly their ability to provide for the patient.

■ Patient functions to maximum ability in a stable and structured environment.

■ Family members describe strategies to help patient cope with chronic confusion.

■ Patient participates in appropriate activities.

■ Family maintains a safe environment in the home.

■ Patient and family members receive adequate information regarding long-term care options to help them make informed decisions regarding patient's future.

■ Patient expresses feelings and receives adequate emotional support before, during, and after relocation to long-term care facility.

■ Care plan is communicated to staff at patient's new residence.

Documentation

■ Assessment of patient's cognitive abilities, behavior, and self-care status

■ Changes in patient's mental status as they occur

■ Assistance given to family to help them cope with patient's confusion

■ Any plans made to move patient to long-term care facility

■ Teaching sessions and referrals

■ Evaluations for expected outcomes

Reference

Rader, J., et al. "The Bathing of Older Adults with Dementia," *AJN* 106(4):40-48, April 2006.

Risk for acute
CONFUSION

Definition

At risk for reversible disturbances of consciousness, attention, cognition, and perception that develop over a short period of time

Assessment

■ Age, gender, level of education, occupation, and recent immigration status

■ Health history, including use of medications, especially with known cognitive and psychotropic adverse effects; recent surgery; allergies; and history of alcoholism, drug abuse, and depression

■ Neurologic status, including level of consciousness (LOC), orientation, thought and speech, mood, affect, memory, visual and spatial ability, judgment and insight, psychomotor activity, and perceptions; delusions, illusions, and hallucinations; pain level; recent behavioral changes; electrolyte imbalances; and history of transient ischemic attacks, head injury, early dementia, acquired immunodeficiency syndrome, or schizophrenia

■ Cardiovascular status, including vital signs, skin color, auscultation of carotid artery and heart sounds, and history of coronary artery disease or hypertension

■ Respiratory status, including rate, depth, and pattern of respirations; auscultation for breath sounds; smoking history; shortness of breath; and history of chronic obstructive pulmonary disease, cancer, or tuberculosis

■ Sensory status, including results of vision and hearing examination, use of corrective lenses or hearing aid, and history of eye or ear disorders

- Nutritional status, including typical daily food intake and weight loss
- Sleep status, including recent change in sleep pattern or environment (recent hospitalization)
- Elimination status, including history of urinary tract infection and patterns of elimination

Risk factors
- Alcohol use
- Decreased mobility
- Decreased restraints
- Dementia
- Fluctuation in sleep-wake cycle
- History of stroke
- Impaired cognition
- Infection
- Male gender
- Medication/drugs:
- Anesthesia
- Anticholinergics
- Diphenhydramine
- Multiple medications
- Opioids
- Psychoactive drugs
- Metabolic abnormalities:
- Azotemia
- Decreased hemoglobin
- Dehydration
- Electrolyte imbalances
- Increased blood urea nitrogen/creatinine
- Malnutrition
- Older than age 60
- Pain
- Sensory deprivation
- Urine retention

Expected outcomes
- Patient will remain free from injury.
- Patient's neurologic status will remain stable.
- Patient will obtain adequate amounts of sleep.
- Patient will maintain optimal hydration and nutrition.
- Family members will report an improved ability to cope with the patient's confused state.
- Patient will begin to participate in activities of daily living (ADLs).
- Patent will report feeling increasingly calm.
- Patient and family will state the causes of acute confusion.
- Patient and family will express an understanding of the importance of informing other health care providers about episodes of acute confusion.

Suggested NOC Outcomes

Cognitive Orientation; Distorted Thought Self-Control; Information Processing; Memory; Neurological Status; Personal Safety Behavior; Sleep

Intervention and rationales

■ Assess patient's LOC and changes in behavior *to provide baseline for comparison with ongoing assessment findings.*

■ Have a staff member stay at patient's bedside, if necessary, *to protect patient from harm.*

■ Enlist the aid of family member *to help calm patient.*

■ Limit noise and environmental stimulation *to prevent patient from becoming more confused.*

■ Monitor neurologic status on a regular basis *to detect improvement or decline in patient's neurologic function.*

■ Use appropriate safety measures *to protect patient from injury.* Avoid physical restraints *to prevent agitating patient.*

■ Address patient by name and tell him your name *to foster his awareness of self and environment.*

■ Give patient short, simple explanations each time you perform a procedure or task *to decrease confusion.*

■ Establish or maintain elimination pattern *to assist in maintaining elimination, orientation, and patient safety.*

■ Schedule nursing care to provide quiet times for patient *to help avoid sensory overload.*

■ Mention time, place, and date frequently throughout day. Have a large clock and a calendar where patient can easily see them. Refer to those aids when orienting him *to foster awareness of self and environment.*

■ Keep patient's possessions in the same place as much as possible. *A consistent, stable environment reduces confusion and frustration and aids completion of ADLs.*

■ Ask family to bring labeled family photos and other favorite articles *to create a more secure environment for patient.*

■ Plan patient's routine, and be as consistent as possible in following it. *A consistent routine aids task completion and reduces confusion.*

■ Speak slowly and clearly and allow patient ample time to respond *to reduce his frustration and promote task completion.*

■ Encourage patient to perform ADLs, dividing tasks into small, critical units. Be patient and specific in providing instructions. Allow time for patient to perform each task. *These measures enhance his self-esteem as well as help prevent complications related to inactivity.*

■ Encourage family to share stories and discuss familiar people and events with patient. *Sharing stories and familiar subjects promotes a sense of continuity, aids memory, and creates a sense of security and comfort.* Note that even if patient's short-term memory is impaired, his remote memory still may be intact.

■ Confer with physician about diagnostic test results, patient's progress in behavior, and patient's LOC. *A collaborative approach to treatment helps ensure high quality care and continuity of care.*

■ Discuss episodes of acute confusion with patient and family members *to make sure they understand the cause of confusion.*

■ Review measures family can take at home to help patient if he begins to exhibit signs of confusion. Tell them to give patient short explanations of activities; remind him of time, place, and date frequently; speak slowly and clearly and allow patient ample time to respond; and provide patient with a consistent routine. *Teaching empowers patient and family to take greater responsibility for their health care needs.*

■ Stress to patient and family that, in the future, they should inform health care providers about episodes of acute confusion *to help ensure continuity of care.*

Suggested NIC Interventions

Behavior Management: Overactivity/Inattention; Cognitive Stimulation; Delirium Management; Hallucination Management; Reality Orientation; Sleep Enhancement

Evaluations for expected outcomes
■ Patient remains free from injury during episodes of acute confusion.
■ Patient exhibits mental status within the normal range.
■ Patient obtains adequate sleep.
■ Patient maintains optimal hydration and nutrition.
■ Family reports an increased ability to cope with patient's confused state.
■ Patient performs ADLs to the extent possible.
■ Patient reports feeling increasingly calm.
■ Patient and family state the causes of acute confusion.
■ Patient and family express an understanding of the importance of telling future health care providers about episodes of acute confusion.

Documentation
■ Description of episodes of acute confusion
■ Factors that precipitate and ameliorate periods of acute confusion
■ Teaching sessions and referrals
■ Evaluations for expected outcomes

Reference
Cacchione, P.Z., et al. "Risk for Acute Confusion in Sensory-impaired, Rural, Long-Term Care Elders," *Clinical Nursing Research* 12(4):340-55, November 2003.

CONSTIPATION
related to insufficient intake of fiber and fluid

Definition
Decrease in normal frequency of defecation accompanied by difficult or incomplete passage of stools and/or passage of excessively dry stools

Assessment
■ History of bowel disorder or surgery

■ GI status, including nausea and vomiting, usual bowel elimination habits, change in bowel elimination habits, laxative use, stools characteristics (color, amount, size, and consistency), pain, inspection of abdomen, auscultation of bowel sounds, palpation for masses and tenderness, and percussion for tympany and dullness

■ Nutritional status, including dietary intake, fiber intake, appetite, current weight, and change from normal weight

■ Fluid status, including fluid intake, urine output, urine specific gravity, and skin turgor

■ Knowledge, including ability and motivation to change current patterns and understanding of relationship between intake, bulk, and constipation

Defining characteristics

■ Abdominal tenderness or pain and feeling of rectal fullness or pressure

■ Borborygmi, hypoactive or hyperactive bowel sounds, or abdominal dullness on percussion

■ Bright red blood with stools; bark-colored or black, tarry stools; or hard, dry stools

■ Change in bowel pattern

■ Changes in mental status, urinary incontinence, unexplained falls, or elevated body temperature in older adults

■ Decreased frequency and volume of stools

■ Distended abdomen and increased abdominal pressure

■ Inability to pass stools

■ General fatigue, anorexia, headache, indigestion, nausea, or vomiting

■ Oozing liquid stools

■ Palpable rectal or abdominal mass

■ Severe flatus

■ Soft, pastelike stools in rectum

■ Straining and possibly pain during defecation

Expected outcomes

■ Patient's elimination pattern will return to normal.

■ Patient will experience bowel movement every ___ day(s).

■ Patient will consume high-fiber or high-bulk diet, unless contraindicated.

■ Patient will maintain oral fluid intake of 2,500 ml daily, unless contraindicated.

■ Patient will state understanding of relationship of dietary intake and bulk to constipation.

■ Patient will list foods needed to prevent recurrence of problem, such as fruit, fruit juices, whole grain bread, and cereals.

Suggested NOC outcomes

Bowel Elimination; Comfort Level; Hydration; Nutritional Status: Food & Fluid Intake; Symptom Control

Interventions and rationales

■ Monitor and record frequency and characteristics of stools. *Careful monitoring forms the basis of an effective treatment plan.*

■ Record intake and output accurately *to ensure correct fluid replacement therapy.*

■ Unless contraindicated, encourage fluid intake of 2,500 ml daily *to ensure correct fluid replacement therapy.*

■ Place patient on bedpan or commode at specific times daily, as close to usual evacuation time (if known) as possible, *to aid adaptation to routine physiologic function.*

■ Administer laxative or enema, as ordered, *to promote elimination of solids and gases from GI tract.* Monitor effectiveness.

■ Teach patient to gently massage along the transverse and descending colon *to stimulate bowel's spastic reflex and aid stools passage.*

■ Consult with dietitian about increasing fiber and bulk in diet to maximum prescribed by physician. *This will improve intestinal muscle tone and promote comfortable elimination.*

■ Instruct patient and family in the relationship of diet, exercise, and fluid intake to constipation. Develop plan and provide for mild exercise periods. *These measures promote muscle tone and circulation and discourage departure from prescribed diet.*

Suggested NIC interventions

Bowel Management; Constipation/Impaction Management; Exercise Promotion; Fluid Management; Nutrition Management

Evaluations for expected outcomes

■ Patient resumes regular bowel elimination schedule.

■ Without using laxatives, enemas, or suppositories, patient has bowel movement every _____ day(s).

■ Patient consumes fruit, bran, and other high-fiber foods.

■ Patient drinks 2,500 ml of fluid daily, unless contraindicated.

■ Patient expresses understanding of the effects of diet and fluid intake on constipation.

■ Patient names foods that will help prevent recurrence of constipation.

Documentation

■ Patient's expressions of concern about constipation, dietary changes, laxative use, and bowel pattern

■ Observations of food and fluid intake and stools characteristics

■ Patient's expression of understanding of relationship between constipation and dietary intake of fluid and bulk

■ Patient's response to nursing interventions

■ Evaluations for expected outcomes

Reference

Hsieh, C. "Treatment of Constipation in Older Adults," *American Family Physician* 72(11):2277-84, December 2005.

CONSTIPATION

related to obstruction

Definition
Decrease in normal frequency of defecation accompanied by difficult or incomplete passage of stools and/or passage of excessively dry or hard stools

Assessment
- History of bowel disorder or surgery
- GI status, including nausea and vomiting, usual bowel elimination habits, change in bowel elimination habits, laxative use, stools characteristics (color, amount, size, and consistency), pain, inspection of abdomen, auscultation of bowel sounds, palpation for masses and tenderness, percussion for tympany and dullness, and results of upper GI series, barium enema, and sigmoidoscopy
- Nutritional status, including dietary intake, fiber intake, appetite, current weight, and change from normal weight
- Fluid and electrolyte status, including intake and output, skin turgor, urine specific gravity, and serum electrolyte level
- History of ingesting nonfood items (in psychiatric patients)

Defining characteristics
- Abdominal tenderness or pain and feeling of rectal fullness or pressure
- Borborygmi, hypoactive or hyperactive bowel sounds, or abdominal dullness on percussion
- Bright red blood with stools; bark-colored or black, tarry stools; or hard, dry, formed stools
- Change in bowel pattern
- Changes in mental status, urinary incontinence, unexplained falls, or elevated body temperature in older adults
- Decreased frequency and volume of stools
- Distended abdomen and increased abdominal pressure
- Inability to pass stools
- Nausea or vomiting
- General fatigue, anorexia, headache, indigestion, nausea, or vomiting
- Oozing liquid stools
- Palpable rectal or abdominal mass
- Severe flatus
- Soft, pastelike stools in rectum
- Straining and possibly pain during defecation

Expected outcomes
- Patient will return to usual bowel pattern.
- Patient will maintain fluid balance; intake equals output.
- Patient will display normal bowel sounds.
- Patient will express pain relief or comfort.
- Patient will stop vomiting through use of antiemetics or GI tube.

■ Patient will state understanding of surgical procedure.

■ Patient or caregiver will demonstrate use of ileostomy or colostomy equipment.

■ Patient will discuss fears and anxieties associated with bowel diversion.

■ Patient or caregiver will discuss effect of bowel diversion on lifestyle.

■ Patient or caregiver will state intention to contact support group.

■ Patient will maintain weight.

■ Patient will perform oral hygiene.

Suggested NOC outcomes

Bowel Elimination; Comfort Level; Hydration; Medication Response; Symptom Control

Interventions and rationales

■ Carefully monitor and record frequency and characteristics of stools *to form basis of effective treatment plan.*

■ Record intake and output accurately *to ensure correct fluid replacement therapy.* Report any imbalance.

■ Auscultate bowel sounds and record every 4 hours. Report significant changes. *Absent or diminished bowel sounds may indicate peritoneal irritation or intestinal obstruction.*

■ Record patient's weight daily *to detect possible fluid retention, food malabsorption, or increased adaptation requirements on body processes.*

■ Administer pain medication and anti-emetics as ordered. Monitor effectiveness *to determine need for alternative treatment.*

■ Promote patient comfort during vomiting episodes by providing oral care and removing vomitus promptly. Carefully record amount and characteristics of vomitus *to ensure accurate intake and output records.*

■ Provide oral and nasal care every 4 hours while GI tube is present. Keep nostrils clean and moist *to prevent irritation.*

■ Prepare patient for surgery:

– Give preoperative instruction for abdominal surgery *to reduce patient's anxiety and increase trust.*

– Inform patient about ileostomy, colostomy, or colectomy, as indicated, *to reduce anxiety.*

■ Instruct patient and caregivers in the use of ileostomy or colostomy equipment *to promote familiarity and establish therapeutic relationship.* Have patient and caregivers demonstrate use of equipment *to encourage feeling of shared responsibility.*

■ Encourage patient and family to express feelings and concerns about changes in body image *to help them learn to cope.*

■ Encourage visits to patient by persons from ileostomy or colostomy support groups *to provide patient with additional health care resources.*

■ Have the patient evaluated for home health care after discharge. The patient and family may need additional support and care after discharge. *Knowing that such help is available may enhance coping as the patient prepares to go home.*

Suggested NIC interventions

Anxiety Reduction; Bowel Management; Fluid/Electrolyte Management; Nutrition Management; Ostomy Care; Skin Surveillance

Evaluations for expected outcomes

■ Patient exhibits a normal bowel elimination pattern.

■ Patient drinks adequate amount of fluids, with intake equal to output.

■ Patient displays normal bowel sounds.

■ Patient states that pain medication is effective.

■ Patient doesn't vomit.

■ Patient expresses understanding of surgical procedure, including need for ileostomy or colostomy.

■ Patient or caregiver demonstrates care, changing, and irrigation of ileostomy or colostomy equipment.

■ Patient states acceptance of bowel diversion.

■ Patient comes to terms with effects of bowel diversion on lifestyle.

■ Patient or caregiver identifies and contacts support group if needed.

■ Patient doesn't exhibit weight loss or gain. Weight is consistent with body weight chart.

■ Patient's mouth is clear and free from odor, and nostrils are clean and moist.

Documentation

■ Patient's expressions of concern about vomiting, GI tube, or surgery

■ Observation of characteristics of vomitus and stools, intake and output, weight, bowel sounds, and condition of oral cavity

■ Patient's reaction and adaptation to ileostomy or colostomy

■ Patient's and caregivers' participation in care and response to instruction

■ Evaluations for expected outcomes

Reference

Amerine, E., and Keirsey, M. "How Should You Respond to Constipation?" *Nursing 2006* 36(10):1-4, October 2006.

Perceived
CONSTIPATION

Definition

Self-diagnosis of constipation and abuse of laxatives, enemas, or suppositories to ensure a daily bowel movement

Assessment

■ Age and gender

■ Family history of constipation

■ History of psychiatric disorders

■ Fluid and electrolyte status, including intake and output, skin turgor, urine specific gravity, and mucous membranes
■ Marital status
■ GI status, including bowel elimination habits, change in bowel elimination habits, stools characteristics (color, amount, size, and consistency), pain, auscultation of bowel sounds, laxative or enema use (time and duration), family habits concerning bowel movements, and rectal examination
■ Nutritional status, including dietary intake and appetite
■ Activity status
■ Psychosocial status, including personality, stressors (finances, job, marital discord, and coping mechanisms), support systems (family and others), lifestyle, and knowledge level

Defining characteristics
■ Expectation of passage of stools at same time each day, with resulting overuse of laxatives, enemas, and suppositories

Expected outcomes
■ Patient will decrease use of laxatives, enemas, or suppositories.
■ Patient will state understanding of normal bowel function.
■ Patient will discuss feelings about elimination pattern.
■ Patient's elimination pattern will return to normal.
■ Patient will experience bowel movement every _____ day(s) without laxatives, enemas, or suppositories.
■ Patient will state understanding of factors causing constipation.
■ Patient will get regular exercise.
■ Patient will describe changes in personal habits to maintain normal elimination pattern.
■ Patient will state intent to use appropriate resources to help resolve emotional or psychological problems.

Suggested NOC outcomes
Adherence Behavior; Bowel Elimination; Health Beliefs; Health Beliefs: Perceived Threat; Knowledge: Health Behavior

Interventions and rationales
■ Modify patient's dietary habits to include adequate fluids, fresh fruits and vegetables, and whole grain cereals and breads, *which supply necessary bulk for normal elimination.*
■ Encourage patient to engage in daily exercise, such as brisk walking, *to strengthen muscle tone and stimulate circulation.*
■ Encourage patient to evacuate at regular times *to aid adaptation and routine physiologic function.*
■ Urge patient to avoid taking laxatives, if possible, or to gradually decrease their use *to avoid further trauma to intestinal mucosa.*
■ Inform patient not to expect a bowel movement every day or even every other day *to avoid use of poor health practices to stimulate elimination.*

■ If not contraindicated, increase patient's fluid intake to about 3 qt (3 L) daily *to increase functional capacity of bowel elimination.*

■ Explain normal bowel elimination habits *so patient can better understand normal and abnormal body functions.*

■ Reassure patient that normal bowel function is possible without laxatives, enemas, or suppositories *to give patient the necessary confidence for compliance.*

■ Give information about self-help groups, as appropriate, *to provide additional resources for patient and family.*

■ Establish and implement an individualized bowel elimination regimen based on patient's needs. *Knowledge of normal body functions will improve patient's understanding of problem.*

■ Instruct patient to avoid straining during elimination *to avoid tissue damage, bleeding, and pain.*

■ Instruct patient that abdominal massage may help relieve discomfort and promote defecation *because it triggers bowel's spastic reflex.*

Suggested NIC interventions

Anxiety Reduction; Bowel Management; Counseling; Health Education; Nutrition Management; Teaching: Individual

Evaluations for expected outcomes

■ Patient decreases use of laxatives, enemas, or suppositories.

■ Patient describes normal bowel function and how fluid consumption, high-fiber diet, and exercise affect function.

■ Patient expresses feelings about changes in elimination pattern.

■ Patient's elimination pattern returns to normal.

■ Without using laxatives, enemas, or suppositories, patient has bowel movement every _____ day(s).

■ Patient lists factors that may cause constipation.

■ Patient engages in regular exercise.

■ Patient states plans to make changes in personal habits to prevent constipation.

■ Patient makes contact with appropriate resources to help resolve psychological conflicts.

Documentation

■ Patient's expressions of concern about change in diet, activity level, laxative and enema use, and bowel pattern

■ Observations of diet, stools characteristics, and activity tolerance

■ Patient teaching about diet, exercise, and constipation management

■ Evaluations for expected outcomes

Reference

Hernando-Harder, A.C., et al. "Intestinal Gas Retention in Patients with Idiopathic Slow-transit Constipation," *Digestive Diseases and Sciences* March 2007. [Epub ahead of print.]

Risk for
CONSTIPATION

Definition
At risk for a decrease in patient's normal frequency of defecation accompanied by difficult or incomplete passage of stools, passage of excessively hard stools, or both

Assessment
- Age and gender
- Vital signs
- Health history, including bowel disorder or surgery, diabetic gastroparesis, immobility or inactivity, chronic debilitating disease, and episodes characterized by inability to swallow food and fluids
- GI status, including nausea and vomiting, usual bowel habits, change in bowel habits, laxative use, stools characteristics (color, amount, size, and consistency), pain, inspection of abdomen, auscultation of bowel sounds, palpation for masses and tenderness, and percussion for tympany and dullness
- Nutritional status, including dietary intake, appetite, current weight, and changes from normal diet
- Fluid status, including intake and output and skin turgor
- Musculoskeletal status, including functional mobility, joint mobility, paralysis, paresis, and activity and exercise status
- Psychosocial status, including understanding of risk of constipation, motivation to change health habits, and understanding of relationship between intake, bulk, activity and mobility, and constipation

Risk factors
- Functional, such as habitual denial and ignoring urge to defecate, recent environmental changes, inadequate toileting (for example, timeliness, positioning for defecation, privacy), irregular defecation habits, insufficient physical activity, and abdominal muscle weakness
- Mechanical, such as rectal abscess or ulcer, pregnancy, rectal anal stricture, postsurgical obstruction, rectal anal fissures, megacolon (Hirschsprung's disease), electrolyte imbalance, tumors, prostate enlargement, rectocele, rectal prolapse, neurologic impairment, hemorrhoids, and obesity
- Pharmacologic, such as phenothiazines, nonsteroidal anti-inflammatory agents, sedatives, aluminum-containing antacids, laxative overuse, iron salts, anticholinergics, antidepressants, anticonvulsants, antilipemic agents, calcium channel blockers, calcium carbonate, diuretics, sympathomimetics, opiates, and bismuth salts
- Physiologic, such as insufficient fiber intake, dehydration, inadequate dentition or oral hygiene, poor eating habits, insufficient fluid intake, change in usual foods and eating patterns, and decreased motility of GI tract
- Psychological, such as emotional stress, mental confusion, and depression

Expected outcomes

- Patient will experience no constipation.
- Patient will maintain bowel movement every _____ day(s).
- Patient will consume a high-fiber or high-bulk diet, unless contraindicated.
- Patient will maintain fluid intake of _____ ml daily (specify).
- Patient will express understanding of the relationship between constipation and dietary intake, bulk, and activity.
- Patient will express understanding of preventive measures, such as eating fruit and whole grain breads and cereals and engaging in mild activity, if appropriate.

Suggested NOC outcomes

Bowel Elimination; Self-Care: Toileting

Interventions and rationales

- Assess bowel sounds and check patient for abdominal distention. Monitor and record frequency and characteristics of stools *to develop an effective treatment plan for preventing constipation and fecal impaction.*
- Record intake and output accurately *to ensure accurate fluid replacement therapy.*
- Encourage fluid intake of 2½ qt (2.5 L) daily, unless contraindicated, *to promote fluid replacement therapy and hydration.*
- Initiate bowel program. Place patient on a bedpan or commode at specific times daily, as close to usual evacuation time (if known) as possible, *to aid adaptation to routine physiologic function.*
- Administer a laxative, an enema, or suppositories, as prescribed, *to promote elimination of solids and gases from GI tract.* Monitor effectiveness.
- Teach patient to gently massage along the transverse and descending colon *to stimulate the bowel's spastic reflex and aid in stools passage.*
- Consult with a dietitian about how to increase fiber and bulk in patient's diet to the maximum amount prescribed by the physician *to improve intestinal muscle tone and promote comfortable elimination.*
- Instruct patient, family member, or caregiver in the relationship between diet, activity and exercise, and fluid intake and constipation *to discourage departure from prescribed diet and assist in promoting elimination.*
- Include a program of mild exercise in your care plan *to promote muscle tone and circulation.*
- Review care plan with patient, family member, or caregiver, emphasizing the relationship between the risk factors for constipation and preventive measures *to foster understanding.*

Suggested NIC interventions

Anxiety Reduction; Bowel Management; Constipation/Impaction Management; Exercise Promotion; Fluid Management; Fluid Monitoring; Nutrition Management

Evaluations for expected outcomes

- Patient doesn't experience constipation.

■ Patient has bowel movement every _____ day(s).
■ Patient consumes a high-fiber or high-bulk diet, unless contraindicated.
■ Patient maintains fluid intake of _____ ml daily (specify).
■ Patient expresses understanding of the relationship between constipation and dietary intake, bulk, and activity.
■ Patient expresses understanding of preventive measures, such as eating fruit and whole grain breads and cereals and engaging in mild activity, if appropriate.

Documentation

■ Patient's, family members', or caregivers' statements regarding risk of constipation
■ Presence of risk factors for constipation
■ Observations of food and fluid intake, urine output, and stools characteristics
■ Instructions regarding preventive care
■ Patient's, family members', or caregivers' statements indicating understanding of instructions
■ Patient's response to preventive interventions
■ Implementation, alteration, or continuation of bowel program
■ Patient's, family members', or caregivers' demonstrated ability to implement preventive measures
■ Evaluations for expected outcomes

Reference

Norton, C. "Constipation in Older Patients: Effects on Quality of Life," *British Journal of Nursing* 15(4):188-92, February-March 2006.

Compromised family
COPING

related to inadequate or incorrect information held by primary caregiver

Definition

A usually supportive primary person (family member or close friend) is providing insufficient, ineffective, or compromised support, comfort, assistance, or encouragement that may be needed by the patient to manage or master adaptive tasks related to his health challenge

Assessment

■ Family status, including normal pattern of interaction among family members, family's understanding and knowledge of patient's present condition, support systems available (financial, social, and spiritual), family's response to past crises, and communication patterns used to express anger, affection, confrontation, and conflict
■ Patient's illness, including progression and severity of illness, patient's perception of health problem, and problem-solving techniques used by patient to cope with life problems

Defining characteristics

■ Family member's displays of protective behavior that's disproportionate (too little or too much) to patient's abilities or need for autonomy

■ Inadequate understanding or knowledge base of family member that interferes with effective assistive or supportive behaviors

■ Preoccupation of family member with personal reaction (such as fear, anticipatory grief, guilt, or anxiety) to patient's illness, disability, or other situational or developmental crisis

■ Family member's withdrawal from or limited communication with patient at time of need

Expected outcomes

■ Family will discuss patient's illness and its impact on family functioning.

■ Family will designate a spokesperson to receive information regarding the patient's illness.

■ Family will establish a visiting routine beneficial to patient and family.

■ Family will state understanding of patient's health status.

■ Family will identify and use available support systems.

Suggested NOC outcomes

Caregiver Emotional Health; Caregiver-Patient Relationship; Caregiver Stressors; Family Coping; Family Normalization

Interventions and rationales

■ Identify the spokesperson for the family *to avoid creating communication conflicts within family.*

■ Facilitate family conferences; help family members identify key issues and select support services, if needed. *Involving patient and family in care planning promotes open communication throughout illness.*

■ Help patient and family establish a visiting routine that won't tax their resources. Each family member may be responsible for a day or period of time, if desired. Use patient's daily routine to aid in planning; for example, no visiting during treatments or periods of uninterrupted sleep. *This enhances family's sense of contributing to patient's overall care.*

■ Encourage family to contact a community agency for continued support if necessary. *This is an effective health-related coping skill.*

■ Provide family with clear, concise information about patient's condition. Be aware of what family has been told and help them interpret information. *This ensures clear, uncluttered communication between patient, family, and caregivers.*

■ Ensure privacy during patient and family visits. *This demonstrates respect and fosters open communication between family members.*

■ Help family support patient's independence. Encourage attendance at therapy sessions, and allow patient to demonstrate new skills and abilities *to help family members learn how they can help promote patient's independence and self-care.*

■ Provide emotional support to family by being available to answer questions. *This demonstrates your willingness to help family seek health-related information.*

Suggested NIC interventions

Caregiver Support; Conflict Mediation; Decision-Making Support; Emotional Support; Family Involvement Promotion

Evaluations for expected outcomes

■ Family members discuss feelings about patient's illness and its impact on family functioning.
■ Family members designate spokesperson to receive and communicate information regarding the patient's illness.
■ Family members agree to follow a consistent visiting routine.
■ Family members accurately describe the patient's health status.
■ Family member contacts at least one support person or group.

Documentation

■ Family's response to patient's illness
■ Family's current understanding of patient's illness
■ Observations about family's interaction with patient and acceptance of current situation
■ Evaluations for expected outcomes

Reference

Stapleton, R.D., et al. "Clinician Statements and Family Satisfaction with Family Conferences in the Intensive Care Unit," *Critical Care Medicine* 34(6):1679-85, June 2006.

Compromised family
COPING

related to prolonged disease

Definition

Behavior of family members that compromises patient's and family's ability to adapt

Assessment

■ Patient's illness, including course and severity and effect on family members
■ Patient's health care resources, including hospital, community resources, health care providers such as therapists, and case manager (outpatient)
■ Family process, including involvement with patient, quality of relationships, communication patterns, coping strategies, demands posed by patient's condition, family's understanding of patient's illness, family's feelings regarding patient's illness, willingness of family members to commit time to patient care, and family's ability to provide care

Defining characteristics

■ Family member's displays of protective behavior that's disproportionate (too little or too much) to patient's abilities or need for autonomy

■ Inadequate understanding or knowledge base of family member that interferes with effective assistive or supportive behaviors

■ Preoccupation of family member with personal reaction (e.g. fear, anticipatory grief, guilt, or anxiety) to patient's illness, disability, or other situational or developmental crisis

■ Family member's withdrawal from or limited communication with patient at time of need

Expected outcomes

■ Family members will express their concerns about coping with patient's illness.
■ Family members will identify their needs.
■ Family members will contact appropriate sources of support.
■ Family members and patient will achieve better cooperation.

Suggested NOC outcomes

Family Coping; Family Normalization

Interventions and rationales

■ Assess effects of patient's disease on family functioning *to plan interventions that enhance long-term well-being of family and patient.*

■ Encourage family members to hold conferences. Help them identify topics appropriate for discussion. Examples of such topics include developing coping strategies for dealing with patient's disease or resolving conflicts between meeting personal needs and meeting patient's health care needs. *Family members may find a group problem-solving approach helpful in correcting dysfunctional behaviors.*

■ Evaluate and rectify any knowledge deficit that family members have about patient's disease and treatment. Experience doesn't guarantee correct knowledge. *Lack of knowledge can exacerbate frustration and tension within the family.*

■ Encourage family members to participate in appropriate support groups *to help them obtain social support and information and to provide an opportunity to express feelings.*

■ Encourage family members to contact and use appropriate community agencies *to help prevent burnout among family members after patient leaves the hospital.* Families may need encouragement to use support and respite care services if past efforts to use such services proved unsuccessful.

Suggested NIC interventions

Family Involvement Promotion; Family Mobilization; Family Support; Normalization Promotion

Evaluations for expected outcomes

■ Family members discuss impact of patient's prolonged disease.
■ Family members communicate their needs regarding the patient's prolonged care.
■ Family members are aware of available sources of support and use them appropriately.

■ Family members and patient negotiate meeting patient's care needs to their mutual satisfaction.

Documentation
■ Assessment of family functioning (including family's level of insight into their behavior)
■ Content of family conferences
■ Community resources used, their effectiveness, and recommendations for future use (indicate family's level of acceptance of nurse's recommendations)
■ Evaluations for expected outcomes

Reference
Nelson, J.E., et al. "When Critical Illness Becomes Chronic: Informational Needs of Patients and Families," *Journal of Critical Care* 20(1):79-89, March 2005.

Defensive
COPING
related to perceived threat to positive self-regard

Definition
Repeated projection of falsely positive self-evaluation based on a self-protective pattern that defends against underlying perceived threats to positive self-regard

Assessment
■ Age and gender
■ Developmental stage
■ Family system, including marital status and sibling position
■ Reason for hospitalization
■ Past experience with illness
■ Patient's perception of health problem
■ Patient's perception of self, including self-worth, body image, problem-solving ability, and coping mechanisms
■ Mental status, including general appearance, affect, mood, cognitive and perceptual functioning, and behavior
■ Social interaction pattern
■ Support systems, such as family and friends

Defining characteristics
■ Denial of obvious problems
■ Difficulty establishing or maintaining relationships
■ Difficulty in reality-testing perceptions
■ Extreme sensitivity to criticism
■ Grandiosity
■ Lack of follow-through or participation in treatment or therapy
■ Projection of blame or responsibility

- Rationalization of failures
- Superior attitude toward and ridicule of others

Expected outcomes

- Patient will state reason for hospitalization.
- Patient will verbally describe self, including concept, body image, successes and positive aspects to live events.
- Patient will participate in self-care.
- Patient will engage in decision making about treatment.
- Patient will accept responsibility for own behavior.
- Patient will demonstrate follow-through in decisions related to health care.
- Patient will interact with others in a socially acceptable manner.

Suggested NOC outcomes

Acceptance: Health Status; Coping; Self-Esteem; Social Interaction Skills

Interventions and rationales

- Encourage patient to evaluate self, possibly by making a written list of positive and negative traits. *This helps patient identify aspects of self and relate changes to specific variables.*
- Have patient perform self-care to the extent possible *to provide a sense of control.*
- Provide a structured daily routine *to provide patient with alternatives to self-absorption.*
- Help patient make treatment-related decisions, and encourage follow-through. *Ability to make decisions is principal component of autonomy.*
- Provide an opportunity for patient to meet with someone who's successfully coping with a similar problem. *This may encourage patient to work toward a positive outcome.*
- Arrange for interaction between patient and others, and observe interaction pattern. *Studying patient's verbal and nonverbal interactions with others gives clues to patient's ability to communicate effectively.*
- Provide positive feedback when patient assumes responsibility for own behavior *to reinforce effective coping behaviors.*

Suggested NIC interventions

Coping Enhancement; Counseling; Emotional Support; Patient Contracting; Self-Awareness Enhancement; Self-Responsibility Facilitation

Evaluations for expected outcomes

- Patient states reason for hospitalization.
- Patient uses at least two positive terms to describe self.
- Patient initiates and completes at least two self-care activities daily.
- Each day, patient makes at least one decision related to activities of daily living, self-care, or treatment.
- Patient expresses responsible attitude toward own behavior.
- Patient reports specific instances of following through on health care decisions.

■ Each day, patient socializes with others in an acceptable manner.

Documentation
■ Patient's perception of self
■ Behavioral responses
■ Social interaction patterns
■ Patient's use of defense mechanisms
■ Interventions used to facilitate effective coping
■ Patient's responses to nursing interventions
■ Evaluations for expected outcomes

Reference
Schwinghammer, S.A., et al. "Different Selves Have Different Effects: Self-activation and Defensive Social Comparison," *Personality and Social Psychology Bulletin* 32(1):27-39, January 2006.

Disabled family
COPING
related to highly ambivalent family relationships

Definition
Behavior of significant person (family members or other primary person) that disables his/her capabilities and the patient's capabilities to effectively address tasks essential to either person's adaptation to the health challenge

Assessment
■ Patient's illness, including its course, severity, and effect on family members
■ Patient's health care resources, including hospital, community resources, and health care providers, such as therapists and case managers
■ Demands on family imposed by patient's condition
■ Family status, including involvement with patient, quality of relationships, communication patterns, coping strategies, family's understanding of patient's illness, family's feelings about patient's illness, willingness of family members to commit time to patient care, and family's ability to provide care

Defining characteristics
■ Intolerance
■ Agitation, depression, aggression, hostility
■ Taking on illness signs of patient
■ Rejection
■ Psychosomaticism
■ Neglectful relationships with other family members
■ Neglectful care of patient in regard to basic human needs
■ Distortion of reality regarding patient
■ Impaired restructuring of a meaningful life for self

■ Decisions and actions by family members that are detrimental to economic or social well-being
■ Carrying on usual routines without regard to patient's needs

Expected outcomes
■ To the extent possible, family members will participate in aspects of patient's care without evidence of increased conflict.
■ Patient will express confidence in his ability to make decisions, despite pressure from family members.
■ Patient will contact appropriate sources of support outside the family.
■ Patient will take steps to ensure that care needs are met despite family's short-comings.
■ Patient will express greater understanding of emotional limitations of family members.

Suggested NOC outcomes
Caregiver Emotional Health; Caregiver-Patient Relationship; Caregiving Endurance Potential; Family Coping

Interventions and rationales
■ Assess effects of patient's disease on family functioning. *A thorough assessment of the family's coping behaviors is necessary to developing a therapeutic action plan.*
■ As possible, encourage family members to participate in patient care. *Family members should have an opportunity to overcome dysfunctional behavior.*
■ Maintain objectivity when dealing with family conflicts. Don't become embroiled in the dynamics of a dysfunctional family *to maintain your ability to intervene objectively and effectively.*
■ If patient and family members appear incapable of taking steps to heal their relationships, focus on being a patient advocate. Reaffirm patient's right to make his own decisions without interference from family members. Provide necessary information to patient to facilitate decision making. *Dysfunctional family coping patterns evolve over many years and are unlikely to change just because patient has a serious illness. Accepting your limitations when working with family members will help you to avoid burnout and better meet patient's needs.*
■ Encourage patient to seek emotional support his family can't provide by participating in a support group. Help patient select support group that best meets his personal needs and outlook. Consider recommending Codependents Anonymous, a group for individuals who have difficulty maintaining healthy relationships as a result of being raised in a dysfunctional family. *Participation in a support group may improve patient's ability to cope as well as provide an opportunity to form meaningful relationships.*
■ Refer patient to a home health care agency, homemaker service, Meals On Wheels, or other appropriate outside agencies for assistance and follow-up. *Use of various community services may help to make up for shortcomings in family's ability to provide care.*
■ Listen openly to patient's expressions of pain over unresolved conflicts with family members. Patient may have to grieve over the fact that he'll never have an "ideal" family, capable of fully meeting his emotional needs. *Therapeutic listening*

helps patient to understand himself and his family better and to understand how conflicts from past affect his behavior.

Suggested NIC interventions
Anger Control Assistance; Caregiver Support; Family Involvement Promotion; Family Mobilization; Family Support

Evaluations for expected outcomes
- Family members demonstrate improved willingness to cooperate in patient's care.
- Patient expresses increased confidence in his ability to make decisions.
- Patient contacts at least one support group in an effort to form meaningful relationships outside family.
- Patient takes steps to meet his own care needs.
- Patient indicates, either verbally or through behavior, a better understanding of family members and an increased ability to accept their emotional limitations.

Documentation
- Family's response to patient's illness
- Observations of patient's interactions with family members
- Referrals made to support groups and community services
- Patient's expressions of grief, anger, and disappointment over unresolved conflicts with family members
- Evaluations for expected outcomes

Reference
Andershed, B. "Relatives in End-of-life Care — Part 1: A Systematic Review of the Literature the Last Five Years, January 1999-February 2004," *Journal of Clinical Nursing* 15(9):1158-69, September 2006.

Ineffective
COPING
related to situational crisis

Definition
Inability to form a valid appraisal of the stressors, inadequate choices of practiced responses, and/or inability to use available resources

Assessment
- Current health status
- Diversional activities
- Financial resources
- Occupation
- Patient's perception of present health problem or crisis
- Family members' understanding of the client's health status

■ Problem-solving techniques usually employed by the family to cope with life problems

■ Support systems, including family, companion, friends, and clergy

Defining characteristics

■ Change in communication patterns

■ Decreased use of social support

■ Destructive behavior toward self or others

■ Difficulty asking for help

■ Fatigue

■ High illness rate

■ Inability to meet basic needs and role expectations

■ Lack of goal-directed behavior, such as inability to focus attention, difficulty organizing information, poor concentration, and poor problem-solving abilities

■ Maladaptive coping behaviors

■ Risk-taking behaviors

■ Sleep disturbance

■ Statements indicating inability to cope

■ Substance abuse

Expected outcomes

■ Patient will communicate feelings about the present situation.

■ Patient will become involved in planning own care.

■ Patient will express feeling of having greater control over present situation.

■ Patient will use available support systems, such as family and friends, to aid in coping.

■ Patient will identify and demonstrate ability to use at least two healthy coping behaviors.

Suggested NOC outcomes

Aggression Self-Control; Coping; Decision-Making; Impulse Self-Control; Information Processing; Role Performance; Social Support

Interventions and rationales

■ If possible, assign a consistent care provider to patient *to provide continuity of care and promote development of therapeutic relationship.*

■ Arrange to spend uninterrupted periods of time with patient. Encourage expression of feelings, and accept what patient says. Try to identify factors that cause or exacerbate patient's inability to cope such as fear of loss of health or job. *Devoting time to listening helps patient express emotions, grasp situation, and cope effectively.*

■ Identify and reduce unnecessary stimuli in environment *to avoid subjecting patient to sensory or perceptual overload.*

■ Initially, allow patient to depend partly on you for self-care. *Patient may regress to a lower developmental level during initial crisis phase.*

■ Explain all treatments and procedures and answer patient's questions *to allay fear and allow patient to regain sense of control.*

■ Encourage patient to make decisions about care *to increase sense of self-worth and mastery over current situation.*

■ Have patient increase self-care performance levels gradually *to allow patient to progress at his own pace.*

■ Praise patient for making decisions and performing activities *to reinforce coping behaviors.*

■ Encourage patient to use support systems to assist with coping, *thereby helping restore psychological equilibrium and prevent crisis.*

■ Help patient look at current situation and evaluate various coping behaviors *to encourage a realistic view of crisis.*

■ Encourage patient to try coping behaviors. A patient in crisis tends to accept interventions and develop new coping behaviors more easily than at other times.

■ Request feedback from patient about behaviors that seem to work *to encourage patient to evaluate effect of these behaviors.*

■ Refer patient for professional psychological counseling. *If patient's maladaptive behavior has high crisis potential, formal counseling helps ease nurse's frustration, increases objectivity, and fosters collaborative approach to patient's care.*

Suggested NIC interventions

Anger Control Assistance; Anxiety Reduction; Coping Enhancement; Impulse Control Training; Learning Facilitation; Role Enhancement

Evaluations for expected outcomes
■ Patient discusses recent stressful event and describes related emotions.
■ Patient cooperates with nurse to plan care.
■ Patient identifies problems, makes plans, and takes action.
■ Patient requests assistance from family and friends.
■ Patient identifies and uses at least two healthy coping behaviors such as relaxation techniques.

Documentation
■ Patient's perception of present situation and what it means
■ Patient's verbal expression of feelings indicating comfort or discomfort
■ Observations of patient's behaviors
■ Interventions to help patient cope
■ Patient's responses to interventions
■ Evaluations for expected outcomes

Reference
Fok, S.K., et al. "Sense of Coherence, Coping and Quality of Life Following a Critical Illness," *Journal of Advanced Nursing* 49(2):173-81, January 2005.

Ineffective
DENIAL
related to fear or anxiety

Definition
Conscious or unconscious attempt to disavow the knowledge or meaning of an event to reduce anxiety or fear to the detriment of health

Assessment
■ Perception of present health state, including awareness of diagnosis, perception of personal relevance or impact on life pattern, and description of symptoms
■ Mental status, including general appearance, affect, mood, memory, orientation, communication, thinking process, perception, abstract thinking, judgment, and insight
■ Coping behaviors
■ Problem-solving strategies
■ Support systems, including family, friends, clergy, and financial resources
■ Belief system, including values, norms, and religion
■ Self-concept, including self-esteem and body image

Defining characteristics
■ Delay in seeking or refusal of medical attention to detriment of health
■ Displacement of fear of condition's impact
■ Displacement of sources of symptoms to other organs
■ Failure to perceive personal relevance or danger of symptoms
■ Inability to admit impact of disease on life pattern
■ Inappropriate affect
■ Minimization of symptoms
■ Refusal to admit fear of death or invalidism
■ Use of dismissive gestures or comments when speaking of distressing events
■ Use of self-treatment to relieve symptoms

Expected outcomes
■ Patient will describe knowledge and perception of present health problem.
■ Patient will describe life pattern and report any recent changes.
■ Patient will express knowledge of stages of grieving.
■ Patient will demonstrate behavior associated with grief process.
■ Patient will discuss present health problem with physician, nurses, and family members.
■ Patient will indicate, either verbally or through behavior, an increased awareness of reality.

Suggested NOC outcomes
Acceptance: Health Status; Anxiety Level; Coping; Fear Self-Control; Health Beliefs; Health Beliefs: Perceived Threat; Symptom Control

Interventions and rationales

■ Provide for a specific amount of uninterrupted, non-care-related time with patient each day. *This allows patient to ventilate knowledge, feelings, and concerns.*

■ Encourage patient to express feelings related to present problem, its severity, and its potential impact on life pattern. *This helps patient express doubts and resolve concerns.*

■ Maintain frequent communication with physician to assess what patient has been told about illness. *This fosters consistent, collaborative approach to patient's care.*

■ Listen to patient with nonjudgmental acceptance *to demonstrate positive regard for patient as person worthy of respect.*

■ Help patient learn the stages of anticipatory grieving *to increase understanding and ability to cope.*

■ Encourage patient to communicate with others, asking questions and clarifying concerns based on readiness. *Patient fixated in denial may isolate and withdraw from others.*

■ Visit more frequently as patient begins to accept reality; alleviate fears when necessary. *This helps reduce patient's fear of being alone and fosters accurate reality testing.*

Suggested NIC interventions

Anxiety Reduction; Behavior Modification; Calming Technique; Coping Enhancement; Counseling; Decision-Making Support; Health Education; Mutual Goal Setting; Reality Orientation; Truth Telling

Evaluations for expected outcomes

■ Patient describes present health problem.

■ Patient describes life pattern and reports recent changes.

■ Patient communicates understanding of stages of grieving.

■ Patient demonstrates behavior appropriate to present phase of grieving process.

■ When ready, patient discusses health problem with physician, nurses, and family members.

■ Patient displays increasing awareness of reality, either verbally or through behavior.

Documentation

■ Patient's perception of health problem

■ Mental status (baseline and ongoing)

■ Patient's knowledge of grief process

■ Patient's behavioral responses

■ Interventions implemented to assist patient

■ Patient's response to nursing interventions

■ Evaluations for expected outcomes

Reference

Telford, K., et al. "Acceptance and Denial: Implications for People Adapting to Chronic Illness: Literature Review," *Journal of Advanced Nursing* 55(4):457-64, August 2006.

DIARRHEA

related to malabsorption, inflammation, or irritation of bowel

Definition

Passage of loose, unformed stools

Assessment

■ History of bowel disorder or surgery
■ GI status, including nausea and vomiting, usual bowel elimination habits, change in bowel elimination habits, stools characteristics (color, amount, size, and consistency), pain, inspection of abdomen, auscultation of bowel sounds, palpation for masses and tenderness, percussion for tympany and dullness, laxative and enema use, medications (especially antibiotics), and results of stool culture, upper GI series, and barium enema
■ Nutritional status, including dietary intake, change from normal diet, appetite, current weight, change from normal weight, food irritants and contaminants, and serum albumin levels
■ Fluid and electrolyte status, including intake and output, urine specific gravity, skin turgor, mucous membranes, serum potassium and sodium levels, and blood urea nitrogen
■ Psychosocial status, including personality, stressors (such as finances, job, marital discord, and disease process), coping mechanisms, support systems, lifestyle, and recent travel

Defining characteristics

■ Abdominal pain and cramping
■ At least three loose, liquid stools per day
■ Hyperactive bowel sounds
■ Urgency
■ High stress levels and anxiety
■ Alcohol abuse
■ Toxins
■ Laxative abuse
■ Radiation
■ Adverse effects of medication
■ Contaminants
■ Travel
■ Inflammation
■ Malabsorption
■ Infectious processes

■ Irritation
■ Parasites

Expected outcomes

■ Patient will control diarrhea with medication.
■ Patient's elimination pattern will return to normal.
■ Patient will regain and maintain fluid and electrolyte balance.
■ Patient's skin will remain intact.
■ Patient will discuss causative factors, preventive measures, and changed body image.
■ Patient will practice stress-reduction techniques daily.
■ Patient will demonstrate skill in using ostomy devices.
■ Patient will seek out persons with similar conditions or join a support group.

Suggested NOC outcomes

Bowel Elimination; Electrolyte & Acid/Base Balance; Fluid Balance; Hydration; Symptom Severity

Interventions and rationales

■ Monitor frequency and characteristics of stools; auscultate bowel sounds and record results at least every shift *to monitor treatment effectiveness.*
■ Tell patient to notify staff of each episode of diarrhea *to promote comfort and maintain communication.*
■ Give antidiarrheal medications, as ordered, *to improve body function, promote comfort, and balance body fluids, salts, and acid-base levels.* Monitor and report efficacy.
■ Monitor and record patient's intake and output, including number of stools. Report imbalances. *Monitoring ensures correct fluid replacement therapy.*
■ Check skin daily *to detect and prevent breakdown.* Report decreased skin turgor or excoriation of perianal area.
■ Weigh patient daily until diarrhea is controlled *to detect fluid loss or retention.*
■ Teach patient about:
– causative and preventive factors *to promote understanding of problem.*
– cleaning of perianal area, including use of powders and lotions, *to promote comfort and skin integrity.*
– dietary restriction *to control diarrhea,* such as a lactose-free diet, *which reduces residual waste and decreases intestinal irritation and spasms.*
■ Teach stress-reduction techniques, and help patient perform them daily by providing time, privacy, and needed equipment. *This temporarily relieves emotional distress.*
■ Prepare patient for surgery and provide preoperative instruction for abdominal surgery *to reassure patient and maintain trust.* Provide information about ileostomy or colostomy, if indicated, *to help patient understand procedure and avoid threat to health equilibrium.*
■ Demonstrate use of ostomy equipment *to encourage understanding and compliance.*
■ Provide support and assistance while patient develops skill in caring for stoma *to improve understanding and reduce anxiety.*

■ Encourage expression of feelings and concerns about impact of changed body image *to allow patient to pinpoint specific fears and promote self-knowledge and growth.*

■ Encourage use of support groups, such as ileostomy clubs, *to provide patient with additional support and health care resources.*

Suggested NIC interventions

Anxiety Reduction; Bowel Management; Diarrhea Management; Fluid/Electrolyte Management; Medication Management; Skin Care: Topical Treatments

Evaluations for expected outcomes

■ Patient doesn't experience diarrhea.
■ Patient's elimination pattern returns to normal.
■ Patient maintains fluid and electrolyte balance.
■ Patient's skin remains intact.
■ Patient explains cause of diarrhea and steps to prevent recurrence.
■ Patient demonstrates successful use of stress-reduction techniques.
■ Patient demonstrates successful use of ostomy devices.
■ Patient attends a support group for individuals with a similar condition.

Documentation

■ Patient's expressions of concern about diarrhea, causative factors, surgery, and adaptation to changes in body image
■ Observations of effects of medications, intake and output, weight, stools characteristics, skin condition, and stoma appearance
■ Evaluations for expected outcomes

Reference

Heitkemper, M., and Jarrett, M. "Overlapping Conditions in Women with Irritable Bowel Syndrome," *Urologic Nursing* 25(1):25-30, February 2005.

DIARRHEA

related to stress and anxiety

Definition

Interruption of normal bowel movements resulting in frequent, loose stools

Assessment

■ History of bowel disorder or surgery
■ GI status, including nausea and vomiting, usual bowel elimination habits, change in bowel elimination habits, stools characteristics (color, amount, size, and consistency), pain and discomfort, inspection of abdomen, auscultation of bowel sounds, palpation for masses and tenderness, and percussion for tympany and dullness

■ Nutritional status, including dietary intake, change from normal diet, appetite, current weight, and change from normal weight

■ Fluid and electrolyte status, including intake and output, urine specific gravity, skin turgor, mucous membranes, serum potassium and sodium levels, and blood urea nitrogen

■ Psychosocial status, including personality, stressors (such as finances, job, and marital discord), coping mechanisms, support systems (family members and others), and lifestyle

Defining characteristics
■ Abdominal pain and cramping
■ At least three loose, liquid stools per day
■ Hyperactive bowel sounds
■ Urgency
■ High stress levels and anxiety
■ Alcohol abuse
■ Toxins
■ Laxative abuse
■ Radiation
■ Tube feedings
■ Adverse effects of medications
■ Contaminants
■ Travel
■ Malabsorption
■ Infectious processes
■ Irritation
■ Parasites

Expected outcomes
■ Patient's diarrheal episodes will decline or disappear.
■ Patient will resume usual bowel pattern.
■ Patient will maintain weight and fluid and electrolyte balance.
■ Patient will keep skin clean and free from irritation or ulcerations.
■ Patient will explain causative factors and preventive measures.
■ Patient will discuss relationship of stress and anxiety to episodes of diarrhea.
■ Patient will state plans to use stress-reduction techniques (specify).
■ Patient will demonstrate ability to use at least one stress-reduction technique.

Suggested NOC outcomes
Bowel Continence; Hydration; Symptom Control

Interventions and rationales
■ Monitor and record frequency and characteristics of stools *to monitor treatment effectiveness.* Instruct patient to record diarrheal episodes and report them to staff *to promote comfort and maintain effective patient-staff communication.*

■ Administer antidiarrheal medications, as ordered, *to improve body function, promote comfort, and balance body fluids, salts, and acid-base levels.* Monitor and report medications' effectiveness.

■ Provide replacement fluids and electrolytes as prescribed. Maintain accurate records *to ensure balanced fluid intake and output.*

■ Monitor perianal skin for irritation and ulceration; treat according to established protocol *to promote comfort, skin integrity, and freedom from infection.*

■ Identify stressors and help patient solve problems *to provide more realistic approach to care.*

■ Encourage patient to ventilate stresses and anxiety; *release of pent-up emotions can temporarily relieve emotional distress.*

■ Teach patient to:

– use relaxation techniques *to reduce muscle tension and nervousness.*

– recognize and reduce intake of diarrhea-producing foods or substances (such as dairy products and fruit) *to reduce residual waste matter and decrease intestinal irritation.*

■ Spend at least 10 minutes with patient twice daily to discuss stress-reducing techniques; *this can help patient pinpoint specific fears.*

■ Encourage and assist patient to practice relaxation techniques *to reduce tension and promote self-knowledge and growth.*

Suggested NIC interventions

Anxiety Reduction; Coping Enhancement; Diarrhea Management; Emotional Support; Energy Management; Nutrition Management; Skin Surveillance; Weight Management

Evaluations for expected outcomes

■ Patient's diarrheal episodes decline by at least 50%.

■ Patient resumes usual bowel elimination pattern.

■ Patient maintains weight and fluid and electrolyte balance.

■ Patient doesn't experience skin breakdown, irritation, or ulcerations.

■ Patient identifies cause of diarrhea and discusses steps to prevent recurrence.

■ Patient explains how stress may contribute to diarrhea.

■ Patient explains plan to use stress-reduction techniques.

■ Patient describes and demonstrates at least one stress-reduction technique.

Documentation

■ Patient's expressions of concern and ability to manage diarrhea produced by stress and anxiety

■ Observations of effects of relaxation and stress-reduction techniques and dietary management on diarrhea

■ Patient's responses and skill level in carrying out stress-reduction techniques and dietary changes

■ Evaluations for expected outcomes

Reference

Fletcher, P.C., and Schneider, M.A. "Is There Any Food I Can Eat? Living with Inflammatory Bowel Disease and/or Irritable Bowel Syndrome," *Clinical Nurse Specialist* 20(5):241-47, September-October 2006.

Risk for compromised human
DIGNITY

Definition
At risk for perceived loss of respect and honor

Assessment
▪ Patient's perception of present health problem and problem-solving techniques used
▪ Patient health status, attitude toward and use of health care services, and beliefs, values, and attitudes about illness
▪ Family status, including family composition, responsibilities assumed in caring for family members (including patient), and ability of family to meet their physical, social, emotional, and economic needs
▪ Support systems, including family members, friends, and clergy
▪ Health history, including medical or mental illness, self-care abilities, and disabilities and deformities
▪ Legal status, including patient's authority to give consent for treatments or procedures
▪ Attitude of health care providers toward the patient
▪ Welfare and health care system and reliance on welfare for support

Risk factors
▪ Cultural incongruity
▪ Disclosure of confidential information
▪ Exposure of the body
▪ Inadequate participation in decision making
▪ Loss of control of body functions
▪ Perceived dehumanizing treatment
▪ Perceived humiliation
▪ Perceived intrusion by clinicians
▪ Perceived invasion of privacy
▪ Stigmatizing label
▪ Use of undefined medical terms

Expected outcomes
▪ Patient and family will express satisfaction with level of respect.
▪ Patient will identify a plan to reduce feelings of powerlessness and vulnerability and increase feelings of autonomy.
▪ Patient and family will develop and implement plans to protect privacy and confidentiality of patient.
▪ Patient and family will evaluate success of plans to protect patient privacy and confidentiality.
▪ Patient and family will report a reduction or elimination of compromised human dignity.

Suggested NOC outcomes

Client Satisfaction: Protection of Rights; Coping; Personal Autonomy; Self-Esteem

Interventions and rationales

■ Assess patient's satisfaction with the health care environment *to determine the extent of positive perception of the nursing staff's concern for the patient.*

■ Work with patient to develop a plan to increase autonomy *to promote feelings of control and independence in making life decisions.*

■ Work closely with patient and health professionals *to promote the positive perception of protection of a patient's legal and moral rights provided by nursing and other staff.*

■ Implement a program to promote patient dignity that involves staff, family, and community *to assist patient in coping to manage the stressors that tax his resources.*

■ Work with various health professionals, families, educators and students *to determine the extent of the problem of protecting human dignity in the delivery of health care.*

■ Encourage health professional groups and religious and social service organizations to feature guest speakers *to provide information on aspects of bioethics and human dignity in the care of patients.*

■ Provide education on the legal and ethical rights of patients to human dignity and have current information available at community and senior centers. *Access to information provides patients and their families with appropriate resources to seek help.*

■ Encourage patient and family to participate in support networks that allow them to discuss care giving and illness pressures and other issues related to the provision of human dignity. *This gives patient and family a chance to express their feelings openly and obtain support.*

■ Develop a referral list for patient and family that includes resources that promote human dignity, including charities, clinics, support groups, and senior centers *to promote family involvement in decision making and delivery and evaluation of care.*

Suggested NIC interventions

Body Image Enhancement; Presence; Self-Awareness Enhancement; Self-Esteem Enhancement

Evaluations for expected outcomes

■ Patient and family express satisfaction with level respect for the patient.

■ Patient and family articulate plan to reduce feelings of powerlessness and vulnerability and increase feelings of patient autonomy.

■ Patient and family develop and implement plan to protect patient privacy and confidentiality.

■ Patient and family report success of plan to protect patient privacy and confidentiality.

■ Patient and family report a reduction or elimination of compromised human dignity.

Documentation

- Patient and family perception of understanding of the need for human dignity
- Community resources that exist to promote human dignity
- Patient and family plans to promote human dignity
- Evaluations for expected outcomes

Reference

Coventry, M.L. "Care with Dignity: A Concept Analysis," *Journal of Gerontological Nursing* 32(5):42-48, May 2006.

Risk for
DISUSE SYNDROME

Definition

State of being at risk for deterioration of body systems as a result of prescribed or unavoidable musculoskeletal inactivity

Assessment

- Condition leading to prolonged inactivity or immobility
- Age
- Neurologic status, including mental status, level of consciousness (LOC), and sensory and motor ability
- Cardiovascular status, including blood pressure, heart rate, temperature, peripheral pulses, capillary refill, clotting profile, skin temperature and color, presence of edema, and chest pain or discomfort
- Respiratory status, including rate and rhythm, depth of inspiration, chest symmetry, use of accessory muscles, cough and sputum, percussion of lung fields, auscultation of breath sounds, chest pain or discomfort, and arterial blood gas (ABG) levels
- GI status, including inspection of abdomen, auscultation of bowel sounds, palpation for tenderness and masses, percussion for areas of dullness, usual bowel habits, change in bowel habits, laxative use, pain or discomfort, and characteristics of stools (color, size, amount, and consistency)
- Nutritional status, including dietary intake, appetite, current weight, and change from normal weight
- Fluid status, including intake and output, urine specific gravity, mucous membranes, serum electrolyte levels, blood urea nitrogen (BUN), and creatinine level
- Genitourinary status, including voiding pattern, characteristics of urine (color, odor, sediment, and amount), history of urinary problems or infections, palpation of bladder, pain or discomfort, use of urinary assistive device, urinalysis, and urine cultures
- Musculoskeletal status, including range of motion (ROM); muscle size, strength, and tone; coordination; and functional mobility scale:
0 = completely independent

1 = requires use of equipment or device
2 = requires help, supervision, or teaching from another person
3 = requires help from another person and equipment or device
4 = dependent; doesn't participate in activity
■ Integumentary status, including skin color, texture, turgor, temperature, elasticity, sensation, moisture, hygiene, and lesions
■ Psychosocial factors, including family support, coping style, current understanding of prescribed inactivity, willingness to cooperate with treatment, mood, behavior, motivation, and stressors (such as inactivity, finances, job, and marital discord)

Risk factors
■ Altered LOC
■ Mechanical immobilization
■ Paralysis
■ Prescribed immobilization
■ Severe pain

Expected outcomes
■ Patient won't display evidence of altered mental, sensory, or motor ability.
■ Patient won't have evidence of thrombus formation, venous stasis, or altered cardiovascular function.
■ Patient won't show evidence of decreased chest movement, cough stimulus, or depth of ventilation.
■ Patient won't show pooling of secretions or signs of infection.
■ Patient won't have evidence of constipation and will maintain normal bowel elimination patterns.
■ Patient will maintain adequate dietary intake, hydration, and weight.
■ Patient won't show evidence of urine retention, infection, or renal calculi.
■ Patient will maintain muscle strength and tone and joint ROM.
■ Patient won't show evidence of contractures.
■ Patient won't show evidence of skin breakdown.
■ Patient will maintain normal neurologic, cardiovascular, respiratory, GI, nutritional, genitourinary, musculoskeletal, and integumentary functioning during period of inactivity.
■ Patient will express feelings about prolonged inactivity.

Suggested NOC outcomes

Comfort Level; Coordinated Movement; Endurance; Immobility Consequences: Physiological; Immobility Consequences: Psycho-Cognitive; Mobility; Pain Level; Risk Control

Interventions and rationales
■ Provide frequent contact with staff, diversionary materials (magazines, radio, and television), and orienting mechanisms (clock and calendar). *Reality orientation fosters patient awareness of environment.*

■ Avoid positions that put prolonged pressure on body parts and compress blood vessels. Patient should change positions at least every 2 hours within prescribed limits. *These measures enhance circulation and help prevent tissue or skin breakdown.*

■ Inspect skin every shift and protect areas subject to irritation. Follow facility policy for prevention of pressure ulcers *to prevent or mitigate skin breakdown.*

■ Use pressure-reducing or pressure-equalizing equipment, as indicated or ordered (flotation pad, air pressure mattress, sheepskin pads, or special bed). *This helps prevent skin breakdown by relieving pressure.*

■ Apply antiembolism stockings; remove for 1 hour every 8 hours. *Stockings promote venous return to heart, prevent venous stasis, and decrease or prevent swelling of lower extremities.*

■ Monitor clotting profile. Administer and monitor anticoagulant therapy, if ordered, and monitor for signs and symptoms of bleeding *because anticoagulant therapy may cause hemorrhage.*

■ Monitor temperature, blood pressure, pulse, and respirations at least every 4 hours *to assess for indications of infection or other complications.*

■ Teach and monitor deep breathing, coughing, and use of incentive spirometer. Maintain regimen every 2 hours. *These measures help clear airways, expand lungs, and prevent respiratory complications.*

■ Encourage fluid intake of 2½ to 3½ qt (2.5 to 3.5 L) daily, unless contraindicated, *to maintain urine output and aid bowel elimination.* Weigh daily and monitor hydration status (serum electrolyte, BUN, creatinine levels, and intake and output).

■ Monitor breath sounds and respiratory rate, rhythm, and depth at least every 4 hours *to rule out respiratory complications.* Monitor ABG levels or pulse oximetry, if indicated, *to assess oxygenation, ventilation, and metabolic status.*

■ Suction airway, as needed and ordered, *to clear airway and stimulate cough reflex;* note secretion characteristics.

■ Establish baseline *to compare elimination patterns and habits.* Elevate head of bed and provide privacy *to allow comfortable elimination.*

■ Instruct patient to avoid straining during bowel movements; administer stool softeners, suppositories, or laxatives, as ordered, and monitor effectiveness. *Straining during bowel movements may be hazardous to patients with cardiovascular disorders and increased intracranial pressure.*

■ Provide small, frequent meals of favorite foods *to increase dietary intake.* Increase fiber content *to enhance bowel elimination.* Increase protein and vitamin C *to promote wound healing.* Limit calcium *to reduce risk of renal and bladder calculi.*

■ Monitor urine characteristics and patient's subjective complaints typical of urinary tract infection (UTI), such as burning, frequency, and urgency. Obtain urine cultures, as ordered. *These measures aid early detection of UTI.*

■ Identify level of functioning to provide baseline for future assessment, and encourage appropriate participation in care *to prevent complications of immobility and increase patient's feelings of self-esteem.*

■ Perform active or passive ROM exercises at least once per shift. Teach and monitor appropriate isotonic and isometric exercises. *These measures prevent joint contractures, muscle atrophy, and other complications of prolonged inactivity.*

■ Provide or help with daily hygiene; keep skin dry and lubricated *to prevent cracking and possible infection.*

■ Encourage patient and family to ventilate frustration. Allow open expression of all feelings associated with prolonged inactivity *to help patient and family cope with treatment.*

Suggested NIC interventions

Activity Therapy; Body Mechanics Promotion; Cognitive Stimulation; Energy Management; Exercise Promotion; Exercise Therapy: Ambulation; Fluid Management; Nutrition Management

Evaluations for expected outcomes

■ Patient doesn't exhibit altered LOC, mental status, sensory ability, or motor ability.

■ Patient doesn't exhibit evidence of thrombus formation, venous stasis, or altered cardiovascular function.

■ Patient shows no evidence of decreased chest movement, cough stimulus, or depth of ventilation.

■ Patient maintains clear breath sounds bilaterally and doesn't show evidence of fever, chills, cough, purulent sputum, pooled secretions, or rapid, shallow respirations.

■ Patient's bowel elimination pattern remains normal.

■ Patient maintains adequate dietary intake, daily fluid intake, and weight.

■ Patient doesn't exhibit evidence of distended bladder, fever, chills, frequent burning or painful urination, urgency, hematuria, flank pain, or urine retention.

■ Patient's muscle strength and tone and joint ROM remain stable.

■ Patient doesn't exhibit evidence of joint contractures.

■ Patient doesn't experience skin breakdown.

■ Patient maintains neurologic, cardiovascular, respiratory, GI, nutritional, genitourinary, musculoskeletal, and integumentary functioning.

■ Patient openly expresses frustration, anger, despondency, and other feelings associated with prolonged inactivity.

Documentation

■ Patient's concerns or perceptions of circumstances necessitating inactivity; willingness to accept and participate in treatment

■ Assessment of body systems at risk for deterioration

■ Interventions to provide preventive or supportive care and prescribed treatment

■ Treatment given to patient and patient's understanding and demonstrated ability to carry out instructions

■ Patient's response to nursing interventions

■ Evaluations for expected outcomes

Reference

Gillis, A., and MacDonald, B. "Deconditioning in the Hospitalized Elderly," *The Canadian Nurse* 101(6):16-20, June 2005.

Deficient
DIVERSIONAL ACTIVITY
related to lack of environmental stimulation

Definition
Decreased stimulation from (or interest or engagement in) recreational or leisure activities

Assessment
■ Physical status, including mobility and activity tolerance
■ Cardiovascular status, including heart rate and rhythm and blood pressure sitting and standing
■ Respiratory status, including respiratory rate and rhythm — resting and with activity
■ Neurologic status, including level of consciousness, orientation, mood, behavior, and memory
■ Psychosocial status, including family and friends, hobbies, and interests; favorite music, television, and reading material; and changes or adaptations needed to carry out activities

Defining characteristics
■ Usual hobbies can't be undertaken in hospital
■ Statements regarding feelings of boredom or wishing for something to do

Expected outcomes
■ Patient will express interest in using leisure time meaningfully.
■ Patient will express interest in activities that can be provided.
■ Patient will participate in chosen activity.
■ Patient will watch selected television program or listen to radio program or selected music daily.
■ Patient will report satisfaction with use of leisure time.
■ Patient or caregiver will modify environment to provide maximum stimulation, such as by hanging posters or cards and moving bed next to a window.

Suggested NOC outcomes
Leisure Participation; Motivation; Social Involvement

Interventions and rationales
■ Encourage discussion of previously enjoyed hobbies, interests, or skills *to direct planning of new activities.* Suggest performing an activity helpful to others or otherwise productive.
■ Obtain radio or television (if desired) and allow patient to select programs. Communicate patient's desires to coworkers. Turn on television set at _____ (time) to _____ (channel). *Selective television or radio use can help pass time.*

■ Ask volunteers (friends, family, or hospital volunteer) to read newspapers, books, or magazines to patient at specific times. *Personal contact helps alleviate boredom.*

■ Engage patient in conversation while carrying out routine care. Discuss patient's favorite topics as much as possible. *Conversation conveys caring and recognition of patient's worth.*

■ Provide supplies and set time to carry out hobby; for example, give crochet hook and yarn to patient daily at _____ (time). *Specifying time for activity indicates its value.*

■ Avoid scheduling procedures during patient's leisure time, *which is integral to quality of life.*

■ Provide talking books or records if available. *These provide low-effort sources of enjoyment for bedridden patient.*

■ Obtain an adapter for television *to provide captions for hearing-impaired patient.*

■ Encourage patient's family or caregiver to bring personal articles (posters, cards, and pictures) to help make environment more stimulating. *Patient may respond better to objects with personal meaning.*

■ Make referral to recreational, occupational, or physical therapist for consultation on adaptive equipment to carry out desired activity; arrange for therapy sessions. *Adaptive equipment allows patient to continue enjoying activities or may stimulate interest in new activities.*

■ Provide plants for patient to tend to. *Caring for live plants may stimulate interest.*

■ Change scenery when possible; for example, take patient outside in wheelchair *to help reduce boredom.*

■ Identify type of music patient prefers; seek help from family and hospital resources to provide selected music daily. *Music may relieve boredom and stimulate interest.*

Suggested NIC interventions
Activity Therapy; Animal-Assisted Therapy; Art Therapy; Energy Management; Recreation Therapy; Self-Responsibility Facilitation

Evaluations for expected outcomes
■ Patient expresses desire to participate in activities during leisure time.
■ Patient discusses recent activity with staff members, family, or others.
■ Patient engages in activity.
■ Patient discusses content of television or radio program.
■ Patient reports reduced feelings of boredom.
■ Patient (or caregiver) has modified environment, thereby increasing stimulation.

Documentation
■ Patient's expression of boredom, frustration, and desire to carry out leisure activity
■ Patient's interests and ability to carry out activity and necessary modifications required to accomplish activity

- Observations of patient's skill level and extent of participation in activity
- Patient's expression of satisfaction with use of unoccupied time
- Evaluations for expected outcomes

Reference
Wheeler, S.L., and Houston, K. "The Role of Diversional Activities in the General Medical Hospital Setting," *Holistic Nursing Practice* 19(2):87-89, March-April 2005.

Deficient
DIVERSIONAL ACTIVITY
related to long-term hospitalization or frequent, lengthy treatments

Definition
Decreased stimulation from (or interest or engagement in) recreational or leisure activities

Assessment
- Physical status, including mobility and activity tolerance
- Cardiovascular status, including heart rate and rhythm and blood pressure sitting and standing
- Respiratory status, including respiratory rate and rhythm
- Neurologic status, including level of consciousness, orientation, mood, behavior, and memory
- Psychosocial status, including family and friends, hobbies, and interests; favorite music, television, and reading material; and changes or adaptations needed to carry out activities

Defining characteristics
- Usual hobbies can't be undertaken in hospital
- Statement regarding feelings of boredom or wishing there was something to do

Expected outcomes
- Patient will express interest in using leisure time meaningfully.
- Patient will participate in chosen activity.
- Patient will state satisfaction with use of leisure time.
- Patient will express interest in activities provided.
- Patient will make decisions about timing and spacing of treatments.
- Patient will express satisfaction with established schedule of treatment routines.

Suggested NOC outcomes
Leisure Participation; Motivation; Social Involvement

Interventions and rationales

■ Schedule time daily for patient to pursue leisure activities; for example, have patient sit at desk daily to use paint-by-number kit. *Diversional activities improve patient's quality of life; scheduling activities indicates their value.*

■ Encourage family members to bring familiar objects. Provide space for favorite plants, cards, reading material, and hobby supplies. For bedridden patients, use ceiling for posters and other objects. *Maintaining personal contacts and involvement relieves boredom and stimulates interest.*

■ Encourage patient to express enjoyment of past hobbies, interests, or skills. *This conveys sense of worth and caring and helps patient think of new activities.*

■ Work with patient and family to find ways to carry out desired activities. Use imagination and creativity; for example, a former carpenter may adapt to carving small objects rather than building large ones. *Adaptive equipment helps patient pursue previous activities within new limits.*

■ Provide radio or television at patient's request *to help relieve boredom and increase enjoyment.*

■ Engage patient in conversation while carrying out procedures, if desired by patient. Discuss favorite topics. *Conversation during treatments reduces discomfort by diverting attention; it also increases patient's sense of self-worth.*

■ Encourage visitors to involve patient in favorite activities through discussion, reading, and attendance at programs, if appropriate, *to reduce boredom.*

■ Keep patient informed of current events through discussion, use of newspapers or books, or by watching television or listening to radio. *Keeping current helps reduce isolation of long-term hospitalization.*

■ Schedule treatments to allow adequate rest periods and pursuit of favorite activity; for example, no treatments between ＿＿＿ and ＿＿＿＿ (time), to allow time for watching television show. *This gives patient more control over environment.*

■ Streamline treatments as much as possible. Have all equipment ready before starting; thoroughly instruct new personnel in routine and plan schedule for minimal interruptions. *Efficiency conveys respect for value of patient's time.*

Suggested NIC interventions

Activity Therapy; Art Therapy; Energy Management; Exercise Promotion; Recreation Therapy; Self-Esteem Enhancement; Socialization Enhancement

Evaluations for expected outcomes

■ Patient expresses desire to participate in activity during leisure hours.
■ Patient engages in chosen activity.
■ Patient reports decreased feelings of boredom.
■ Patient discusses recent activity with staff members, family, or others.
■ Patient makes decisions about timing and spacing of treatments.
■ Patient expresses a positive attitude about treatment schedule.

Documentation

■ Patient's expressions of boredom, desire to carry out leisure activity, and frustration at being restricted

- Patient's interests, skills, and abilities to carry out activity
- Observations of patient's skill level and extent of participation in activity
- Patient's expression of satisfaction with use of non-treatment-related time
- Evaluations for expected outcomes

Reference
Wheeler, S.L., and Houston, K. "The Role of Diversional Activities in the General Medical Hospital Setting," *Holistic Nursing Practice* 19(2):87-89, March-April 2005.

ENERGY FIELD DISTURBANCE
related to blocking of energy fields

Definition
Disruption of the flow of energy surrounding a person's being that results in disharmony of the body, mind, or spirit

Assessment
- Psychological status, including anxiety, fatigue, depression, somatic complaints, and recent lifestyle changes (death of loved one, conflict in a relationship, or loss of job)
- Health status, including presence of disorder that's life-threatening or requires surgery
- Sensory status, including pain and disorders that may affect senses
- Spiritual status, including religious beliefs and affiliation; available support systems; and feelings of helplessness, hopelessness, anger, and withdrawal
- Caregiver's readiness to provide therapeutic healing, including education and training in therapeutic touch or similar treatment technique

Defining characteristics
Perceptions of changes in patterns of energy flow, such as:
- Movement (wave, spike, tingling, dense, flowing, sounds [tones, words])
- Temperature change (warmth, coolness)
- Visual changes (image, color)
- Disruption of field (deficit, hole, spike, bulge, obstruction, congestion, diminished flow in energy field)

Expected outcomes
- Patient will feel increasingly relaxed as demonstrated by slower and deeper breathing, skin flushing in treated area, audible sighing, or verbal reports of feeling more relaxed.
- Patient will visualize images that relax him.
- Patient will report feeling less tension or pain.
- Patient will use self-healing techniques, such as meditation, guided imagery, yoga, and prayer.

■ Patient will express increased sense of well-being.

Suggested NOC outcomes

Comfort Level; Health Beliefs; Personal Health Status; Personal Well-Being; Spiritual Health

Interventions and rationales

■ Implement measures to promote therapeutic healing. Place your hands 4″ to 6″ (10 to 15 cm) above patient's body. Pass your hands over entire skin surface. *This technique helps you become attuned to patient's energy field, which is the flow of energy that surrounds a person's being.* With experience and training in therapeutic touch or similar treatment, you can identify sensory cues to energy field disturbances, such as heat, cold, tingling, and an electric sensation.

■ Try to gain patient's cooperation as you perform healing techniques, such as therapeutic touch, *to enhance effectiveness of healing techniques and foster participation in spiritual aspects of care.*

■ Continue to treat patient using therapeutic healing techniques. *One treatment rarely restores a full sense of inner well-being.*

■ Suggest that patient use self-healing techniques, such as meditation, guided imagery, yoga, and prayer, *to encourage patient to participate in his care.*

Suggested NIC interventions

Communication Enhancement; Energy Management; Environmental Management; Pain Management; Spiritual Support

Evaluations for expected outcomes

■ Patient shows evidence of relaxation, such as slower and deeper breathing, flushing in treated area, audible sighing, or verbal reports of feeling more relaxed.

■ Patient reports experiencing relaxing visual images.

■ Patient reports reduction in tension or pain.

■ Patient uses self-healing techniques, such as meditation, guided imagery, yoga, and prayer.

■ Patient reports an increased sense of well-being.

Documentation

■ Summary of patient's psychosocial status

■ Patient's progress in learning techniques that enhance relaxation

■ Patient's perceptions of benefits of healing and self-healing techniques

■ Evaluations for expected outcomes

References

Burden, B., et al. "The Increasing Use of Reiki as a Complementary Therapy in Specialist Palliative Care," *International Journal of Palliative Care* 11(5):248-53, May 2005.

Robb, W.J. "Self-healing: A Concept Analysis," *Nursing Forum* 41(2):60-77, April-June 2006.

Impaired
ENVIRONMENTAL INTERPRETATION SYNDROME
related to dementia

Definition
Consistent lack of orientation to time, place, person, or circumstances that lasts more than 3 to 6 months and necessitates placement in a protective environment

Assessment
■ Cultural status, including age, sex, level of education, occupation, living arrangements, nationality, race, ethnic group, religion, and personal habits
■ Family status, including marital status, family composition, and family members' ability to meet patient's needs
■ Cardiovascular status, including vital signs; skin color (especially lips and nails); chest pain, fatigue on exertion, dyspnea, and dizziness; and electrocardiography or echocardiography results
■ Neurologic status, including level of consciousness (LOC), motor activity, thought and speech, mood and affect, memory, attention span, judgment, orientation, comprehension, and perception; cerebellar function, cranial nerve function, sensation, reflexes, and pupillary response; and medications
■ Psychological status, including changes in appearance, appetite, energy level, motivation, personal hygiene, self-image, self-esteem, sleep patterns, or LOC; alcohol and drug use; and life changes, such as recent divorce, separation, job loss, death of a loved one, or relocation
■ Psychiatric history, including age at onset of illness, severity of symptoms, impact on functioning, and type of treatment and response
■ Self-care status, including functional ability (muscle tone, size, and strength; range of motion; and coordination); daily activities (dressing, grooming, bathing, toileting, and hygiene); and use of adaptive equipment
■ Social status, including interaction with others and ability to function in social or occupational roles
■ Sensory status, including presence of vision or hearing deficits and use of hearing aid or eyeglasses

Defining characteristics
■ Consistent disorientation to environment
■ Chronic confusion
■ Inability to reason, concentrate, or follow simple directions or instructions
■ Loss of occupation or social function resulting from memory decline
■ Slow response to questions

Expected outcomes
■ Staff members will communicate clear, concise goals for coping with disorientation to patient and caregiver.
■ Patient will acknowledge and respond to efforts by others to establish communication.

■ Patient will remain oriented to environment to fullest extent possible.

■ Family members will participate in efforts to help patient cope with disorientation.

■ Patient will remain free from injury.

■ Caregiver will describe measures for helping patient cope with disorientation.

■ Caregiver will demonstrate reorientation techniques.

■ Caregiver will describe ways to ensure that home is made safe for patient.

■ Caregiver will describe plans to continue to help patient cope with disorientation in least restrictive way possible.

■ Caregiver, in cooperation with patient, will identify and contact appropriate support services.

Suggested NOC outcomes

Cognitive Orientation; Concentration; Fall Prevention Behavior; Memory; Safe Home Environment

Interventions and rationales

■ Spend time with patient and caregiver *to establish a trusting relationship.*

■ Be clear, concise, and direct in establishing goals and skills for coping with disorientation *so patient and caregiver can understand them.*

■ Consider performing the following interventions *to effect successful communication:*

– Assess patient's sight and hearing, and assist him with glasses or a hearing aid, as necessary.

– Minimize distractions by turning off radio or television.

– When speaking to patient, face him, maintain eye contact, and smile.

– Speak slowly in clear, low tones, using simple, direct language. Repeat your remarks, as needed.

– Be aware that patient may be especially sensitive to your unspoken feelings about him.

These measures will help foster trust and communication with patient.

■ Orient patient to reality, as needed, *to improve his awareness of himself and his environment:*

– Call him by name.

– Tell him your name.

– Provide background information (place, time, and date) frequently throughout the day. Reinforce this information verbally and by also using a reality orientation board.

– Orient him to his environment.

■ Place patient's photograph or name on room door *to aid memory and help him find his room.*

■ Keep items in same places. *A consistent, stable environment reduces confusion, decreases frustration, and aids successful completion of activities of daily living.*

■ Ask family members to provide patient with photographs (labeled with name and relationship on back) and favorite belongings *to spark his memory and promote a sense of security.*

■ Have someone accompany a patient who wanders *to prevent patient injury.*

■ Place patient in a room close to nursing station, clear area of as many hazards as possible, make sure he wears an identification bracelet, and provide hospital security with a recent photograph of him *to prevent patient from getting lost or being injured.*

■ Encourage patient to interact with others *to increase social activity and ease feelings of isolation that may result from disorientation.*

■ Provide reassurance and praise patient for completing simple tasks *to increase patient's self-esteem.*

■ Help patient and caregiver identify feelings associated with disorientation *to help improve their ability to cope.*

■ Work with patient and caregiver to establish goals for coping with disorientation in least restrictive way *to maximize independence and reduce feelings of loneliness.*

■ Demonstrate reorientation techniques to caregiver and provide time for supervised return demonstrations *to prepare caregiver to cope with patient when he returns home.*

■ Instruct caregiver on how to maintain a safe home environment for patient. *Patient may be unable to consider his own safety needs.*

■ Refer patient and caregiver to appropriate social service and mental health care agencies *to ensure continued care.*

Suggested NIC interventions

Anxiety Reduction; Behavior Management; Dementia Management; Emotional Support; Energy Management; Mood Management; Reality Orientation; Sleep Enhancement

Evaluations for expected outcomes

■ Staff members communicate clear, concise goals for coping with disorientation to patient and caregiver.

■ Patient acknowledges and responds to efforts by others to establish communication.

■ Patient remains oriented to environment to fullest extent possible.

■ Family members participate in efforts to help patient cope with disorientation.

■ Patient remains free from injury.

■ Caregiver describes measures for helping patient cope with disorientation.

■ Caregiver demonstrates reorientation techniques.

■ Caregiver describes measures to improve safety of home for patient.

■ Caregiver describes plans to help patient cope with disorientation in least restrictive way possible.

■ Caregiver, in cooperation with patient, identifies and contacts appropriate support services.

Documentation

■ Assessment of patient's level of orientation

■ Assessment of patient's response to various interventions

■ Instructions to caregiver on how to reorient patient and how to maintain a safe home environment

■ Referrals to community agencies
■ Evaluations for expected outcomes

Reference
Patton, D. "Reality Orientation: Its Use and Effectiveness Within Older Person Mental Health Care," *Journal of Clinical Nursing* 15(11):1440-49, November 2006.

Interrupted
FAMILY PROCESSES
related to power shift of family members

Definition
Change in family relationships or functioning

Assessment
■ Family status, including normal patterns of interaction among family members, family members' and patient's understanding of present situation, and support systems available (financial, social, and spiritual)
■ Family's past response to crises, including coping patterns and communication patterns to express anger, affection, and confrontation

Defining characteristics
Changes in the following:
■ assigned tasks and effectiveness in completing those tasks
■ availability for affective responsiveness and intimacy
■ availability for emotional support
■ communications patterns
■ expressions of conflict with or isolation from community resources
■ expressions of conflict within family
■ mutual support
■ participation in problem solving and decision making
■ patterns and rituals
■ power alliances
■ satisfaction with family
■ somatic complaints
■ stress-reduction behaviors.

Expected outcomes
■ Family members will agree on who's the primary decision maker.
■ Family members will develop adaptive responses by assuming duties carried out by ill member; for example, meal preparation, transportation, shopping, laundry, cleaning, and providing emotional support to other family members.
■ Family members will identify support systems to assist them and will participate in mobilizing those systems.

■ Family members will contact a community agency or support group for continued assistance (depending on type, severity, and prognosis of illness); for example, American Cancer Society, American Lung Association, Arthritis Foundation, Hospice, Myasthenia Gravis Foundation, Multiple Sclerosis Society, or National Kidney Foundation.

■ Family members will share feelings about illness.

Suggested NOC outcomes

Coping; Decision Making; Family Coping; Family Environment: Internal; Family Functioning; Family Normalization; Family Resiliency; Family Social Climate; Social Involvement

Interventions and rationales

■ Identify individual assuming role as head of family *to establish family hierarchy and functional ability.*

■ Provide head of family with information necessary for decision making, such as updated information on patient's condition. *This avoids potential for misinterpretation and places responsibility for communication within family unit.*

■ Help head of family decide which support systems need to be mobilized and used. *This allows opportunity to evaluate head of family's management ability and family's problem-solving ability.*

■ Provide emotional support to head of family regarding altered role and additional responsibilities. *This encourages family member to express feelings, ask questions, seek help, and make decisions.*

■ Expedite communication within family to allow members to express their feelings about present situation. *This encourages supportive behavior to meet reciprocal needs in a crisis.*

■ Arrange for and participate in family conferences, if appropriate.

– Whenever possible, ensure privacy to family members for their discussions or conferences.

– Include patient in family conferences and family interaction as often as possible.

These measures allow you to help family identify and work toward mutual goals and facilitate effective family coping.

■ Make referrals to social services or community agencies, as appropriate, *to provide family with access to additional coping resources.*

Suggested NIC interventions

Coping Enhancement; Counseling; Family Mobilization; Family Process Maintenance; Family Support; Family Therapy; Normalization Promotion; Spiritual Support; Support System Enhancement

Evaluations for expected outcomes

■ Family members identify family member to be primary decision maker, serving as head of family.

■ Family members assume responsibilities formerly carried out by ill member.

■ Family members identify and contact available resources, as needed.

■ Family members contact community support groups and associations and attend at least two meetings.
■ Family members openly share feelings about present situation.

Documentation
■ Observations of family's reactions to situation
■ Interventions to assist family and family's responses to those interventions
■ Referrals to outside agencies
■ Evaluations for expected outcomes

Reference
Badger, J.M. "Factors that Enable or Complicate End-of-Life Transitions in Critical Care," *American Journal of Critical Care* 14(6):513-21, November 2005.

FATIGUE

related to poor physical condition

Definition
Overwhelming sustained sense of exhaustion and decreased capacity for physical and mental work, regardless of adequate sleep

Assessment
■ History of underlying disease process
■ Respiratory status, including dyspnea on exertion and respiratory rate and depth
■ Cardiovascular status, including skin color, temperature, turgor, and blood pressure
■ Age
■ Sleep pattern, including hours slept at night and amount of time awake before becoming tired
■ Nutritional status, including appetite, dietary intake, current weight, and change from normal weight
■ Neurologic status, including headaches
■ Activity status, including type and duration of exercise, occupation, and use of leisure time
■ Psychosocial status, including personality stressors (finances, job, or marital discord), coping mechanisms, support systems (family members and others), and lifestyle
■ Menstrual history, including length of menses and amount of menstrual flow

Defining characteristics
■ Decreased libido
■ Decreased performance
■ Disinterest in surroundings
■ Drowsiness

- Failure of sleep to restore energy
- Lack of energy
- Guilt for not meeting responsibilities
- Inability to maintain usual routines
- Impaired concentration
- Increased need for rest
- Increased physical complaints
- Lethargy or listlessness
- Perceived need for more energy for routine tasks
- Verbalization of overwhelming lack of energy

Expected outcomes

- Patient will identify measures to prevent or modify fatigue.
- Patient will incorporate as part of daily activities those measures necessary to modify fatigue.
- Patient will explain relationship of fatigue to disease process and activity level.
- Patient will verbally express increased energy.
- Patient will articulate plan to resolve fatigue problems.
- Patient will employ measures to prevent and modify fatigue.

Suggested NOC outcomes

Activity Tolerance; Comfort Level; Endurance; Energy Conservation; Nutritional Status: Energy; Psychomotor Energy; Pain Level; Personal Health Status; Personal Well-Being

Interventions and rationales

- Prevent unnecessary fatigue; for example, avoid scheduling two energy-draining procedures on same day. *Using energy-conserving techniques avoids overexertion and potential for exhaustion.*
- Conserve energy through rest, planning, and setting priorities *to prevent or alleviate fatigue.*
- Alternate activities with periods of rest. Encourage activities that can be completed in short periods or divided into several segments; for example, read one chapter of a book at a time. *Scheduling regular rest periods helps decrease fatigue and increase stamina.*
- Discuss effect of fatigue on daily living and personal goals. Explore with patient relationship between fatigue and disease process *to help increase patient compliance with schedule for activity and rest.*
- Reduce demands placed on patient; for example, ask one family member to call at specified times and relay messages to friends and other family members *to reduce physical and emotional stress.*
- Structure patient's environment; for example, set up daily schedule based on patient's needs and desires. *This encourages compliance with treatment regimen.*
- Encourage patient to eat foods rich in iron and minerals, unless contraindicated. *This helps avoid anemia and demineralization.*
- Postpone eating when patient is fatigued *to avoid aggravating condition.*
- Provide small, frequent feedings *to conserve patient's energy and encourage increased dietary intake.*

■ Establish a regular sleeping pattern. *Getting 8 to 10 hours of sleep nightly helps reduce fatigue.*
■ Avoid highly emotional situations, *which aggravate patient's fatigue.*
■ Encourage patient to explore feelings and emotions with a supportive counselor, clergy, or other professional *to help cope with illness.*

Suggested NIC interventions
Activity Therapy; Coping Enhancement; Energy Management; Exercise Promotion; Nutrition Management; Mood Management; Mutual Goal Setting; Sleep Enhancement

Evaluations for expected outcomes
■ Patient describes at least three measures to prevent or modify fatigue.
■ Patient incorporates at least three measures to modify fatigue into daily routine.
■ Patient discusses relationship of fatigue to disease process and activity level; for example, in heart disease, fatigue is a sign that the heart can't meet increased oxygen demands.
■ Patient states that his fatigue level is reduced.
■ Patient describes plan to resolve fatigue problems, including both physiologic and emotional remedies.
■ Patient follows measures to prevent and modify fatigue.

Documentation
■ Patient's ability to describe fatigue and its relationship to disease process and condition
■ Patient's ability to decrease fatigue by using various effective methods
■ Patient's level of activity in relation to fatigue
■ Patient's dietary intake
■ Evaluations for expected outcomes

Reference
Barsevick, A.M., et al. "Cancer-Related Fatigue, Depressive Symptoms, and Functional Status: A Mediation Model," *Nursing Research* 55(5):366-72, September-October 2006.

FEAR
related to separation from support system

Definition
Response to a perceived threat that is consciously recognized as a danger

Assessment
■ History of experience with illness, hospitalization, and surgery
■ Availability of support systems, including family members, friends, and clergy

- Financial resources
- History of coping with fear
- Physiologic manifestations of fear, including changes in pulse rate, respiratory rate, blood pressure, skin temperature, and quality and pitch of voice
- Psychological manifestations of fear, including changes in behavior, appetite, and sleep pattern

Defining characteristics

- Aggression
- Decreased self-assurance
- Feelings of alarm, apprehension, dread, horror, panic, and terror
- Focus of attention on "something out there"
- Identification of and concentration on object of fear
- Impulsive behavior
- Increased alertness
- Increased heart rate, anorexia, nausea, vomiting, diarrhea, muscle tightness, fatigue, increased respiratory rate, shortness of breath, pallor, increased perspiration, increased blood pressure
- Increased tension, worrying, and wariness
- Jitteriness
- Wide-eyed appearance
- Withdrawal

Expected outcomes

- Patient will identify source of fear.
- Patient will communicate feelings about separation from support systems.
- Patient will communicate feelings of comfort or satisfaction.
- Patient will use situational supports to reduce fear.
- Patient will integrate into daily behavior at least one fear-reducing coping mechanism, such as asking questions about treatment progress or making decisions about care.

Suggested NOC outcomes

Anxiety Control; Comfort Level; Coping; Fear Control; Pain Level

Interventions and rationales

- Ask patient to identify source of fear; try to assess patient's understanding of situation. *Patient's perceptions may be erroneously based.*
- If patient has no visitors, spend an extra 15 minutes each shift in casual conversation; encourage other staff members to stop for brief visits *to help patient cope with separation.*
- Help patient maintain daily contact with family:
- Arrange for telephone calls.
- Help write letters.
- Promptly convey messages to patient from family and vice-versa.
- Encourage patient to have pictures of loved ones.
- Provide privacy for visits; take patient to day room or other quiet area.
These measures help patient reestablish and maintain social relationships.

■ Involve patient in planning care and setting goals *to renew confidence and give sense of control in a crisis situation.*

■ Instruct patient in relaxation techniques, such as imagery and progressive muscle relaxation, *to reduce symptoms of sympathetic stimulation.*

■ Administer antianxiety medications, as ordered, and monitor effectiveness. *Drug therapy may be needed to manage high anxiety levels or panic disorders.*

■ Answer questions and help patient understand care *to reduce anxiety and correct misconceptions.*

■ When feasible and where policies permit, relax visiting restrictions *to reduce patient's sense of isolation.*

■ Allow a close family member or friend to participate in care *to provide an additional source of support.*

■ Support family and friends in their efforts to understand patient's fear and to respond accordingly *to help them understand that patient's emotions are appropriate in context of situation.*

Suggested NIC interventions

Active Listening; Anxiety Reduction; Cognitive Restructuring; Counseling; Coping Enhancement; Decision-Making Support; Security Enhancement; Presence; Support Group

Evaluations for expected outcomes

■ Patient states causes of fear.

■ Patient expresses distress caused by separation from support systems.

■ Patient reports feeling less fearful.

■ Patient reaches out to others for support through phone calls, letters, or other means.

■ Patient demonstrates use of at least one coping mechanism daily to reduce fear.

Documentation

■ Patient's expressions of concern about illness, hospitalization, and separation from support system, and overt expressions of fear

■ Observations of physiologic and behavioral manifestations of patient's fear

■ Interventions performed to allay patient's fears and encourage healthy coping mechanisms

■ Patient's response to interventions

■ Evaluations for expected outcomes

Reference

Cookman, C. "Attachment in Older Adulthood: Concept Clarification," *Journal of Advanced Nursing* 50(5):528-35, June 2005.

FEAR

related to unfamiliarity with environmental experience

Definition
Response to a perceived threat that's consciously recognized as a danger

Assessment
- History of experience with illness, hospitalization, and surgery
- Availability of support systems, including family members, friends, and clergy
- Financial resources
- History of coping with fear
- Neurologic status, including mental status, orientation, and sensory status
- Physiologic manifestations of fear, including changes in pulse rate, blood pressure, respiratory rate, skin temperature, and quality and pitch of voice
- Psychological manifestations of fear, including changes in behavior, appetite, and sleep pattern

Defining characteristics
- Aggression
- Decreased self-assurance
- Feelings of alarm, apprehension, dread, horror, panic, and terror
- Focus of attention on "something out there"
- Identification of and concentration on object of fear
- Impulsive behavior
- Increased alertness
- Increased heart rate and blood pressure, increased respiratory rate, shortness of breath, pallor, increased perspiration, anorexia, nausea, vomiting, diarrhea, muscle tightness, and fatigue
- Increased tension, worrying, and wariness
- Jitteriness
- Wide-eyed appearance
- Withdrawal

Expected outcomes
- Patient will identify source of fear.
- Patient will state understanding of procedures.
- Patient will verbally express comfort with surroundings.
- Patient will manifest no physical signs or symptoms of fear.
- Patient will use available support systems to assist in coping with fear.
- Patient will integrate into daily behavior at least one fear-reducing coping mechanism, such as asking questions about treatment progress and making decisions about care.

Suggested NOC outcomes
Anxiety Self-Control; Fear Control; Pain Level; Comfort Level

Interventions and rationales

- Encourage patient to identify source of fear. *Patient's perceptions may be erroneously based.*
- Explain all treatments and procedures, answering any questions patient might have. Present information at patient's level of understanding or acceptance *to reduce patient's anxiety and enhance cooperation.*
- Orient patient to surroundings. Make any adaptations to compensate for sensory deficits. *This enhances patient's ability to orient to time, place, person, and events.*
- Assign same nurse to care for patient whenever possible *to provide consistency of care, enhance trust, and reduce threat commonly associated with multiple caregivers.*
- Spend time with patient each shift *to allow time for expression of feelings, provide emotional outlet, and promote feeling of acceptance.*
- Involve patient in planning care and setting goals *to give patient some control over situation and restore sense of self-esteem.*
- Orient family to patient's specific needs, allowing family members to participate in giving care. *This helps them provide effective support.*
- Request that family bring pictures and other small, personal objects to patient. *This helps alleviate patient's altered mental state by familiarizing the environment.*
- Arrange for family member or friend to stay with patient *to help patient cope with fears.*
- If a language barrier is the source of fear, use family and other resources in hospital (such as an interpreter) *to help reduce patient's fear and aid effective communication.*

Suggested NIC interventions

Active Listening; Anticipatory Guidance; Coping Enhancement; Counseling; Support System Enhancement

Evaluations for expected outcomes

- Patient identifies causes of fear.
- Patient demonstrates comprehension of procedures.
- Patient reports feeling comfortable in hospital.
- Patient's blood pressure, pulse rate, and respirations remain within set limits.
- Patient requests assistance from support systems to diminish fears (specify).
- Patient uses at least one effective fear-reducing behavior each day.

Documentation

- Patient's verbal expressions of fear
- Behavioral and physiologic manifestations of fear
- Interventions performed to reduce patient's fear
- Patient's response to interventions
- Family's involvement in patient care
- Patient's response to family involvement
- Evaluations for expected outcomes

Reference
Cuningham, C. "Understanding Challenging Behavior in Patients with Dementia," *Nursing Standard* 20(47):42-45, August 2006.

Deficient
FLUID VOLUME
related to active fluid volume loss

Definition
Decreased intravascular, interstitial, or intracellular fluid; water loss alone without change in sodium

Assessment
- History of fluid loss, including vomiting, nasogastric tube drainage, diarrhea, or hemorrhage
- Pulse, blood pressure, respirations, and temperature
- Fluid and electrolyte status, including weight, intake and output, urine specific gravity, skin turgor, and mucous membranes
- Laboratory studies, including serum electrolyte, blood urea nitrogen, hemoglobin levels, hematocrit, and stool cultures

Defining characteristics
- Changes in mental status
- Decreased pulse volume and pressure
- Decreased urine output
- Decreased venous filling
- Dry skin and mucous membranes
- Increased body temperature
- Increased hematocrit
- Increased pulse rate
- Increased urine concentration
- Low blood pressure
- Poor turgor of skin or tongue
- Sudden weight loss
- Thirst
- Weakness

Expected outcomes
- Patient's vital signs will remain stable.
- Patient's skin color will be normal.
- Patient's electrolyte levels will stay within normal range.
- Patient's fluid volume will remain adequate.
- Patient will produce adequate urine volume.
- Patient will have normal skin turgor and moist mucous membranes.
- Patient's urine specific gravity will remain between 1.005 and 1.010.

- Patient's fluid and blood volume will return to normal.
- Patient will express understanding of factors that caused fluid volume deficit.

Suggested NOC outcomes

Electrolyte & Acid-Base Balance; Fluid Balance; Hydration; Nausea & Vomiting Severity; Nutritional Status: Appetite; Nutritional Status: Food & Fluid Intake; Urinary Elimination

Interventions and rationales

- Monitor and record vital signs every 2 hours or as often as necessary until stable. Then monitor and record vital signs every 4 hours. *Tachycardia, dyspnea, or hypotension may indicate fluid volume deficit or electrolyte imbalance.*
- Cover patient lightly. Avoid overheating *to prevent vasodilation, blood pooling in extremities, and reduced circulating blood volume.*
- Measure intake and output every 1 to 4 hours. Record and report significant changes. Include urine, stools, vomitus, wound drainage, nasogastric drainage, chest tube drainage, and any other output. *Low urine output and high specific gravity indicate hypovolemia.*
- Administer fluids, blood or blood products, or plasma expanders *to replace fluids and whole blood loss and facilitate fluid movement into intravascular space.* Monitor and record effectiveness and any adverse effects.
- Weigh patient daily at same time to give more accurate and consistent data. *Weight is a good indicator of fluid status.*
- Assess skin turgor and oral mucous membranes every 8 hours *to check for dehydration.* Give meticulous mouth care every 4 hours *to avoid dehydrating mucous membranes.*
- Test urine specific gravity every 8 hours. *Elevated specific gravity may indicate dehydration.*
- Don't allow patient to sit or stand up quickly as long as circulation is compromised *to avoid orthostatic hypotension and possible syncope.*
- Measure abdominal girth every shift *to monitor for ascites and third-space shift.* Report changes.
- Administer and monitor medications *to prevent further fluid loss.*
- Explain reasons for fluid loss, and teach patient how to monitor fluid volume; for example, by recording daily weight and measuring intake and output. *This encourages patient involvement in personal care.*

Suggested NIC interventions

Acid-Base Management; Electrolyte Monitoring; Fluid Management; Hypovolemia Management; Nutrition Management; Swallowing Therapy; Vital Signs Monitoring

Evaluations for expected outcomes

- Patient's pulse rate, blood pressure, respirations, and body temperature remain within set limits.
- Patient's skin color remains normal.
- Patient's electrolyte values remain within normal range.

- Patient's fluid volume remains adequate.
- Patient's urine output remains at volume established for patient.
- Patient's skin turgor and mucous membranes remain normal.
- Patient's specific gravity remains between 1.005 and 1.010, unless specified otherwise.
- Patient's fluid volume returns to normal and remains normal, as evidenced by stable vital signs.
- Patient and caregiver demonstrate understanding of factors precipitating fluid volume deficit.

Documentation
- Patient's complaints of thirst, weakness, dizziness, and palpitations
- Observations of physical findings
- Intake and output (amount and type)
- Patient's weight and abdominal girth
- Interventions performed to control fluid loss
- Patient's response to interventions
- Evaluations for expected outcomes

Reference
Kelley, D.M. "Hypovolemic Shock: An Overview," *Critical Care Nursing Quarterly* 28(1):2-19, January-March 2005.

Excess
FLUID VOLUME
related to compromised regulatory mechanisms

Definition
Increased isotonic fluid retention

Assessment
- Neurologic status, including level of consciousness, orientation, and mental status
- Cardiovascular status, including skin color, temperature, and turgor; central venous pressure and pulmonary artery pressure (if available); heart rate and rhythm; blood pressure; heart sounds, electrocardiogram (ECG) results; and hemoglobin (Hb) level and hematocrit (HCT)
- Respiratory status, including rate, depth, and pattern of respiration; breath sounds; chest X-ray; and arterial blood gas levels
- Renal status, including intake and output, urine specific gravity, weight, serum electrolyte and serum and urine osmolality levels, and blood urea nitrogen (BUN), creatinine, and serum protein levels
- Endocrine status, including general appearance, size and body proportions, skin color and condition, and distribution of body hair

Defining characteristics

- Altered mental status
- Altered respiratory pattern
- Anasarca
- Azotemia
- Changes in blood pressure, pulmonary artery pressure, urine specific gravity, and electrolyte levels
- Crackles
- Decreased Hb level and HCT
- Dyspnea
- Edema
- Increased central venous pressure
- Intake greater than output
- Jugular vein distention
- Oliguria
- Orthopnea
- Pleural effusion
- Positive hepatojugular reflex
- Pulmonary congestion
- Rapid weight gain
- Restlessness and anxiety
- S_3 heart sound

Expected outcomes

- Patient's blood pressure will remain no lower than _____ mm Hg and no higher than _____ mm Hg.
- Patient will demonstrate no signs of hyperkalemia on ECG.
- Patient will maintain fluid intake of no more than ___ ml and output of no less than _____ ml.
- Patient's urine specific gravity will remain between _____ and _____.
- Patient's HCT will stay above _____ %.
- Patient's BUN, creatinine, sodium, and potassium levels will stay within acceptable range.
- Patient will plan 24-hour fluid intake, as prescribed.
- Patient will tolerate restricted intake with no physical or emotional discomfort.
- Patient's skin will remain intact and infection-free.
- Patient will assist with activities of daily living (ADLs), without undue fatigue.
- Patient will ambulate and carry out ADLs safely and comfortably.
- Patient will demonstrate skill in selecting permitted foods, such as those low in sodium and potassium.
- Patient will describe signs and symptoms that require medical treatment.

Suggested NOC outcomes

Electrolyte & Acid-Base Balance; Fluid Balance; Fluid Overload Severity; Hydration; Kidney Function; Knowledge: Disease Process; Knowledge: Treatment Regimen; Vital Signs

Interventions and rationales

■ Monitor blood pressure, pulse rate, heart rhythm, temperature, and breath sounds at least every 4 hours; record and report changes. *Changed parameters may indicate altered fluid or electrolyte status.*

■ Carefully monitor intake, output, and urine specific gravity at least every 4 hours. *Intake greater than output and elevated specific gravity may indicate fluid retention or overload.*

■ Monitor BUN, creatinine, electrolyte, and Hb levels and HCT. *BUN and creatinine levels indicate renal function; electrolyte and Hb levels and HCT help indicate fluid status.*

■ Weigh patient daily before breakfast, as ordered, *to provide consistent readings.* Check for signs of fluid retention, such as dependent edema, sacral edema, and ascites.

■ Give fluids, as ordered. Monitor I.V. flow rate carefully *because excess I.V. fluids can worsen patient's condition.*

■ If oral fluids are allowed, help patient make a schedule for fluid intake. *Patient involvement encourages compliance.*

■ Explain reasons for fluid and dietary restrictions *to enhance patient's understanding and compliance.*

■ Learn patient's food preferences and plan accordingly within prescribed dietary restrictions *to enhance compliance.*

■ Provide mouth care every 4 hours. Keep mucous membranes moist with water-soluble lubricant *to prevent them from dehydrating.*

■ Provide sour hard candy *to decrease thirst and improve taste.*

■ Support patient with positive feedback about adherence to restrictions *to encourage compliance.*

■ Give skin care every 4 hours. Change patient's position at least every 2 hours. Elevate edematous extremities. *These measures enhance venous return, reduce edema, and prevent skin breakdown.*

■ Examine skin daily for signs of bruising or other discoloration. *Edema may cause decreased tissue perfusion with skin changes.*

■ Encourage patient to help in performing ADLs. *This boosts self-image and helps mobilize fluid from edematous areas.*

■ Alternate periods of rest and activity *to avoid worsening fatigue caused by electrolyte imbalance.*

■ Increase patient's activity level, as tolerated; for example, ambulate and increase self-care measures performed by patient. *Gradually increasing activity helps body adjust to increased tissue oxygen demand and possible increased venous return.*

■ Apply antiembolism stockings or intermittent pneumatic compression stockings *to increase venous return.* Remove for 1 hour and inspect skin every 8 hours or according to facility policy.

■ Assess skin turgor *to monitor for dehydration.*

■ Measure abdominal girth every shift and report changes *to monitor for ascites.*

■ Have dietitian see patient *to teach or reinforce dietary restrictions.*

■ Educate patient regarding:
– environmental safety measures
– fluid restriction and diet
– signs and symptoms requiring immediate medical treatment

– medications (name, dosage, frequency, therapeutic effects, and adverse effects)
– activity level
– ways to prevent infection.
   These measures encourage patient and family members to participate more fully in care.

Suggested NIC interventions
Acid-Base Management; Electrolyte Management; Fluid Management; Fluid Monitoring; Medication Management; Nutrition Management; Weight Management

Evaluations for expected outcomes
■ Patient's blood pressure remains within established limits.
■ Signs of hyperkalemia (peaked or elevated T waves, prolonged PR intervals, widened QRS complexes, or depressed ST segments) don't appear on ECG.
■ Patient's fluid intake and output remain within established limits.
■ Patient's urine specific gravity remains within established limits.
■ Patient's HCT remains above specified level.
■ Patient's electrolyte levels remain within established limits.
■ Patient plans 24-hour fluid intake.
■ Patient doesn't indicate discomfort with restricted fluid intake, either verbally or through behavior.
■ Patient's skin remains intact and free from infection.
■ Patient assists caregiver with ADLs without undue fatigue.
■ Patient ambulates and carries out ADLs comfortably and safely.
■ Patient plans own menu and selects foods low in sodium and potassium. Patient follows other dietary restrictions (specify).
■ Patient and caregiver list signs and symptoms that require medical attention.

Documentation
■ Expression of patient's needs, desires, or perceptions of situation
■ Specific changes in patient's physical status
■ Observations about patient's response to treatment
■ Observations about how patient appears to be coping with fluid and dietary restrictions
■ Condition of skin and mucous membranes
■ Interventions performed to alleviate or resolve diagnosis
■ Evaluations for expected outcomes

Reference
Ancheta, I.B. "A Retrospective Pilot Study: Management of Patients with Heart Failure," *Dimensions of Critical Care Nursing* 25(5):228-33, September-October 2006.

Excess
FLUID VOLUME
related to excess fluid intake or retention, or excess sodium intake or retention

Definition
Increased isotonic fluid retention

Assessment
■ Neurologic status, including level of consciousness, orientation, and mental status

■ Cardiovascular status, including skin color, temperature, and turgor; jugular venous pressure; central venous pressure (CVP) and pulmonary artery pressure (if available); heart rate and rhythm; blood pressure; heart sounds; electrocardiogram results; hemoglobin (Hb) level; and hematocrit (HCT)

■ Respiratory status, including breath sounds, chest X-ray, arterial blood gas levels, and rate, depth, and pattern of respiration

■ Renal status, including intake and output, urine specific gravity, weight, serum electrolyte levels, serum and urine osmolality, blood urea nitrogen, urine and serum creatinine, and serum protein levels

Defining characteristics
■ Altered mental status
■ Altered respiratory pattern
■ Anasarca
■ Azotemia
■ Changes in blood pressure, pulmonary artery pressure, urine specific gravity, and electrolyte levels
■ Crackles
■ Decreased Hb level and HCT
■ Dyspnea
■ Edema
■ Increased CVP
■ Intake greater than output
■ Jugular vein distention
■ Oliguria
■ Orthopnea
■ Pleural effusion
■ Positive hepatojugular reflex
■ Pulmonary congestion
■ Rapid weight gain
■ Restlessness and anxiety
■ S_3 heart sound

Expected outcomes
■ Patient will state ability to breathe comfortably.
■ Patient will maintain fluid intake at ___ ml/day.

- Patient will return to baseline weight.
- Patient will maintain vital signs within normal limits (specify).
- Patient will exhibit urine specific gravity of 1.005 to 1.010.
- Patient will have normal skin turgor.
- Patient will show electrolyte level within normal range (specify).
- Patient will avoid complications of excess fluid.
- Patient will state understanding of health problem.
- Patient will demonstrate skill in health-related behaviors.

Suggested NOC outcomes

Electrolyte Balance; Fluid Balance; Fluid Overload Severity; Kidney Function; Nutritional Status: Food & Fluid Intake; Urinary Elimination; Weight: Body Mass

Interventions and rationales

- Help patient into a position that aids breathing, such as Fowler's or semi-Fowler's, *to increase chest expansion and improve ventilation.*
- Administer oxygen, as ordered, *to enhance arterial blood oxygenation.*
- Restrict fluids to _____ ml per shift. *Excessive fluids will worsen patient's condition.*
- Monitor and record vital signs at least every 4 hours. *Changes may indicate fluid or electrolyte imbalances.*
- Measure and record intake and output. Intake greater than output may indicate fluid retention and possible overload.
- Weigh patient at same time each day *to obtain consistent readings.*
- Administer diuretics *to promote fluid excretion.* Record effects.
- Test urine specific gravity every 8 hours and record results. Monitor laboratory values and report significant changes to physician. *High specific gravity indicates fluid retention. Fluid overload may alter electrolyte levels.*
- Assess patient daily for edema, including ascites and dependent or sacral edema. *Fluid overload or decreased osmotic pressure may result in edema, especially in dependent areas.*
- Maintain patient on sodium-restricted diet, as ordered, *to reduce excess fluid and prevent reaccumulation.*
- Reposition patient every 2 hours, inspect skin for redness with each turn, and institute measures as needed *to prevent skin breakdown.*
- Apply antiembolism stockings or intermittent pneumatic compression stockings *to increase venous return.* Remove for 1 hour every 8 hours or according to facility policy.
- Encourage patient to cough and deep breathe every 2 to 4 hours *to prevent pulmonary complications.*
- Educate patient regarding maintenance of daily weight record, daily measuring and recording of intake and output, diuretic therapy, and dietary restrictions, especially sodium. *These measures encourage patient and caregivers to participate more fully.*

Suggested NIC interventions

Electrolyte Management; Fluid Management; Fluid Monitoring; Nutrition Management; Urinary Elimination Management; Vital Signs Monitoring; Weight Management

Evaluations for expected outcomes

■ Patient indicates, verbally and through behavior, ability to breathe comfortably.
■ Patient's fluid intake remains at established daily limit (specify).
■ Patient's weight returns to baseline and remains stable.
■ Patient's pulse and respiratory rates, blood pressure, and temperature remain within established limits.
■ Patient's urine specific gravity remains between 1.005 and 1.010.
■ Patient's skin turgor remains normal.
■ Patient's electrolyte levels remain within established range.
■ Complications of excess fluid don't occur.
■ Patient expresses understanding of health problem.
■ Patient demonstrates skill in health-related behaviors, such as maintaining weight and monitoring intake and output.

Documentation

■ Patient's perceptions of situation
■ Observations of physical findings
■ Interventions to correct fluid volume excess
■ Patient's responses to fluid and dietary restrictions
■ Patient's demonstration of skills
■ Evaluations for expected outcomes

Reference

Bennett, S.J., et al. "Medication and Dietary Compliance Beliefs in Heart Failure," *Western Journal of Nursing Research* 27(8):977-93, December 2005.

Risk for deficient
FLUID VOLUME
related to excessive loss

Definition
At risk for experiencing vascular, cellular, or intracellular dehydration

Assessment

■ History of problems that can cause fluid loss, such as vomiting, diarrhea, indwelling tubes, and hemorrhage
■ Pulse, blood pressure, respirations, and temperature
■ Fluid and electrolyte status, including weight, intake and output, urine specific gravity, skin turgor, and mucous membranes

■ Laboratory studies, including serum electrolyte, blood urea nitrogen, and hemoglobin (Hb) levels and hematocrit (HCT)

Risk factors
■ Conditions that influence fluid needs (such as a hypermetabolic state)
■ Excessive loss of fluid from normal routes (such as from diarrhea)
■ Extremes of age or weight
■ Factors that affect intake of, absorption of, or access to fluids (such as immobility)
■ Knowledge deficit related to fluid volume
■ Loss of fluid through abnormal routes (such as a drainage tube)
■ Medications that cause fluid loss

Expected outcomes
■ Patient's vital signs will remain stable.
■ Patient's skin color will remain normal.
■ Patient will maintain urine output of at least ___ ml/hour.
■ Patient's electrolyte values will remain within normal range.
■ Patient will maintain intake at _____ ml/24 hours.
■ Patient's intake will equal or exceed output.
■ Patient will express understanding of need to maintain adequate fluid intake.
■ Patient will demonstrate skill in weighing himself accurately and recording weight.
■ Patient will measure and record own intake and output.
■ Patient will return to normal, appropriate diet.

Suggested NOC outcomes

Electrolyte & Acid-Base Balance; Fluid Balance; Hydration; Nausea & Vomiting Severity; Nutritional Status: Food & Fluid Intake; Risk Detection; Self-Care Status; Swallowing Status; Urinary Elimination

Interventions and rationales
■ Monitor and record vital signs every 4 hours. *Fever, tachycardia, dyspnea, or hypotension may indicate hypovolemia.*
■ Maintain accurate record of intake and output *to aid estimation of patient's fluid balance.*
■ Measure urine output every hour. Record and report an output of less than ____ ml/hour. *Decreased urine output may indicate reduced fluid volume.*
■ Measure and record drainage from all tubes and catheters *to take such losses into account when replacing fluid.*
■ When copious drainage appears on dressings, weigh dressings every 8 hours and record with other output sources. *Excessive wound drainage causes significant fluid imbalances (1 kg dressing equals about 1 qt [1 L] of fluid).*
■ Test urine specific gravity each shift. Monitor laboratory values and report abnormal findings to physician. *Increased urine specific gravity may indicate dehydration. Elevated HCT and Hb level also indicate dehydration.*

■ Monitor serum electrolyte levels and report abnormalities. *Fluid loss may cause significant electrolyte imbalance.*

■ Obtain and record patient's weight at same time every day to help ensure accurate data. *Daily weighing helps estimate body fluid status.*

■ Monitor skin turgor each shift to check for dehydration; report any decrease in turgor. *Poor skin turgor is a sign of dehydration.*

■ Examine oral mucous membranes each shift. *Dry mucous membranes are a sign of dehydration.*

■ Cover wounds *to minimize fluid loss and prevent skin excoriation.*

■ Determine patient's fluid preferences *to enhance intake.*

■ Keep oral fluids at bedside within patient's reach and encourage patient to drink. *This gives patient some control over fluid intake and supplements parenteral fluid intake.*

■ Instruct patient in maintaining appropriate fluid intake, including recording daily weight, measuring intake and output, and recognizing signs of dehydration. *This encourages patient and caregiver participation and enhances patient's sense of control.*

■ Force oral fluids when possible and indicated *to enhance replacement of lost fluids.* (Bowel sounds should be present and patient awake before giving oral fluids.)

■ Administer parenteral fluids, as prescribed, *to replace fluid losses.* Maintain parenteral fluids or blood transfusions at prescribed rate *to prevent further fluid loss or overload.*

■ Progress patient to appropriate diet, as prescribed, *to help achieve fluid and electrolyte balance.*

Suggested NIC interventions

Acid-Base Management; Fluid Management; Fluid Monitoring; Hypovolemia Management; Nutrition Management; Intravenous (IV) Therapy; Hypovolemia Monitoring; Surveillance

Evaluations for expected outcomes

■ Patient's temperature, pulse rate, blood pressure, and respirations are within set limits (specify).

■ Patient's skin color remains normal.

■ Patient's urine output remains at specified volume.

■ Patient's electrolyte values remain normal.

■ Patient's daily fluid intake remains within established limits (specify).

■ Patient's cumulative intake equals or exceeds cumulative output.

■ Patient demonstrates understanding of importance of maintaining fluid balance.

■ Patient weighs himself with same scale at same time each day and records results.

■ Patient measures fluid intake and output; records are reviewed to ensure accuracy.

■ Patient returns to normal, appropriate diet.

Documentation

- Observations of physical findings
- Intake and output
- Drainage from indwelling tubes and catheters, including amount, color, and consistency
- Amount, color, and odor of drainage on dressings
- Patient teaching about fluid intake and diet
- Patient's response to interventions
- Evaluations for expected outcomes

Reference

Mentes, J. "Oral Hydration in Older Adults: Greater Awareness is Needed in Preventing, Recognizing, and Treating Dehydration," *AJN* 106(6):40-49, June 2006.

Impaired
GAS EXCHANGE

related to alveolar-capillary changes

Definition

Excess or deficit in oxygenation or carbon dioxide at the alveolar-capillary level

Assessment

- Neurologic status, including level of consciousness, orientation, and mental status
- Respiratory status, including respiratory rate and depth, symmetry of chest expansion, use of accessory muscles, cough, sputum, palpation for fremitus, percussion of lung fields, auscultation of breath sounds, arterial blood gas (ABG) levels, and pulmonary function studies
- Cardiovascular status, including skin color and temperature, heart rate and rhythm, blood pressure, and complete blood count
- Activity status, including such functional capabilities as range of motion and muscle strength, activities of daily living (ADLs), and occupation

Defining characteristics

- Abnormal pH and ABG levels
- Abnormal respiratory rate, rhythm, and depth
- Confusion
- Cyanosis (in neonates)
- Diaphoresis
- Dyspnea
- Headache upon awakening
- Hypoxia and hypoxemia
- Increased or decreased carbon dioxide levels
- Irritability
- Nasal flaring

- Pale, dusky skin
- Restlessness or somnolence
- Tachycardia
- Vision disturbances

Expected outcomes

- Patient will maintain respiratory rate within 5 breaths of baseline.
- Patient will express feelings of comfort in maintaining air exchange.
- Patient will cough effectively.
- Patient will expectorate sputum.
- Patient will sustain sufficient fluid intake to prevent dehydration: ___ ml/24 hours.
- Patient will perform ADLs to level of tolerance.
- Patient will have normal breath sounds.
- Patient's ABG levels will return to baselines: ___ pH; ____ partial pressure of arterial oxygen (Pa_{O_2}); ____ partial pressure of arterial carbon dioxide (Pa_{CO_2}).
- Patient will perform relaxation techniques every 4 hours.
- Patient will use correct bronchial hygiene.

Suggested NOC outcomes

Cognition; Electrolyte & Acid-Base Balance; Respiratory Status: Gas Exchange; Respiratory Status: Ventilation; Tissue Perfusion: Pulmonary; Vital Signs

Interventions and rationales

- Assess and record pulmonary status every 4 hours or more frequently if patient's condition is unstable. *Poor pulmonary status may result in hypoxemia.*
- Monitor vital signs and heart rhythm at least every 4 hours *to detect tachycardia and tachypnea, which could indicate hypoxemia.*
- Place patient in position that best facilitates chest expansion *to enhance gas exchange.*
- Change patient's position at least every 2 hours *to mobilize secretions and allow aeration of all lung fields.*
- Perform bronchial hygiene, as ordered, including coughing, percussion, postural drainage, and suctioning. *These measures promote drainage and keep airways clear.*
- Give medications, as ordered, *to improve oxygenation.* Monitor and record efficacy and adverse reactions *to guide treatment.*
- Monitor oxygen therapy, *which increases alveolar oxygen concentration and enhances arterial blood oxygenation.*
- Record intake and output *to monitor patient's fluid status.*
- Report signs of dehydration or fluid overload immediately. *Dehydration may hinder tissue perfusion and secretion mobilization; fluid overload may cause pulmonary edema.*
- Assist patient with ADLs *to decrease tissue oxygen demand.*
- Include periods of rest in care plan *to reduce patient's tissue oxygen demand.*

■ Monitor ABG levels and notify physician immediately if Pao_2 or arterial oxygen saturation drops or $Paco_2$ rises. Administer endotracheal intubation and mechanical ventilation if needed. *This helps increase ventilation and gas exchange.*
■ Teach patient relaxation techniques *to reduce tissue oxygen demand.*
■ Have patient perform relaxation techniques every 4 hours *to establish routine and reduce oxygen demand.*

Suggested NIC interventions
Airway Management; Airway Suctioning; Anxiety Reduction; Cough Enhancement; Energy Management; Mechanical Ventilation; Positioning

Evaluations for expected outcomes
■ Patient's respiratory rate remains within established limits.
■ Patient doesn't experience dyspnea.
■ Patient demonstrates ability to cough and produce sputum.
■ Patient expectorates sputum produced by coughing and deep breathing.
■ Patient's fluid intake remains sufficient to prevent dehydration.
■ Patient performs ADLs without exhibiting dyspnea or other signs of abnormal ABG levels.
■ Patient has normal breath sounds.
■ Patient's pH, Pao_2, and $Paco_2$ return to and remain within established limits.
■ Patient performs relaxation techniques every 4 hours.
■ Patient uses correct bronchial hygiene.

Documentation
■ Patient's complaints of dyspnea, headache, and restlessness
■ Patient's expression of well-being
■ Observations of physical findings
■ Effectiveness of medications
■ Other treatments performed by nurse
■ Evaluations for expected outcomes

Reference
Considine, J. "The Role of Nurses in Preventing Adverse Events Related to Respiratory Dysfunction: Literature Review," *Journal of Advanced Nursing* 49(6):624-33, March 2005.

Impaired
GAS EXCHANGE
related to ventilation-perfusion imbalance

Definition
Excess or deficit in oxygenation or carbon dioxide at the alveolar-capillary level

Assessment

■ Neurologic status, including level of consciousness, orientation, and mental status

■ Respiratory status, including respiratory rate and depth, symmetry of chest expansion, accessory muscle use, cough, sputum, palpation for fremitus, percussion of lung fields, auscultation of breath sounds, arterial blood gas (ABG) levels, and pulmonary function studies

■ Cardiovascular status, including skin color and temperature, heart rate and rhythm, blood pressure, hemoglobin (Hb) level and hematocrit (HCT), red blood cell count, white blood cell count, platelet count, prothrombin time (PT), partial thromboplastin time (PTT), and serum iron level

■ Activity status, including such functional capabilities as range of motion and muscle strength, activities of daily living (ADLs), and occupation

Defining characteristics

■ Abnormal pH and ABG levels
■ Abnormal respiratory rate, rhythm, and depth
■ Confusion
■ Cyanosis (in neonates)
■ Diaphoresis
■ Dyspnea
■ Headache upon awakening
■ Hypoxia and hypoxemia
■ Increased or decreased carbon dioxide levels
■ Irritability
■ Nasal flaring
■ Pale, dusky skin
■ Restlessness or somnolence
■ Tachycardia

Expected outcomes

■ Patient will carry out ADLs without weakness or fatigue.
■ Patient won't have signs of active bleeding.
■ Patient's Hb level and HCT will return to normal (specify).
■ Patient's clotting profile will remain within normal limits (specify).
■ Patient will maintain adequate ventilation.
■ Patient will communicate understanding of precautions needed to prevent bleeding.

Suggested NOC outcomes

Cognition; Electrolyte & Acid-Base Balance; Respiratory Status: Gas Exchange; Respiratory Status: Ventilation; Tissue Perfusion: Pulmonary; Vital Signs

Interventions and rationales

■ Encourage patient to alternate periods of rest and activity. *Activity increases tissue oxygen demand; rest enhances tissue oxygen perfusion.*

■ If patient is on bed rest, help him into a comfortable position and raise side rails *to prevent falls.*

■ Have patient turn, cough, and deep-breathe every 4 hours *to prevent atelectasis or fluid buildup in lungs and to enhance blood oxygen level.*

■ Move patient slowly *to avoid orthostatic hypotension.*

■ Assist patient when out of bed in case of dizziness. Avoid bumps and scratches *to avoid possible trauma and tissue bleeding.*

■ Plan patient's activities within level of tolerance *to avoid fatigue.*

■ Provide gentle oral hygiene *to avoid injuring oral mucosa.*

■ Check all urine and stools for blood *to detect internal bleeding.* Check for evidence of bleeding at least once every 8 hours. *Hemorrhage or bleeding may cause anemia.*

■ Administer blood or blood products and monitor for adverse reactions *to restore fluid volume and prevent complications.*

■ Consolidate laboratory work *to avoid multiple needle sticks and reduce chance of hematoma or hemorrhage in patients with altered clotting mechanisms.*

■ Apply pressure for at least 1 minute after puncture *to promote clotting.*

■ Auscultate lungs every 4 hours and report abnormalities *to detect decreased or adventitious breath sounds.*

■ Monitor vital signs, heart rhythm, and ABG and Hb levels *to detect impaired gas exchange.* Report abnormalities.

■ Teach patient about safety at home and work, including:
– use of soft toothbrush
– use of an electric razor for shaving
– careful use of sharp objects, such as knives, tweezers, and scissors
– monitoring of urine, stools, and sputum for blood and reporting results immediately if blood is present
– disadvantages and risks of smoking
– using medications (name, dosage, therapeutic effect, adverse effects, and precautions).
These measures encourage patient and caregivers to participate in care.

Suggested NIC interventions

Acid-Base Management; Airway Management; Airway Suctioning; Anxiety Reduction; Chest Physiotherapy; Energy Management; Exercise Promotion; Fluid Management; Oxygen Therapy; Respiratory Monitoring

Evaluations for expected outcomes

■ Patient carries out ADLs without fatigue or weakness.

■ Patient doesn't exhibit signs of active bleeding, such as oozing from wounds or puncture site, bruising, petechiae, and occult blood in stools or urine.

■ Patient's Hb level and HCT remain within established limits.

■ Patient's clotting profile, including platelet count, PTT, PT, fibrinogen, and fibrin split products, remains within normal limits.

■ Patient maintains adequate ventilation.

■ Patient communicates understanding of precautions needed to prevent bleeding.

Documentation
- Patient's expression of personal feelings
- Observations about physical findings
- Results of laboratory studies that significantly affect nursing care
- Patient's response to interventions
- Evaluations for expected outcomes

Reference
Marklew, A. "Body Positioning and its Effect on Oxygenation—A Literature Review," *Nursing in Critical Care* 11(1):16-22, January-February 2006.

GRIEVING

Definition
A normal, complex process that includes emotional, physical, spiritual, social, and intellectual responses and behaviors by which individuals, families, and communities incorporate an actual, anticipated, or perceived loss into their daily lives

Assessment
- Age, gender, developmental stage
- Patient's perceived value of loss
- Emotional status including anger, denial, or hostility
- Patient's usual pattern of coping with loss
- Changes in activity level, appetite, libido or sleep pattern
- Emotional and spiritual support systems

Defining characteristics
- Alterations in activity level, immune function, neuroendocrine function, sleep patterns, dream patterns
- Anger
- Blame
- Detachment
- Despair
- Disorganization
- Experiencing relief
- Maintaining connection to the deceased
- Making meaning of the loss
- Pain
- Panic behavior
- Personal growth
- Psychological distress
- Suffering

Expected outcomes
- Patient will identify and acknowledge the loss.
- Patient will accepts that grief is a natural response to loss and understands the grief process.
- Patient will express his or her grief in a nondestructive manner.
- Patient will seek emotional or spiritual support.
- Patient will progress through the various stages of the grieving process.
- Patient will establish plans for the future.

Suggested NOC outcomes

Coping; Family Coping; Grief Resolution; Life Change; Psychosocial Adjustment

Interventions and rationales
- Assist patient to understand grieving process and accept feelings; *this enhances patient's understanding and ability to cope.*
- Provide time for the patient to express his feelings about death or terminal illness; *active listening helps decrease feelings of loneliness and isolation.*
- Encourage expression of grief in a support group; *comfort is received in knowing that the pain from grief is normal.*
- Involve the interdisciplinary team in patient care; *each team member offers unique training to meet patient's needs.*
- Help patient make a specific plan for coping *to enable patient to integrate the loss and adjust to new lifestyle.*

Suggested NIC interventions

Active Listening; Emotional Support; Family Support; Grief Work Facilitation; Presence; Touch

Evaluations for expected outcomes
- Patient identifies and acknowledges loss.
- Patient accepts that grief is a natural response to loss and understands the grief process.
- Patient is able to express his grief in a nondestructive manner.
- Patient will participate in organized spiritual or emotional support systems.
- Patient progresses through the stages of grief.
- Patient describes plans for the future.

Documentation
- Patient's verbal expression of grief
- Observations of emotional responses at attempts at coping
- Interventions to assist coping with loss
- Patient's response to nursing interventions
- Evaluations for expected outcomes

References

Doka, K.J. "Grief: The Constant Companion of Illness," *Anesthesiology Clinician* 24(1):205-12, March 2006.

Krueger, G. "Meaning-making in the Aftermath of Sudden Infant Death Syndrome," *Nursing Inquiry* 13(3):163-71, September 2006.

Complicated
GRIEVING
related to predisposition for anxiety and feelings of inadequacy

Definition
Disorder that occurs after the death of a significant other, in which the experience of distress accompanying bereavement fails to follow normative expectations and manifests in functional impairment

Assessment
- History of loss
- Length of grief process
- Pattern of coping (grief delayed or avoided)
- Self-destructive behaviors
- Sleep assessment
- Nutritional assessment
- Changes in presentation of self
- Social or spiritual support
- Ability to maintain roles at occupation and within family

Defining characteristics
- Decreased functioning in life roles
- Decreased sense of well-being
- Depression
- Fatigue
- Grief avoidance
- Longing for the deceased
- Low levels of intimacy
- Persistent emotional distress
- Preoccupation with thoughts of the deceased
- Rumination
- Searching for the deceased
- Verbalization of anxiety; distress about the deceased; feeling dazed, empty, in shock, or stunned; detachment from others; disbelief, mistrust, or lack of acceptance of the death; persistent painful memories; self-blame

Expected outcomes
- Patient will express appropriate feelings of loss, guilt, fear, anger, or sadness.
- Patient will identify the loss and describe what it means to him.

- Patient will appropriately move through stages of grief.
- Patient will maintain healthy patterns of sleep, activity, and eating.
- Patient will verbalize understanding that grief is normal.
- Patient will use healthy coping mechanisms and social support systems.
- Patient will seek fulfillment through preferred spiritual practices.
- Patient will begin planning for future.

Suggested NOC outcomes

Coping; Family Coping; Grief Resolution; Life Change; Psychosocial Adjustment

Interventions and rationales

- Encourage patient to express grief and feelings of anger, guilt, and sadness. *Inability to express these feelings may result in maladaptive behaviors.*
- Encourage journaling to express grief and loss. *Writing and exploring feelings is an active process, which may assist in grieving.*
- Help patient to identify an area of hope in his life. *Focusing on a life purpose may decrease anger and feelings of frustration.*
- Refer patient to community support systems *to help him deal with his bereavement and grief process*
- Contact patient's preferred spiritual leader, if patient desires; *this may provide relief from spiritual distress.*
- Help patient to focus realistically on changes the loss has brought about. *This will assist patient in forming plans for the future and improving social relationships.*
- Encourage patient and family to engage in reminiscing; *this will give purpose and meaning to the loss and assist in maintenance of self-esteem.*
- Help patient to formulate goals for the future, *this helps patient to place loss in perspective and to move on to new situations and relationships.*
- Identify previous losses and assess for depression; *in the elderly, losses frequently occur without adequate recovery time before the next loss.*

Suggested NIC interventions

Calming Technique; Coping Enhancement; Counseling; Emotional Support; Family Therapy; Grief Facilitation Work

Evaluations for expected outcomes

- Patient expresses feelings, which may include grief, guilt, anger, or sadness.
- Patient verbalizes feelings and behaviors related to the grieving process and applies these behaviors and feelings to his life.
- Patient appropriately moves through stages of grief.
- Patient maintains healthy patterns of sleep, activity, and eating.
- Patient communicates understanding that grieving is an appropriate response to loss and comes to terms with own grief response.
- Patient uses coping mechanisms and discusses loss with others, including support group and family.
- Patient experiences satisfaction and support from chosen religious practices.
- Patient begins planning for future.

Documentation

- Patient's verbal expression of grief
- Observations of emotional responses, attempts at coping, and interactions with family and staff
- Interventions to assist coping with loss
- Patient's response to nursing interventions
- Evaluations for expected outcomes

References

Ferrell, B.R., and Coyle, N. *Textbook of Palliative Nursing,* 2nd ed. New York: Oxford University Press, 2006.

Szanto, K., et al. "Indirect Self-destructive Behavior and Overt Suicidality in Patients with Complicated Grief," *Journal of Clinical Psychiatry* 67(2):233-39, February 2006.

Ineffective
HEALTH MAINTENANCE
related to lack of motor skills

Definition

Inability to identify, manage, or seek out help to maintain a healthy state

Assessment

- Neuromuscular status, including muscle strength and mass, gross and fine motor skills, joint mobility, and electromyelogram and EEG
- Abilities and limitations, including turning, transferring, ambulating, wheelchair use, driving, and activities of daily living
- Knowledge of health practices, including body maintenance, preventive health care needs, health care team follow-up, and safety measures
- Psychosocial support, including lifestyle, communication status (verbal, nonverbal, phone, and written), family members, and finances

Defining characteristics

- Demonstrated lack of knowledge regarding basic health practices
- Demonstrated lack of adaptive behaviors to internal or external environmental changes
- Reported or observed inability to take responsibility for meeting basic health practices in any or all functional areas
- History of lack of health seeking behaviors
- Expressed interest in improving health behaviors
- Reported or observed lack of equipment, financial, or other resources
- Reported or observed impairment of personal support systems

Expected outcomes

- Patient will identify necessary health maintenance activities.

■ Patient will make decisions about daily schedule.

■ Patient will perform health maintenance activities according to level of ability (specify).

■ Patient will communicate understanding of necessity for continuous self-monitoring of body functions.

■ Patient will maintain muscle strength and joint mobility.

■ Patient will demonstrate specific motor skills, such as brushing teeth.

■ Family members will demonstrate skill in carrying out activities patient can't perform.

■ Patient will identify community and social resources available to help with health maintenance.

Suggested NOC outcomes

Coping; Decision-Making; Health Beliefs: Perceived Resources; Health Promoting Behavior; Health Seeking Behaviors; Knowledge: Health Behavior; Knowledge: Health Promotion; Motivation; Self-Care Status; Social Support; Spiritual Health

Interventions and rationales

■ Discuss health maintenance needs with patient while carrying out routine activities *to reinforce their importance.*

■ Involve patient in decision making by allowing choices in determining where, when, and how activities are to be carried out. Ask, for example, "Would you like a bath or shower in the morning or evening?" *Participation in decision making increases feelings of independence.*

■ Help patient perform health maintenance activities, such as daily skin inspection and weekly catheterization for residual urine. *Encouraging skill development in patient promotes continued use of those skills after discharge.*

■ Instruct patient in specific skills needed in monitoring health status *to prompt participation in self-care.* Allow patient to carry out skills *to encourage independence.*

■ Perform or help patient perform passive and active range-of-motion exercises *to help maintain joint mobility and muscle strength.*

■ Identify level of mobility (independent in feeding and bathing; needs assistance to brush teeth; dependent in use of wheelchair) and communicate skill level to all personnel *to provide continuity and preserve level of independence.*

■ Educate family members in skills that patient can't perform unassisted, such as bathing, maintaining hygiene, driving to appointments, transferring, or using walker. *This allows patient and family members to take active role in care.*

■ Consult with social services or other health care team members to identify health care resources (for example, Meals On Wheels or homemaker services), and help patient contact and arrange for follow-up. *These resources can help patient maintain independence after discharge.*

Suggested NIC interventions

Anticipatory Guidance; Behavior Modification; Decision-Making Support; Health Education; Health System Guidance; Referral; Support System Enhancement; Teaching: Disease Process

Evaluations for expected outcomes

- Patient identifies health maintenance activities.
- Patient plans daily schedule.
- Patient's functional level is appropriate to capability level.
- Patient communicates understanding of importance of monitoring body functions, such as blood glucose levels, blood pressure, and pulse rate.
- Patient maintains muscle strength and joint mobility.
- Patient demonstrates motor skills correctly without prompting.
- Family members demonstrate skill in carrying out activities patient can't perform.
- Patient identifies and contacts community resources to assist with health maintenance, if needed.

Documentation

- Patient's identified health needs and perceptions and limitations in achieving them
- Patient's willingness to make decisions and participate in health maintenance activities
- Observations of motor abilities, level of skill performance, and health status
- Patient's response to nursing interventions
- Evaluations for expected outcomes

Reference

Schumacher, K., et al. "Family Caregivers: Caring for Older Adults, Working with their Families," *AJN* 106(8):40-49, August 2006.

Ineffective
HEALTH MAINTENANCE
related to perceptual or cognitive impairment

Definition

Inability to identify, manage, or seek out help to maintain health

Assessment

- Age
- Current health status
- History of neurologic, sensory, or psychological impairment
- Neurologic status, including level of consciousness, orientation, cognition (memory, insight, and judgment), sensory ability, and motor ability
- Personal habits, such as smoking and alcohol consumption

■ Psychosocial status, including support systems, personality, coping mechanisms, drug use, and communication status (verbal, nonverbal, phone, or written)

Defining characteristics
■ Demonstrated lack of knowledge regarding basic health practices
■ Demonstrated lack of adaptive behaviors to internal or external environmental changes
■ Reported or observed inability to take responsibility for meeting basic health practices in any or all functional areas
■ History of lack of health seeking behaviors
■ Expressed interest in improving health behaviors
■ Reported or observed lack of equipment, financial, or other resources
■ Reported or observed impairment of personal support systems

Expected outcomes
■ Patient will maintain current health status.
■ Patient will sustain no harm or injury.
■ Patient and family members will verbalize feelings and concerns.
■ Patient and family members will explain health maintenance program.
■ Patient and family members will demonstrate health maintenance program.
■ Patient and family members will identify available health resources.
■ Patient and family members will demonstrate appropriate coping skills.

Suggested NOC outcomes
Coping; Decision-Making; Health Beliefs: Perceived Resources; Health Promoting Behavior; Social Support; Spiritual Health

Interventions and rationales
■ Determine patient's ability to maintain health, degree of support available from family or others, degree of motivation, and level of dependence. Report any changes. *Comprehensive assessment provides a basis for evaluating future functional changes.*
■ Perform prescribed treatment for condition causing perceptual or cognitive impairment. Monitor progress and report favorable and adverse responses. *Evaluating patient's responses to treatment and collaborating with physician fosters appropriate care planning.*
■ Help patient and family members identify strengths and weaknesses in maintaining health (such as self-care deficits) *to provide focus for interventions.* Also help family members communicate with patient and understand what patient's behaviors mean. *This reduces patient's feelings of helplessness and gives a sense of control over situation.*
■ Plan a health maintenance program with patient and family members, addressing current disabilities.
– Reorient patient as often as necessary *to enhance reality testing and mental status.* Adapt environment to appear somewhat familiar to patient. Display such personal objects as pictures and clocks from patient's home.
– Provide a structured care program in writing *to give patient sense of security.*
– Have same person provide care on an ongoing basis *to provide stability.*

– Fully describe all aspects of care to patient and family members *to elicit patient's cooperation.*

– When discussing care, give short, simple explanations geared to patient's level of understanding *to enhance cooperation.*

– If possible, prepare patient for any unexpected change *to minimize disruption.*

– Provide ample time for patient to perform health maintenance tasks *to reduce frustration and encourage success.*

■ Instruct family members to carry out health maintenance practices. Demonstrate such necessary skills as bathing, feeding, and reality orientation; then have family members perform them under supervision. *Involving family members allows them to solve problems with supervision and support.*

■ Instruct family members on how to maintain a safe environment *to reduce risk of patient injury.*

■ Encourage patient and family members to verbalize feelings and concerns related to health maintenance *to help them develop greater understanding and better manage their health.*

■ Help family members develop coping skills necessary to deal with patient. *If patient's illness is prolonged, family members could develop maladaptive coping strategies.*

■ Help family members identify available social and community resources, such as stroke support group and Alzheimer's family support group. *This helps them gain social support and factual information and allows them to express feelings associated with patient's disorder.*

■ Make referrals, as appropriate, to psychiatric liaison nurse and social services *to help prevent burnout among family members.*

Suggested NIC interventions

Anticipatory Guidance; Coping Enhancement; Counseling; Discharge Planning; Health Education; Health System Guidance; Physician Support; Referral; Support System Enhancement

Evaluations for expected outcomes

■ Patient maintains health.

■ Patient doesn't show signs of injury.

■ Patient discusses impact of illness and self-care needs on others' lives. Family members voice feelings about patient's illness.

■ Patient and family members state at least three health maintenance strategies.

■ Patient performs health maintenance practices to extent possible. Family members assist patient, as needed.

■ Patient and family members identify and contact sources of support.

■ Patient copes with current situation without experiencing severe emotional upset. Family members also display effective coping.

Documentation

■ Expressions of concern by patient and family members about patient's inability to maintain health

■ Observations of patient's impaired ability to perform self-care and response to treatment

■ Patient's response to nursing interventions
■ Instructions given to patient and family members, their level of understanding, and demonstrated skill in carrying out health maintenance program
■ Referrals made for patient and family members
■ Evaluations for expected outcomes

Reference

Cole, C.S., et al. "Assessment and Discharge Planning for Hospitalized Older Adults with Delirium," *Medsurg Nursing* 15(2):71-76, April 2006.

Impaired
HOME MAINTENANCE

related to impaired cognitive or emotional functioning

Definition

Inability to independently maintain a safe growth promoting environment

Assessment

■ Home environment
■ Financial resources
■ Patient's and family's knowledge of self-care requirements
■ Patient's and family's psychological status, including perception of reality, communication patterns, assignment of responsibilities, degree of awareness and concern, and history of psychiatric illness
■ Drug or alcohol abuse
■ Support systems, including close friends, organizations with which patient is affiliated, and community resources

Defining characteristics

■ Difficulty in maintaining home in a comfortable fashion
■ Outstanding debts or financial crises
■ Request for assistance with home maintenance
■ Disorderly surroundings
■ Unwashed or unavailable cooking equipment, clothes, or linens
■ Accumulation of dirt, food wastes, or hygienic wastes
■ Offensive odors
■ Inappropriate household temperatures
■ Lack of necessary equipment or aids
■ Presence of vermin or rodents
■ Repeated hygienic disorders, infestations, or infections

Expected outcomes

■ Patient and family members will express concern about poor home maintenance.

■ Patient and family members will verbalize plan to correct health and safety hazards in home.

■ Patient and family members will identify community resources available to help maintain home.

Suggested NOC outcomes

Family Functioning; Role Performance; Self-Care: Instrumental Activities of Daily Living (IADL)

Interventions and rationales

■ Discuss obstacles to effective home maintenance management with patient and family *to develop understanding of potential and actual health and safety hazards.*

■ Help family members assign responsibilities for household care and establish appropriate expectations *to aid communication and help set realistic goals.*

■ Help family members establish daily and weekly home maintenance activities and assignments *to impose structure on family's routine and set standards for measuring progress.*

■ Encourage weekly discussions about progress in maintaining home maintenance *schedule to develop family unity and allow members to address problems before they become overwhelming.*

■ Help family members contact community resources that can assist them in their efforts to improve home maintenance management, such as self-help groups, cleaning services, and exterminators. *Community resources can lessen family's burden while members learn to function independently.*

Suggested NIC interventions

Counseling; Emotional Support; Family Integrity Promotion; Family Support; Home Maintenance Assistance

Evaluations for expected outcomes

■ Patient and family members establish and follow daily and weekly schedule for home maintenance.

■ With help of appropriate community resources, as needed, patient and family members clear home of clutter, debris, and waste.

■ Patient and family members contact community resources.

Documentation

■ Patient's and family members' expressions of difficulty in maintaining household

■ Patient's and family members' mental status

■ Presence of health hazards, such as filth, rodents, and waste matter

■ Presence of safety hazards, such as faulty wiring

■ Presence of offensive odors

■ Patient's and family members' understanding of home maintenance management and resources

■ Interventions to improve home maintenance skills

■ Patient's and family members' responses to nursing interventions

■ Evaluations for expected outcomes

Reference

Horvath, K.J., et al. "Caregiver Competence to Prevent Home Injury to the Care Recipient with Dementia," *Rehabilitation Nursing* 30(5):189-96, September-October 2005.

Impaired
HOME MAINTENANCE
related to inadequate support system

Definition
Inability to independently maintain a safe growth promoting environment

Assessment
■ Psychosocial status
■ Support systems, including family, close friends, and organizations with which patient is affiliated; if patient lives alone, access to family, friends, and pets
■ Financial resources
■ Home environment
■ Patient's and family members' knowledge of disease and self-care requirements

Defining characteristics
■ Difficulty in maintaining home in a comfortable fashion
■ Outstanding debts or financial crises
■ Request for assistance with home maintenance
■ Disorderly surroundings
■ Unwashed or unavailable cooking equipment, clothes, or linens
■ Accumulation of dirt, food wastes, or hygienic wastes
■ Offensive odors
■ Inappropriate household temperatures
■ Lack of necessary equipment or aids
■ Presence of vermin or rodents
■ Repeated hygienic disorders, infestations, or infections

Expected outcomes
■ Patient and family members will express need to make adjustments in home to help manage patient's condition.
■ Patient and family members will identify individuals or organizations that may provide assistance.

Suggested NOC outcomes
Family Functioning; Role Performance; Self-Care: Activities of Daily Living (ADL)

Interventions and rationales

■ Help patient and family members explore available *resources to help identify discharge problems and ease transition from hospital to home.*

■ Provide sufficient information to patient and family members *to ensure knowledge necessary for them to make appropriate decisions.*

■ Refer patient to social service department *to assist with follow-up care after discharge.*

■ Suggest referral to home health agency, homemaker service, Meals On Wheels, or other appropriate outside agencies for assistance and follow-up. *Patient may need a range of community services to meet various needs.*

Suggested NIC interventions

Caregiver Support; Family Support; Home Maintenance Assistance; Role Enhancement; Support System Enhancement

Evaluations for expected outcomes

■ Patient and family members describe changes needed to promote maximum health and safety at home.

■ Patient and family members list agencies that can assist with home care.

Documentation

■ Patient's and family members' perception of problem
■ Observations regarding problem's magnitude
■ Interventions performed to alleviate problem
■ Responses of others asked to assist with problem
■ Evaluations for expected outcomes

Reference

King, R.B., and Semik, P.E. "Stroke Caregiving: Difficult Times, Resource Use, and Needs During the First 2 Years," *Journal of Gerontological Nursing* 32(4):37-44, April 2006.

HOPELESSNESS

related to failing or deteriorating physiologic condition

Definition

Subjective state in which an individual sees few or no available alternatives or personal choices and can't mobilize energy on own behalf

Assessment

■ Nature of current medical diagnosis
■ Patient's and family members' knowledge of diagnosis and prognosis
■ Actual or perceived self-care deficits (specify)
■ Mental status, including cognitive functioning, affect, and mood

■ Communication, including verbal (speech content, quality, and quantity) and nonverbal (body positioning, eye contact, and facial expression)
■ Available support systems, including clergy, family, and friends
■ Past experience with loss, including body part or function, death, residence, and employment
■ Coping mechanisms and decision-making ability
■ Nutritional status, including changes in appetite or body weight
■ Sleep pattern
■ Motivation level for personal hygiene, therapies (physical and occupational therapy), and diversional activities
■ Developmental stage (Erikson's model), including age and role in family

Defining characteristics
■ Decreased affect
■ Decreased appetite
■ Decreased response to stimuli
■ Decreased verbalization
■ Increased or decreased sleep
■ Lack of involvement in self-care
■ Nonverbal cues, such closing eyes, shrugging in response to questions, and turning away from speaker
■ Passivity and lack of initiative
■ Verbal cues, including sighing and despondent comments such as "I can't"

Expected outcomes
■ Patient will identify feelings of hopelessness regarding current situation.
■ Patient will demonstrate more effective communication skills, including direct verbal responses to questions and increased eye contact.
■ Patient will resume appropriate rest and activity pattern.
■ Patient will participate in self-care activities and in decisions regarding care planning.
■ Patient will use diversional activities (specify).
■ Patient will identify factors that make him feel more hopeful.
■ Patient will identify social and community resources for continued assistance.

Suggested NOC outcomes
Acceptance: Health Status; Adaptation to Physical Disability; Decision Making; Depression Control; Hope; Quality of Life

Interventions and rationales
■ Follow medical regimen *to manage patient's physiologic condition and increase potential for patient's physiologic recovery.*
■ Allow specific amount of uninterrupted, non-care-related time each shift to talk with patient. If patient chooses not to talk, spend time in silence. *This time together establishes rapport with depressed patient even if patient talks little.*
■ Encourage patient to talk about personal assets and accomplishments and about improvements in condition, no matter how small. Give positive feedback.

Conversation helps you evaluate patient's self-concept and adaptive abilities; positive feedback reinforces patient's healthy perceptions.

■ Direct patient's focus beyond current state. For example, "Your nasogastric tube will come out tomorrow and you'll feel more comfortable." *This helps instill hope in a depressed patient with no time perspective.*

■ Encourage patient to identify enjoyable diversions and to participate in them. *Pleasurable activity decreases potential hazard of crisis situation.*

■ Keep patient informed of what to expect and when to expect it. *Accurate information reduces patient's anxiety.*

■ Involve patient and family members in care planning, and allow patient to choose degree of self-involvement. Begin by offering patient a choice between two alternatives. Increase alternatives as initiative improves. *Cognitive disturbances associated with anxiety or depression usually prevent patient from making healthy decisions.*

■ Use comfort measures (give back rub, dim room light, reduce noise level, and minimize procedures) in addition to prescribed sleep medication *to help induce sleep.*

■ Refer patient and family members to other caregivers (such as dietitian, social worker, clergy, and mental health clinical nurse specialist) or support groups (such as I Can Cope, Ostomy Support Group, and Reach For Recovery), as necessary. *These groups give patient chance to discuss illness with others similarly afflicted.*

■ Help patient mobilize resources before discharge, including contacting family and scheduling follow-up appointments with referral groups. *This helps give patient a sense of future direction.*

■ If not contraindicated medically, allow patient to use therapies practiced in his culture in conjunction with normal treatment *to increase his sense of control.*

Suggested NIC interventions

Coping Enhancement; Decision-Making Support; Energy Management; Mutual Goal Setting; Sleep Enhancement; Spiritual Growth Facilitation; Support Group

Evaluations for expected outcomes

■ Patient voices feelings of hopelessness.

■ Patient responds to questions and, at least once each day, participates in a conversation.

■ Patient sleeps at least 6 hours per night and remains awake during day, except for two rest periods.

■ Patient performs self-care measures and makes decisions related to care.

■ Patient engages in diversional activity (specify) at least twice daily.

■ Patient identifies factors that make him feel more hopeful (specify).

■ Patient seeks out help from social support groups and professional agencies.

Documentation

■ Patient's and family's knowledge of current condition

■ Patient's mental status

■ Patient's verbal and nonverbal behaviors

■ Interventions to increase patient's feelings of hope, self-worth, and initiative in self-care
■ Patient's and family's responses to nursing interventions
■ Evaluations for expected outcomes

Reference

Kronenwetter, C., et al. "A Qualitative Analysis of Interviews of Men with Early Stage Prostate Cancer: The Prostate Cancer Lifestyle Trial," *Cancer Nursing* 28(2):99-107, March-April 2005.

HOPELESSNESS

related to lost belief in transcendent values

Definition

Subjective state in which an individual sees few or no available alternatives or personal choices and can't mobilize energy on own behalf

Assessment

■ Nature of chronic illness
■ Patient's and family members' knowledge of illness
■ Mental status, including cognitive functioning, affect, mood, and stage in grieving process
■ Communication, including verbal (speech content, quality, and quantity), nonverbal (body positioning, eye contact, and facial expression), and quality of interactions with others
■ Nutritional status, including alteration in appetite or body weight
■ Motivation level, including personal hygiene, therapies (physical and occupational), use of diversional activities, and sense of control over current life situation
■ Developmental stage, including age and role in family
■ Disruption in usual roles and activities and losses (real and perceived)
■ Actual or perceived self-care deficits (specify)
■ Number and types of stressors
■ Coping mechanisms and decision-making ability
■ Support systems, including clergy, family, and friends
■ Spiritual values or religious beliefs

Defining characteristics

■ Decreased affect
■ Decreased appetite
■ Decreased response to stimuli
■ Decreased verbalization
■ Increased or decreased sleep
■ Lack of involvement in self-care
■ Nonverbal cues, such closing eyes, shrugging in response to questions, and turning away from speaker

■ Passivity and lack of initiative

■ Verbal cues, including sighing and despondent comments such as "I can't"

Expected outcomes

■ Patient will express feelings of hopelessness.

■ Patient will recognize and accept limitations of chronic illness.

■ Patient will work through stages of grieving.

■ Patient will develop coping mechanisms to deal with feelings of hopelessness.

■ Patient will recognize benefit of positive social interactions.

■ Patient will participate in self-care activities and in decisions regarding care planning.

■ Patient will resume and maintain as many former roles as possible.

■ Patient will regain and maintain self-esteem.

■ Patient will begin to develop feelings of hope.

Suggested NOC outcomes

Comfort Level; Coping; Decision Making; Depression Control; Depression Level; Hope; Mood Equilibrium; Quality of Life; Will to Live; Spiritual Health

Interventions and rationales

■ Assess for evidence of self-destructive behavior. *Assessment for suicide potential in a depressed patient is a nursing care priority.*

■ If possible, assign a primary nurse to patient *to encourage establishment of a therapeutic relationship between patient and nurse.*

■ Allow for specific amount of uninterrupted, non-care-related time each shift to talk with patient. Encourage verbal response with open-ended statements and questions. If patient chooses not to talk, spend time in silence. *This establishes rapport with depressed patient even if patient talks little.*

■ Provide for appropriate physical outlets for expression of feelings (punching bag, walking) *to help patient release hostilities, thereby decreasing tension and anxiety.*

■ Convey belief in patient's ability to develop and use coping skills *to increase patient's self-esteem and reduce feelings of dependence.*

■ Acknowledge patient's pain. Encourage patient to express feelings of depression, anger, guilt, and sadness. Convey to patient that all these feelings are appropriate. *This will help patient work through stages of coming to terms with chronic illness.*

■ Identify patient's strengths and encourage putting strengths to use *to maintain optimal functioning.*

■ Encourage patient's participation in self-care to fullest extent possible *to reduce feelings of helplessness.*

■ Help patient to participate in usual activities as strength, energy, and time permit *to maintain a sense of being connected to others.*

■ Encourage patient to identify enjoyable diversions and to participate in them *to decrease negative thinking and enhance self-esteem.*

■ Encourage positive thinking. Convey a sense of confidence in patient's ability to cope with illness *to promote an optimistic outlook.*

■ Provide positive reinforcement for patient's efforts to participate in self-care activities *to encourage patient to participate in self-care.* Encourage patient to establish self-care schedule *to enhance feelings of usefulness and control.*

■ Assist patient with hygiene and grooming needs *to help enhance patient's self-esteem.*

■ Offer patient and family a realistic assessment of situation, and communicate hope for immediate future. *This facilitates acceptance, helps promote patient safety and security, and allows planning of future health care.*

■ Encourage patient to identify spiritual needs and facilitate fulfillment of those needs *to help patient come to terms with chronic illness and its limitations.*

■ Involve patient and family members in care planning, and allow patient to choose degree of self-involvement on a continuing basis. Begin by offering patient a choice between two alternatives. Increase alternatives as initiative improves. *Cognitive disturbances associated with anxiety or depression usually prevent patient from making healthy decisions.*

■ Teach patient and family members how to manage illness, prevent complications, and control factors in the environment that affect patient's health. *Education enables family members to become resources in patient's care.*

■ Refer patient and family members to other caregivers (such as dietitian, social worker, clergyman, and mental health clinical nurse specialist) or support groups, as necessary. *Referrals to outside specialists ensure continuity of care. Support groups give patient chance to discuss illness with others similarly affected.*

Suggested NIC interventions
Coping Enhancement; Counseling; Decision-Making Support; Family Mobilization; Hope Instillation; Spiritual Growth Facilitation

Evaluations for expected outcomes
■ Patient talks about negative feelings instead of acting on them.

■ Patient expresses understanding of lifestyle changes imposed by chronic illness.

■ Patient discusses impact of illness and sees future realistically.

■ Patient demonstrates at least ___(specify) coping mechanisms.

■ Patient interacts with others and regains involvement in life experiences.

■ Patient demonstrates understanding that involvement in self-care is necessary to maintain optimal functioning.

■ Patient demonstrates involvement in as many former roles as possible.

■ Patient acknowledges a belief in himself and demonstrates increased energy and will to live.

■ Patient states that feelings of hopelessness are less frequent and expresses feelings of hope.

Documentation
■ Patient's perception of chronic illness

■ Patient's responses to treatment regimen

■ Patient's mental and emotional status (baseline and ongoing)

■ Patient education, counseling, and precautions taken to maintain or enhance patient's level of functioning

■ Interventions to help patient deal with daily stressors

- Interventions to protect patient from harming himself
- Patient's response to nursing interventions
- Evaluations for expected outcomes

Reference
Sun, F.K., et al. "A Theory for the Nursing Care of Patients at Risk of Suicide," *Journal of Advanced Nursing* 53(6):680-90, March 2006.

HYPERTHERMIA
related to increased metabolic rate

Definition
Elevation of body temperature above normal range

Assessment
- History of present illness
- History of exposure to communicable disease
- Health history, including chronic disease or disability, pathologic conditions known to cause dehydration, recent traumatic event, exposure to sources of infection, exposure to communicable diseases, and other related events
- Medications
- Physiologic manifestations of fever, including vital signs and skin temperature and color
- Fluid and electrolyte status, including skin turgor, intake and output, mucous membranes, serum electrolyte levels, and urine specific gravity
- Laboratory studies, including white blood cell count and culture and sensitivity findings
- Neurologic status, including level of consciousness (LOC) and orientation
- Skin integrity, including open lesions and rashes

Defining characteristics
- Fever
- Flushed, warm skin
- Increased heart and respiratory rate
- Seizures

Expected outcomes
- Patient will remain afebrile.
- Patient will maintain adequate hydration:
- Intake and output will be balanced and within normal limits.
- Urine specific gravity will range from 1.005 to 1.015.
- Patient will exhibit moist mucous membranes.
- Patient will exhibit good skin turgor.
- Patient will remain alert and responsive.

Suggested NOC outcomes

Comfort Level; Hydration; Infection Severity; Thermoregulation; Vital Signs

Interventions and rationales

■ Take temperature every 1 to 4 hours *to obtain an accurate core temperature.* Identify route and record measurements.

■ Administer antipyretics, as prescribed, and record effectiveness. *Antipyretics act on hypothalamus to regulate temperature.*

■ Use nonpharmacologic measures to reduce excessive fever, such as removing sheets, blankets, and most clothing; placing ice bags on axillae and groin; and sponging with tepid water. Explain these measures to patient. *Nonpharmacologic measures lower body temperature and promote comfort. Sponging reduces body temperature by increasing evaporation from skin. Tepid water is used because cold water increases shivering, thereby increasing metabolic rate and causing temperature to rise.*

■ Use a hypothermia blanket if patient's temperature rises above 103° F (39.4° C). Monitor vital signs every 15 minutes for 1 hour and then as indicated. Turn off blanket if shivering occurs. *Shivering increases metabolic rate, increasing temperature.*

■ Monitor heart rate and rhythm, blood pressure, respiratory rate, LOC and level of responsiveness, and capillary refill time every 1 to 4 hours *to evaluate effectiveness of interventions and monitor for complications.*

■ Determine patient's preferences for oral fluids, and encourage patient to drink as much as possible, unless contraindicated. Monitor and record intake and output, and administer I.V. fluids, if indicated. *Because insensible fluid loss increases by 10% for every 1.8° F (1° C) increase in temperature, patient must increase fluid intake to prevent dehydration.*

Suggested NIC interventions

Environmental Management; Fever Treatment; Fluid Management; Temperature Regulation

Evaluations for expected outcomes

■ Patient remains afebrile.

■ Patient maintains adequate hydration:

– Intake and output are balanced and within normal limit for age.

– Urine specific gravity ranges from 1.005 to 1.015.

■ Patient exhibits moist mucous membranes.

■ Patient exhibits good skin turgor.

■ Patient remains alert and responsive.

Documentation

■ Observations of physical findings

■ Nursing interventions and patient's response to interventions

■ Administration of medication, such as antipyretics, and patient's response

■ Evaluations for expected outcomes

Reference

Kayser-Jones, J. "Preventable Causes of Dehydration: Nursing Home Residents are Especially Vulnerable," *AJN* 106(6): 45, June 2006.

HYPOTHERMIA

related to exposure to cold or cold environment

Definition

State in which body temperature is reduced below normal range

Assessment

- History of present illness
- Circumstances surrounding development of hypothermia
- Age
- Medication history
- Neurologic status, including level of consciousness, mental status, motor status, and sensory status
- Cardiovascular status, including blood pressure, capillary refill time, electrocardiogram results, heart rate and rhythm, pulses (apical, peripheral), and temperature
- Respiratory status, including arterial blood gas analysis, breath sounds, and rate, depth, and character of respirations
- Integumentary status, including color, temperature, and turgor
- Nutritional status, including current (and normal) weight and dietary pattern
- Fluid and electrolyte status, including blood urea nitrogen level, intake and output, serum electrolyte levels, and urine specific gravity
- Psychosocial status, including behavior, financial resources, mood, and occupation

Defining characteristics

- Body temperature below normal range
- Cool, pale skin
- Cyanotic nail beds
- Increased blood pressure and heart rate
- Increased capillary refill time
- Piloerection
- Shivering

Expected outcomes

- Patient's body temperature will remain within normal range.
- Patient's skin will feel warm and dry.
- Patient's heart rate and blood pressure will remain within normal range.
- Patient won't shiver.
- Patient will express feelings of comfort.

■ Patient will show no complications associated with hypothermia, such as soft-tissue injury, fracture, dehydration, and hypovolemic shock, if warmed too quickly.

■ Patient will understand how to prevent further episodes of hypothermia.

Suggested NOC outcomes

Comfort Level; Neurological Status: Autonomic; Thermoregulation; Vital Signs

Interventions and rationales

■ Monitor body temperature at least every 4 hours or more frequently, if indicated, *to evaluate effectiveness of interventions.* Record temperature and route *to allow accurate data comparison.* Baseline temperatures vary, depending on route used. If temperature drops below 95° F (35° C), use a low-reading thermometer *to obtain accurate reading.*

■ Monitor and record neurologic status at least every 4 hours. *Falling body temperature and metabolic rate reduce pulse rate and blood pressure, which reduces blood perfusion to brain, resulting in disorientation, confusion, and unconsciousness.*

■ Monitor and record heart rate and rhythm, blood pressure, and respiratory rate at least every 4 hours. *Blood pressure and pulse decrease in hypothermia. During rewarming, patient may develop hypovolemic shock. During warming, ventricular fibrillation and cardiac arrest may occur, possibly signaled by irregular pulse.*

■ Provide supportive measures, such as placing patient in warm bed and covering with warm blankets, removing wet or constrictive clothing, and covering metal or plastic surfaces that contact patient's body. *These measures protect patient from heat loss.*

■ Follow prescribed treatment regimen for hypothermia:

– As ordered, administer medications *to prevent shivering to avoid overheating.* Monitor and record effectiveness.

– As ordered, administer analgesic *to relieve pain associated with warming.* Monitor and record effectiveness.

– Use hyperthermia blanket *to warm patient* if temperature drops below 95° F (35° C). Warm patient to 97° F (36.1° C).

– As appropriate, administer fluids during rewarming *to prevent hypovolemic shock.* If administering large volumes of I.V. fluids, consider using a fluid warmer *to avoid heat loss.*

■ Discuss precipitating factors with patient, if indicated. *Patient may require community outreach assistance with certain precipitating factors, including inadequate living conditions, insufficient finances, and abuse of medications (such as sedatives and alcohol).*

■ Instruct patient in precautionary measures to avoid hypothermia, such as dressing warmly even when indoors, eating proper diet, and remaining as active as possible. *Precautions help to prevent accidental hypothermia.*

Suggested NIC interventions

Comfort Level; Fluid Management; Hypothermia Treatment; Temperature Regulation; Vital Signs Monitoring

Evaluations for expected outcomes

- Patient's temperature remains within normal range.
- Patient's skin is warm and dry.
- Patient's heart rate and blood pressure remain within normal range.
- Patient doesn't shiver.
- Patient voices feelings of comfort.
- Patient doesn't develop complications associated with hypothermia.
- Patient describes measures to prevent further episodes of hypothermia.

Documentation

- Patient's shivering and complaints of coldness
- Observations of physical findings
- Nursing interventions and patient's response to interventions, including physiologic, behavioral, and cognitive
- Evaluations for expected outcomes

Reference

Good, K.K., et al. "Postoperative Hypothermia — The Chilling Consequences," *AORN Journal* 83(5):1055-66, May 2006.

Functional urinary
INCONTINENCE
related to impaired cognition

Definition

Inability of usually continent person to reach toilet in time to avoid unintentional loss of urine

Assessment

- History of mental illness
- Age
- Gender
- Vital signs
- Genitourinary status, including frequency and voiding pattern
- Fluid and electrolyte status, including blood urea nitrogen level, creatinine level, intake and output, mucous membranes, serum electrolyte levels, and skin turgor
- Neuromuscular status, including activities of daily living, mental status, mobility, and sensory ability to perceive bladder fullness
- Psychosocial status, including behavior before and after voiding, support from family members, impact of incontinence on himself and others, and stressors (family, job, and change in environment)

Defining characteristics

■ Amount of time needed to reach toilet exceeding length of time between sensing urge to void and uncontrolled voiding
■ Loss of urine before reaching toilet
■ May only be incontinent in morning
■ Able to empty bladder completely

Expected outcomes

■ Patient will void at appropriate intervals.
■ Patient won't void in unacceptable situations.
■ Patient will have minimal, if any, complications.
■ Patient and family members will demonstrate skill in managing incontinence.
■ Patient will discuss impact of incontinence on himself and family members.
■ Patient and family members will identify resources to assist with care following discharge.

Suggested NOC outcomes

Coordinated Movement; Self-Care: Toileting; Symptom Control; Urinary Continence; Urinary Elimination

Interventions and rationales

■ Monitor and record patient's voiding patterns *to ensure correct fluid replacement therapy.*
■ Assist with specific bladder elimination procedures, such as:
– bladder training. Place patient on commode or toilet every 2 hours while awake and once during night. *Successful bladder training revolves around adequate fluid intake, muscle-strengthening exercises, and carefully scheduled voiding times.*
– rigid toilet regimen. Place patient on toilet at specific intervals (every 2 hours or after meals). Note whether patient was wet or dry and whether voiding occurred at each interval. *This helps patient adapt to routine physiologic function.*
– behavior modification. Reward continence or voiding in lavatory. Don't punish unwanted behavior such as voiding in wrong place. Reinforce behavior consistently, using social or material rewards. *This helps patient learn alternatives to maladaptive behaviors.*
– use of external catheter. Apply according to established procedure and maintain patency. Observe condition of perineal skin and clean with soap and water at least twice daily. *This ensures effective therapy and prevents infection and skin breakdown.*
– application of protective pads and garments. Use only when interventions have failed *to prevent infection and skin breakdown and promote social acceptance.* Allow at least 4 to 6 weeks for trial period. *Establishing continence requires prolonged effort.*
■ Maintain continence based on patient's voiding patterns and limitations.
– Use reminders. *Reminders help limit amount of information patient must retain in his memory.*
– Orient patient to toileting environment: time, place, and activity. *A structured environment offers security and helps patient with elimination problems.*

– Stimulate patient's voiding reflexes (give patient drink of water while on toilet; stroke area over bladder; or pour water over perineum). *External stimulation triggers bladder's spastic reflex.*

– Provide hyperactive patient with distraction, such as a magazine, to occupy attention while on toilet. *This reduces anxiety and eases voiding.*

– Provide privacy and adequate time to void *to allow patient to void easily without anxiety.*

– Praise successful performance *to give patient a sense of control and to encourage compliance.*

– Change wet clothes *to accustom patient to dry clothes.*

– Teach family members and support personnel to assist, *thus reducing anxiety that results from noninvolvement and increasing chances for successful treatment.*

– Respond to patient's call light promptly *to avoid delays in voiding routine.*

– Choose patient's clothing to promote easy dressing and undressing. (For example, use Velcro fasteners and gowns instead of pajamas.) *This reduces patient's frustration with voiding routine.*

■ Schedule patient's fluid intake to encourage voiding at convenient times. Maintain adequate hydration up to 3,000 ml daily, unless contraindicated. *Scheduling fluid intake promotes regular bladder distention and optimal time intervals between voidings.* Limit fluid intake to 150 ml after dinner *to reduce need to void at night.*

■ Instruct patient and family members on continence techniques to use at home *to increase chances of successful bladder retraining.*

■ Encourage patient and family members to share feelings related to incontinence. *This allows specific problems to be identified and resolved. Attentive listening conveys recognition and respect.*

■ Refer patient and family members to psychiatric liaison nurse, home health care agency, or support group *to provide access to additional community resources.*

Suggested NIC interventions

Environmental Management; Pelvic Muscle Exercise; Prompted Voiding; Self-Care Assistance; Urinary Elimination Management; Urinary Habit Training

Evaluations for expected outcomes

■ Patient voids at appropriate intervals, with minimal episodes of incontinence.

■ Patient recognizes urge to void, undresses without assistance, and uses toilet.

■ Patient doesn't experience urinary tract infection, skin breakdown, or other complications related to incontinence.

■ Patient and family members demonstrate proper procedures for managing incontinence.

■ Patient expresses feelings about condition and its effect on family. Patient and family members are neither overwhelmed nor excessively optimistic about patient's condition.

■ Patient and family members contact support group or home health care agency, if needed.

Documentation

- Observations of incontinence and response to treatment regimen
- Interventions to provide supportive care and patient's response to supportive care
- Instructions given to patient and family members; return demonstration of knowledge and skills needed to carry out continence management techniques
- Patient's expression of concern about incontinence and motivation to participate in self-care
- Evaluations for expected outcomes

References

Dowd, T., and Dowd, E.T. "A Cognitive Therapy Approach to Promote Continence," *Journal of Wound, Ostomy, and Continence Nursing* 33(1):63-68, January-February 2006.

Zarowitz, B.J., and Ouslander, J.G. "Management of Urinary Incontinence in Older Persons," *Geriatric Nursing* 27(5):265-70, September-October 2006.

Reflex urinary
INCONTINENCE
related to sensory or neuromuscular impairment

Definition

Involuntary loss of urine, controlled by spinal cord reflex, occurring at somewhat predictable intervals when a specific bladder volume is reached

Assessment

- History of sensory or neuromuscular impairment
- History of urinary tract disease, trauma, surgery, or infection
- Genitourinary status, including bladder palpation, residual urine volume after voiding, urinalysis, urine characteristics, urine culture and sensitivity, and voiding patterns
- Neuromuscular status, including anal sphincter tone, motor ability to start and stop urine stream, neuromuscular function, sensory ability to perceive bladder fullness and voiding, and involuntary voiding after stimulation of skin on abdomen, thighs, or genitals
- Fluid and electrolyte status, including blood urea nitrogen level, creatinine level, intake and output, medication history, mucous membranes, serum electrolyte levels, skin turgor, and urine specific gravity
- Sexuality status, including capability, concerns, and habits
- Psychosocial status, including coping skills, self-concept, and perception of problem by patient and family members

Defining characteristics

- Complete emptying (with lesion above pontine micturition center) or incomplete emptying (with lesion above sacral micturition center) of bladder

- Either inability to sense full bladder, urge to void, or voiding, or ability to sense urge to void without ability to voluntarily inhibit bladder contraction
- Inability to voluntarily inhibit or initiate voiding
- Predictable pattern of voiding
- Sensations associated with full bladder (sweating, restlessness, and abdominal discomfort)

Expected outcomes

- Patient will maintain fluid balance, with intake approximately equaling output.
- Patient will have minimal, if any, complications.
- Patient will achieve urinary continence.
- Patient and family members will demonstrate skill in managing urinary incontinence.
- Patient will discuss impact of incontinence on himself and family.
- Patient and family members will identify resources to assist with care following discharge.

Suggested NOC outcomes

Knowledge: Treatment Regimen; Nutritional Status: Food & Fluid Intake; Tissue Integrity: Skin & Mucous Membranes; Urinary Continence; Urinary Elimination

Interventions and rationales

- Monitor intake and output *to ensure correct fluid replacement therapy.* Report output greater than intake.
- Implement and monitor effectiveness of specific bladder elimination procedure, such as:
- stimulating reflex arc. Patient who voids at somewhat predictable intervals may be able to regulate voiding by reflex arc stimulation. Trigger voiding at regular intervals (for example, every 2 hours) by stimulating skin of abdomen, thighs, or genitals to initiate bladder contractions. Avoid stimulation at nonvoiding times. Stimulate primitive voiding reflexes by giving patient water to drink while he sits on toilet or pouring water over perineum. *External stimulation triggers bladder's spastic reflex.*
- applying external catheter according to established procedure and maintaining patency. Observe condition of perineal skin and clean with soap and water at least twice daily. *Cleanliness prevents skin breakdown and infection. External catheter protects surrounding skin, promotes accurate output measurement, and keeps patient dry. Applying foam strip in spiral fashion increases adhesive surface and cuts risk of impaired circulation.*
- inserting indwelling catheter. Monitor patency and keep tubing free from kinks *to avoid drainage pooling and ensure accurate therapy.* Keep drainage bag below level of bladder *to avoid urine reflux into bladder.* Perform catheter care according to established procedure. Maintain closed drainage system *to prevent bacteriuria.* Secure catheter to leg (female) or abdomen (male) *to avoid tension on bladder and sphincter.*
- applying suprapubic catheter. Change dressing according to established procedure *to avoid skin breakdown.* Monitor patency and keep tubing free from kinks *to*

avoid drainage pooling in loops of catheter. Keep drainage bag below bladder level *to avoid urine reflux into bladder.* Maintain closed drainage system *to prevent bacteriuria.*

– changing wet clothes *to prevent patient from becoming accustomed to wet clothes.*

■ Encourage high fluid intake (3,000 ml daily, unless contraindicated) *to stimulate micturition reflex.* Limit fluid intake after 7 p.m. *to prevent nocturia.*

■ Instruct patient and family members on continence techniques to use at home. Have patient and family members return demonstrations until they can perform procedure well. *Patient education begins with assessment and depends on nurse's therapeutic relationship with patient and family.*

■ Encourage patient and family members to share feelings and concerns regarding incontinence. *A trusting environment allows nurse to make specific recommendations to resolve patient's problems.*

■ Refer patient and family members to psychiatric liaison nurse, home health care agency, support group, or other resources, as appropriate. *Community resources typically provide health care not available from other health agencies.*

Suggested NIC interventions

Pelvic Muscle Exercise; Urinary Bladder Training; Urinary Elimination Management; Urinary Incontinence Care

Evaluations for expected outcomes

■ Patient maintains fluid balance, with intake approximately equaling output.

■ Patient avoids complications associated with incontinence, such as infections, swelling of penis (because of external catheter), skin breakdown, catheter obstruction, and urine odor.

■ Patient achieves urinary continence.

■ Patient and family members successfully demonstrate chosen technique for bladder control.

■ Patient expresses both positive and negative feelings about condition. Patient can cope with dependence brought on by condition.

■ Patient and family members initiate contact with support group or visiting nurse.

Documentation

■ Observations of urologic condition and response to treatment regimen

■ Interventions to provide supportive care and patient's response

■ Instructions given to patient and family members; return demonstration of knowledge and skills needed to carry out continence management techniques

■ Patient's expression of concern about incontinence and its impact on body image and lifestyle; patient's motivation to participate in self-care

■ Evaluations for expected outcomes

Reference

Zarowitz, B.J., and Ouslander, J.G. "Management of Urinary Incontinence in Older Persons," *Geriatric Nursing* 27(5):265-70, September-October 2006.

Stress urinary
INCONTINENCE
related to weak pelvic musculature

Definition
Loss of urine (less than 50 ml) resulting from increased abdominal pressure

Assessment
- History of long-term use of tranquilizers, multiple pregnancies, prolonged or difficult labor, surgery, trauma, and vaginal infections
- Age
- Gender
- Vital signs
- Genitourinary status, including inspection of abdomen for scars from previous surgeries, rectal examination, vaginal examination, voiding pattern, and leakage of urine during sneezing, laughing, vomiting, coughing, defecating, physical exertion, or change from prone to upright position
- Fluid and electrolyte status, including creatinine level, blood urea nitrogen level, estrogen levels, intake and output, mucous membranes, serum electrolyte levels, and skin turgor
- Nutritional status, including appetite, dietary habits, and present weight
- Neuromuscular status, including degree of neuromuscular function, motor ability to start or stop urine stream, and sensory ability to perceive fullness
- Sexuality status, including capability, concerns, habits, and patterns
- Psychosocial status, including coping skills, self-concept, stressors (such as finances, family, and job), and perception of problem by family members

Defining characteristics
- Dribbling with increased abdominal pressure
- Frequency
- Urgency

Expected outcomes
- Patient will maintain continence.
- Patient will state increased comfort.
- Patient will state understanding of treatment.
- Patient will state understanding of surgical procedure.
- Patient and family members will demonstrate skill in managing urinary elimination problems.
- Patient and family members will identify resources to assist with care following discharge.

Suggested NOC outcomes
Comfort Level; Referral; Tissue Integrity: Skin & Mucous Membranes; Urinary Continence; Urinary Elimination

Interventions and rationales

■ Observe patient's voiding patterns, time of voiding, amount voided, and whether voiding is provoked by stimuli. *Accurate, thorough assessment forms basis of an effective treatment plan.*

■ Provide appropriate care for patient's urologic condition, monitor progress, and report patient's responses to treatment. *Patient expects to receive adequate care and to participate in decisions regarding care.*

■ Help patient to strengthen pelvic floor muscles by Kegel exercises for sphincter control. *Exercises increase muscle tone and restore cortical control.*

■ Promote patient's awareness of condition through education *to help patient understand illness as well as treatment.*

■ Help patient reduce intra-abdominal pressure by:
− losing weight
− avoiding heavy lifting
− avoiding chairs or beds that are too high or too low.
These measures reduce intra-abdominal pressure and bladder pressure.

■ Provide supportive measures:
− Respond to call bell quickly, assign patient to bed next to bathroom, put night-light in bathroom, and have patient wear easily removable clothing (gown rather than pajamas and Velcro fasteners rather than buttons or zippers). *Early recognition of problems promotes continence; easily removed clothing reduces patient frustration and helps achieve continence.*
− Provide privacy during toileting *to reduce anxiety and promote elimination.*
− Have patient empty bladder before meals, at bedtime, and before leaving accessible bathroom area *to promote elimination, avoid accidents, and help relieve intra-abdominal pressure.*
− Limit fluids to 150 ml after dinner *to reduce need to void at night.*
− Encourage high fluid intake, unless contraindicated, *to moisten mucous membranes and maintain hydration.*
− Suggest patient eat increased amount of salty food before going on a long trip (unless contraindicated). *Increased sodium decreases urine production.*
− Make protective pads available for patient's undergarments, if needed, *to absorb urine, protect skin, and control odors.*

■ If surgery is scheduled, give attentive, appropriate preoperative and postoperative instructions and care *to reduce patient's anxiety and build trust in caregivers.*

■ Encourage patient to express feelings and concerns related to urologic problems. *This helps patient focus on specific problem.*

■ Refer patient and family members to psychiatric liaison nurse, support group, or other resources, as appropriate. *Community resources typically provide health care not available from other health agencies.*

■ Alert patient and family members about need for toilet schedule. Prepare for discharge according to individual needs *to ensure that patient will receive proper care.*

Suggested NIC interventions

Pelvic Muscle Exercise; Teaching: Individual; Urinary Elimination Management; Urinary Habit Training; Urinary Incontinence Care

Evaluations for expected outcomes

■ Patient maintains continence.

■ Patient expresses satisfaction with progress in overcoming stress incontinence.

■ Patient expresses understanding of techniques to reduce intra-abdominal pressure and other supportive measures.

■ Patient explains surgical procedure, including risks and expected outcome.

■ Patient and family members demonstrate all procedures and supportive measures to enable patient to remain continent. They also make arrangements for home care, such as providing bedroom near bathroom and purchasing easily removable clothing.

■ Patient and family members contact appropriate community resources.

Documentation

■ Observations of urologic condition and patient's response to treatment regimen

■ Interventions to provide supportive care and patient's response to interventions

■ Instructions given to patient and family members on patient's urologic problem, their response to instructions, and demonstrated ability to carry out self-care management

■ Patient's expression of concern about urologic problem and its impact on body image and lifestyle

■ Patient's motivation to participate in self-care

■ Evaluations for expected outcomes

Reference

Anders, K. "Recent Developments in Stress Urinary Incontinence in Women," *Nursing Standard* 20(35):48-54, May 2006.

Total urinary
INCONTINENCE
related to neurologic dysfunction

Definition

Continuous and unpredictable passage of urine

Assessment

■ History of trauma, sensory or neuromuscular impairment, surgery, and congenital anomalies

■ Vital signs

■ Age

■ Gender

■ Genitourinary status, including palpation of bladder, previous bladder elimination procedures, urinalysis, urine characteristics, use of urinary assistive devices, and voiding pattern

■ Fluid and electrolyte status, including blood urea nitrogen level, creatinine level, intake and output, mucous membranes, skin turgor, and serum electrolyte levels

■ Neuromuscular status, including degree of neuromuscular function, motor ability to start or stop urine stream, and sensory ability to perceive bladder fullness

■ Sexuality status, including capability, concerns, and sexual partner

■ Psychosocial status, including patient's perception of health problem, coping skills, family, and self-concept

Defining characteristics

■ Constant flow of urine that occurs at unpredictable times without distention or uninhibited bladder contractions or spasms

■ Incontinence refractory to treatments

■ Lack of awareness of incontinence, perineal fullness, or bladder filling

■ Nocturia

Expected outcomes

■ Patient will maintain fluid balance, with intake approximately equaling output.

■ Patient will state increased comfort.

■ Patient will have minimal, if any, complications.

■ Patient will maintain continence with assistive devices.

■ Patient and family members will demonstrate skill in managing incontinence.

■ Patient and family members will discuss impact of incontinence on their lives.

■ Patient and family members will identify resources to assist with care following discharge.

Suggested NOC outcomes

Adaptation to Physical Disability; Referral; Symptom Control; Symptom Severity; Tissue Integrity: Skin & Mucous Membranes; Urinary Continence; Urinary Elimination

Interventions and rationales

■ Monitor patient's voiding pattern; document and report intake and output *to ensure correct fluid replacement therapy.*

■ Assist with specific bladder elimination devices, such as:

– external catheter. Apply according to established procedure and maintain patency. Avoid constriction. Observe condition of perineal area and clean with soap and water at least twice daily. Reusable penile sheaths are available for long-term use. *Cleanliness prevents skin breakdown or infection. External catheter protects surrounding skin, promotes accurate output measurement, and keeps patient dry. Applying foam strip in spiral fashion increases adhesive surface and cuts risk of impaired circulation.*

– indwelling catheter. Monitor patency and keep tubing free from kinks *to avoid drainage pooling and ensure accurate therapy.* Keep drainage bag below level of bladder *to avoid urine reflux into bladder.* Clean urinary meatus according to established procedure *to reduce risk of infection.* Maintain closed drainage system *to prevent bacteriuria.* Secure catheter to leg (female) or abdomen (male) *to avoid tension on bladder and sphincter.*

– suprapubic catheter. Monitor patency, change dressing, and clean catheter site according to established policy *to avoid skin breakdown.* Keep tubing free from kinks; keep drainage bag below level of bladder *to prevent urine reflux into bladder.* Maintain closed drainage system *to prevent bacteriuria.*

– body-worn appliances. These body-worn "urinals" fit over penis and have a drainage bag and waist and leg straps for body attachment *to protect skin and keep patient dry.* Selection depends on patient's self-help skills. Appliances need regular, careful washing *to protect skin and keep patient dry.*

– incontinence aids. As needed, provide patient with absorbent pad and pants with protective waterproof shield, a drip collector (an absorbent pouch that fits over penis), and absorbent pad that protects patient's bed. *These aids trap urine to keep it away from patient's skin.*

■ Disguise urine bag by placing it in shopping bag or tote bag *to enhance patient's self-image.*

■ Provide supportive measures:

– Regulate fluid intake on a specific schedule *to encourage voiding at convenient times.* Maintain adequate hydration up to 3,000 ml daily, unless contraindicated. Limit fluid intake to 150 ml after dinner *to reduce need to void at night.*

– Clothe patient to promote ease in dressing and undressing and to accommodate appliance. (For example, use Velcro fasteners and gowns rather than pajamas.) *Unwieldy clothing increases patient frustration with voiding routine.*

– Keep skin as clean and dry as possible *to promote skin integrity.* Treat urea burns by cleaning with mild soap and water.

■ Instruct patient and family members on continence techniques for home use. Provide for return demonstrations. *Patient education begins with assessment and depends on nurse's establishing therapeutic relationship with patient and family.*

■ Encourage patient and family members to share feelings and concerns related to incontinence. *A trusting environment allows nurse to make specific recommendations to resolve patient's problems.*

■ Refer patient and family members to psychiatric liaison nurse, home health care agency, support group, or other resources, as appropriate. *Community resources typically provide health care not available from other health agencies.*

Suggested NIC interventions

Environmental Management; Fluid Management; Perineal Care; Urinary Catheterization; Urinary Incontinence Care

Evaluations for expected outcomes

■ Patient takes in enough fluid to void approximately eight times each day.

■ Patient expresses increased comfort.

■ Patient has minimal, if any, complications.

■ Patient maintains continence, using assistive devices.

■ Before discharge, patient and family members demonstrate skill in managing incontinence.

■ Patient and family members discuss impact of incontinence on their lives.

■ Patient and family members identify two resources in community to assist with care following discharge.

Documentation
■ Observations of incontinence and response to treatment regimen
■ Interventions to provide supportive care and patient's response to interventions
■ Instructions given to patient and family members, their understanding of information, and their demonstrated ability to carry out continence management techniques
■ Patient's expressions of concern about incontinence and motivation to participate in self-care
■ Evaluations for expected outcomes

Reference
Milne, J.L., and Moore, K.N. "Factors Impacting Self-care for Urinary Incontinence," *Urologic Nursing* 26(1):41-51, February 2006.

Urge urinary
INCONTINENCE
related to decreased bladder capacity

Definition
Involuntary passage of urine occurring shortly after a strong sense of urgency to void

Assessment
■ History of stroke, urinary tract disease, spinal cord injury, surgery, or infection
■ Medication history
■ Vital signs
■ Genitourinary status, including cystometrogram, pain or discomfort, urinalysis, urine specific gravity, use of urinary assistive devices, and voiding pattern
■ Fluid and electrolyte status, including blood urea nitrogen level, creatinine level, intake and output, mucous membranes, postvoiding residual volume, skin turgor, and serum electrolyte levels
■ Neuromuscular status, including ambulation ability, degree of neuromuscular function, dexterity, and sensory ability to perceive fullness
■ Sexuality status, including capability, concerns, habits, and sexual partner
■ Psychosocial status, including coping skills, self-concept, stressors (such as finances, family, and job), and perception of health problem by patient and family members

Defining characteristics
■ Bladder contraction or spasm
■ Frequency
■ Inability to reach toilet in time
■ Increased or decreased volume

- Nocturia
- Urgency

Expected outcomes
- Patient will have fewer episodes of incontinence.
- Patient will state increased comfort.
- Patient will state understanding of treatment.
- Patient will have minimal, if any, complications.
- Patient will discuss impact of disorder on himself and family members.
- Patient and family members will demonstrate skill in managing incontinence.

Suggested NOC outcomes
Knowledge: Treatment Regimen; Self-Esteem; Tissue Integrity: Skin & Mucous Membranes; Treatment Behavior: Illness or Injury; Urinary Continence; Urinary Elimination

Interventions and rationales
- Observe voiding pattern; document intake and output. *This ensures correct fluid replacement therapy and provides information about patient's ability to void adequately.*
- Provide appropriate care for patient's urologic condition, monitor progress, and report patient's responses to treatment. *Patient should receive adequate care and take part in decisions about care as much as possible.*
- Provide supportive measures:
– Administer pain medication and monitor effectiveness. *Patient's knowledge that pain can be alleviated reduces tension and anxiety.*
– Prepare pleasant toilet environment that's warm, clean, and free from odors *to promote continence.*
– Place commode next to bed, or assign patient bed next to bathroom. *A bedside commode or convenient bathroom requires less energy expenditure than bedpan.*
– Keep bed and commode at same level *to facilitate patient's movements.*
– Provide good lighting from bed to bathroom *to reduce sensory misinterpretation.*
– Remove all obstacles between bed and bathroom *to reduce chance of falling.*
– Provide clock *to help patient maintain voiding schedule through self-monitoring.*
– Unless contraindicated, maintain fluids to 3,000 ml daily *to moisten mucous membranes and ensure hydration;* limit patient to 150 ml after dinner *to reduce need to void at night.*
– Have patient wear easily removable clothes (gown instead of pajamas and Velcro fasteners instead of buttons or zippers) *to reduce frustration and delay in voiding routine.*
– If patient loses control on way to bathroom, instruct patient to stop and take a deep breath. *Anxiety and rushing may strengthen bladder contractions.*
- Assist with specific bladder elimination procedures, such as:
– bladder training. Place patient on commode every 2 hours while awake and once during night. Provide privacy. Gradually increase intervals between toileting. *These measures aim to restore a regular voiding pattern.*

– rigid toilet regimen. Place patient on toilet at specific times. *This aids adaptation to routine physiologic function.* Keep baseline micturition record for 3 to 7 days *to monitor toileting effectiveness.*

■ Encourage patient to express feelings and concerns related to his urologic problem *to identify patient's fears.*

■ Explain urologic condition to patient and family members; include instructions on preventive measures and established bladder schedule. *Patient education begins with educational assessment and depends on establishing a therapeutic relationship with patient and family.* Prepare patient for discharge according to individual needs *to allow patient to practice under supervision.*

■ Instruct patient and family members on continence techniques for home use. *This reduces fear and anxiety resulting from lack of knowledge of patient's condition and reassures patient of continuing care.*

■ Refer patient and family members to psychiatric liaison nurse, support group, or other resources, as appropriate. *Community resources typically provide health care not available from other health agencies.*

Suggested NIC interventions
Bathing; Environmental Management; Fluid Monitoring; Perineal Care; Self-Care Assistance: Toileting; Urinary Elimination Management; Urinary Habit Training; Urinary Incontinence Care

Evaluations for expected outcomes
■ Patient maintains continence.
■ Patient expresses increased comfort.
■ Patient expresses understanding of treatment.
■ Patient doesn't experience nighttime incontinence or other complications.
■ Patient expresses feelings about condition.
■ Patient and family members discuss treatment of urologic condition and home bladder schedule; they also demonstrate necessary skills.

Documentation
■ Observations of urologic condition and patient's response to treatment regimen
■ Interventions to provide supportive care
■ Patient's response to nursing interventions
■ Instructions given to patient and family members on urologic problem, their response to instructions, and their demonstrated ability to carry out self-care management
■ Patient's expression of concern about urologic problem and its impact on body image and lifestyle; patient's motivation to participate in self-care
■ Evaluations for expected outcomes

Reference
Dingwall, L., and McLafferty, E. "Do Nurses Promote Urinary Continence in Hospitalized Older People?: An Exploratory Study," *Journal of Clinical Nursing* 15(10):1276-86, October 2006.

Risk for
INFECTION
related to external factors

Definition
At risk for being invaded by pathogenic organisms

Assessment
- Health history, including accidents, allergies, falls, hyperthermia, hypothermia, poisoning, seizures, trauma, and exposure to pollutants
- Sensory or perceptual changes (auditory, gustatory, kinesthetic, olfactory, tactile, and visual)
- Circumstances of present situation that could lead to infection
- Neurologic status, including level of consciousness, mental status, and orientation
- Laboratory studies, including clotting factors, hemoglobin level, hematocrit, platelet count, serum albumin level, white blood cell (WBC) count, and cultures of blood, body fluid, sputum, urine, and wound drainage

Risk factors
- Altered immune function
- Amniotic membrane rupture
- Chronic illness
- Drug use
- Environmental exposure to pathogens
- Invasive procedures
- Lack of knowledge about causes of infection
- Lack of primary (such as skin) or secondary (such as inflammatory response) defenses
- Malnutrition
- Tissue destruction
- Trauma

Expected outcomes
- Patient's temperature will stay within normal range.
- Patient's WBC count and differential will stay within normal range.
- Patient's cultures won't show evidence of pathogens.
- Patient will maintain good personal and oral hygiene.
- Patient's respiratory secretions will be clear and odorless.
- Patient's urine will remain clear, yellow, odorless, and free from sediment.
- Patient won't show evidence of diarrhea.
- Patient's wounds and incisions will appear clean, pink, and free from purulent drainage.
- Patient's I.V. sites won't show signs of inflammation.
- Patient won't show evidence of skin breakdown.
- Patient will take ___ ml of fluid and ___ g of protein daily.

■ Patient will state infection risk factors.

■ Patient will identify signs and symptoms of infection.

■ Patient will remain free from signs and symptoms of infection.

Suggested NOC outcomes

Immune Status; Infection Status; Knowledge: Treatment Procedure(s); Nutritional Status; Risk Control; Risk Detection; Wound Healing: Primary Intention

Interventions and rationales

■ Minimize patient's risk of infection by:

– washing hands before and after providing care. *Hand washing is the single best way to avoid spreading pathogens.*

– wearing gloves to maintain asepsis when providing direct care. *Gloves offer protection when handling wound dressings or carrying out various treatments.*

■ Monitor temperature at least every 4 hours and record on graph paper. Report elevations immediately. *Sustained temperature elevation after surgery may signal onset of pulmonary complications, wound infection or dehiscence, UTI, or thrombophlebitis.*

■ Monitor WBC count, as ordered. Report elevations or depressions. *Elevated total WBC count indicates infection. Markedly decreased WBC count may indicate decreased production resulting from extreme debilitation or severe lack of vitamins and amino acids. Any damage to bone marrow may suppress WBC formation.*

■ Culture urine, respiratory secretions, wound drainage, or blood according to facility policy and physician's order. *This identifies pathogens and guides antibiotic therapy.*

■ Help patient wash hands before and after meals and after using bathroom, bedpan, or urinal. *Hand washing prevents spread of pathogens to other objects and food.*

■ Assist patient when necessary to ensure that perianal area is clean after elimination. *Cleaning perineal area by wiping from area of least contamination (urinary meatus) to area of most contamination (anus) helps prevent genitourinary infections.*

■ Instruct patient to report incidents of loose stools or diarrhea. Inform physician immediately. *Diarrhea or loose stools may indicate need to discontinue or change antibiotic therapy. It may also indicate need to test for Clostridium difficile.*

■ Offer oral hygiene to patient every 4 hours to prevent colonization of bacteria and reduce risk of descending infection. *Disease and malnutrition may reduce moisture in mucous membranes of mouth and lips.*

■ Use strict sterile technique when suctioning lower airway, inserting indwelling urinary catheters, inserting I.V. catheters, and providing wound care *to avoid spreading pathogens.*

■ Change I.V. tubing and give site care every 24 to 48 hours or as facility policy dictates *to help keep pathogens from entering body.*

■ Rotate I.V. sites every 48 to 72 hours or as facility policy dictates *to reduce chances of infection at individual sites.*

■ Have patient cough and deep-breathe every 4 hours after surgery *to help remove secretions and prevent pulmonary complications.*

■ Provide tissues and disposal bags for expectorated sputum. *Convenient disposal encourages expectoration; sanitary disposal reduces spread of infection.*

■ Help patient turn every 2 hours. Provide skin care, particularly over bony prominences, *to help prevent venous stasis and skin breakdown.*

■ Use sterile water for humidification or nebulization of oxygen. *This prevents drying and irritation of respiratory mucosa, impaired ciliary action, and thickening of secretions within respiratory tract.*

■ Encourage fluid intake of 3,000 to 4,000 ml daily, unless contraindicated, *to help thin mucus secretions.*

■ Ensure adequate nutritional intake. Offer high-protein supplements, unless contraindicated. *This helps stabilize weight, improves muscle tone and mass, and aids wound healing.*

■ Arrange for protective isolation if patient has compromised immune system. Monitor flow and number of visitors. *These measures protect patient from pathogens in environment.*

■ Teach patient about:
– good hand-washing technique
– factors that increase infection risk
– signs and symptoms of infection.

   These measures allow patient to participate in care and help patient modify lifestyle to maintain optimum health.

Suggested NIC interventions

Incision Site Care; Infection Protection; Teaching: Procedure/Treatment; Wound Care

Evaluations for expected outcomes

■ Patient's temperature remains within normal range.
■ Patient's WBC count and differential remain within normal range.
■ Patient's cultures don't exhibit pathogen growth.
■ Patient demonstrates appropriate personal and oral hygiene.
■ Patient's respiratory secretions remain clear and odorless.
■ Patient's urine remains clear, yellow, odorless, and free from sediment.
■ Patient's bowel patterns remain normal.
■ Patient's incisions or wounds remain clear, pink, and free from purulent drainage.
■ Patient's I.V. sites don't show signs of inflammation.
■ Patient's skin doesn't exhibit signs of breakdown.
■ Patient's fluid and protein intake remains at specified levels.
■ Patient lists risk factors for infection.
■ Patient lists signs and symptoms of infection.
■ Patient remains free from signs and symptoms of infection.

Documentation

■ Temperature
■ Dates, times, and sites of all cultures
■ Dates, times, and sites of all catheter insertions
■ Appearance of all invasive catheter sites, tube sites, and wounds

- Interventions performed to reduce infection risk
- Patient's response to nursing interventions
- Evaluations for expected outcomes

Reference
Marrs, J.A. "Care of Patients with Neutropenia," *Clinical Journal of Oncology Nursing* 10(2):164-66, April 2006.

Risk for
INFECTION
related to surgical incision

Definition
At risk for being invaded by pathogenic organisms

Assessment
- Age, gender, weight
- Type of surgery, reason for surgery
- Anticipated length of surgery
- Mobility status
- Current health status, including vital signs, nutritional status, and integumentary status
- Laboratory studies, including hematocrit and hemoglobin level, complete blood count, electrolyte studies, urinalysis, blood cultures, blood coagulation studies, immunologic and serologic tests, and liver function tests
- Presence of infection (urinary, respiratory, or oral)
- Health history, including drug allergies, recent infection, substance abuse, and chronic metabolic or systemic disease (diabetes mellitus; cardiovascular, hepatic, or renal disease; coagulation disorders; and splenic or bone marrow disorders)
- Current medical treatments, including radiation therapy, chemotherapy, antibiotic or antifungal therapy, steroid treatment, anticoagulant or thrombolytic therapy, and immunosuppressive therapy
- Presence of invasive devices, including indwelling urinary catheter, endotracheal tube, tracheostomy tube, I.V. lines, central venous and arterial lines, drains, and gastric feeding tubes
- Wound classification (clean, clean-contaminated, contaminated, or dirty)

Risk factors
- Altered immune function
- Amniotic membrane rupture
- Chronic illness
- Drug use
- Environmental exposure to pathogens
- Invasive procedures
- Lack of knowledge about causes of infection

■ Lack of primary (such as skin) or secondary (such as inflammatory response) defenses
■ Malnutrition
■ Tissue destruction
■ Trauma

Expected outcomes

■ Patient's vital signs and laboratory values will remain within normal limits.
■ Patient's incision site will remain free from signs and symptoms of infection.
■ Patient's won't experience dehiscence.

Suggested NOC outcomes

Immune Status; Infection Severity; Wound Healing: Secondary Intention

Interventions and rationales

■ Document and report results of preoperative nursing assessment. Identify risk factors predisposing patient to infection. *A complete nursing assessment allows development of an individualized care plan.*
■ Make sure all surgical team members wear appropriate operating room attire. *The human body is a major source of microbial contamination.*
■ Inspect operating room for cleanliness before opening supplies and instruments *to provide a safe environment.*
■ Perform a surgical hand scrub. Put on sterile gown and gloves. Place sterile drapes on patient, furniture, and equipment. *Surgical hand scrub minimizes number of microorganisms on skin. Sterile gown and gloves protect against contamination. Sterile drapes create sterile field.*
■ Check package integrity, chemical indicator, and, if appropriate, expiration date on all sterile items before dispensing them onto sterile field. *All items used within field must be sterile or field will become contaminated.*
■ Closely monitor sterile field and initiate corrective measures when a break in technique occurs. *Contamination of sterile field may lead to wound contamination and subsequent infection.*
■ Use proper technique when opening items onto sterile field *to avoid contamination.*
■ Perform preoperative skin preparation of surgical site. *Skin preparation reduces resident microbial count to subpathogenic amounts and inhibits rapid rebound growth of microbes.*
■ Keep operating room doors closed at all times and minimize traffic in and out. *Air turbulence caused by movement and mixing of corridor air with room air can sharply increase bacterial counts in operating room.*
■ Maintain room temperature of 68° to 75° F (20° to 23.9° C) and relative humidity at 50% + 10, unless contraindicated. *Cooler air temperature and lower humidity inhibit microbial growth.*
■ Classify surgical wound according to degree of contamination of wound and surrounding tissue. *Classification helps to assess risk of wound infection from an endogenous source and determine need for antibiotic therapy.*

■ Wash hands following contact with patient or any object contaminated with blood or body fluids. *Hand washing is the most effective means for preventing microbial transmission.*

■ Administer antibiotics, as ordered. *Intraoperative administration of antibiotics can decrease incidence of wound infection and lessen its severity.*

■ Disinfect and sterilize all instruments and equipment before and immediately after surgical procedure. All instruments and equipment used during surgery must be free from microorganisms. *Sterilizing instruments and equipment after use prevents growth and spread of microorganisms during storage.*

■ Promptly clean areas outside sterile field that become contaminated by blood, tissue, or body fluids with an approved disinfectant *to prevent distribution of microbes into environment.*

■ Apply sterile dressing to surgical wound before removing surgical drapes *to avoid wound contamination and subsequent infection.*

Suggested NIC interventions

Infection Control; Infection Protection; Nutrition Therapy; Wound Care

Evaluations for expected outcomes

■ Patient's oral temperature remains below 100° F (37.8° C). Postoperative vital signs and laboratory values (especially white blood cell count) are consistent with preoperative values.

■ Patient's incision site remains free from erythema, edema, undue tenderness, warmth, induration, foul odor, purulent drainage, and other signs and symptoms of infection.

■ Patient's wound edges are approximated, and evidence of dehiscence is absent.

Documentation

■ Results of preoperative nursing assessment
■ Operative procedure
■ Type of anesthesia
■ Surgical times (time patient entered operating room, time incision was made, time incision was closed, and time patient left operating room)
■ Wound classification
■ Intraoperative administration of antibiotics
■ Presence of packing, drains, indwelling urinary catheter, or other invasive devices
■ Intraoperative insertion of permanent or temporary implants
■ Type of wound closure method
■ Type of dressing applied
■ Estimated intraoperative blood loss
■ Evaluations for expected outcomes

Reference

Haycock, C., et al. "Implementing Evidence-Based Practice Findings to Decrease Postoperative Sternal Wound Infections Following Open Heart Surgery," *The Journal of Cardiovascular Nursing* 20(5):299-305, September-October 2005.

| Risk for |
| **INJURY** |
| related to lack of awareness of environmental hazards |

Definition
At risk for injury as a result of environmental conditions interacting with the individual's adaptive and defensive resources

Assessment
- Age
- Health history, including accidents, falls, and exposure to environmental hazards
- Environmental factors, including household layout, electrical wiring, lighting, utilities, fire precautions, presence of toxic or noxious substances, medications, special safety needs, and childproofing
- Mental status, including mood, affect, thought processes, thought content, orientation, judgment, and ability to perform activities of daily living
- Knowledge level, including understanding of household safety precautions and automobile safety
- Participation in recreational activities, such as swimming, diving, motorcycling, bicycling, and contact sports

Risk factors
- Mode of transportation
- Physical (design structure of home environment)
- Nutrients
- Abnormal blood profile
- Altered mobility
- Confusion
- Disorientation
- Exposure to biological or chemical hazards
- Malnutrition
- Skin breakdown

Expected outcomes
- Patient and family will acknowledge presence of environmental hazards in their everyday surroundings.
- Patient and family will take safety precautions in and out of home.
- Adults in household will instruct children in safety habits.
- Adults in household will childproof house to ensure safety of young children and cognitively impaired adults.

Suggested NOC outcomes
Immune Status; Risk Control; Safety Behavior: Home Physical Environment; Safety Behavior: Personal; Safety Status: Physical Injury

Interventions and rationales

■ Help patient identify situations and hazards that can cause accidents *to increase patient's awareness of potential dangers.*

■ Encourage patient to make repairs and remove potential safety hazards from environment *to decrease possibility of injury.*

■ Encourage adults to discuss safety rules with children. For example:
– Don't play with matches.
– Use electrical equipment carefully.
– Know location of fire escape route.
– Don't speak to strangers.
– Dial 911 in an emergency.
Teaching by parents fosters household safety.

■ Arrange environment of patient with dementia to minimize risk of injury:
– Place furniture against walls.
– Don't use throw rugs.
– Maintain lighting so that patient can find his way around room and to bathroom.
Arranging patient's environment helps prevent injury.

■ Refer patient to appropriate community resources for more information about identifying and removing safety hazards. *This enables patient and family to alter environment to achieve optimal safety level.*

Suggested NIC interventions

Environmental Management; Fall Prevention; Health Education; Surveillance: Safety

Evaluations for expected outcomes

■ Patient and family identify and eliminate safety hazards in their surroundings.
■ Patient and family members demonstrate prevention and safety precautions.
■ Children describe safety measures they have learned.
■ Patient and family point out evidence of childproofing measures in home.

Documentation

■ Patient's statements about situations that cause accidents and injuries
■ Patient's lack of awareness of, or disregard for, safety hazards
■ Patient's cognitive deficits that inhibit learning or attention to safety hazards
■ Interventions to help patient recognize and eliminate safety hazards
■ Patient's or family's response to nursing interventions
■ Evaluations for expected outcomes

References

Bright, L. "Strategies to Improve the Patient Safety Outcome Indicator: Preventing or Reducing Falls," *Home Healthcare Nurse* 23(1):29-36, January 2005.

Yuan, J.R., & Kelly, J. "Falls Prevention, or "I Think I Can, I Think I Can": An Ensemble Approach to Falls Management," *Home Healthcare Nurse* 24(2):103-11, February 2006.

| Risk for |
| **INJURY** |
| related to sensory or motor deficits |

Definition
At risk for injury as a result of environmental conditions interacting with the individual's adaptive and defensive resources

Assessment
- Age
- Nature of sensory or motor deficit
- Pain or fatigue
- Health history, including cerebral function, mobility, sensory function, and use of adaptive devices
- Psychological status, including substance abuse, familiarity with surroundings, mental status, coping skills, and self-concept
- Medication history and use, including understanding of medications, compliance with prescribed regimen, use of over-the-counter medications, and interactions
- Knowledge level, including understanding of safety precautions
- Laboratory studies, including complete blood count and differential and coagulation studies
- Diagnostic tests, including chest X-ray and brain scan
- Sensory status, including hearing, vision, touch, and taste

Risk factors
- Abnormal blood profile
- Altered mobility
- Confusion
- Disorientation
- Exposure to biological or chemical hazards
- Malnutrition
- Skin breakdown

Expected outcomes
- Patient will identify factors that increase potential for injury.
- Patient will help identify and apply safety measures to prevent injury.
- Patient and family members will develop strategy to maintain safety.
- Patient will optimize activities of daily living within sensorimotor limitations.

Suggested NOC outcomes
Immune Status; Risk Control; Safe Home Environment: Personal Safety Behavior: Fall Prevention

Interventions and rationales

■ Observe for factors that may cause or contribute to injury *to increase awareness of patient, family members, and caregivers.*

■ Improve environmental safety, as needed:

– Orient patient to environment. Assess patient's ability to use call bell, side rails, and bed positioning controls. Keep bed at lowest level, and conduct close night watch. *These measures will help patient cope with unfamiliar surroundings.*

– Teach patient and family about need for safe illumination. Advise patient to wear sunglasses to reduce glare. Advise using contrasting colors in household furnishings. *These measures will enhance visual discrimination.*

– Test heating pads and bath water before using; assess extremities daily for injury *to assist patient with decreased tactile sensitivity.*

– For patient with hearing loss, encourage use of hearing aid *to minimize deficit.*

– Teach patient with unstable gait correct use of adaptive devices *to decrease potential for injury.*

■ Provide additional patient teaching, as needed. Possible topics may include household, automobile, and pedestrian safety. Refer patient to appropriate resources (police, fire, and home health care agency) for more information. *Health education can help patient take steps to prevent injury.*

Suggested NIC interventions

Environmental Management: Safety; Fall Prevention; Health Education; Home Maintenance Assistance; Surveillance: Safety

Evaluations for expected outcomes

■ Patient identifies two factors that increase risk of injury.

■ Patient applies safety measures.

■ Patient and family members describe and demonstrate preventive measures to minimize potential for injury.

■ Patient increases self-care activities within limits posed by sensorimotor limitations.

Documentation

■ Statements by patient and family members about potential for injury due to sensory or motor deficits

■ Manifestations of deficit

■ Observation or knowledge of unsafe practices

■ Interventions to decrease risk of injury to patient

■ Patient's responses to nursing interventions

■ Evaluations for expected outcomes

Reference

McCullagh, M.C. "Home Modification," *AJN* 106(10):54-63, October 2006.

Risk for perioperative-positioning
INJURY

Definition
At risk for inadvertent anatomical and physical changes as a result of posture on equipment used during an invasive/surgical procedure

Assessment
- Reason for surgery
- Type of surgery and its expected length
- Health status, including age, weight, vital signs, nutritional status, integumentary status, musculoskeletal status, hydration status, temperature, peripheral vascular status, neurologic status, and smoking history
- Laboratory studies, including hematocrit and hemoglobin levels, complete blood count, electrolyte levels, urinalysis, blood coagulation studies, and liver function tests
- Mobility status, including range of motion (ROM), presence of prosthesis, and limb abnormality, impairment, or injury
- Current medical treatments, including radiation therapy, chemotherapy, and steroid therapy

Risk factors
- Disorientation
- Edema
- Emaciation
- Immobilization
- Muscle weakness
- Obesity
- Sensory-perceptual disturbances from anesthesia

Expected outcomes
- Patient will maintain effective breathing patterns.
- Patient will maintain adequate cardiac output.
- Patient's surgical positioning will facilitate gas exchange.
- Patient won't show evidence of neurologic, musculoskeletal, or vascular compromise.
- Patient will maintain tissue integrity.

Suggested NOC outcomes

Blood Coagulation; Circulation Status; Cognitive Orientation; Neurological Status; Respiratory Status: Ventilation; Thermoregulation; Tissue Integrity: Skin & Mucous Membranes; Tissue Perfusion: Peripheral

Interventions and rationales

■ Document and report the results of the preoperative nursing assessment. Identify factors predisposing patient to tissue injury. *This information guides interventions.*

■ Use the appropriate mode of patient transportation (stretcher, patient bed, wheelchair, or crib) *to ensure patient safety.*

■ Make sure an adequate number of staff members assist with transferring patient—at least two for moving patient onto an operating room bed and at least four for moving anesthetized patient off operating room bed. *Adequate staffing enhances safety.*

■ Check the operating room bed before surgery for proper functioning. *Intraoperative bed malfunction can result in increased anesthesia time and a more difficult surgical approach.*

■ Ensure proper positioning.

Supine position

– Check patient's neck and spine for proper alignment *to avoid trauma.*

– Check that patient's legs are straight and ankles uncrossed. *Crossed ankles cause pressure on tissue, vessels, and nerves.*

– Place a safety strap 2″ (5 cm) above patient's knees, tight enough to restrain without compromising superficial venous return. *Applied too tightly, the safety strap may cause venous thrombosis or compression of tibial, peroneal, or sciatic nerves.*

– Secure patient's arms at his sides with a drawsheet, with palms down, making sure no part of the arm or hand extends over the mattress. Alternatively, secure his arms on padded arm boards at less than a 90-degree angle from his body, with palms supinated. *Hyperextension can cause injury to the brachial plexus. Supination of palms minimizes pressure.*

– Apply eye pads if patient's eyelids won't remain closed or if surgery is being performed on his head, neck, or chest. If allowed to remain open, the eye may dry out and become infected. *Corneal abrasions may result from drapes and other foreign material rubbing against the eye.*

– If surgery is expected to last more than 2 hours or if patient is predisposed to a pressure injury, place padding under his occiput, scapulae, olecranon, sacrum, coccyx, and calcaneus *to protect potential pressure points.* Apply a padded footboard *to support patient's feet, avoid plantar flexion, and prevent stretching of the tibial nerve and subsequent footdrop.*

– Unless contraindicated, place a foam doughnut or small pillow under patient's head *to prevent stretching of the neck muscles.*

Prone position

– Make sure at least four staff members assist when turning patient *to ensure safety.*

– Place a foam doughnut or small pillow under patient's head. Check the lower eye and ear for excessive pressure. Apply eye pads. *Head support helps maintain cervical and thoracic spine alignment. Checking the dependent ear and eye lowers the risk of pressure injury. Pads protect the eyes.*

– Place patient's arms on arm boards extended in front beside his head with the elbows slightly flexed and palms pronated *to prevent strain on the shoulder, elbows, and wrist joints.*

– Check for proper alignment of the neck and spine *to avoid trauma.*

– Check a female patient's breasts and male patient's genitalia for excessive pressure from chest rolls or a laminectomy brace *to avoid soft-tissue and nerve injury.*

– Check the bilateral pulses of upper and lower extremities. *The top and bottom edges of chest rolls or a laminectomy brace may compress radial and femoral arteries.*

– Place padding under patient's knees *to avoid injury to soft tissue and knee joint.*

– Place a pillow under patient's ankles *to avoid putting pressure on toes and feet, stretching the tibial nerve, or causing plantar flexion.*

– Place a safety strap 2″ above patient's knees, securely but not too tightly, *to restrain patient without compromising superficial venous return.*

– If surgery is expected to last more than 2 hours or if patient is predisposed to a pressure injury, place padding under his acromion process, olecranon, and anterior iliac spine *to protect pressure points.*

Lateral position

– Make sure at least four staff members assist when turning patient *to ensure safety.*

– Check patient's neck and spine for proper alignment *to avoid trauma.*

– Place a foam doughnut or small pillow under patient's head. Check his dependent eye and ear for excessive pressure. Apply eye pads. *Head supports help maintain cervical and thoracic spine alignment. Checking the dependent ear and eye lowers the risk of pressure injury. Pads protect patient's eyes.*

– Place a small roll under patient's dependent lower axilla t*o relieve pressure on chest and axilla, allow for adequate chest expansion, and prevent compression of the brachial plexus by the humeral head.*

– Place patient's lower arm on arm board at less than 90-degree angle from his body, with palm supinated. Place his upper arm on an elevated padded support at less than a 90-degree angle from his body, with palm pronated, and apply restraints *to avoid injury to brachial plexus.*

– Place his bottom leg flexed at the hip and knee and the top leg straight. *Flexing the bottom leg provides greater stability for the torso, decreases pressure on the lateral aspect of the lower leg, and prevents the bony areas of the knees and ankles from pressing against each other.*

– Place pillows between patient's knees and ankles *to support his top leg, prevent strain on the top hip, and pad pressure points on the medial aspects of both legs.*

– Place padding under the lateral aspects of patient's bottom knee and ankle *to reduce the risk of tissue injury to the area over the lateral malleolus of the ankle and peroneal nerve damage (footdrop).*

– Place a safety strap across patient's upper thighs or wide tape over his hips. Attach a strap or tape to the bed *to ensure safety.*

– If surgery is expected to last more than 2 hours or if patient is predisposed to a pressure injury, place padding under his acromion process, ilium, and greater trochanter *to protect pressure points.*

Lithotomy position
– Secure patient's arms on arm boards or at his sides. If his arms are placed at his sides, position his fingers away from the break in the table *to prevent the fingers from becoming compressed in the bed mechanism.*
– Check patient's neck and spine for proper alignment *to avoid trauma.*
– Position the stirrups at equal height and attach them to the bed securely to prevent accidental movement. *Uneven leg flexion and hip abduction can cause strain on the lumbar and sacral areas.*
– Place the loop straps of the post stirrup behind patient's ankle and under his foot. Pad the post portion of the stirrup if it could come in contact with his leg. *Loop straps support and secure the legs.*
– Pad popliteal knee support stirrups *to prevent possible thrombosis of superficial vessels and pressure injury to femoral and obturator nerves.*
– If surgery is expected to last more than 2 hours or if patient is predisposed to a pressure injury, place padding under his occiput, scapulae, olecranon, and sacrum *to protect potential pressure points.*
– With the help of a coworker, raise and lower patient's legs simultaneously and slowly *to prevent ankle and knee injury and hip dislocation. Lowering legs too quickly may cause sudden hypotension.*
■ Assess patient position following each positional change *to ensure proper body alignment and adequate padding and support.*
■ Apply restraints after positioning patient *to prevent falls and injury.*

Suggested NIC interventions

Aspiration Precautions; Bleeding Reduction: Wound; Circulatory Care: Arterial Insufficiency; Circulatory Care: Venous Insufficiency; Embolus Care: Pulmonary; Fluid Management; Hemodynamic Regulation; Infection Control: Intraoperative; Positioning: Intraoperative; Skin Surveillance; Surgical Precautions; Temperature Regulation: Intraoperative

Evaluations for expected outcomes
■ Patient maintains effective breathing patterns. Patient's position doesn't restrict ventilation. Patient has adequate chest expansion.
■ Patient maintains adequate cardiac output. Patient doesn't experience any significant episodes of hypertension or hypotension.
■ Patient's positioning allows for adequate gas exchange, as evidenced by patient's ventilation-perfusion ratio and oxygen saturation.
■ Patient shows no evidence of neurologic, musculoskeletal, or vascular compromise. Patient's mobility status and ROM remain at preoperative levels. Patient doesn't experience pain, numbness, tingling, or weakness in positioned body parts.
■ Patient's tissue integrity remains intact; skin doesn't become reddened, discolored, ulcerated, edematous, or excoriated.

Documentation
■ Results of preoperative nursing assessment
■ Operative procedure, type of anesthesia, and surgical positioning

- Surgical times, including time patient entered operating room, time incision was made, time incision was closed, and time patient left operating room
- Method of patient transport and transfer
- Estimated intraoperative blood loss
- Types and placement of padding, restraints, and positional devices
- Intraoperative repositioning of patient
- Intraoperative insertion of permanent or temporary implants
- Peripheral pulses
- Evaluations for expected outcomes

Reference
Millsaps, C.C. "Pay Attention to Patient Positioning!" *RN* 69(1):59-63, January 2006.

INSOMNIA
related to anxiety

Definition
A disruption in the amount and quality of sleep that impairs functioning

Assessment
- Age
- Daytime activity and work patterns
- Normal bedtime
- Number of hours of sleep patient usually needs to feel rested
- Problems associated with sleep, including early morning awakening, difficulty falling and staying asleep, nightmares, and sleepwalking
- Quality of sleep
- Sleeping environment
- Activities associated with sleep, including bath, drink, food, and medication
- Personal beliefs about sleep

Defining characteristics
- Observed changes in affect
- Observed lack of energy
- Increased work or school absenteeism
- Reports changes in mood
- Reports decreased health status
- Reports decreased quality of life
- Reports difficulty concentrating
- Reports difficulty falling asleep
- Reports difficulty staying asleep
- Reports dissatisfaction with sleep (current)
- Reports early morning awakening
- Reports nonrestorative sleep
- Reports sleep disturbances that produce next-day consequences

Expected outcomes

- Patient will identify factors that prevent or disrupt sleep.
- Patient will sleep ___ hours a night.
- Patient will express feeling well rested.
- Patient won't show physical signs of sleep deprivation.
- Patient won't exhibit sleep-related behavioral symptoms, such as restlessness, irritability, lethargy, and disorientation.
- Patient will perform relaxation exercises at bedtime.

Suggested NOC outcomes

Anxiety Level; Anxiety Self-Control; Medication Response; Personal Well-Being; Rest; Sleep; Stress Level

Interventions and rationales

- Allow patient to discuss any concerns that may be preventing sleep. *Active listening helps you determine causes of difficulty with sleep.*
- Plan nursing care routines to allow _____ hours of uninterrupted sleep. *This allows consistent nursing care and gives patient uninterrupted sleep time.*
- Provide patient with usual sleep aids, such as pillows, bath before sleep, food or drink, and reading materials. *Milk and some high-protein snacks, such as cheese and nuts, contain L-tryptophan, a sleep promoter. Personal hygiene and prebedtime rituals preceed and promote sleep in many patients.*
- Create quiet environment conducive to sleep; for example, close curtains, adjust lighting, and close door. *These measures promote rest and sleep.*
- Administer medications that promote normal sleep patterns, as ordered. Monitor and record adverse effects and effectiveness. *Hypnotic agents induce sleep; tranquilizers reduce anxiety.*
- Promote involvement in diversional activities or exercise program during day. Discuss and relate exercise and activity to improved sleep. Discourage excessive napping. *Activity and exercise promote sleep by increasing fatigue and relaxation.*
- Ask patient to describe in specific terms each morning the quality of sleep during the previous night. *This helps detect sleep-related behavioral symptoms.*
- Educate patient in such relaxation and stress-reducing techniques, such as guided imagery, progressive muscle relaxation, aromatherapy, relaxation music, and meditation. *Purposeful relaxation efforts usually help promote sleep.*

Suggested NIC interventions

Calming Technique; Coping Enhancement; Energy Management; Medication Management; Positioning; Simple Relaxation Therapy; Sleep Enhancement

Evaluations for expected outcomes

- Patient identifies factors that prevent or disrupt sleep.
- Patient sleeps specified number of hours nightly.
- Patient expresses feeling well rested.
- Patient doesn't exhibit signs of sleep deprivation.
- Patient doesn't exhibit sleep-related behavioral symptoms.

■ Patient performs relaxation exercises at bedtime.

Documentation
■ Patient's complaints about sleep disturbances
■ Patient's report of improvement in sleep patterns
■ Observations of physical and behavioral sleep-related disturbances
■ Interventions to alleviate sleep disturbances
■ Patient's response to nursing interventions
■ Evaluations for expected outcomes

Reference
Turkoski, B.B. "Managing Insomnia," *Orthopedic Nursing* 25(5):339-45, September-October 2006.

INSOMNIA
related to unfamiliar sleep surroundings, noise, light

Definition
A disruption in the amount and quality of sleep that impairs functioning

Assessment
■ Daytime activity and work patterns
■ Travel history
■ Normal bedtime
■ Detailed sleep history, including number of hours of sleep required
■ Problems associated with sleep, including early morning awakening, difficulty falling and staying asleep, nightmares, and sleepwalking
■ Quality of sleep
■ Sleeping environment
■ Activities associated with sleep
■ Personal beliefs about sleep
■ Chemical ingestion, including alcohol, caffeine, hypnotics, and nicotine
■ Use of herbal or dietary products used to facilitate sleep
■ Any illness or injury related to lack of sleep

Defining characteristics
■ Observed changes in affect
■ Observed lack of energy
■ Increased work or school absenteeism
■ Reports changes in mood
■ Reports decreased health status
■ Reports decreased quality of life
■ Reports difficulty concentrating
■ Reports difficulty falling asleep
■ Reports difficulty staying asleep

- Reports dissatisfaction with sleep (current)
- Reports early morning awakening
- Reports nonrestorative sleep
- Reports sleep distrubances that produce next-day consequences

Expected outcomes

- Patient will identify factors that prevent or promote sleep.
- Patient will sleep ___ hours without interruption.
- Patient will express feeling well rested.
- Patient won't show physical signs of sleep deprivation.
- Patient will alter diet and habits to promote sleep, such as reducing caffeine and alcohol intake before bedtime.
- Patient won't exhibit sleep-related behavioral symptoms, such as restlessness, irritability, lethargy, and disorientation.
- Patient will perform relaxation exercises at bedtime.

Suggested NOC outcomes

Anxiety Level; Fear Level; Mood Equilibrium; Personal Well-Being; Rest; Sleep

Interventions and rationales

- Ask patient what environmental factors make sleep difficult. *Sleeping in strange or new environment tends to influence both REM and non-REM sleep.*
- Ask patient what changes would promote sleep *to allow patient to take an active role in treatment.*
- Make whatever immediate changes are possible to accommodate patient; for example, reduce noise pollution, change lighting, and close door. *These measures promote rest and sleep.*
- Plan medication administration schedules to allow for maximum rest. If patient requires diuretics in the evening, give far enough in advance *to allow peak effect before bedtime. Other medications that may interfere with sleep include beta-adrenergic blockers, MAO inhibitors, and phenytoin.*
- Make a detailed plan to provide patient with a set number of hours of uninterrupted sleep, if possible. *This allows consistent nursing care and gives patient uninterrupted sleep time.*
- Provide patient with usual sleep aids, such as pillows, bath before sleep, food or drink, and reading materials. *Milk and some high-protein snacks, such as cheese and nuts, contain L-tryptophan, a sleep promoter. Personal hygiene and prebedtime rituals preceed and promote sleep in many patients.*
- Ask patient to keep a sleep log describing sleep disturbances and the impact on daytime functioning, such as with cognition, mood, coping skills, and physical complaints. *This allows increased awareness of potential sleep distrubances.*
- Ask patient to describe in specific terms each morning the quality of sleep during the previous night. *This helps detect the presence of sleep-related behavioral symptoms.*
- Teach patient such relaxation techniques as guided imagery, meditation, aromatherapy, and progressive muscle relaxation. Practice them with patient at bedtime. *Purposeful relaxation efforts usually help promote sleep.*

■ Instruct patient to eliminate or reduce caffeine and alcohol intake and avoid foods that interfere with sleep (for example, spicy foods). *Foods and beverages containing caffeine consumed fewer than 4 hours before bedtime may interfere with sleep. Alcohol disrupts normal sleep, especially when ingested immediately before retiring.*

Suggested NIC interventions

Biofeedback; Calming Technique; Coping Enhancement; Energy Management; Security Enhancement; Simple Relaxation Therapy; Sleep Enhancement

Evaluations for expected outcomes

■ Patient describes factors that prevent or promote sleep.
■ Patient sleeps specified number of hours without interruption.
■ Patient expresses feeling well rested.
■ Patient shows no physical signs of sleep deprivation.
■ Patient reports changing diet habits and making lifestyle changes to promote sleep.
■ Patient doesn't exhibit sleep-related behavioral symptoms.
■ Patient performs relaxation exercises at bedtime.

Documentation

■ Patient's complaints about sleep disturbances
■ Patient's verbalization of feelings about sleep
■ Observations of behavior that indicate sleep deprivation
■ Interventions to alleviate sleep disturbance
■ Patient's response to nursing interventions
■ Evaluations for expected outcomes

Reference

Holcomb, S.S. "Recommendations for Assessing Insomnia," *The Nurse Practitioner* 31(2):55-60, February 2006.

Decreased
INTRACRANIAL ADAPTIVE CAPACITY

Definition

A state in which physiologic mechanisms that normally compensate for increased intracranial volumes are compromised, resulting in disproportionate increases in intracranial pressure (ICP) in response to stimuli

Assessment

■ Cardiovascular status, including vital signs, skin color and temperature, carotid and apical pulses, heart sounds, jugular vein distention, electrocardiography, and history of hypertension

■ GI status, including bowel elimination patterns, dietary intake, and abdominal inspection, palpation, and auscultation

■ Musculoskeletal status, including range of motion (ROM); joint and muscle symmetry; muscle size, strength, and tone; functional mobility; contractures, subluxation, dislocation, and atrophy; previous trauma; and degenerative joint diseases

■ Neurologic status, including mental status; cranial nerve function; cerebellar function; reflexes (deep tendon, superficial, and pathologic [Babinski's reflex]); peripheral sensory system (pain, position, and vibration); pupillary size and reactivity; use of anticonvulsant, neuroleptic, antidepressant, antimanic, analgesic, or illicit drugs; history of head injury; alcohol abuse; history of lethargy, restlessness, stupor, headaches, seizures, tremors, paresthesia, paresis, incoordination, ticks, fasciculation, pain, psychiatric disorders, or abnormal posturing (decorticate or decerebrate); and tests such as computed tomography scan, magnetic resonance imaging, cerebral arteriography, EEG, evoked potential studies, and Glasgow Coma Scale

■ Respiratory status, including chest expansion; rate, depth, and pattern of respirations; tracheal position; fremitus; auscultation of lung fields; arterial blood gas (ABG) analysis, pulse oximetry, and mixed venous oxygen saturation; history of lung disease; tobacco use; and use of bronchodilators, antibiotics, or diuretics

■ Sensory status, including visual and auditory acuity, use of hearing aid or eye glasses, tactile sensitivity eye disorders, and hearing loss

Defining characteristics

■ Baseline ICP equal to or greater than 10 mm Hg; wide amplitude ICP waveform

■ Disproportionate increase in ICP following single nursing maneuver

■ Elevated P2 ICP waveform

■ Repeated increases in ICP exceeding 10 mm Hg for more than 5 minutes following external stimuli

■ Volume pressure response test variation (volume-pressure ratio greater than 2, pressure-volume index less than 10)

Expected outcomes

■ Patient will maintain patent airway, effective breathing patterns, and normal ABG levels.

■ Patient will show no evidence of fever.

■ Patient's position will promote venous drainage from brain.

■ Patient won't experience sustained rise in ICP in response to stimulation.

■ Patient's environment will be modified to reduce noxious stimuli.

■ Patient will maintain regular bowel function.

■ Patient will maintain skin integrity.

■ Patient will remain free from signs and symptoms of infection.

■ Patient won't show evidence of neurologic compromise.

■ Patient and family members will express feelings about treatment and recovery.

Suggested NOC outcomes

Electrolyte & Acid-Base Balance; Fluid Balance; Neurological Status; Neurological Status: Consciousness; Wound Healing: Primary Intention

Interventions and rationales

■ Perform thorough nursing history and head-to-toe assessment and document *to establish baseline of patient's condition for future comparison and to ensure continuity and consistency of care among nursing staff.*

■ Monitor neurologic status, including level of consciousness, pupillary size and reactivity, eye movement, selected reflexes, and motor and sensory function *to identify changes that indicate increased ICP.*

■ Monitor vital signs and hemodynamic parameters (mean arterial blood pressure and pulmonary artery pressure) *to assess hemodynamic stability and to note trends.*

■ Maintain ICP monitoring systems, if used. Use sterile technique for dressing changes. Maintain closed system. *Sterile technique prevents contamination of equipment and subsequent infections.*

■ Monitor ICP waveforms for trends over time (A waves, B waves, C waves). Assess intracranial pulse waves (P1 percussion waves, P2 tidal waves, P3 dicrotic waves). Monitor for damped waveforms, absent waveforms, or abnormally high or low readings. *Waveforms provide information about cerebral compliance. Cerebral compliance is the body's attempt to cope with changes in intracranial content (brain tissue, blood volume, and cerebral spinal fluid). Compliance is expressed as a mathematic ratio between volume and pressure changes within the skull.*

■ Assess cerebral perfusion pressure. *Adequate cerebral perfusion pressure is critical to prevent cerebral ischemia.* Cerebral perfusion pressure is calculated by taking mean arterial pressure and subtracting ICP.

■ Assess temperature every 2 hours. *Fever increases cerebral metabolic demands, cerebral blood flow, and ICP.*

■ Maintain patent airway. Assess rate, depth, and rhythm of respirations *to monitor lung expansion and presence of abnormal sounds.*

■ Suction patient only if needed. Limit suctioning to 10 to 15 seconds per pass of catheter. *Suctioning stimulates coughing and Valsalva's maneuver; Valsalva's maneuver increases intrathoracic pressure, decreases cerebral venous drainage, and increases cerebral blood volume, resulting in increased ICP.*

■ Administer 100% oxygen for 1 minute before and after suctioning. Hypercapnia results in cerebral vasodilation, increased cerebral blood volume, and increased ICP. *Giving supplemental oxygen helps avoid hypoxemia and tissue ischemia.*

■ Administer lidocaine, if prescribed, I.V. or into endotracheal (ET) tube before suctioning. *Lidocaine suppresses cough reflex, thereby preventing increases in ICP.*

■ Monitor ABG levels. Observe for signs and symptoms of respiratory distress. *Hypercapnia results in vasodilation, increased cerebral blood volume, and increased ICP. Hypoxia may contribute to tissue ischemia.*

■ Elevate head of bed 15 to 30 degrees or as ordered. Keep patient's head and neck straight. Use sandbags, rolled towels, or small pillows to keep head in neutral position. Avoid hip flexion of 90 degrees or more. *Neutral head position promotes venous drainage from head. Some positions cause increased intra-abdominal and intrathoracic pressure that can interfere with venous drainage from head.*

■ When performing neurologic assessment, use minimal amount of stimuli required to obtain a response. *Unpleasant or painful stimuli increase ICP.*

■ Limit environmental noise as much as possible. *Auditory stimuli can contribute to increased ICP.*

■ Monitor for seizure activity. Maintain seizure precautions. Administer anticonvulsant drugs, as prescribed. *Tonic-clonic seizures increase intrathoracic pressure, decrease cerebral venous outflow, and increase cerebral blood volume, thereby raising ICP.*

■ Maintain intake and output. Maintain fluid restriction, if ordered. *Fluid restriction helps decrease extracellular fluid, thereby decreasing ICP.*

■ Administer osmotic diuretics, if prescribed. Monitor for signs and symptoms of dehydration (increased sodium, serum osmolality, and decreased urine output). *Osmotic diuretics pull fluid from nonedematous areas of brain, thereby decreasing ICP.*

■ Administer loop diuretics, if prescribed, *to decrease water in injured brain tissue and to decrease overall body water, thereby reducing cerebral edema and lowering ICP.* Monitor for signs of dehydration and hypokalemia, which are adverse effects of diuretics.

■ Turn and reposition patient every 2 hours and as needed *to prevent pressure ulcer formation.*

■ While turning, keep patient's head in neutral position *to promote venous drainage from head.*

■ Use a draw sheet to reposition patient. Instruct patient to exhale, if conscious, when turning or moving in bed *to avoid Valsalva's maneuver, which can increase ICP by increasing intrathoracic and intra-abdominal pressures.*

■ Monitor and record bowel movements. Administer stool softeners, as prescribed. Instruct patient not to hold his breath or strain on defecation. *Straining associated with constipation can cause Valsalva's maneuver, thereby increasing ICP.*

■ Instruct patient, if he can follow simple commands, to avoid pushing against footboard or digging heels into mattress when moving up in bed. Remove footboard if possible, especially if patient has decerebrate or abnormal posturing. *Isometric muscle contraction can increase ICP.*

■ Perform passive ROM exercises *to maintain muscle tone and prevent atrophy and contractures.*

■ Maintain normothermia. Administer antipyretics if ordered. Apply hypothermia blanket. Assess rectal temperature every 30 minutes while patient is on blanket. Control shivering. Administer chlorpromazine, if prescribed. *Shivering causes isometric muscle contraction, which can increase ICP.*

■ Continue frequent neurologic assessment. Compare results with previous findings. *Frequent assessment allows detection of subtle changes in neurologic signs that indicate improvement or deterioration in patient's status.*

■ Try to limit painful procedures, if possible. Avoid unnecessary tension or pulling on tubes (such as ET tube or indwelling urinary catheter). *Unpleasant or painful stimuli increase ICP.*

■ Involve family members in gentle stroking of patient's face, hand, or arm. *Touch provided by family members may lower ICP in some patients.*

■ Speak in a low, soft voice. Provide nursing care in calm, reassuring manner. Explain all procedures before touching patient. *Explanations can help prevent emotional upsets that may increase ICP.*

■ Avoid discussion of upsetting topics near patient's bedside. Patient may be upset by discussion of his prognosis, treatment procedures, or his level of pain. Instruct patient's family members not to discuss upsetting topics within patient's hearing range. *Emotional upsets may increase ICP.*

■ Ask family members to bring in audiotapes of familiar voices and patient's favorite music. Play audiotapes through earphones if appropriate. *Family members' voices and preferred music have been shown to decrease ICP in some patients.*

■ Provide uninterrupted rest periods as much as possible. Avoid awakening patient during rapid eye movement (REM) sleep. *Cerebral blood flow increases during REM sleep.* Don't carry out nursing activities known to increase ICP during that time. *Nursing procedures performed during REM sleep may cause additional elevations in patient's ICP.*

■ Schedule sufficient time, at least 10 minutes, between nursing care activities (such as bathing, turning, and suctioning) *to allow patient to rest and to avoid cumulative effects of continuous activity on ICP.* Close spacing of activities has been known to cause sustained increases of ICP.

■ Encourage patient and family to express feelings associated with diagnosis, treatment, and recovery. *Expression of feelings helps patient and family cope with treatment.*

■ Refer patient and family to appropriate support groups *to assist them in dealing with the injury, diagnosis, or recovery.*

Suggested NIC interventions

Acid-Base Management; Bedside Laboratory Testing; Cerebral Edema Management; Fluid-Electrolyte Management; Intracranial Pressure (ICP) Monitoring; Respiratory Monitoring

Evaluations for expected outcomes

■ Patient maintains effective breathing patterns, patent airway, and normal ABG levels.

■ Patient shows no evidence of fever.

■ Patient maintains proper positioning to promote venous drainage from brain.

■ Patient shows no evidence of sustained increase in ICP in response to stimulation.

■ Patient's environment contains fewer noxious stimuli as a result of modifications.

■ Patient is free from constipation.

■ Patient has intact skin.

■ Patient has no signs or symptoms of infection.

■ Patient shows no evidence of neurologic compromise.

■ Patient and family members openly express fear, anxiety, anger, and other feelings associated with treatment and recovery.

Documentation
- Results of initial nursing assessment
- Monitoring procedures and results
- Nursing interventions and patient's response
- Instructions to patient, family, or caregiver and their demonstrated understanding of those instructions
- Evaluations for expected outcomes

Reference
Littlejohns, L., and Bader, M.K. "Prevention of Secondary Brain Injury: Targeting Technology," *AACN Clinical Issues* 16(4):501-14, October-December 2005.

Deficient
KNOWLEDGE
related to cognitive limitation

Definition
Absence or deficiency of cognitive information related to a specific subject

Assessment
- Psychosocial status, including age, learning ability (affective, cognitive, and psychomotor domains), decision-making ability, developmental stage, financial resources, interest in learning, knowledge and skills related to current health problem, obstacles to learning, support systems (willingness and ability of others to help patient), and usual coping pattern
- Neurologic status, including level of consciousness, memory, mental status, and orientation

Defining characteristics
- Inability to follow through with instruction
- Inability to perform well on test
- Inappropriate or exaggerated behaviors (hysteria, hostility, agitation, apathy)
- Verbalization of problem

Expected outcomes
- Patient will demonstrate ability to perform simple self-care measures, such as feeding, maintaining hygiene, dressing, and toileting.
- Family members will communicate understanding of patient's cognitive impairment.
- Family members will express willingness to help patient maintain maximum independence.
- Family members will demonstrate method being used to teach patient.

Suggested NOC outcomes

Cognition; Concentration; Information Processing; Knowledge: Disease Process; Knowledge: Health Behaviors; Knowledge: Health Resources; Knowledge: Illness Care; Stress Level

Interventions and rationales

■ Provide all equipment needed for each self-care measure patient must learn. *This reduces frustration, aids learning, and minimizes dependence by promoting self-care.*

■ When teaching self-care measures, go slowly and repeat frequently. Offer small amounts of information and present it in various ways. *By building cognition, patient will be better able to complete self-care measures.*

■ Have patient practice each task. Provide positive reinforcement each time patient performs task correctly. *This encourages desired behavior.*

■ Discuss patient's limitations with family members. *Communication promotes working relationship and reduces fear and anxiety.*

■ Demonstrate to family members how each self-care measure is broken down into simple tasks *to enhance patient's success and foster sense of control.*

■ Encourage family members to participate in patient's learning process *to help create an encouraging, therapeutic climate after discharge.*

■ Have family members give return demonstration of patient's methods of performing self-care measures. *This provides hands-on experience with equipment, builds confidence, and encourages compliance.*

■ Refer family members to outside agencies, such as a home health care organization, for assistance after patient's discharge. *This ensures continuity of care and assistance with follow-up after discharge.*

Suggested NIC interventions

Behavior Management; Behavior Modification; Decision-Making Support; Energy Management; Family Support; Health Education; Learning Facilitation; Support System Enhancement

Evaluations for expected outcomes

■ Patient practices simple self-care measures and demonstrates ability to perform activities of daily living.

■ Family members describe cause of patient's cognitive impairment.

■ Family members demonstrate willingness to help patient learn to perform self-care measures.

■ Family members provide return demonstration of patient's methods of performing self-care measures.

Documentation

■ Patient's abilities and limitations in performing self-care measures

■ Progress made by patient in learning each specific task

■ Information given to family members concerning patient's limitations and progress in learning tasks

■ Family members' participation in learning process

- Referrals to outside agencies
- Evaluations for expected outcomes

Reference

Shen, Q., et al. "Evaluation of a Medication Education Program for Elderly Hospital In-patients," *Geriatric Nursing* 27(3):184-92, May-June 2006.

Deficient
KNOWLEDGE
related to lack of exposure

Definition
Absence or deficiency of cognitive information related to a specific topic

Assessment
- Psychosocial status, including age, learning ability (affective, cognitive, and psychomotor domains), decision-making ability, developmental stage, financial resources, health beliefs and attitudes, interest in learning, knowledge and skill regarding current health problem, obstacles to learning, support systems (willingness and ability of others to help patient), and usual coping pattern
- Neurologic status, including level of consciousness, memory, mental status, and orientation

Defining characteristics
- Inability to follow through with instruction
- Inability to perform well on test
- Inappropriate or exaggerated behaviors (hysteria, hostility, agitation, apathy)
- Verbalization of problem

Expected outcomes
- Patient will communicate need to know.
- Patient will state or demonstrate understanding of what has been taught.
- Patient will demonstrate ability to perform new health-related behaviors as they're taught and will list specific skills and realistic target dates for each.
- Patient will set realistic learning goals.
- Patient will state intention to make needed changes in lifestyle, including seeking help from health professional, when needed.

Suggested NOC outcomes

Client Satisfaction: Teaching; Concentration; Knowledge: Diet; Knowledge: Disease Process; Knowledge: Energy Conservation; Knowledge: Health Behaviors; Motivation

Interventions and rationales

■ Establish environment of mutual trust and respect to ⌐
fort with growing self-awareness, ability to share this awar⌐
tiveness to new experiences, and consistency between actio⌐
trusting relationship.

■ Negotiate with patient to develop goals for learning. ⌐
ning meaningful goals encourages follow-through.

■ Select teaching strategies (such as discussion, demon⌐
visual materials) appropriate for patient's individual le⌐
hance teaching effectiveness.

■ Teach skills that patient must incorporate into daily ⌐
return demonstration of each new skill to help gain co⌐

■ Have patient incorporate learned skills into daily routine during hospitalization
(specify skills). This allows patient to practice new skills and receive feedback.

■ Provide patient with names and telephone numbers of resource people or organizations to provide continuity of care and follow-up after discharge.

■ As needed, arrange for interpreter. Patient who doesn't speak English may understand health-related behaviors but may need interpreter to express them.

Suggested NIC interventions

*Behavior Modification; Discharge Planning; Health Education; Learning
Readiness Enhancement; Teaching: Prescribed Diet*

Evaluations for expected outcomes

■ Patient expresses desire to overcome lack of knowledge.
■ Patient states understanding of what he has learned.
■ Patient demonstrates newly learned health-related behaviors.
■ Patient develops realistic learning goals and performs new skills by target date.
■ Patient identifies specific changes in lifestyle needed to promote optimal health.

Documentation

■ Patient's statements of information and skills he knows and doesn't know
■ Expressions of need to know and motivation to learn
■ Learning objectives
■ Methods used to teach patient
■ Information imparted
■ Skills demonstrated
■ Patient's responses to teaching
■ Evaluations for expected outcomes

Reference

Toth, P.E. "Ostomy Care and Rehabilitation in Colorectal Cancer," *Seminars in
Oncology Nursing* 22(3):174-77, August 2006.

Deficient

KNOWLEDGE

related to lack of interest in learning

Definition

Absence or deficiency of cognitive information related to a specific topic

Assessment

■ Psychosocial status, including age, learning ability (affective, cognitive, and psychomotor domains), decision-making ability, developmental stage, financial resources, interest in learning, knowledge and skills related to current health problem, obstacles to learning, support systems (willingness and ability of others to help patient), and usual coping pattern

■ Neurologic status, including level of consciousness, memory, mental status, and orientation

Defining characteristics

■ Inability to follow through with instruction

■ Inability to perform well on test

■ Inappropriate or exaggerated behaviors (hysteria, hostility, agitation, apathy)

■ Verbalization of problem

Expected outcomes

■ Patient will express interest in learning new behaviors.

■ Patient will gradually set realistic learning objectives (specify).

■ Patient will strive to meet each objective by target date.

■ Patient will practice new health-related behaviors during hospitalization (for example, selecting appropriate diet, self-medicating, weighing self daily, and monitoring intake and output).

■ Patient will develop realistic plan for maintaining new skills at home.

Suggested NOC outcomes

Client Satisfaction: Teaching; Cognition; Knowledge: Diabetes Management; Knowledge: Disease Process; Knowledge: Health Behavior; Memory; Motivation

Interventions and rationales

■ Provide uninterrupted time for patient to state reasons for not wanting to learn or practice new health-related behaviors. *Attentive listening conveys caring attitude, encouraging patient to talk.*

■ Avoid nonconstructive criticism. Rather, encourage expression of feelings. *Nonjudgmental approach encourages patient to express feelings more freely.*

■ Ascertain what patient knows to determine what patient needs to know. *Building on known information leads to successful learning.*

■ Explore with patient impact of behavior on self and family members. *Learning is more effective if patient recognizes need to know.*

■ Urge patient to ask questions *to help clarify information and evaluate patient's comprehension.*

■ Determine whether patient enjoys learning through such media as videotapes, audiotapes, books, and discussions *to discover most effective teaching tools.*

■ Begin negotiating learning objectives with patient. *Involving patient in defining goals increases understanding and encourages compliance.*

■ Be patient; offer praise when patient attempts new behaviors *to motivate patient to learn more.*

■ Provide emotional support as patient attempts to perform distasteful or anxiety-producing behaviors. *Support will help patient perform tasks successfully.*

■ Suggest that patient discuss situation with someone who has developed skill in managing a similar health problem *to encourage patient to air feelings and concerns.*

■ Help patient plan realistically for continuing new behaviors; include teaching family members, as needed. *Setting realistic goals increases probability of compliance. Involving others adds support after discharge.*

Suggested NIC interventions

Active Listening; Family Support; Health Education; Learning Readiness Enhancement; Self-Responsibility Facilitation; Support Group; Values Clarification

Evaluations for expected outcomes

■ Patient expresses desire to change behavior.
■ Patient participates in developing educational goals.
■ Patient displays motivation to attain each goal by target date.
■ Patient practices new health-related behaviors.
■ Patient states plans for inclusion of new activities into daily routine after discharge.

Documentation

■ Statements of motivation or lack of interest in learning
■ Observations that indicate readiness or lack of readiness to learn
■ Goals set by patient
■ Methods used to teach patient
■ Information imparted
■ Skills demonstrated
■ Patient's responses to trying new behaviors
■ Evaluations for expected outcomes

Reference

Eldh, A.C., et al. "Conditions for Patient Participation and Non-participation in Health Care," *Nursing Ethics* 13(5):503-14, September 2006.

Sedentary

LIFESTYLE

related to physical deconditioning

Definition
Habit of life that's characterized by a low physical activity level

Assessment
- Age, gender, cognitive status
- Daytime activity and work patterns
- Possible precipitating factors
- Height, weight, body mass index (BMI), and muscle and weight bearing
- Underlying conditions or medications
- Overall quality and duration of sleep
- Situational daily stressors
- Nutritional status and opportunity for exercise and social interaction
- Convenience of exercise facilities and safety of environment
- Recent changes in health status or lifestyle
- Dietary and medication history
- Culturally determined expectations of body image or dietary intake
- Risk assessment for substance abuse, smoking, and high-risk behaviors
- Disabilities

Defining characteristics
- Daily routine lacking physical exercise
- Physical deconditioning
- Preference for activities low in physical activity

Expected outcomes
- Older adult will maintain independent living status with reduced risk for falling.
- Patient will identify barriers to increasing physical activity level.
- Patient will identify health benefits to increasing physical activity level.
- Patient will increase physical activity and limit inactive forms of diversion, such as television and computer games.
- Patient will seek professional consultation to develop an appropriate plan to increase physical activity.
- Patient will identify factors that enhance readiness for sleep.
- Patient will demonstrate readiness for enhanced sleep through the use of appropriate sleep hygiene measures.
- Patient's amount of sleep and rapid-eye-movement (REM) sleep will be congruent with developmental needs.
- Patient will express a feeling of being rested after sleep.
- Patient will increase lean muscle and bone strength and decrease body fat.
- Patient will demonstrate weight control and, if appropriate, weight loss.

■ Patient will demonstrate enhanced psychological well-being and reduced risk of depression.

■ Patient will have reduced depression and anxiety and an improved mood.

■ Patient with certain chronic, disabling conditions will have increased ability to perform activities of daily living.

Suggested NOC outcomes

Activity Intolerance; Adherent Behavior; Client Satisfaction: Teaching; Endurance; Energy Conservation; Health-promoting Behavior; Immobility Consequences: Physiological and Psycho-cognitive; Knowledge: Diet; Knowledge: Rest; Knowledge: Risk Control; Knowledge: Sleep

Interventions and rationales

■ Provide counseling tailored to patient's risk factors, needs, preferences, and abilities *to enhance emotional well-being and motivation for physical activity.*

■ Discuss behavioral risk factors in lack of motivation to increase physical activity, such as ingestion of carbohydrates, caffeine, nicotine, alcohol, sedatives, and hypnotics, and fluid intake, *to focus behavior on positive outcomes of increased physical activity.*

■ Instruct patient to keep a daily activity and dietary log *to help him achieve a more objective view of his behavior.*

■ Identify barriers and enhancers to increasing physical activity, including time management, access to facilities, and safe environments in which to be active. *Breaking down barriers and building opportunities for activity increases the probability of consistent physical activity.*

■ Educate patient about how sedentary lifestyle affects cardiovascular risk factors (such as hypertension, dyslipidemia, hyperinsulinemia, insulin resistance) *to motivate patient to be more active.*

■ Discuss the need for activity that will improve psychosocial well-being *to encourage compliance with activities.*

■ Develop a behavior modification plan based on patient's condition, history, and precipitating factors *to maximize physical activity and compliance.*

■ Provide education about community resources available to increase physical activity *to decrease barriers to activity.*

■ Teach exercises for increasing strength and endurance *to maintain mobility and prevent musculoskeletal degeneration.*

■ Educate patient about using the bedroom only for sleep or sexual activity and avoiding other activities such as watching television, reading, and eating *to increase sleep efficiency.*

Suggested NIC interventions

Activity Therapy; Body Mechanics Promotion; Energy Management; Risk Identification; Sleep Enhancement; Teaching: Prescribed Activity/Exercise

Evaluations for expected outcomes

■ Patient seeks professional consultation to develop a plan to increase physical activity and limit inactive forms of diversion, such as watching television.

- Patient's BMI is appropriate for his height and weight.
- Patient verbalizes how sedentary lifestyle impacts morbidity and mortality.
- Patient reduces high-risk behaviors.
- Patient demonstrates increased ability to perform activities of daily living and, if appropriate, to maintain independent living status.
- Patient demonstrates motivation to increase physical activity.
- Patient demonstrates readiness for enhanced sleep through the use of appropriate sleep hygiene measures.
- Patient's amount of sleep and REM sleep matches developmental needs.
- Patient demonstrates behaviors of psychological well-being and reduced risk for developing depression.
- Patient experiences reduced depression and anxiety and improved mood.
- Change in sedentary lifestyle is congruent with cultural expectations.
- Facility policies and staff behaviors reflect opportunities to provide physical activity for patients and limit inactive forms of diversion, such as television watching and computer games.

Documentation
- Daytime activity and work patterns
- Behavioral modification plan
- Dietary and drug history
- Height, weight, and BMI
- High-risk behavior assessment
- Sleep hygiene behaviors
- Culturally determined expectations
- Nursing interventions to increase patient's physical activity
- Response to nursing interventions
- Evaluations for expected outcomes

Reference
Zabinski, M.F., et al. "Patterns of Sedentary Behavior Among Adolescents," *Health Psychology* 26(1):113-20, January 2007.

Risk for
LONELINESS
related to physical isolation

Definition
At risk for experiencing vague dysphoria

Assessment
- Family status, including family composition, presence of a spouse, ability of family to meet patient's physical and emotional needs, conflicts between patient's needs and family's ability to meet them, and family members' feelings of self-worth

■ Psychological status, including changes in appetite, behavior, energy level, mood, motivation, self-image, self-esteem, or sleep patterns; alcohol and drug consumption; recent death, job loss, loss of loved one, or relocation; and psychiatric history

■ Social status, including interpersonal skills, size of social network, quality of relationships, degree of trust in others, level of self-esteem, and ability to function in social and occupational roles

■ Health history, including medical illness, disabilities, and deformities

■ Spiritual status, including religious or church affiliation, description of faith and religious practices, and support network (family, clergy, and friends)

Risk factors
■ Affectional deprivation
■ Cathetic deprivation
■ Physical isolation
■ Social isolation

Expected outcomes
■ Patient will identify feelings of loneliness and will express desire to socialize more.

■ Patient will identify behaviors that lead to loneliness.

■ Patient will identify people who will likely support and accept him.

■ Patient will spend time with others.

■ Patient will be comfortable in social settings, will interact with peers, and will receive support from others.

■ Patient will make specific plans to continue involvement with others, such as through recreational activities or social interaction groups.

Suggested NOC outcomes
Grief Resolution; Loneliness Severity; Risk Control; Social Involvement; Social Support

Interventions and rationales
■ Spend sufficient time with patient to allow him to express his feelings of loneliness *to establish trusting relationship.*

■ Inform patient that you'll help him express feelings of loneliness and identify ways to increase social activity *to bring issue into open and help patient understand that you want to help him.*

■ Work with patient to identify factors and behaviors that have contributed to loneliness *to begin changing behaviors that may have alienated others.*

■ Help patient identify feelings associated with loneliness *to lessen their impact and mobilize energy to counteract them.*

■ Help patient curb feelings of loneliness by encouraging one-on-one interaction with others who are likely to accept him — for example, church members or patients with similar health problems — *to promote feelings of acceptance and support.*

■ Encourage patient to address his needs assertively. *By being assertive, patient assumes responsibility for meeting his needs, without anger or guilt.*

■ As patient's comfort level improves, encourage him to attend group activities and social functions *to promote use of social skills.*

■ Help patient identify social activities he can initiate, such as becoming active in a support group or volunteer organization, *to foster feelings of control and increase social contacts.*

■ Help patient accept that other people may view him differently because of his illness, and explore ways of coping with their reactions *to help patient learn to cope with stigma associated with illness.*

■ Work with patient to establish goals for reducing feelings of loneliness after he leaves health care setting *to focus energy on specific objectives.*

■ Refer patient and family to social service agencies, mental health center, and appropriate support groups *to ensure continued care and maintain social involvement.*

Suggested NIC interventions

Activity Therapy; Anxiety Reduction; Counseling; Emotional Support; Energy Management; Socialization Enhancement; Spiritual Support; Visitation Facilitation

Evaluations for expected outcomes

■ Patient expresses feelings of loneliness.
■ Patient describes behaviors that lead to loneliness.
■ Patient lists at least __ (specify) people who will likely support and accept him.
■ Patient initiates conversations with peers.
■ Patient participates in group activities.
■ Patient describes plans to continue involvement with others.

Documentation

■ Patient's statements of loneliness
■ Observations of patient's behaviors and problems associated with loneliness
■ Patient's choice of activities to end isolation
■ Teaching of new coping methods
■ Goals established by patient
■ Evidence of efforts to use new coping mechanisms
■ Referral
■ Evaluations for expected outcomes

Reference

Perese, E.F., and Wolf, M. "Combating Loneliness Among Persons with Severe Mental Illness: Social Network Interventions' Characteristics, Effectiveness, and Applicability," *Issues in Mental Health Nursing* 6(6):591-609, July 2005.

Impaired
MEMORY
related to neurologic disturbance

Definition
Inability to remember or recall fragments of information or behavioral skills

Assessment
■ Age, gender, level of education, occupation, and living arrangements
■ Cardiovascular status, including vital signs, apical pulse, pulse rate and rhythm, and heart sounds; color of skin, lips, and nails; fatigue on exertion, dyspnea, and dizziness; history of hypertension, chest pain, or anoxia; and complete blood count and differential, thyroid studies, electrocardiography, and echocardiography
■ Family status, including household composition and marital status (presence of a spouse, length of marriage, divorce, or death of spouse)
■ Neurologic status, including mental status (abstract thinking, insight about present situation, judgment, long-term and short-term memory, cognition, and orientation to time, place, and person); level of consciousness; sensory ability; fine and gross motor functioning; history of neurologic disorder, head injury, or psychiatric illness; medication use; and computed tomography scan, magnetic resonance imaging, cerebral angiography, EEG, toxicology studies, thyroid function, and serotonin levels
■ Psychological status, including changes in appetite, behavior, energy level, mood, motivation, self-image, self-esteem, and sleep patterns; alcohol and drug consumption; recent divorce, separation, death, job loss, loss of loved one, relocation, or physical or emotional trauma; and psychiatric history
■ Self-care status, including ability to carry out voluntary activities and use of adaptive equipment

Defining characteristics
■ Inability to determine whether a behavior was performed
■ Inability to learn new skills or information or to perform previously learned skills
■ Inability to recall factual information and recent or past events
■ Incidences of forgetting, including forgetting to perform a behavior at a scheduled time

Expected outcomes
■ Patient will express feelings about memory impairment.
■ Patient will acknowledge need to take measures to cope with memory impairment.
■ Patient will identify coping skills to deal with memory impairment.
■ Patient and family members will state specific plans to modify lifestyle.
■ Patient and family members will establish realistic goals to deal with further memory loss.

Suggested NOC outcomes

Cognition; Cognitive Orientation; Concentration; Depression Level; Memory; Neurological Status

Interventions and rationales

■ Observe patient's thought processes during every shift. Document and report any changes. *Changes may indicate progressive improvement or a decline in patient's underlying condition.*

■ Implement appropriate safety measures to protect patient from injury. *He may be unable to provide for his own safety needs.*

■ Call patient by name and tell him your name. Provide background information (place, time, and date) frequently throughout the day *to provide reality orientation.* Use a reality orientation board *to visually reinforce reality orientation.*

■ Spend sufficient time with patient to allow him to become comfortable discussing memory loss *to establish a trusting relationship.*

■ Inform patient that you're aware of his memory loss and that you'll help him cope with his condition *to bring the issue into the open and help patient understand that your goal is to help him.*

■ Be clear, concise, and direct in establishing goals *so that patient can maximize the use of his remaining cognitive skills.*

■ Offer short, simple explanations to patient each time you carry out any medical or nursing procedure *to avoid confusion.*

■ Label patient's personal possessions and photos, keeping them in the same place as much as possible, *to reduce confusion and create a secure environment.*

■ Encourage patient to develop a consistent routine for performing activities of daily living *to enhance his self-esteem and increase his self-awareness and awareness of his environment.*

■ Teach patient ways to cope with memory loss — for example, using a beeper to remind him when to eat or take medications, using a pillbox organized by days of the week, keeping lists in notebooks or a pocket calendar, and having family members or friends remind him of important tasks. *Reminders help limit the amount of information patient must maintain in his memory.*

■ Encourage patient to interact with others t*o increase social involvement, which may decline with memory loss.*

■ Encourage patient to express the feelings associated with impaired memory *to reduce the impact of memory impairment on patient's self-image and lessen anxiety.*

■ Help patient and family members establish goals for coping with memory loss. Discuss with family members the need to maintain the least restrictive environment possible. Instruct them on how to maintain a safe home environment for patient. *This helps ensure that patient's needs are met and promotes his independence.*

■ Demonstrate reorientation techniques to family members and provide time for supervised return demonstrations *to prepare them to cope with patient with memory impairment.*

■ Help family members identify appropriate community support groups, mental health services, and social service agencies *to assist in coping with the effects of patient's illness or injury.*

Suggested NIC interventions

Anxiety Reduction; Calming Technique; Cerebral Perfusion Promotion; Dementia Management; Fluid/Electrolyte Management; Memory Training; Neurologic Monitoring; Reality Orientation

Evaluations for expected outcomes

- Patient expresses feelings about memory impairment.
- Patient acknowledges need to take measures to cope with memory impairment.
- Patient describes mechanisms for coping with memory loss.
- Patient and family members describe plans to modify lifestyle.
- Patient and family members set realistic goals to cope with further memory loss.

Documentation

- Description of patient's mental status, including documentation of changes from shift to shift
- Outline of goals for helping patient cope with memory loss
- Response of family members to techniques for keeping patient functioning at maximal level
- Referrals to community support groups
- Evaluations for expected outcomes

Reference

Parahoo, K., et al. "Expert Nurses' Use of Implicit Memory in the Care of Patients with Alzheimer's Disease," *Journal of Advanced Nursing* 54(5):563-71, June 2006.

Impaired physical
MOBILITY

related to musculoskeletal, neuromuscular impairment

Definition

Limitation in independent, purposeful physical movement of the body or of one or more extremities

Assessment

- History of neuromuscular disorder or dysfunction
- Musculoskeletal status, including coordination, gait, muscle size and strength, muscle tone, range of motion (ROM), and functional mobility scale:

0 = completely independent

1 = requires use of equipment or device

2 = requires help, supervision, or teaching from another person

3 = requires help from another person and equipment or device

4 = dependent; doesn't participate in activity

- Neurologic status, including level of consciousness, motor ability, and sensory ability

Defining characteristics

- Difficulty turning
- Gait changes (for instance, shuffling gait and exaggerated lateral postural sway)
- Limited fine and gross motor skills
- Limited ROM
- Movement-induced tremor
- Postural instability when performing routine activities of daily living
- Shortness of breath
- Slowed movement
- Slowed reaction time
- Substitution of other behaviors for impaired mobility (for instance, increased attention to other's activity and controlling behavior)
- Uncoordinated or jerky movements

Expected outcomes

- Patient will maintain muscle strength and joint ROM.
- Patient will show no evidence of complications, such as contractures, venous stasis, thrombus formation, skin breakdown, and hypostatic pneumonia.
- Patient will achieve highest level of mobility (will transfer independently, will be wheelchair-independent, or will ambulate with such assistive devices as walker, cane, and braces).
- Patient or family member will carry out mobility regimen.
- Patient or family member will make plans to use resources to help maintain level of functioning.

Suggested NOC outcomes

Ambulation; Ambulation: Wheelchair; Discharge Readiness: Independent Living: Discharge Readiness: Supported Living; Joint Movement: Hip; Joint Movement: Shoulder; Mobility; Transfer Performance

Interventions and rationales

- Perform ROM exercises to joints, unless contraindicated, at least once every shift. Progress from passive to active, as tolerated. *This prevents joint contractures and muscular atrophy.*
- Turn and position patient every 2 hours. Establish a turning schedule for dependent patients; post at the bedside and monitor frequency of turning. *This prevents skin breakdown by relieving pressure.*
- Place joints in functional position, use trochanter roll along the thigh, abduct the thighs, use high-top sneakers, and put a small pillow under patient's head. *These measures maintain joints in a functional position and prevent musculoskeletal deformities.*
- Identify the level of functioning using a functional mobility scale (see Assessment). Communicate patient's skill level to all staff members *to provide continuity and preserve identified level of independence.*
- Encourage independence in mobility by helping patient to use a trapeze and side rails, to use his unaffected leg to move his affected leg, and to perform such

self-care activities as combing hair, feeding, and dressing. *This increases muscle tone and patient's self-esteem.*

■ Place items within reach of the unaffected arm if patient has one-sided weakness or paralysis *to promote patient's independence.*

■ Monitor and record daily any evidence of immobility complications (such as contractures, venous stasis, thrombus, pneumonia, and urinary tract infection). *Patients with a history of neuromuscular disorders or dysfunction may be more prone to develop complications.*

■ Carry out a medical regimen to manage or prevent complications; for example, administer prophylactic heparin for venous thrombosis. *This promotes patient's health and well-being.*

■ Provide progressive mobilization to the limits of patient's condition (bed mobility to chair mobility to ambulation) *to maintain muscle tone and prevent complications of immobility.*

■ Refer patient to a physical therapist for development of mobility regimen *to help rehabilitate musculoskeletal deficits.*

■ Encourage attendance at physical therapy sessions, and support activities on the unit by using the same equipment and technique. Request written mobility plans and use as reference. *All members of the health care team should reinforce learned skills in the same manner.*

■ Instruct patient and family members in ROM exercises, transfers, skin inspection, and mobility regimen *to help prepare patient for discharge.*

■ Demonstrate the mobility regimen, and note date. Have patient and family members return mobility regimen demonstration, and note date. *This ensures continuity of care and use of proper technique.*

■ Assist in identifying resources to carry out the mobility regimen, such as American Heart Association and National Multiple Sclerosis Society. *These resources help provide a comprehensive approach to rehabilitation.*

Suggested NIC interventions

Activity Therapy; Energy Management; Exercise Promotion: Strength Training; Exercise Therapy: Joint Mobility; Exercise Therapy: Muscle Control; Positioning: Wheelchair; Surveillance: Safety

Evaluations for expected outcomes

■ Patient maintains muscle strength and joint ROM.

■ Patient shows no evidence of contractures, venous stasis, thrombus formation, skin breakdown, hypostatic pneumonia, or other complications.

■ Patient achieves highest mobility level possible identified by health care team (specify).

■ Patient or family member carries out mobility regimen.

■ Patient or family member identifies and contacts at least one resource person or group to help maintain level of functioning.

Documentation

■ Patient's expression of concern about loss of mobility, current status of functional abilities, and goals set for self

■ Observations of patient's mobility status, presence of complications, and response to mobility regimen
■ Instruction and demonstration of skills in carrying out mobility regimen
■ Patient's response to nursing interventions
■ Evaluations for expected outcomes

Reference
Gillis, A., and MacDonald, B. "Deconditioning in the Hospitalized Elderly," *The Canadian Nurse* 101(6):16-20, June 2005.

Impaired physical
MOBILITY

related to pain or discomfort

Definition
Limitation of physical movement

Assessment
■ History of recent surgery, injury, or disorder causing pain or discomfort
■ Medication history
■ Musculoskeletal status, including coordination, gait, muscle size and strength, muscle tone, range of motion (ROM), and functional mobility scale:
0 = completely independent
1 = requires use of equipment or device
2 = requires help, supervision, or teaching from another person
3 = requires help from another person and equipment or device
4 = dependent; doesn't participate in activity
■ Pain, including environmental and cultural influences, intensity, location, quality, and temporal factors
■ Psychosocial status, including coping mechanisms, family members, lifestyle, personality, and stressors (disease process, finances, job, and marital discord)

Defining characteristics
■ Difficulty turning
■ Gait changes (for instance, shuffling gait and exaggerated lateral postural sway)
■ Limited fine and gross motor skills
■ Limited ROM
■ Movement-induced tremor
■ Postural instability when performing routine activities of daily living
■ Shortness of breath
■ Slowed movement
■ Slowed reaction time
■ Substitution of other behaviors for impaired mobility (such as focusing on one's pre-illness activities or on another person's activities)
■ Uncoordinated or jerky movements

Expected outcomes

- Patient will state relief from pain.
- Patient will display increased mobility.
- Patient will show no evidence of such complications as contractures, venous stasis, thrombus formation, skin breakdown, and hypostatic pneumonia.
- Patient or family member will demonstrate mobility regimen.
- Patient will begin to accept limitations imposed by immobility and accompanying lifestyle changes.
- Patient will express willingness to participate in care.

Suggested NOC outcomes

Joint Movement: Elbows; Joint Movement: Hips; Joint Movement: Shoulders; Mobility; Transfer Performance

Interventions and rationales

- Observe patient's functional ability daily; document and report any changes using the functional mobility scale (see "Assessment"). *Changes may indicate progressive decline or improvement in underlying disorder.*
- Encourage patient to verbalize pain and discomfort. Observe for nonverbal cues of pain, including favoring a body part and grimacing. *This aids assessment of location, quality, and intensity of pain.*
- Perform the prescribed treatment regimen for the underlying condition producing pain or discomfort. Monitor progress and report favorable and adverse responses to treatment *to assess effectiveness of treatment.*
- Administer pain medication and assess nonverbal cues, verbal reports, and vital signs *to monitor effectiveness.*
- Ensure patient comfort by padding extremities prone to skin breakdown (such as heels and elbows), ensuring correct measurement of crutches, and using a convoluted foam mattress on the bed. *These measures prevent skin breakdown.*
- Encourage patient's active movement by using assistive devices *to increase muscle tone and increase patient's feelings of self-esteem;* promote joint rest between activities.
- Implement ROM exercises every shift after pain medication, unless medically contraindicated; progress from passive to active, as tolerated. *This prevents joint contracture and muscle atrophy.*
- Reposition patient every 2 hours and provide meticulous skin care *to prevent skin breakdown.*
- Promote progressive mobilization to maximum, within the limits of patient's tolerance for pain (bed mobility to chair mobility to ambulation). *This maintains muscle tone and prevents complications of immobility.*
- Discuss the use of distraction and other nonpharmacologic pain-relief methods with patient. Instruct patient and family members on the preferred method and monitor effectiveness. Encourage patient to choose an alternative if a method is ineffective. Document the response. *In addition to providing pain relief, nonpharmacologic techniques may help patient achieve a sense of control. Documentation helps ensure the continuity of care.*
- Explain the necessity of movement even during painful periods, unless contraindicated, to prevent greater pain such as occurs in arthritic conditions and af-

ter surgery. Let patient know when to expect to move; provide pain-relief measures before moving patient. *Movement alleviates the effects of immobility. Medication alleviates pain and maintains patient's functional activity level.*

■ Instruct patient and family members in ROM exercises, transfers, skin inspection, and mobility regimen. Have patient and family members return a mobility demonstration under supervision. *Education will enable patient and family members to prevent complications of immobility.*

■ Encourage patient to discuss feelings and concerns about his altered state of mobility *to reduce anxiety and promote compliance.*

■ Encourage adherence to other aspects of health care management to control or minimize effects on mobility. *This promotes health and well-being by alleviating pain and preventing complications.*

■ Refer patient to psychiatric liaison nurse, social service agency, support group, or other resources, as appropriate, *to provide patient with alternative approaches to care.*

Suggested NIC interventions
Body Mechanics Promotion; Energy Management; Exercise Therapy: Balance; Exercise Therapy: Joint Mobility

Evaluations for expected outcomes
■ Patient expresses relief from pain.
■ Patient demonstrates increased mobility.
■ Patient shows no evidence of contractures, venous stasis, thrombus formation, skin breakdown, hypostatic pneumonia, or other complications.
■ Patient attains highest mobility level possible as determined by health care team (specify).
■ Patient or family member carries out mobility regimen.
■ Patient begins to accept limitations imposed by immobility and accompanying lifestyle changes.
■ Patient expresses willingness to participate in care.

Documentation
■ Patient's expression of feelings and concerns about immobility, impact on lifestyle, and willingness to participate in care
■ Observations of patient's impaired mobility, pain, and response to treatment
■ Interventions to provide supportive care
■ Instructions to patient and family members, their understanding of instructions, and demonstrated skill in carrying out prescribed mobility and pain-relief program
■ Patient's response to nursing interventions
■ Evaluations for expected outcomes

Reference
DiNucci, E.M. "Energy Healing: A Complementary Treatment for Orthopaedic and Other Conditions," *Orthopedic Nursing* 24(4):259-69, July-August 2005.

NAUSEA

related to irritation to the GI system

Definition

Subjective, wavelike sensation in the back of the throat, epigastrium, or throughout the abdomen that may lead to vomiting

Assessment

- Health history, including illnesses, pregnancy, and medication use
- Nutritional status, including height, weight, fluctuations in weight, food preferences, and usual dietary patterns
- Psychosocial status, including ethnic background, family dynamics, lifestyle, perception of self, recent stressful events, and coping skills

Defining characteristics

- Gagging sensation
- Sour taste in mouth
- Gastric stasis
- Increased salivation
- Reports "nausea" or "sick to stomach"
- Increased swallowing

Expected outcomes

- Patient will state reasons for nausea and vomiting.
- Patient will take steps to manage episodes of nausea and vomiting.
- Patient will ingest sufficient nutrients to maintain health.
- Patient will take steps to ensure adequate nutrition when nausea abates.
- Patient will maintain weight within specified range.

Suggested NOC outcomes

Appetite; Comfort Level; Fluid Balance; Hydration; Nausea & Vomiting Control; Nutritional Status: Food & Fluid Intake; Suffering Severity; Symptom Control

Interventions and rationales

- Ask patient his reasons for nausea or inability to eat and document his explanation in his own words *to plan interventions.*
- Observe patient's fluid and food intake and document the findings *to assess nutrient consumption and the need for supplements.*
- Encourage patient to eat dry, bland foods (such as dry toast or crackers) during periods of nausea *to make it possible for him to eat.*
- Suggest that patient avoid offensive foods and food odors, shorten food preparation time, and eat and drink slowly. *These measures may help to prevent nausea from getting worse.*
- Administer antinausea medications, as prescribed, *to provide relief from nausea and allow patient to eat.*

■ Teach relaxation techniques and help patient use such techniques during meal-time *to reduce stress and divert attention from nausea, thereby helping patient eat and drink.*

■ Encourage patient to make a list of best-tolerated and least-tolerated foods *to help him choose foods wisely when nausea abates.*

■ When nausea abates, encourage patient to eat larger amounts of food *to help patient consume adequate nutrients over time.*

Suggested NIC interventions

Diet Staging; Fluid/Electrolyte Management; Fluid Monitoring; Medication Management; Nausea Management

Evaluations for expected outcomes

■ Patient states reasons for nausea and vomiting.
■ Patient takes steps to manage episodes of nausea and vomiting.
■ Patient ingests sufficient nutrients to maintain health.
■ Patient takes steps to ensure adequate nutrition when nausea abates.
■ Patient maintains weight within specified range.

Documentation

■ Patient's statements regarding nausea and its causes
■ Episodes of nausea or vomiting
■ Intake and output measurements
■ Types of food and fluids ingested and patient's tolerance
■ Nursing interventions, including teaching provided to patient
■ Patient's response to nursing interventions
■ Evaluations for expected outcomes

Reference

Mamaril, M.E., et al. "Prevention and Management of Postoperative Nausea and Vomiting: A Look at Complementary Techniques," *Journal of Perianesthesia Nursing* 21(6):404-10, December 2006.

Unilateral
NEGLECT

related to neurologic illness or trauma

Definition
Lack of awareness and attention to one side of the body

Assessment
■ History of neurologic impairment
■ Age
■ Neurologic status, including awareness of body parts, cognition, level of consciousness, mental status, memory, sensory function, orientation, position sense,

visual acuity, visual fields, ability to communicate (verbally and nonverbally), and bowel and bladder control
■ Musculoskeletal status, including coordination, muscle size and strength, muscle tone, range of motion (ROM), and functional mobility scale:
0 = completely independent
1 = requires use of equipment or device
2 = requires help, supervision, or teaching from another person
3 = requires help from another person and equipment or device
4 = dependent; doesn't participate in activity
■ Integumentary status, including color, texture, turgor, temperature, elasticity, sensation, moisture, hygiene, and lesions
■ Psychosocial status, including coping mechanisms, support systems (family and others), lifestyle, and understanding of physical condition
■ Self-care abilities, including preparation of equipment and supplies, technical or mechanical skills, and use of assistive devices

Defining characteristics
■ Consistent inattention to stimuli on affected side
■ Failure to eat food on plate on affected side
■ Inadequate self-care
■ Need for positioning and safety precautions to protect affected side

Expected outcomes
■ Patient will avoid injury to affected body part.
■ Patient will avoid skin breakdown.
■ Patient will avoid contractures.
■ Patient will recognize neglected body part.
■ Patient and family members will demonstrate exercises for affected body part.
■ Patient and family members will demonstrate measures for maximum functioning and arrange environment to protect affected body part.
■ Patient and family members will express feelings about altered state of health and neurologic deficits.
■ Patient and family members will identify community resources and support groups to help cope with the effects of illness.

Suggested NOC outcomes
Adaptation to Physical Disability; Body Image; Body Mechanics Performance; Body Positioning: Self-Initiated; Self-Care: Activities of Daily Living (ADL)

Interventions and rationales
■ Place a sling on the affected arm *to prevent dangling or injury.* Support the affected leg and foot while in bed, place a foot strap on the wheelchair, and perform other measures, as appropriate, *to keep patient's limbs in functional position and avoid contractures.* Use a drawsheet to move patient up in bed *to avoid skin abrasions.*

■ Touch and rub the affected limb. Describe it in conversation with patient *to remind patient of neglected body part.*

■ Direct patient to perform activities that require the use of the affected limb. *A patient who uses a paretic or paralyzed limb will more easily integrate the affected limb into his body image.*

■ Encourage patient to check the position of the affected body part with each repositioning or transfer *to reestablish awareness of the body part.*

■ Establish and follow a regular turning schedule *to maintain skin integrity.*

■ Request consultations with occupational and physical therapists about adaptive equipment, exercise program, and other recommendations *to increase patient's awareness of the affected limb.*

■ Use safety belts or protective devices according to facility policy. *Safety devices remind patient of his limitations and help prevent falls.*

■ Remove splints and other devices at least every 2 hours. Inspect the skin for pressure areas. Reapply the splint. *Proper use of splints and other devices prevents deformities and maintains skin integrity.*

■ Perform ROM exercises on the affected side at least once every shift, unless medically contraindicated, *to maintain joint flexibility and prevent contractures.*

■ Instruct family and nursing personnel to observe the position of the affected body part frequently. Remove food or drainage from the face if unnoticed by patient. Place the arm or leg in the proper position as often as necessary *to prevent injury.*

■ Arrange the environment for maximum functioning; for example, place water, television controls, and the call bell within reach. *These measures enhance orientation and encourage independence.*

■ Assist with ADLs or provide supervision, as appropriate, *to protect patient's affected side.*

■ Encourage patient and family members to express their feelings regarding patient's condition and level of functioning *to release tension and enhance coping.*

■ Refer patient and family members to appropriate support groups and other community resources *to assist patient and family in adjusting to patient's altered state of health.*

Suggested NIC interventions

Anticipatory Guidance; Body Image Enhancement; Coping Enhancement; Exercise Therapy: Joint Mobility; Mutual Goal Setting; Self-Care Assistance; Unilateral Neglect Management

Evaluations for expected outcomes

■ Patient doesn't experience injury.

■ Patient's skin doesn't show signs of breakdown.

■ Patient doesn't show evidence of contractures.

■ Patient recognizes and protects neglected body part when carrying out ADLs.

■ Patient and family members demonstrate exercise routine for affected body part.

■ Patient and family members demonstrate measures for maximum functioning and arrange environment to protect affected body part.

■ Patient and family members openly express fear and other feelings associated with patient's neurologic deficits and altered level of functioning.
■ Patient and family members identify and contact appropriate community resources and support groups.

Documentation
■ Patient's expressions of feelings about neglected side of body
■ Safety measures taken to prevent injury
■ Patient's ability to perform ADLs and nursing measures taken to overcome deficits
■ Observations of patient's and family's coping skills
■ Patient's response to nursing interventions, including verbal expressions or behavior that indicates increased awareness of affected limb
■ Evaluations for expected outcomes

Reference
Macko, R.F., et al. "Task-oriented Aerobic Exercise in Chronic Hemiparetic Stroke: Training Protocols and Treatment Effects," *Topics in Stroke Rehabilitation* 12(1): 45-57, Winter 2005.

NONCOMPLIANCE
related to patient's value system

Definition
Behavior of person or caregiver that fails to coincide with a health-promoting or therapeutic plan agreed on by the person (or family or community) and health care professional, possibly leading to clinically ineffective outcomes

Assessment
■ Age
■ Health beliefs
■ Patient's perceptions of health problem, treatment regimen, and importance of complying with treatment regimen
■ Patient's ability to learn and perform prescribed treatment (activity, diet, and medications)
■ Financial resources
■ Cultural and ethnic influences
■ Religious influences
■ Educational and language background

Defining characteristics
■ Behavior indicative of failure to adhere (by direct observation or by statements of patient or significant other)
■ Complications or evidence of exacerbation of signs and symptoms
■ Failure to keep appointments and adhere to treatment regimen

■ Failure to progress
■ Objective indications (such as physiologic tests) of failure to progress

Expected outcomes

■ Patient will identify factors that influence noncompliance.
■ Patient will demonstrate level of compliance that doesn't interfere with physiologic safety.
■ Patient will contract with nurse to perform ___ (specify behavior and frequency).
■ Patient will use support systems to modify noncompliant behavior.

Suggested NOC outcomes

Acceptance: Health Status; Adherence Behavior; Compliance Behavior; Health Beliefs: Perceived Resources; Health Orientation; Symptom Control; Treatment Behavior: Illness or Injury

Interventions and rationales

■ Listen to patient's reasons for noncompliance. *Active listening may reveal concerns not clearly stated in words and helps individualize the teaching process.*
■ Approach patient in nonjudgmental manner. *This demonstrates unconditional positive regard for patient.*
■ Identify specific areas of patient's noncompliant behavior *to help develop appropriate interventions.*
■ Attempt to identify influencing factors associated with noncompliant behaviors, such as lack of understanding, unrealistic expectations, and cultural differences. *Reasons for noncompliance may range widely and include lack of knowledge, forgetting, feeling better or worse, and getting contradictory advice from family, friends, and health care providers.*
■ Emphasize the positive aspects of compliance. *Understanding that compliance can reduce risk factors, prevent complications, and help manage certain chronic diseases may encourage patient to comply.*
■ Help patient clarify his values *to allow him to explore the intellectual and emotional components of the values that form the basis for his behavior.*
■ Acknowledge patient's right to choose against carrying out prescribed regimen. *Patient's autonomy must be respected; control over patient's action is legitimate only if needed to prevent harm to patient, to others, or to yourself.*
■ Contract with patient to practice only nonthreatening behaviors. *This involves both patient and caregiver in a formal commitment and gives patient a sense of personal control.*
■ Use support systems to enforce or reinforce negotiated behaviors. *Support from patient's family helps foster compliance.*
■ Give positive reinforcement for compliant behavior *to encourage patient to continue such behavior.*
■ As medically appropriate, support patient who chooses to follow Eastern therapies instead of traditional Western medical practices. *Such support demonstrates your respect for patient's beliefs.*
■ Determine whether patient's perceived noncompliance actually stems from a lack of financial resources. Contact appropriate agencies to help patient meet the

costs of medical treatment and supplies and other financial needs. *Helping patient meet the financial requirements of treatment improves compliance.*

Suggested NIC interventions

Coping Enhancement; Counseling; Decision-Making Support; Health Education; Patient Contracting; Self-Modification Assistance; Self-Responsibility Facilitation

Evaluations for expected outcomes

- Patient describes factors that influence noncompliance with health care regimen.
- Patient performs daily self-care in compliance with health care regimen.
- Patient performs behaviors agreed upon in contract with nurse.
- Patient uses available support resources, as needed.

Documentation

- Patient's statements that indicate noncompliant behavior
- Direct observation of noncompliant behavior
- Statements by patient that provide insight into causes of noncompliant behavior
- Terms agreed on by patient in performing negotiated behaviors
- Patient's daily progress in complying with treatment regimen
- Evaluations for expected outcomes

Reference

Riegel, B., et al. "A Motivational Counseling Approach to Improving Heart Failure Self-care: Mechanisms of Effectiveness," *The Journal of Cardiovascular Nursing* 21(3):232-41, May-June 2006.

Imbalanced
NUTRITION: LESS THAN BODY REQUIREMENTS
related to inability to digest or absorb nutrients because of biological factors

Definition

Intake of nutrients insufficient to meet metabolic needs

Assessment

- GI assessment, including antibiotic therapy, auscultation of bowel sounds, change in bowel habits, stool characteristics (color, amount, size, and consistency), history of GI disorder or surgery, inspection of abdomen, pain or discomfort, usual bowel elimination pattern, palpation for masses and tenderness, percussion for tympany and dullness, and nausea and vomiting
- Nutritional status, including change in type of food tolerated, financial resources, height and weight, meal preparation, serum albumin level, sociocultural influences, usual dietary pattern, and weight fluctuations over past 10 years

■ Change in intrapersonal or interpersonal factors, including internal or external cues that trigger desire to eat, rate of food consumption, and stated food preference

■ Psychosocial status

■ Activity level

■ Coping behaviors

■ Body image, including perception of observer and self-perception

Defining characteristics

■ Abdominal pain or cramping, with or without disease

■ Altered taste sensation

■ Aversion to or lack of interest in eating

■ Body weight 20% or more under ideal weight

■ Diarrhea and steatorrhea

■ Evidence of lack of food

■ Excessive hair loss

■ Fragile capillaries

■ Hyperactive bowel sounds

■ Inadequate food intake (less than recommended daily allowances)

■ Lack of information or misinformation about nutrition

■ Loss of body weight despite adequate food intake

■ Pale conjunctivae and mucous membranes

■ Perceived inability to ingest food

■ Poor muscle tone

■ Satiety immediately after eating

■ Sore, inflamed buccal cavity

■ Weakness of muscles required for chewing or swallowing

Expected outcomes

■ Patient will show no further evidence of weight loss.

■ Patient will tolerate oral, tube, or I.V. feedings without adverse effects.

■ Patient will take in _____ calories daily.

■ Patient will gain _____ lb weekly.

■ Patient and family members will communicate understanding of preoperative instructions.

■ Patient and family members will communicate understanding of special dietary needs.

■ Patient and family members will demonstrate ability to plan diet after discharge.

Suggested NOC outcomes

Nutritional Status; Nutritional Status: Nutrient Intake; Symptom Severity; Weight Control

Interventions and rationales

■ Obtain and record patient's weight at the same time every day *to obtain accurate readings.*

■ Monitor fluid intake and output *because body weight may decrease as a result of fluid loss.*

■ Maintain parenteral fluids, as ordered, *to provide patient with needed fluids and electrolytes.*

■ Provide a diet prescribed for patient's specific condition *to improve patient's nutritional status and increase weight.*

■ Determine food preferences and provide them within the limitations of patient's prescribed diet. *This enhances compliance with diet regimen.*

■ Monitor electrolyte levels and report abnormal values. *Poor nutritional status may cause electrolyte imbalances.*

■ If patient vomits, record amount, color, and consistency. Keep a record of all stools. *Vomitus and stool characteristics indicate status of nutrient absorption.*

■ Refer patient to a dietitian or nutritional support team for dietary management (possible regimens include yogurt feedings and low-bulk diet). *Dietitian or nutritional support team can help patient and health care team individualize patient's diet within prescribed restrictions.*

■ If patient is receiving tube feeding:

– Add food coloring if patient has an altered state of consciousness or diminished gag reflex *to help detect aspiration.*

– If possible, use a continuous infusion pump for tube feeding *to avoid diarrhea.*

– Begin the tube feeding regimen with a small amount and diluted concentration *to decrease diarrhea and improve absorption.* Increase the volume and concentration, as tolerated.

– Keep the head of the bed elevated during tube feeding *to reduce the risk of aspiration.*

– Check the feeding tube placement each shift *to verify placement in the GI tract rather than in the lungs.*

■ If patient is receiving total parenteral nutrition:

– Ensure delivery, as prescribed. *Electrolytes, amino acids, and other nutrients must be tailored to patient's needs.*

– Monitor blood glucose levels and urine specific gravity at least once each shift. *Because glucose is the main component of total parenteral nutrition, patient may become hyperglycemic if not carefully monitored.*

■ Monitor bowel sounds once per shift. *Normal active bowel sounds may indicate readiness for enteral feedings; hyperactive sounds may indicate poor absorption and may be accompanied by diarrhea.*

■ Reinforce the medical regimen by explaining to patient and family members the reasons for the present regimen. *Collaborative practice enhances patient's overall care.*

■ Teach the principles of good nutrition for patient's specific condition. *This encourages patient and family members to participate in patient's care.*

■ Provide or assist with oral hygiene *to help keep patient comfortable.*

■ Provide preoperative teaching, if needed, *to reduce patient's fear and anxiety and promote understanding.*

■ Involve family members in meal planning *to encourage them to help patient comply with the diet regimen after discharge.*

Suggested NIC interventions

Energy Management; Nutritional Counseling; Nutrition Management; Nutrition Therapy; Weight Gain Assistance

Evaluations for expected outcomes

■ Patient remains at or above specified weight.
■ Patient doesn't develop adverse reactions from feedings, such as aspiration of food particles into lungs, diarrhea, and hyperglycemia.
■ Patient consumes specified number of calories daily.
■ Patient's weight increases by specified amount weekly.
■ Patient and family communicate understanding of preoperative instructions, either verbally or through behavior.
■ Patient and family communicate understanding of special dietary needs, either verbally or through behavior.
■ Patient and family plan appropriate diet for patient to follow after discharge.

Documentation

■ Daily weight
■ Mouth care
■ Maintenance of nasogastric tube
■ Intake and output
■ Bowel sounds
■ Blood glucose levels
■ Urine specific gravity
■ Patient's ability to eat
■ Incidence of vomiting or diarrhea
■ Presence of other complications
■ Patient's statements of understanding of dietary education
■ Evaluations for expected outcomes

Reference

Bowman, A., et al. "Implementation of an Evidence-based Feeding Protocol and Aspiration Risk Reduction Algorithm," *Critical Care Nursing Quarterly* 28(4): 324-33, October-December 2005.

Imbalanced
NUTRITION: LESS THAN BODY REQUIREMENTS

related to inability to ingest foods

Definition

Intake of nutrients insufficient to meet metabolic needs

Assessment

■ GI assessment, including auscultation of bowel sounds, change in bowel habits, characteristics of stools (color, amount, size, and consistency), history of GI disor-

der or surgery, inspection of abdomen, pain or discomfort, palpation for masses and tenderness, percussion for tympany and dullness, nausea and vomiting, and usual bowel pattern
■ Nutritional status, including financial resources, height, meal preparation, serum albumin level, sociocultural influences, usual dietary pattern, weight, and weight fluctuations over past 10 years
■ Intrapersonal and interpersonal factors, including internal and external cues that trigger desire to eat, rate of food consumption, and stated food preference
■ Psychosocial status
■ Activity level
■ Coping behaviors
■ Body image, including self-perception and perception of observer

Defining characteristics
■ Abdominal pain or cramping, with or without disease
■ Altered taste sensation
■ Aversion to or lack of interest in eating
■ Body weight 20% or more under ideal weight
■ Diarrhea and steatorrhea
■ Evidence of lack of food
■ Excessive hair loss
■ Fragile capillaries
■ Hyperactive bowel sounds
■ Inadequate food intake (less than recommended daily allowances)
■ Lack of information or misinformation about nutrition
■ Loss of body weight despite adequate food intake
■ Pale conjunctivae and mucous membranes
■ Perceived inability to ingest food
■ Poor muscle tone
■ Satiety immediately after eating
■ Sore, inflamed buccal cavity
■ Weakness of muscles required for chewing or swallowing

Expected outcomes
■ Patient will show no further evidence of weight loss.
■ Patient will tolerate ___ ml of nasogastric (NG) or gastrostomy tube feedings.
■ Patient will avoid aspiration, diarrhea, and hyperglycemia.
■ Patient will gain ___ lb weekly.
■ Patient will consume ___ calories daily.
■ Patient will avoid skin breakdown and infection around tube site.
■ Patient and family members will communicate understanding of special dietary needs.
■ Patient and family members will demonstrate correct tube feeding procedures.

Suggested NOC outcomes
Nutritional Status; Nutritional Status: Food & Fluid Intake; Nutritional Status: Nutrient Intake; Weight Control

Interventions and rationales

■ Obtain and record patient's weight at the same time every day *to obtain accurate readings.*

■ Monitor fluid intake and output *because body weight may increase as result of fluid retention.*

■ Administer the prescribed amount of food *to provide patient with needed nutrition.*

– Begin the regimen with a small amount and diluted concentration *to decrease diarrhea and improve absorption.* Increase the volume and concentration, as tolerated.

– Elevate the head of the bed during tube feeding *to reduce the risk of aspiration.*

– Check the feeding tube placement at least once every shift *to verify placement in the GI tract rather than in the lungs.*

– Give water and juices, as needed, *to maintain adequate hydration.*

– If possible, use a continuous infusion pump *to prevent diarrhea.*

– Put food coloring in the food *to monitor for aspiration.*

■ Provide nares care every 4 hours to prevent ulceration and skin breakdown. Tape the NG tube *to prevent visual obstruction.* Use hypoallergenic tape *to minimize skin reactions.*

■ Change a gastrostomy dressing daily or according to facility protocol *to prevent infection.*

■ Ensure the proper temperature of each feeding (room temperature); change the feeding tube bags and tubing according to facility protocol *to maximize tolerance and minimize infection.*

■ Assess and record bowel sounds once per shift *to monitor for increase or decrease.*

■ Auscultate and record breath sounds every 4 hours *to monitor for aspiration.* Report wheezes, rhonchi, crackles, or decreased breath sounds. If aspiration is suspected, stop tube feeding. Keep suction apparatus at the bedside and suction, as needed. Turn patient on his side *to avoid further aspiration.*

■ Instruct patient and family members in tube feeding procedures. Supervise return demonstrations until competency is achieved. *This encourages patient and family members to participate in patient's care.*

Suggested NIC interventions

Bowel Management; Enteral Tube Feeding; Fluid/Electrolyte Management; Fluid Monitoring; Nutrition Management; Positioning

Evaluations for expected outcomes

■ Patient shows no further evidence of weight loss.

■ Patient tolerates NG or gastrostomy tube feedings without adverse effects.

■ Patient doesn't exhibit signs of aspiration, diarrhea, or hyperglycemia.

■ Patient gains specified amount of weight weekly.

■ Patient consumes specified amount of calories daily.

■ Patient avoids skin breakdown and infection around tube site.

■ Patient and family members communicate understanding of special dietary needs and plan appropriate diet.

■ Patient and family members demonstrate correct tube-feeding procedures.

Documentation
- Daily weight
- Intake and output
- Tolerance of tube feeding
- Incidents of vomiting, aspiration, and diarrhea
- Bowel sounds
- Breath sounds
- Response to instructions
- Demonstration of feeding procedures
- Evaluations for expected outcomes

References
Corcoran, L. "Nutrition and Hydration Tips for Stroke Patients with Dysphagia," *Nursing Times* 101(48):24-27, November-December 2005.

Ellett, M.L. "Important Facts about Intestinal Feeding Tube Placement," *Gastroenterology Nursing* 29(2):112-24, March-April 2006.

Imbalanced
NUTRITION: LESS THAN BODY REQUIREMENTS
related to psychological factors

Definition
Intake of nutrients insufficient to meet metabolic needs

Assessment
- History of eating disorders
- Nutritional history, including financial resources, height and weight, hereditary influences, meal preparation, sociocultural influences, usual dietary pattern, and weight fluctuations over past 10 years
- Change in intrapersonal or interpersonal factors, including internal and external cues that trigger desire to eat, rate of food consumption, and stated food preference
- Activity level
- Coping behaviors
- Body image, including self-perception and perception of observer

Defining characteristics
- Abdominal pain or cramping, with or without disease
- Altered taste sensation
- Aversion to or lack of interest in eating
- Body weight 20% or more under ideal weight
- Diarrhea and steatorrhea
- Evidence of lack of food
- Excessive hair loss
- Fragile capillaries

- Hyperactive bowel sounds
- Inadequate food intake (less than recommended daily allowances)
- Lack of information or misinformation about nutrition
- Loss of body weight despite adequate food intake
- Pale conjunctivae and mucous membranes
- Perceived inability to ingest food
- Poor muscle tone
- Satiety immediately after eating
- Sore, inflamed buccal cavity
- Weakness of muscles required for chewing or swallowing

Expected outcomes

- Patient will consume at least _____ calories daily.
- Patient will gain _____ lb weekly.
- Patient will eat independently, without being prodded.
- Patient will identify emotional and psychological factors that interfere with eating.
- Patient will develop plan to monitor and maintain target weight at discharge.
- Patient will plan to use mental health resources to help resolve psychological problems.

Suggested NOC outcomes

Adherence Behavior; Body Image; Depression Level; Nutritional Status; Nutritional Status: Food & Fluid Intake; Nutritional Status: Nutrient Intake; Weight Control

Interventions and rationales

- Provide opportunities for patient to discuss reasons for not eating *to help assess causes of eating disorder.*
- Observe and record patient's intake (both liquid and solid) *to assess what nutrients patient consumes and what supplements she needs.*
- Determine patient's food preferences and attempt to obtain these foods. Offer foods that appeal to olfactory, visual, and tactile senses *to enhance patient's appetite.*
- Offer high-protein, high-calorie supplements, such as milk shakes, custard, and ice cream. *Such foods prevent body protein breakdown and provide caloric energy.*
- Serve foods that require little cutting or chewing *to help prevent malingering at meals.*
- Provide a pleasant environment at mealtime *to enhance patient's appetite.*
- Keep snacks at the bedside *to give patient some control over eating time.*
- With some patients, begin with nutritious liquids and gradually introduce solid food. *Severely malnourished patient may not be able to chew solid foods immediately.*
- Avoid asking whether patient is hungry or wants to eat. Be positive in offering food. *A positive, undemanding attitude avoids confrontation with patient.*
- Whenever possible, sit with patient for a predetermined length of time during each meal. *This inhibits patient from dawdling during the meal and from hiding or hoarding food.*

■ Monitor and record elimination patterns. *Patient may be taking laxatives or diuretics to keep her weight low in spite of eating.*

■ Weigh patient at the same time every day. *This yields accurate data and gives patient some control over foods eaten and privileges or rewards gained.*

■ Set a target weight and have patient record daily weight *to involve patient in treatment.*

■ Refer patient and family members to appropriate mental health professional as most eating disorders are psychological. *Patient and family members require treatment and follow-up to prevent recurrence.*

Suggested NIC interventions

Diet Staging; Eating Disorders Management; Fluid Monitoring; Mutual Goal Setting; Referral; Weight Gain Assistance

Evaluations for expected outcomes

■ Patient consumes specified number of calories daily.

■ Patient gains specified amount of weight weekly.

■ Patient eats independently without constant encouragement.

■ Patient lists emotional and psychological factors that interfere with eating.

■ Patient states plan to monitor and maintain specific target weight after discharge.

■ Patient contacts support groups and mental health resources, as needed.

Documentation

■ Patient's expressed attitudes toward food and eating at present time

■ Patient's expressed feelings about weight, body image, and emotional status

■ Patient's daily intake (liquid and solid) and output (urine, stools, and vomitus)

■ Daily weight and progression of weight gain

■ Interventions to feed patient adequately

■ Emotional support provided

■ Patient's response to nursing interventions

■ Evaluations for expected outcomes

Reference

Harris, M., and Cumella, E.J. "Eating Disorders Across the Life Span," *Journal of Psychological Nursing and Mental Health Services* 44(4):20-26, April 2006.

Imbalanced
NUTRITION: MORE THAN BODY REQUIREMENTS

related to excessive intake in relation to metabolic needs

Definition

Intake of nutrients that exceed metabolic needs

Assessment

- Nutritional history, including financial resources, height and weight, weight fluctuations over past 10 years, hereditary influences, history of obesity, meal preparation, sociocultural influences, and usual dietary pattern
- Change in intrapersonal or interpersonal factors, including internal and external cues that trigger desire to eat, motivation to lose weight, rate of food consumption, and stated food preference
- Psychosocial status
- Activity level
- Coping patterns
- Body image, including self-perception and perception of observer

Defining characteristics

- Body weight 20% or more over ideal weight
- Dysfunctional eating patterns, such as concentrating food intake at end of day, eating in response to internal cue other than hunger (such as anxiety), eating in response to external cues (such as social situations), and pairing food with other activities
- Sedentary lifestyle
- Triceps skin fold greater than 15 mm in men and 25 mm in women

Expected outcomes

- Patient will voice feelings about present weight.
- Patient will identify internal and external cues that increase food consumption.
- Patient will state need to lose weight.
- Patient will set a weight-loss goal of _____ lb weekly.
- Patient will plan menus appropriate to prescribed diet.
- Patient will adhere to prescribed diet.
- Patient will lose at least ___ lb weekly.
- Patient will set target weight before discharge.
- Patient will state plan to monitor and maintain target weight.
- Patient will participate in selected exercise program _____ times weekly.

Suggested NOC outcomes

Adherence Behavior; Knowledge: Diet; Motivation; Nutritional Status; Nutritional Status: Nutrient Intake; Risk Control; Risk Detection; Stress Level; Weight Control

Interventions and rationales

- Help patient identify the problem, feelings associated with eating, and circumstances in which patient turns to food. *Permanent weight loss starts with examination of factors contributing to weight gain.*
- Discuss patient's normal food preferences *to evaluate eating habits and include preferred foods (if nutritious) in patient's diet.*
- Have a dietitian calculate caloric intake patient will require to reach a desirable weight *to allow planning of appropriate diet.*

■ Have a dietitian discuss meal planning with patient during hospitalization *to help patient plan nutritious, satisfying meals.*

■ If the resource is available, refer patient to a mental health professional for behavior modification *to help patient change poor eating habits and ensure permanent weight loss.*

■ Teach patient about low-calorie, nutritious foods. This encourages patient *to eat foods that provide energy without causing weight gain.*

■ Help patient set realistic goals for losing weight. *This aids positive reinforcement and reduces frustration.*

■ Give patient emotional support and positive feedback for adhering to the prescribed dietary regimen *to promote compliance.* Encourage nondietary rewards, such as the purchase of a new accessory or book, *to promote continuation of the dietary plan and help patient avoid using food as a reward.*

■ Weigh patient weekly, or as prescribed, *to monitor the effectiveness of the diet plan.*

■ Set a target weight with patient and have patient record his weight. *This involves patient in the plan and provides positive reinforcement.*

■ Explore the feasibility of having patient participate after discharge in Weight Watchers, Overeaters Anonymous, or another group or individual diet therapies. *Such resources provide reinforcement and information.*

■ Help patient select an exercise program (such as walking, jogging, aerobics, or swimming) appropriate to his age and physical condition. *Besides aiding weight loss, such activities offer an alternative to eating to alleviate stress.*

Suggested NIC interventions

Behavior Management; Behavior Modification; Coping Enhancement; Eating Disorders Management; Exercise Promotion; Limit Setting; Nutrition Management; Weight Reduction Assistance

Evaluations for expected outcomes
■ Patient expresses feelings about present weight.
■ Patient identifies cues that increase food consumption.
■ Patient expresses desire to lose weight.
■ Patient and health care professional establish weekly weight loss goal.
■ Patient and family plan menus within parameters of prescribed diet.
■ Patient adheres to prescribed diet.
■ Patient loses specified amount of weight weekly.
■ Patient and health care professional set target weight before discharge.
■ Patient summarizes plan to monitor and maintain specified target weight.
■ Patient participates in specified number of selected exercise activities weekly.

Documentation
■ Patient's expressions of feelings about weight, eating, food, and dieting
■ Goals set by patient
■ Record of weight
■ Foods consumed by patient
■ Behaviors that promote or impede weight reduction
■ Evaluations for expected outcomes

Reference

Daggett, L.M., and Rigdon, K.L. "A Computer-assisted Instructional Program for Teaching Portion Size versus Serving Size, " *Journal of Community Health Nursing* 23(1):29-35, Spring 2006.

Risk for imbalanced
NUTRITION: MORE THAN BODY REQUIREMENTS
related to excessive intake

Definition
At risk for intake of nutrients that exceeds metabolic needs

Assessment
■ Nutritional history, including financial resources, height and weight, hereditary influences, history of obesity, meal preparation, sociocultural influences, usual dietary pattern, and weight fluctuations over past year
■ Eating patterns, including internal and external cues that trigger desire to eat, rate of food consumption, and stated food preferences
■ Psychosocial status, including behavior, mood, stressors (finances, job, and marital discord), coping mechanisms, sources of support (family, friends, and others), lifestyle, knowledge level, hobbies, and interests
■ Activity levels
■ Body image, including self-perception and perception of observer
■ Additional circumstances that may lead to excessive intake

Risk factors
■ Consumption of solid food as major food source before age 5 months
■ Dysfunctional eating patterns, such as concentrating food intake at end of day, using food as reward or comfort measure, eating in response to internal cues other than hunger (such as anxiety), and eating in response to external cues (such as social situations)
■ High baseline weight at beginning of each pregnancy
■ Obesity in one or both parents
■ Rapid movement across growth percentiles (in infant or child)

Expected outcomes
■ Patient will express need to maintain or stabilize weight within 5 to 10 lb (2.5 to 4.5 kg) of target weight.
■ Patient will plan to monitor weight and sustain target weight.
■ Patient will express feelings regarding dietary regimen and current weight.
■ Patient will identify internal and external cues that lead to increased food consumption.
■ Patient will plan menus appropriate for prescribed diet.
■ Patient will adhere to prescribed diet.
■ Patient will participate in selected exercise program every week (specify).

■ Patient will achieve weight goal.

Suggested NOC outcomes

Knowledge: Diet; Nutritional Status; Nutritional Status: Nutrient Intake; Risk Control; Stress Level; Weight Control

Interventions and rationales

■ Weigh patient weekly or as prescribed *to monitor the effectiveness of the diet.*
■ Work with patient to establish a realistic target weight. Instruct patient how to record his weight. *Involvement in the nursing care plan improves compliance.*
■ Instruct patient to keep a food diary. *This helps patient confront actual intake, break through denial, and achieve a more objective view of eating habits.*
■ Monitor fluid intake and output and assess for edema. *Fluid retention may increase body weight.*
■ Encourage patient to express feelings about dietary restrictions *to assess his perception of the problem.* Help patient identify emotions associated with food and situations that trigger eating episodes. *Permanent weight maintenance requires an understanding of the risk factors that contribute to weight gain.*
■ Determine patient's food preferences *to evaluate eating habits and to include preferred foods, if nutritious, in patient's diet.*
■ Encourage consumption of foods low in calories and fat and high in complex carbohydrates and fiber. Have patient meet with a dietitian to discuss meal planning. *These steps will help patient plan nutritious, well-balanced meals.*
■ Refer patient to an appropriate resource for behavior modification and cognitive therapy *to prevent relapse into high-risk eating behaviors.*
■ Give patient emotional support and positive feedback for adhering to the prescribed diet. *This will foster compliance and help ensure adherence to the regimen.*
■ Recommend that patient explore group diet therapies, such as Weight Watchers and Overeaters Anonymous, *to provide additional sources of information and encouragement.*
■ Discuss the importance of incorporating exercise into lifestyle. Help patient select a program with various activities (such as swimming, walking, aerobics, and biking) appropriate for his age and physical condition. *Exercise burns calories, offers an alternative to eating to alleviate stress, and fosters a sense of accomplishment.*

Suggested NIC interventions

Behavior Management; Exercise Promotion; Nutritional Counseling; Nutrition Management; Teaching: Prescribed Diet

Evaluations for expected outcomes

■ Patient expresses need to maintain or stabilize weight.
■ Patient states plan to maintain food diary, weighs self weekly, and expresses motivation to sustain current weight.
■ Patient expresses feelings regarding dietary regimen and current weight.
■ Patient identifies at least three internal and three external cues that lead to increased food consumption.

■ When filling out menus, patient selects low-fat, high-fiber foods that are high in complex carbohydrates.

■ Patient adheres to prescribed diet, as evidenced by selection of well-balanced meals and low-calorie snacks.

■ Patient selects at least two activities for exercise program.

■ Patient achieves weight goal.

Documentation

■ Patient's expression of feelings about weight, eating, and dietary regimen
■ Patient's weight
■ Ability of patient to maintain target weight
■ Foods consumed by patient
■ Behaviors that promote or impede weight maintenance
■ Evaluations for expected outcomes

Reference

Werrij, M.Q., et al. "Overweight and Obesity: The Significance of a Depressed Mood," *Patient Education and Counseling* 62(1):126-31, July 2006.

Impaired
ORAL MUCOUS MEMBRANE
related to dehydration

Definition

Disruption of the lips and soft tissue of the oral cavity

Assessment

■ History of pathologic conditions known to cause dehydration such as diabetes mellitus
■ Medications, such as diuretics and antihistamines
■ Vital signs
■ Fluid and electrolyte status, including blood urea nitrogen level, creatinine level, intake and output, mucous membranes, serum electrolyte levels, skin turgor, and urine specific gravity
■ Oral status, including inspection of oral cavity (gums and tongue), pain or discomfort, and salivation
■ Nutritional status, including current weight, change from normal weight, and dietary pattern
■ Psychosocial status, including change in financial status, coping skills, habits (smoking and alcohol intake), patient's perception of health problem, and recent traumatic event

Defining characteristics

■ Bleeding
■ Coated tongue

- Desquamation
- Difficulty eating, speaking, or swallowing
- Diminished, absent, or bad taste
- Dry mouth
- Edema
- Enlarged tonsils
- Fissures and chelitis
- Gingival hyperplasia or recession (pockets deeper than 4 mm)
- Gingival or mucosal pallor
- Halitosis
- Mucosal denudation
- Oral lesions, ulcers, pain, or discomfort
- Purulent drainage or exudate; presence of pathogens
- Smooth, atrophic, sensitive tongue
- Spongy patches or white, curdlike exudate
- Stomatitis
- Vesicles, nodules, or papules
- White patches and plaque

Expected outcomes
- Patient will maintain fluid balance (intake equals output).
- Patient will state increased comfort.
- Patient will have pink, moist oral mucous membranes.
- Patient will have minimal, if any, complications.
- Patient will correlate precipitating factors with appropriate oral care.
- Patient will demonstrate oral hygiene practices.

Suggested NOC outcomes
Oral Hygiene; Tissue Integrity: Skin & Mucous Membranes

Interventions and rationales
- Inspect patient's oral cavity every shift. Describe and document condition; report any change in status. *Regular assessments can anticipate or alleviate problems.*
- Perform the prescribed treatment regimen, including administering I.V. or oral fluids, *to improve the condition of patient's mucous membranes.* Monitor progress, reporting favorable and adverse responses to the treatment regimen.
- Provide supportive measures, as indicated:
– Assist with oral hygiene before and after meals *to promote a feeling of comfort and well-being.*
– Use a toothbrush with suction if patient can't spit out water *to minimize risk of aspiration.*
– Provide mouthwash or gargles, as ordered, *to increase patient comfort and maintain moisture in his mouth.*
– Lubricate patient's lips frequently with water-based lubricant *to prevent cracked, irritated skin.*
- Instruct patient in oral hygiene practices, if necessary. Have patient return a demonstration of the oral care routine.
– Use a soft-bristled toothbrush.

– Brush with a circular motion away from the gums.

– Include the tongue when brushing.

– Review the need for routine visits to a dentist (annually for adults).

These measures increase patient's awareness of oral hygiene practices and reduce discomfort, resulting in increased nutrition and hydration.

■ Tell patient to chew gum or suck on sugarless hard candy *to stimulate salivation.*

■ Discuss precipitating factors, if known, and work to prevent future episodes. For example, encourage patient to avoid exercising in heat and to report effects of medication. *Patient's increased awareness of causative factors will help prevent recurrence.*

■ Encourage adherence to other aspects of health care management (controlling diabetes, changing dietary habits, and avoiding alcoholic beverages) *to control or minimize effects on mucous membranes.*

Suggested NIC interventions

Fluid/Electrolyte Management; Oral Health Maintenance; Oral Health Restoration

Evaluations for expected outcomes

■ Patient's total daily fluid intake equals total output.

■ Patient chews and swallows without discomfort.

■ Patient's mucous membranes remain moist, pink, and free from cuts and abrasions.

■ Patient doesn't develop complications related to extended dehydration of mucous membranes.

■ Patient discusses possible causes of alteration in oral mucous membranes, such as heat exhaustion and reactions to medication.

■ Patient discusses and demonstrates preventive measures such as regular oral hygiene.

Documentation

■ Observations of condition, healing, and response to treatment

■ Interventions to provide supportive care and patient's response to supportive care

■ Instructions given, patient's understanding of instructions, and patient's demonstrated skill in carrying out prescribed oral care measures

■ Evaluations for expected outcomes

Reference

Bailey, R., et al. "The Oral Health of Older Adults: An Interdisciplinary Mandate," *Journal of Gerontological Nursing*, 31(7):11-17, July 2005.

| Impaired |
| **ORAL MUCOUS MEMBRANE** |
| related to mechanical trauma |

Definition
Altered mouth integrity

Assessment
- History of oral surgery, dentures, braces, or dental problems
- Medications, such as diuretics and antihistamines
- Vital signs
- Fluid and electrolyte status, including blood urea nitrogen level, creatinine level, intake and output, mucous membranes, serum electrolyte levels, skin turgor, and urine specific gravity
- Oral status, including inspection of oral cavity (with gums and tongue), pain or discomfort, and salivation
- Nutritional status, including current weight, change from normal weight, and dietary pattern
- Psychosocial status, including coping skills, patient's perception of health problem, and recent traumatic event

Defining characteristics
- Bleeding
- Coated tongue
- Desquamation
- Difficulty eating, speaking, or swallowing
- Diminished, absent, or bad taste
- Dry mouth
- Edema
- Enlarged tonsils
- Fissures and chelitis
- Gingival hyperplasia or recession (pockets deeper than 4 mm)
- Gingival or mucosal pallor
- Halitosis
- Mucosal denudation
- Oral lesions, ulcers, pain, or discomfort
- Purulent drainage or exudate; presence of pathogens
- Smooth, atrophic, sensitive tongue
- Spongy patches or white, curdlike exudate
- Stomatitis
- Vesicles, nodules, or papules
- White patches and plaque

Expected outcomes
- Patient will maintain fluid balance (intake equals output).
- Patient will have pink, moist oral mucous membranes.

■ Patient will state increased comfort.

■ Patient will have minimal, if any, complications.

■ Patient will correlate precipitating factors with appropriate oral care.

■ Patient will demonstrate correct oral hygiene practices.

Suggested NOC outcomes

Oral Hygiene; Pain Level; Tissue Integrity: Skin & Mucous Membranes

Interventions and rationales

■ Inspect patient's oral cavity every shift. Describe and document the condition and report any status change. *Ill-fitting dentures, jagged teeth, braces, oral surgery, and insertion of an endotracheal tube may cause mechanical trauma. Regular assessments can anticipate or alleviate problems.*

■ Establish and follow a routine oral hygiene schedule. For example, soak dentures every evening, clean with denture cream, rinse, and keep them in a properly labeled container at patient's bedside. *Routine oral hygiene can improve the condition of mucous membranes.*

■ Provide supportive measures, as indicated:

– Assist with oral hygiene before and after meals *to promote a feeling of comfort and well-being.*

– Use a toothbrush with suction if patient can't spit out water *to minimize the risk of aspiration.*

– Provide mouthwash or gargles, as ordered, *to increase patient comfort.*

– Lubricate patient's lips frequently with water-based lubricant. *Fluid and food intake increases when patient is more comfortable.*

■ Instruct patient in oral hygiene practices, if necessary. Have patient return a demonstration of the oral care routine. Tell patient to stimulate saliva by chewing gum or sucking on sugarless hard candy. *These measures increase patient's awareness of oral hygiene practices and reduce discomfort, resulting in increased nutrition and hydration.*

■ Discuss precipitating factors, if known, and work to prevent future episodes (for example, weight loss may change the contours of the oral cavity). *Patient's increased awareness of causative factors will help prevent recurrence.*

■ Encourage adherence to other aspects of health care management *to control or minimize the effects on mucous membranes.* For example, encourage patients with braces to avoid popcorn, chewing gum, and caramels. *These measures reduce the risk of trauma to oral mucous membrane.*

■ Refer patient to a dentist, dental hygienist, or other appropriate resource to correct ill-fitting dentures, modify braces, and adjust jaw wires as needed. *Regularly scheduled dental follow-up reduces the risk of trauma to oral mucous membranes.*

Suggested NIC interventions

Fluid/Electrolyte Management; Oral Health Maintenance; Oral Health Restoration; Nutrition Management; Pain Management

Evaluations for expected outcomes

■ Patient's total daily fluid intake equals output.

■ Patient's mucous membranes remain moist, pink, and free from cuts and abrasions.

■ Patient chews and drinks without discomfort.

■ Patient doesn't exhibit complications related to trauma to oral mucous membranes.

■ Patient discusses possible causes of alteration in oral mucous membranes, such as ill-fitting dentures or braces.

■ Patient discusses preventive measures such as regular oral hygiene, which includes cleaning of dentures.

Documentation

■ Observations of condition, healing, and response to treatment

■ Interventions to provide supportive care and patient's response to supportive care

■ Instructions given, patient's understanding of instructions, and demonstrated skill in carrying out prescribed oral care measures

■ Evaluations for expected outcomes

Reference

Cawley, M.M., and Benson, L.M. "Current Trends in Managing Oral Mucositis," *Clinical Journal of Oncology Nursing* 9(5):584-92, October 2005.

Impaired
ORAL MUCOUS MEMBRANE
related to pathologic condition

Definition

Disruption of the lips and soft tissue of the oral cavity

Assessment

■ History of oral cavity disorder or surgery

■ Medication history

■ Oral status, including condition of teeth, inspection of oral cavity (including gums and tongue), oral hygiene routine, pain or discomfort, palpation of buccal mucosa, and salivation

■ Nutritional status, including current weight, change from normal weight, dietary pattern, and vitamin intake

■ Psychosocial status, including coping skills, family members' habits (smoking and alcohol intake), patient's perception of health problem, self-concept, and stressors (finances, family, and job)

Defining characteristics

■ Bleeding

■ Coated tongue

■ Desquamation

- Difficulty eating, speaking, or swallowing
- Diminished, absent, or bad taste
- Dry mouth
- Edema
- Enlarged tonsils
- Fissures and chelitis
- Gingival hyperplasia or recession (pockets deeper than 4 mm)
- Gingival or mucosal pallor
- Halitosis
- Mucosal denudation
- Oral lesions, ulcers, pain, or discomfort
- Purulent drainage or exudate; presence of pathogens
- Smooth, atrophic, sensitive tongue
- Spongy patches or white, curdlike exudate
- Stomatitis
- Vesicles, nodules, or papules
- White patches and plaque

Expected outcomes

- Patient's lesions or wounds will show improvement or heal.
- Patient will have minimal, if any, complications.
- Patient will voice increased comfort.
- Patient will demonstrate understanding of surgical measures.
- Patient will voice feelings about condition.
- Patient will explain oral care routine.
- Patient will demonstrate oral hygiene practices.

Suggested NOC outcomes

Hydration; Oral Hygiene; Self-Care: Oral Hygiene; Tissue Integrity: Skin & Mucous Membranes

Interventions and rationales

- Inspect patient's oral cavity every shift. Describe and document its condition, reporting any status change. *Regular assessment prevents recurrence or exacerbation of problems.*
- Perform the prescribed treatment regimen for the underlying pathologic condition. Report favorable and adverse responses to the treatment regimen. *Treating the underlying condition improves the condition of the oral mucous membranes.*
- Encourage patient to state feelings and concerns about oral condition and its impact on body image *to help him accept changes in body image.*
- Provide supportive measures, as indicated:
- Assist with oral hygiene before and after meals. Use a soft-bristled toothbrush or cotton applicator and nonalcoholic mouthwash *to minimize trauma to damaged tissues.*
- Lubricate patient's lips frequently *to prevent cracking and irritation.*
- Use artificial saliva solution if the mouth remains dry *to restore normal moisture.*

– Avoid serving hot, cold, spicy, fried, or citrus foods *to avoid irritating damaged tissue.*

– Suction the oral cavity to prevent drooling and aspiration of accumulated secretions. *Aspiration may lead to pneumonia or coughing and further trauma.*

– Give soft or pureed foods, which don't irritate tissues, *to reduce pain.*

■ If oral surgery is scheduled, give the appropriate preoperative and postoperative instruction and care. Document the response. *Instruction enhances compliance with therapy.*

■ Instruct patient in oral hygiene practices, and have patient give a return demonstration. Suggest a referral to a dentist or dental hygienist. *This increases patient's awareness of oral hygiene and reduces discomfort, resulting in increased nutrition and hydration.*

■ Encourage patient to stop smoking. *Smoking has been linked to mucous membrane breakdown and cancer.*

■ Refer patient to a psychiatric liaison nurse or support group *to help patient cope with altered body image.*

Suggested NIC interventions

Fluid/Electrolyte Management; Infection Protection; Nutrition Management; Oral Health Restoration; Pain Management

Evaluations for expected outcomes

■ Patient has no lesions or wounds, or they cause patient less discomfort.

■ Patient doesn't exhibit complications related to trauma to oral mucous membranes.

■ Patient chews and swallows without discomfort.

■ Patient discusses impending surgical procedures.

■ Patient discusses fear of oral surgery and outcome.

■ Patient discusses postoperative oral care routine.

■ Patient demonstrates oral hygiene practices, including treatments and medications.

Documentation

■ Patient's expression of concern about oral condition and its impact on body image

■ Patient's willingness to join in own care

■ Observations of condition, healing, and response to treatment

■ Interventions to provide supportive care and patient's response to supportive care

■ Instructions given, patient's understanding of instructions, and demonstrated skill in carrying out prescribed oral care measures

■ Evaluations for expected outcomes

Reference

Cohn, J.L., and Fulton, J.S. "Nursing Staff Perspectives on Oral Care for Neuroscience Patients," *The Journal of Neuroscience Nursing* 38(1):22-30, February 2006.

Acute
PAIN

related to physical, biological, or chemical agents

Definition

An unpleasant sensory and emotional experience arising from actual or potential tissue damage or described in terms of such damage; pain may be of sudden or slow onset, vary in intensity from mild to severe, and be constant or recurring; pain lasts less than 6 months; and period of pain has an anticipated or predictable end

Assessment

■ Descriptive characteristics of pain, including location, quality, intensity on a scale of 1 to 10, temporal factors, and sources of relief
■ Physiologic variables, such as age and pain tolerance
■ Psychological variables, such as body image, personality, previous experience with pain, anxiety, and secondary gain
■ Sociocultural variables, including cognitive style, culture or ethnicity, attitude and values, sex, and birth order
■ Environmental variables, such as setting and time

Defining characteristics

■ Alteration in muscle tone (may range from listless to rigid)
■ Autonomic responses (diaphoresis; blood pressure, pulse rate, and respiratory rate changes; and dilated pupils)
■ Changes in appetite and eating
■ Communication (verbal or coded) of pain
■ Distracting behavior (such as pacing, seeking out other people, and performing repetitive activities)
■ Expressions of pain (such as moaning and crying)
■ Facial mask of pain (grimacing)
■ Guarding or protective behavior
■ Narrowed focus (including altered time perception, withdrawal from social contact, and impaired thought process)
■ Self-focusing
■ Sleep disturbance

Expected outcomes

■ Patient will rate pain on a scale of 1 to 10.
■ Patient will articulate factors that intensify pain and will modify behavior accordingly.
■ Patient will state and carry out appropriate interventions for pain relief.
■ Patient will report more than 4 hours of sleep nightly.
■ Patient will decrease amount and frequency of pain medication needed.
■ Patient will express feeling of comfort and relief from pain.

Comfort Level; Pain Control; Pain: Disruptive Effects; Pain Level; Sleep

Interventions and rationales

■ Assess patient's signs and symptoms of pain and administer pain medication, as prescribed. Monitor and record the medication's effectiveness and adverse effects. *Assessment allows for care plan modification, as needed.*

■ Perform comfort measures to promote relaxation, such as massage, bathing, repositioning, and relaxation techniques. *These measures reduce muscle tension or spasm, redistribute pressure on body parts, and help patient focus on non-pain–related subjects.*

■ Plan activities with patient to provide distraction, such as reading, crafts, television, and visits, *to help patient focus on non-pain–related matters.*

■ Provide patient with information to help increase pain tolerance; for example, reasons for pain and length of time it will last. *This educates patient and encourages compliance in trying alternative pain-relief measures.*

■ Manipulate the environment to promote periods of uninterrupted rest. This promotes health, well-being, and increased energy level important to pain relief.

■ Apply heat or cold as ordered (specify), *to minimize or relieve pain.*

■ Help patient into a comfortable position and use pillows to splint or support painful areas, as appropriate, *to reduce muscle tension or spasm and to redistribute pressure on body parts.*

■ Collaborate with patient in administering prescribed analgesics when alternative methods of pain control are inadequate. *Gaining patient's trust and involvement helps ensure compliance and may reduce medication intake.*

■ When possible, allow patient to use alternative pain treatments from his culture (such as acupuncture) as a substitute for or complement to Western treatments *to promote nonpharmacologic pain management.*

Suggested NIC interventions

Coping Enhancement; Emotional Support; Medication Management; Pain Management; Positioning; Sleep Enhancement

Evaluations for expected outcomes

■ Patient's pain rating is documented (using a scale of 1 to 10) before administering medication and 30 to 45 minutes afterward.

■ Patient articulates factors that intensify pain and modifies behavior accordingly.

■ Patient carries out alternative pain-control measures such as heat or cold applications.

■ Patient reports more than 4 hours sleep nightly (reports of less than 4 hours require further assessment).

■ Patient decreases amount and frequency of pain medication within 72 hours.

■ Patient expresses feeling of comfort.

Documentation

■ Patient's description of physical pain, pain relief, and feelings about pain

■ Observations of patient's physical, psychological, and sociocultural responses to pain

■ Comfort measures and medications provided to reduce pain and effectiveness of interventions

■ Information provided to patient about pain and pain relief

■ Other interventions performed to assist patient with pain control

■ Evaluations for expected outcomes

Reference

de Jong, A.E., and Gamel, C. "Use of Simple Relaxation Technique in Burn Care: Literature Review," *Journal of Advanced Nursing* 54(6):710-21, June 2006.

Acute
PAIN

related to psychological factors

Definition

An unpleasant sensory and emotional experience arising from actual or potential tissue damage or described in terms of such damage; pain may be of sudden or slow onset, vary in intensity from mild to severe, and be constant or recurring; pain lasts less than 6 months; and period of pain has an anticipated or predictable end

Assessment

■ History of exposure to physical, biological, or chemical agents as a cause of pain

■ Descriptive characteristics of pain, including location, quality, intensity on a scale of 1 to 10, temporal factors, and sources of provocation or relief

■ Physiologic variables, such as age and pain tolerance

■ Psychological variables, such as body image, personality, previous experience with pain, anxiety, and secondary gain

■ Sociocultural variables, including cognitive style, culture and ethnicity, attitude and values, sex, and birth order

■ Environmental variables, such as time and setting

Defining characteristics

■ Alteration in muscle tone (may range from listless to rigid)

■ Autonomic responses (diaphoresis; blood pressure, pulse rate, and respiratory rate changes; and dilated pupils)

■ Changes in appetite and eating

■ Communication (verbal or coded) of pain

■ Distracting behavior (such as pacing, seeking out other people, and performing repetitive activities)

■ Expressions of pain (such as moaning and crying)

■ Facial mask of pain (grimacing)

■ Guarding or protective behavior

■ Narrowed focus (including altered time perception, withdrawal from social contact, and impaired thought process)
■ Self-focusing
■ Sleep disturbance

Expected outcomes
■ Patient will identify specific characteristics of pain.
■ Patient will express relief from pain within a reasonable time after taking prescribed medication.
■ Patient will help develop a plan for pain control.
■ Patient will articulate possibility of physical pain being associated with emotional stressors.
■ Patient will require less pain medication (specify).
■ Patient will state satisfaction with pain-management regimen.
■ Patient will use available resources to understand pain phenomenon and will cooperate with treatment plan.

Suggested NOC outcomes

Comfort Level; Pain Control; Pain: Disruptive Effects; Pain Level

Interventions and rationales
■ Assess physical symptoms that require pain medication, and administer medication, as prescribed. *Continuous reassessment documents patient's subjective complaints and behavior with organic pathology.*
■ Return to patient in 30 minutes to check the medication's effectiveness. *This establishes trusting-caring relationship that encourages accurate communication.*
■ Discuss with patient possible association between exacerbation of pain and patient's identified stressors. *This helps patient explore exacerbating emotional or environmental factors that may affect pain.*
■ Ask patient to help establish goals and develop plan for pain control. *This gives patient a sense of control.*
■ Provide patient with positive feedback about his progress toward reaching goals *to improve motivation and encourage compliance.*
■ Spend at least 15 minutes per shift allowing patient to express feelings, *which will help give patient a sense of control.*
■ Consider the services of a psychiatric mental health professional to help patient and staff members establish a realistic plan to resolve the problem. *Patients who remain helpless, unmotivated, uncooperative, and manipulative are self-destructive. Underlying causes should be explored.*
■ Plan activities to distract patient, such as reading, television, and family visits, *to help keep patient from focusing on pain.*

Suggested NIC interventions

Anxiety Reduction; Coping Enhancement; Emotional Support; Hope Instillation; Medication Management; Pain Management; Sleep Enhancement

Evaluations for expected outcomes

■ Patient discusses characteristics of pain, including location, duration, and frequency.

■ Patient reports achieving pain relief with analgesia or other measures.

■ Patient participates in development of health care plan and discusses modifications.

■ Patient acknowledges that pain may be related to emotional factors and lists stressors that may exacerbate pain.

■ Patient achieves reduction in use of pain medication.

■ Patient states satisfaction with pain-management regimen.

■ Patient displays motivation by seeking out resources to explain pain phenomenon and cooperating with treatment plan.

Documentation

■ Patient's expressions of physical pain and well-being and emotional pain and well-being

■ Observations of patient's physical well-being

■ Interventions performed to help patient control pain and patient's response

■ Evaluations for expected outcomes

Reference

Siedlecki, S.L., and Good, M. "Effect of Music on Power, Pain, Depression, and Disability," *Journal of Advanced Nursing* 54(5):553-62, June 2006.

Chronic
PAIN
related to physical disability

Definition

An unpleasant sensory and emotional experience arising from actual or potential tissue damage or described in terms of such damage; pain may be of sudden or slow onset, vary in intensity from mild to severe, and be constant or recurring; pain lasts more than 6 months; and period of pain doesn't have an anticipated or predictable end

Assessment

■ Descriptive characteristics of pain, including location, quality, intensity on a scale of 1 to 10, temporal factors, duration, precipitating factors (food, alcohol, activity, and stress), and comfort factors

■ Physiologic variables, such as general health state, length of pain, organ system involvement, pain tolerance, disability (work, family, or social), and pain interventions (such as injection, traction, ice, physical therapy, and transcutaneous electrical nerve stimulation)

■ Psychological variables, such as age, self-esteem, self-worth, role (worker, husband, breadwinner), coping behavior (appropriate or inappropriate), secondary

gains (disability insurance, workmen's compensation, litigation), suffering (emotional component), manipulative behavior, dependence on others or on system, and previous hospital experience
- Sociocultural variables, including educational level, motivation, culture or ethnicity, sex, values and beliefs, pain behaviors, financial distress, and religion
- Environmental variables, such as setting and time
- Pharmacologic variables, including type of drugs, amount used in one day, use of illicit drugs, and use of alcohol

Defining characteristics
- Altered ability to continue previous activities
- Atrophy of involved muscle group
- Changes in sleep pattern
- Depression
- Facial mask
- Fatigue
- Fear of reinjury
- Irritability
- Protective or guarding behavior
- Reduced social interaction
- Restlessness
- Self-focusing
- Sympathetic-mediated responses (such as change in temperature and hypersensitivity)
- Weight gain or loss

Expected outcomes
- Patient will identify characteristics of pain and pain behaviors.
- Patient will develop pain management program that includes activity and rest schedule, exercise program, and medication regimen that isn't pain-contingent.
- Patient will carry out resocialization behavior and activities.
- Patient will state relationship of increasing pain to stress, activity, and fatigue.
- Patient will state importance of self-care behavior or activities.

Suggested NOC outcomes
Comfort Level; Depression Level; Depression Self-Control; Pain Control; Pain Level; Quality of Life; Sleep; Symptom Control

Interventions and rationales
- Assess patient's physical symptoms of pain, physical complaints, and daily activities. Administer pain medication, as prescribed. Monitor and record the effectiveness and adverse effects of medication. (Keep in mind that pain behavior and pain talk may be inconsistent.) *Correlating patient's pain behavior with activities, time of day, and visits may be useful in modifying tasks.*
- Develop a behavior-oriented care plan; for instance, set up a plan to follow the activity schedule. *Behavioral-cognitive measures can help patient modify learned pain behaviors.*

■ Teach patient how to use relaxation techniques, guided imagery, massage, or music therapy to relieve pain. *These methods work as an adjunct to medications, increase self-help, and foster independence.*

■ Teach patient and family members such techniques as massage, application of ice, and exercise *to relieve pain and foster independence.*

■ Work closely with staff and patient's family *to achieve pain-management goals and maximize patient's cooperation.*

■ Use behavior modification; for example, spend time with patient only if the discussion includes no pain talk. Use contingency rewards for decreasing pain talk and pain behavior. *Reducing pain talk helps patient refocus on other, more important matters.*

■ Encourage self-care activities. Develop a schedule. *This helps patient gain a sense of control and reduces dependence on caregivers and society.*

■ Establish a specific time to talk with patient about pain and its psychological and emotional effects *to establish a trusting, supportive relationship that encompasses patient's physiologic, emotional, social, sexual, and financial concerns.*

Suggested NIC interventions

Analgesic Administration; Behavior Modification; Biofeedback; Emotional Support; Mood Management; Pain Management; Patient Contracting; Simple Massage

Evaluations for expected outcomes

■ Patient maintains activity diary and pain-level chart that rates severity of pain on a scale of 1 to 10.

■ Patient maintains pain-management program that includes activity and rest schedule, exercise program, and medication regimen.

■ Patient demonstrates resocialization behavior and activities.

■ Patient states that stress, activity, and fatigue may increase pain.

■ Patient states that self-care activities are important.

Documentation

■ Patient's description of physical pain, pain relief, and feelings about pain

■ Pain talk and pain behavior and affect

■ Relationship of reports of pain to activities

■ Treatments and pain talk

■ Time out of bed

■ Comfort measures initiated by nurse, patient, or family members

■ Response to interventions

■ Response to pharmacologic agents

■ Interaction with staff

■ Evaluations for expected outcomes

Reference

Siedlecki, S.L. "Predictors of Self-rated Health Status in Patients with Chronic Nonmalignant Pain," *Pain Management Nursing* 7(3):109-16, September 2006.

Risk for
PERIPHERAL NEUROVASCULAR DYSFUNCTION

Definition
Accentuated risk of disruption in circulation or sensation in or motion of an extremity

Assessment
- History of trauma or vascular injuries
- Inspection of extremities, including signs of soft-tissue injury, such as abrasions, lacerations, and contusions
- Pain sensation, including characteristics (sharp, dull, constant, or intermittent) of pain, precipitating factors, and reaction to passive stretching of affected muscles
- Tactile sensation in areas innervated by major nerves of upper extremities, including deltoid, radial side of forearm, palmar surface of thumb, fingers, palmar surface of little finger, and webbed space between thumb and index finger
- Tactile sensation in lower extremities, including medial side of foot and leg, medial side of thigh, sole of foot, and lateral aspect of leg below the knee
- Motor nerve function of upper extremities, including arm abduction at shoulder, arm flexion at elbow, thumb and little finger opposition, abduction and adduction of fingers, and extension of wrist and fingers
- Motor nerve function of lower extremities, including knee extension, thigh adduction, plantar flexion and dorsiflexion of ankle, and flexion and extension of toes
- Pulses in upper and lower extremities, including radial, ulnar, brachial, femoral, popliteal, posterior tibial, and dorsalis pedis; perform bilateral comparison and rank quality using following scale:
0 = absent
1 = very weak, barely palpable
2 = weak, reduced
3 = slightly weak, easily located
4 = normal, easily located
- Vascular status, including capillary refill time, blanching, skin temperature, and skin color
- Point tenderness, especially over bony prominences
- Edema
- Increased intracompartmental pressure
- Cranial nerves (if patient has halo cast)

Risk factors
- Burns
- Fractures
- Immobilization

■ Mechanical compression (such as tourniquet, cast, brace, dressing, and restraint)
■ Orthopedic surgery
■ Trauma
■ Vascular obstruction

Expected outcomes

■ Patient won't experience disability related to peripheral neurovascular dysfunction after injury or treatment.
■ Patient will maintain circulation in extremities.
■ Patient will feel and move each toe or finger after application of cast, brace, or splint.
■ Patient will demonstrate correct body positioning techniques.
■ Patient and family members will express understanding of risk of altered neurovascular status and need to report symptoms of impaired circulation.
■ Patient will enroll in smoking-cessation program, as appropriate.
■ Patient will not exhibit symptoms of neurovascular compromise.

Suggested NOC outcomes

Circulation Status; Coordinated Movement; Neurological Status: Spinal Sensory/Motor Function; Risk Control; Risk Detection; Tissue Perfusion: Peripheral

Interventions and rationales

■ Note if patient will undergo surgery or a procedure that increases his risk of peripheral neurovascular dysfunction *to anticipate complications.*
■ Immobilize the joints directly above and below the suspected fracture site, leaving room for pulse assessment *to facilitate monitoring of circulatory status.*
■ As appropriate, assess circulation before the application of the cast, brace, or splint. After application of the cast, brace, or splint, have patient move his fingers and toes every 4 hours until discharge *to detect signs of impaired circulation.*
■ Remove the clothing around the suspected fracture site, clean the site, apply sterile dressings to open wounds, and carefully apply a cast, brace, or splint *to avoid further infection and trauma.*
■ Follow facility guidelines for the application of such devices as tourniquets, restraints, and tape *to ensure adequate circulation in affected extremity.*
■ If you suspect nerve compression, assess the position of the extremity that has a cast, brace, or splint. *Positioning of the extremity may affect circulation.*
■ Elevate the limb above heart level after surgery or trauma *to reduce the risk of edema.* If increased intracompartmental pressure is evident, maintain the affected limb at heart level *to reduce pressure.*
■ If edema appears in the affected extremity, split, bivalve, slit, or cut a window in the cast and padding according to facility protocol *to avoid neurovascular impairment.*
■ Inject prescribed neurotoxic agents (such as penicillin G, hydrocortisone, tetanus toxoid, and diazepam) away from the affected extremity and major nerves *to avoid injury.*

■ Avoid flexing the affected extremity. *Flexion may reduce venous circulation, increasing the risk of neurovascular complications.*

■ If patient smokes, encourage him to enroll in a smoking-cessation program. *Quitting smoking may enhance oxygenation, decreasing the risk of peripheral neurovascular dysfunction.*

■ Take steps to ease patient's anxiety. *Stress may lead to vasoconstriction.*

■ Administer and monitor the effectiveness of vasodilators, as ordered, *to control vasospasm.*

■ If patient requires a fasciotomy to restore circulation, provide educational material that explains this emergency procedure *to reduce patient anxiety.*

■ Instruct patient and family members in proper positioning when lying in bed and when sitting and in methods of obtaining pressure relief *to avoid pooling of blood and pressure ulcers.*

■ If appropriate, discuss the cause of the injury and safety precautions *to avoid further injury.* Injuries to upper extremities usually result from industrial accidents; injuries to lower extremities, from automobile accidents.

■ Instruct patient and family members in recognizing the symptoms of peripheral neurovascular dysfunction, including numbness, pain, and tingling. Emphasize the need to report these symptoms to a physician *to prevent onset of neurovascular damage after discharge.*

Suggested NIC interventions

Circulatory Precautions; Exercise Promotion: Strength Training; Exercise Therapy: Joint Mobility; Peripheral Sensation Management; Positioning: Neurologic; Pressure Ulcer Prevention; Skin Surveillance; Splinting

Evaluations for expected outcomes

■ Patient doesn't experience disability related to peripheral neurovascular dysfunction.

■ Patient maintains circulation in extremities.

■ Patient demonstrates ability to move each toe or finger after application of cast, brace, or splint.

■ Patient demonstrates correct body positioning techniques.

■ Patient and family members express understanding of risk of altered neurovascular status.

■ Patient enrolls in smoking-cessation program, as appropriate.

■ Patient shows no symptoms of neurovascular compromise.

Documentation

■ Results of neurovascular assessment (baseline and ongoing)

■ Nature of injury or treatment

■ History of illnesses and surgeries

■ Symptoms of neurovascular dysfunction reported by patient and family members

■ Patient's turning schedule

■ Instructions provided to patient and family members at discharge

■ Evaluations for expected outcomes

Reference

Oka, R.K. "Peripheral Arterial Disease in Older Adults: Management of Cardiovascular Disease Risk Factors," *The Journal of Cardiovascular Nursing* 21(5 Supp 1):S15- S20, September-October 2006.

Risk for
POISONING

related to external factors

Definition

Accentuated risk of accidental exposure to or ingestion of drugs or dangerous products in doses sufficient to cause poisoning

Assessment

■ Health history, including accidents, allergies, exposure to pollutants, falls, hyperthermia, hypothermia, poisoning, sensory or perceptual changes (auditory, gustatory, kinesthetic, olfactory, tactile, and visual), and trauma
■ Circumstances surrounding present situation that might lead to injury
■ Neurologic status, including level of consciousness (LOC), mental status, and orientation
■ Psychosocial history, including age, habits (drug or alcohol use), occupation, and personality
■ Laboratory studies, including clotting factors, hemoglobin levels and hematocrit, platelet count, white blood cell count, and toxicology screening

Risk factors

■ Atmospheric pollutants
■ Chemical contamination of food or water
■ Dangerous products or drugs stored within reach of children or confused people
■ Flaking or peeling paint or plaster in presence of young children
■ Poisonous plants
■ Storing of large amounts of drugs in home
■ Unprotected contact with heavy metals or chemicals
■ Use of illegal drugs contaminated with poisonous additives
■ Use of paint, lacquer, or similar materials in poorly ventilated area or without effective protection

Expected outcomes

■ Patient won't ingest or be exposed to dangerous substances.
■ Patient will communicate an understanding of need for self-protection.
■ Patient and family members will state method for safekeeping of potentially dangerous products.

Suggested NOC outcomes

Safe Home Environment

Interventions and rationales

■ Observe, record, and report falls, seizures, and unsafe practices to ensure implementation of appropriate interventions. *Overdose of certain medications (such as phenothiazines) can cause such neurologic problems as seizures.*

■ Monitor and record patient's respiratory status *because certain poisons can cause respiratory depression.*

■ Monitor and record neurologic status *because excessive toxic exposure can cause coma.* Patient may have pinpoint or dilated pupils, depending on the type of drug ingested and the length of time patient has been hypoxic.

■ Monitor vital signs, intake and output, and LOC. Record and report any changes. *Severe hypotension may develop following overdose. It may be related to central nervous system defect, direct myocardial depression, or vasodilation. Marked hyperthermia can occur with salicylate overdose, which affects the metabolic rate. Dehydration may develop in some patients from an increased respiratory rate, sweating, vomiting, and urine losses.*

■ Remove dangerous or potentially dangerous products from the environment *to avoid injury.*

■ Check the settings on oxygen flow meters every hour on patients known to retain carbon dioxide (for example, some patients with chronic obstructive pulmonary disease). *This avoids carbon dioxide narcosis from excessive oxygen therapy in poorly ventilated patients; if unchecked, patient may stop breathing.*

■ Provide patient and family members with information about such specific products as medications, oxygen, and total parenteral nutrition. Tailor instructions to a specific product and patient's ability to learn self-care. *This enables patient and family members to identify and alter environmental or lifestyle factors to achieve optimum health level.*

Suggested NIC interventions

Environmental Management: Safety; Environmental Risk Protection; Health Education; Home Maintenance Assistance; Surveillance: Safety; Vital Signs Monitoring

Evaluations for expected outcomes

■ Patient doesn't report or exhibit signs or symptoms resulting from exposure to or ingestion of dangerous substances.

■ Patient requests information on protection from dangerous products.

■ Patient and family members describe method for safekeeping of potentially dangerous products.

Documentation

■ Patient's statements that indicate potential for injury
■ Physical findings
■ Observations or knowledge of unsafe practices
■ Interventions performed to prevent injury

- Patient's response to nursing interventions
- Evaluations for expected outcomes

References

Kendall, P.A., et al. "Food Safety Guidance for Older Adults," *Clinical Infectious Diseases* 42(9):1298-304, May 2006.

Todd, B. "The Increasing Risk of Salmonella Infections. Food Industry Practices, Inadequate Regulation, and Antimicrobial Resistance Heighten Concerns," *AJN* 106(7):35-37, July 2006.

Risk for
POISONING
related to internal factors (biological, psychological, developmental)

Definition
Accentuated risk of accidental exposure to or ingestion of drugs or dangerous products in doses sufficient to cause poisoning

Assessment
- Health history, including accidents, allergies, exposure to pollutants, falls, hyperthermia, hypothermia, poisoning, seizures, trauma, and sensory-perceptual changes (auditory, gustatory, kinesthetic, olfactory, tactile, and visual)
- Circumstances of present situation that might lead to injury
- Neurologic status, including level of consciousness (LOC), mental status, and orientation
- Psychosocial history, including age, habits (drug or alcohol use), occupation, and personality
- Laboratory studies, including clotting factors, hemoglobin levels and hematocrit, platelet count, white blood cell count, and toxicology screening

Risk factors
- Cognitive or emotional difficulties
- Insufficient resources
- Lack of drug education
- Lack of safety precautions
- Occupational setting without adequate safeguards
- Reduced vision

Expected outcomes
- Patient won't ingest or be exposed to dangerous products.
- Patient will communicate understanding of need for self-protection.
- Patient and family members will explain method for safekeeping of dangerous products.

Suggested NOC outcomes

Risk Control: Drug Use; Risk Detection; Safe Home Environment

Interventions and rationales

■ Observe, record, and report falls, seizures, and unsafe practices to ensure implementation of appropriate interventions. *Overdose of certain medications can cause such neurologic problems as seizures.*

■ Monitor and record patient's respiratory status *because certain poisons can cause respiratory depression.*

■ Monitor and record neurologic status *because excessive toxic exposure can cause coma.* Patient may have pinpoint or dilated pupils, depending on the type of drug ingested and the length of time patient has been hypoxic.

■ Remove dangerous or potentially dangerous products from the environment *to avoid injury.*

■ Monitor vital signs, intake and output, and LOC. Record and report changes. *Severe hypotension may develop following overdose. It may be related to central nervous system defect, direct myocardial depression, or vasodilation. Marked hyperthermia can occur with salicylate overdose, which affects metabolic rate. Dehydration may develop in some patients from an increased respiratory rate, sweating, vomiting, and urine losses.*

■ Provide patient and family members with information about such specific products as medications, oxygen, and total parenteral nutrition. Tailor instructions to a specific product and patient's ability to learn self-care. *This enables patient and family members to identify and alter environmental or lifestyle factors to achieve optimum health level.*

Suggested NIC interventions

Home Maintenance Assistance; Medication Management; Risk Identification; Surveillance: Safety

Evaluations for expected outcomes

■ Patient doesn't report or exhibit signs or symptoms related to exposure to or ingestion of dangerous products.

■ Patient requests information on self-protection from dangerous products.

■ Patient and family members state method for safekeeping of potentially dangerous products.

Documentation

■ Patient's statements about situation that indicate potential for injury
■ Physical findings
■ Record of falls, seizures, and unsafe practices
■ Interventions that reduce risk of injury
■ Patient's response to nursing interventions
■ Evaluations for expected outcomes

Reference
Daly, F.F., et al. "A Risk-Assessment–Based Approach to the Management of Acute Poisoning," *Emergency Medicine Journal* 23(5):396-99, May 2006.

POSTTRAUMA SYNDROME
related to accidental injury

Definition
Sustained maladaptive response to a traumatic, overwhelming event

Assessment
- History and circumstances of accident
- Physical injuries sustained, including cardiopulmonary, musculoskeletal, genitourinary, and integumentary
- Neurologic status
- Emotional reactions, including grief reaction, self-concept, and sleep pattern
- Cognitive reactions, including concentration, memory, and orientation
- Behavioral reactions, including available support systems, clergy, coping patterns, family members, problem-solving ability, and social interactions

Defining characteristics
- Aggression, anxiety, anger, rage
- Avoidance, alienation, altered moods
- Compulsive behavior
- Denial, grief, fear, depression
- Detachment
- Exaggerated startle response, flashbacks
- Guilt
- Headaches
- Hypervigilance
- Intrusive dreams, nightmares, or thoughts; difficulty concentrating
- Irritability
- Numbness
- Panic attacks
- Psychogenic amnesia
- Repression
- Shame
- Substance abuse

Expected outcomes
- Patient will recover or be rehabilitated from physical injuries to extent possible.
- Patient will state feelings and fears related to traumatic event.
- Patient will express feelings of safety.
- Patient will use available support systems.
- Patient will use effective coping mechanisms to reduce fear.

■ Patient will maintain or reestablish adaptive social interactions with family members.

Suggested NOC outcomes

Anxiety Self-Control; Body Image; Coping; Depression Level; Fear Self-Control; Hope; Impulse Self-Control; Quality of Life; Self-Esteem; Stress Level

Interventions and rationales

■ Follow the medical regimen to manage physical injuries. *Attention to physical needs remains primary, according to Maslow's hierarchy.*
■ Provide emotional support:
– Visit patient frequently *to reduce his fear of being alone.*
– Be available to listen *to respond empathetically to patient's feelings.*
– Accept and encourage the statement of patient's feelings *to reassure patient that feelings are appropriate and valid.*
– Assure patient of his safety, and take the measures needed to ensure it. *Frequent nightmares or flashbacks may cause patient to question the safety of his environment.*
– Avoid care-related activities or environmental stimuli that may intensify symptoms associated with trauma (loud noises, bright lights, abrupt entrances to patient's room, or painful procedures or treatment). *Environmental stimuli can easily intensify flashbacks to a traumatic event.*
– Reorient patient to surroundings and reality as frequently as necessary. *Posttrauma psychic numbing impairs orientation, memory, and reality perception.*
– Instruct patient in at least one fear-reducing behavior such as seeking support from others when frightened. *As patient learns to reduce fears, coping skills will increase.*
■ Support patient's family members:
– Provide time for them to express feelings.
– Help them understand patient's reactions.
This reduces their anxiety and gives them a chance to help patient.
■ Offer referrals to other support persons or groups, including clergy, mental health professionals, and trauma support groups. *Referrals help patient to regain a sense of universality, reduce isolation, share fears, and deal constructively with feelings.*
■ Recognize that patient's culture may affect his response to trauma; remain supportive and nonjudgmental *to show patient that you support and accept his response to trauma.*

Suggested NIC interventions

Active Listening; Anxiety Reduction; Coping Enhancement; Counseling; Forgiveness Facilitation; Mood Management; Security Enhancement; Socialization Enhancement; Support Group

Evaluations for expected outcomes

■ Patient resumes usual activities of daily living to extent possible.
■ Patient expresses feelings associated with traumatic event.

- Patient expresses feeling of safety.
- Patient interacts with supportive people to alleviate distress.
- Patient demonstrates use of at least one fear-reducing behavior (specify).
- Patient interacts with family members in beneficial manner.

Documentation
- Patient's perception of traumatic event
- Observations of patient's behavior
- Observations of patient's social interaction with others
- Interventions
- Patient's responses to nursing interventions
- Referrals to other support persons or groups
- Evaluations for expected outcomes

Reference
Olszewski, T.M., and Varrasse, J.F. "The Neurobiology of PTSD: Implications for Nurses," *Journal of Psychological Nursing and Mental Health Services* 43(6):40-47, June 2005.

Risk for
POSTTRAUMA SYNDROME

Definition
At risk for sustained maladaptive response to traumatic, overwhelming event

Assessment
- Age and gender
- History of traumatic event, including circumstances, losses incurred (financial, property, physical integrity, close relationships), effect of trauma on social interactions, and grief reaction
- Health history, including previous traumatic events, patient's characteristic perception of such events and coping responses, and alcohol or substance abuse
- Mental status, including cognitive and emotional function, problems with concentration, memory, orientation, mood, and behavior
- Changes in appetite, self-image, sleep pattern, or sexual drive
- Available sources of support, including friends, family, caregivers, and community resources

Risk factors
- Diminished ego strength
- Displacement for home
- Duration of the event
- Exaggerated sense of responsibility
- Inadequate social support

- Nonsupportive environment
- Occupation
- Perception of event
- Survivor's role in the event

Expected outcomes

- Patient won't develop chronic posttrauma response, substance abuse, or other mental health disorders.
- Patient will express understanding of posttrauma response.
- Patient's response to trauma won't be characterized by avoidance, numbness, or intrusiveness.
- Patient will express feelings of safety.
- Patient will employ effective coping skills and will reach out to appropriate sources of support to reduce fear.

Suggested NOC outcomes

Coping; Depression Level; Depression Self-Control; Risk Detection; Social Support; Spiritual Health; Stress Level

Interventions and rationales

- Follow the medical regimen *to treat medical problems associated with the traumatic event.*
- Assess patient's baseline mental status and monitor changes in cognitive and psychosocial function *to detect the need for intervention as soon as possible.*
- Listen actively to patient's statements about the traumatic event *to encourage a trusting relationship and open discussion.*
- Communicate to patient that you accept his fears and feelings related to the traumatic event *to reassure patient that his feelings are appropriate and valid.*
- Reassure patient that he's in a safe environment. *Patient may be reluctant to express lingering fears and require reassurance.*
- Avoid nursing care or environmental stimuli that may worsen or initiate symptoms (such as loud noise, bright lights, and painful procedures) *to avoid triggering flashbacks to the traumatic event.* Also, warn patient to avoid disruptive stimuli.
- Caution patient before you touch him and avoid approaching him from behind *to avoid actions that may be misinterpreted and trigger reexperience of the traumatic event.*
- Explore with patient strategies to reduce the traumatic response, such as having a support person call patient on a regular basis and using stress-reducing techniques when experiencing increased fear and anxiety, *to strengthen coping skills and foster a sense of control.*
- Teach patient that a posttrauma response may occur immediately or days, weeks, or years after a trauma *to alert him to the risk of posttrauma response.*
- Help patient to increase his awareness of people, places, and events that trigger or reduce a posttrauma response *to encourage him to take an active role in treatment.*

■ Provide opportunities for patient to discuss the trauma periodically, based on patient's needs and his willingness to talk *to prevent the development of posttrauma response.*

■ Encourage family members and friends to express their perceptions and feelings about the traumatic event and reactions they see in patient *to aid assessment.*

■ Provide teaching to family members, friends, and caregivers about the signs and symptoms of posttrauma response and interventions they can use *to promote involvement with rather than withdrawal from patient.*

■ Explore uses of appropriate community resources and make referrals according to patient's and family members' needs *to ensure continuity of care and decrease patient's isolation.*

Suggested NIC interventions

Coping Enhancement; Hope Instillation; Mood Management; Self-Awareness Enhancement

Evaluations for expected outcomes

■ Patient doesn't develop chronic posttrauma response, substance abuse, or other mental health disorders.

■ Patient expresses understanding of posttrauma response.

■ Patient's response to trauma isn't characterized by avoidance, numbness, or intrusiveness.

■ Patient expresses feelings of safety.

■ Patient employs effective coping skills and reaches out to appropriate sources of support to reduce fear.

Documentation

■ Patient's perception of the traumatic event
■ Observation of patient's behavior, coping skills, and use of support systems
■ Patient's response to nursing care activities
■ Patient's communication patterns with friends, family, and others and their responses
■ Teaching provided to patient and family
■ Referrals for ongoing support
■ Evaluations for expected outcomes

Reference

Guess, K.F. "Posttraumatic Stress Disorder: Early Detection is Key," *The Nurse Practitioner* 31(3):26-33, March 2006.

POWERLESSNESS

related to health care environment

Definition

Perception that one's own action will not significantly affect an outcome; a perceived lack of control over a current situation or immediate perceived loss of control over what happens to oneself and one's environment

Assessment

- Nature of the medical diagnosis
- Mobility
- Behavioral responses (verbal and nonverbal), including calmness or agitation, anger, independence or dependence, interest or apathy, and satisfaction or dissatisfaction
- Usual coping strategies
- Past experiences with hospitalization
- Knowledge, including current understanding of physical condition and physical, mental, and emotional readiness to learn
- Environment, including equipment and supplies, health care professionals and personnel, lighting, location of patient's personal belongings, noise, privacy, and space

Defining characteristics

- Apathy
- Depression over physical deterioration
- Expressed dissatisfaction over inability to perform previous tasks
- Expressed lack of control over self-care, current situation, and outcome
- Expressed self-doubt
- Failure to defend self-care practices
- Failure to monitor progress
- Failure to seek information about care
- Irritability because of dependence on others
- Passivity
- Reluctance to express true feelings because of fear of alienating caregivers
- Reluctance to participate in decisions about health
- Resentment, anger, and guilt
- Uncertainty about fluctuating energy levels

Expected outcomes

- Patient will identify feelings of powerlessness associated with the environment.
- Patient will describe modifications or adjustments to the environment that allow feelings of control.
- Patient will participate in self-care activities (specify).
- Patient will state feelings of regained control.

Suggested NOC outcomes

Anxiety Level; Decision-Making; Depression Self-Control; Family Participation in Professional Care; Fear Level; Health Beliefs; Self-Esteem; Social Involvement; Social Support

Interventions and rationales

■ Visit with patient 15 minutes each shift *to allow patient to express concerns and feelings.*
■ Acknowledge the importance of patient's space:
– Verbally delineate patient's space.
– Orient patient to his space.
– If patient is immobilized, ask for instructions regarding placement of personal belongings.
– If possible, allow patient to walk around the space and arrange personal belongings.
These measures enhance patient's potential for regaining sense of power.
■ Place the call bell, television controls, bedside table, telephone, urinal, and other items within easy reach. Improvise wherever possible to give patient control over the use of these objects. Attend to patient's ability or inability to use his hands and arms. *These measures help reduce patient's frustration over his inability to reach items in his immediate area.*
■ Reduce irritating noises, if possible, and explain the reasons for alarms and other disturbances. *Excessive sensory stimuli can cause disorientation, hallucinations, and delusional thinking.*
■ Explain treatments and procedures, and encourage patient to participate in planning his care. Provide choices for when and how activities will occur (such as bathing, eating, and getting out of bed). *This increases patient's feeling of powerfulness and reduces passivity and dependence on caregiver.*
■ Provide as many situations as possible where patient can take control (such as positioning, choosing an injection site, and visiting) *to help reduce potential for maladaptive coping behaviors.*
■ Encourage participation in self-care. Provide positive reinforcement for patient's activities *to encourage increasing participation in self-care in the future.*
■ Help patient learn as much about his current health problem as possible. *The greater his understanding, the more patient will feel in control.*

Suggested NIC interventions

Anxiety Reduction; Cognitive Restructuring; Decision-Making Support; Family Presence Facilitation; Mutual Goal Setting; Presence; Self-Esteem Enhancement; Values Clarification

Evaluations for expected outcomes

■ Patient expresses feelings of lack of control.
■ Patient's environment is adjusted to enhance his feelings of control.
■ Patient performs self-care measures to extent possible.
■ Patient expresses feelings of regained control.

Documentation
- Patient's expressions of anger, frustration, and sense of lack of control over environment
- Patient's interest in surroundings, participation in self-care, verbalization of understanding, and demonstration of skill in relation to medical diagnosis
- Interventions to promote patient's control over environment
- Patient's response to nursing interventions
- Evaluations for expected outcomes

Reference
Erlen, J.A. "Who Speaks for the Vulnerable?" *Orthopedic Nursing* 25(2):133-36, March-April 2006.

POWERLESSNESS
related to illness-related regimen

Definition
Perception that one's own action won't significantly affect an outcome; a perceived lack of control over a current situation or immediate happening

Assessment
- Nature of medical diagnosis
- Mobility
- Behavioral responses (verbal and nonverbal), including calmness or agitation, anger, anxiety, depression, independence or dependence, interest or apathy, and satisfaction or dissatisfaction
- Coping strategies, including passage through grieving process
- Past experiences with illness
- Knowledge, including current understanding of physical condition and physical, mental, and emotional readiness to learn
- Environment, including equipment and supplies, health care professionals and personnel, lighting, location of patient's personal belongings, noise, privacy, and space
- Number and types of stressors
- Social factors
- Spiritual beliefs and value system

Defining characteristics
- Apathy
- Depression over physical deterioration
- Expressed dissatisfaction over inability to perform previous tasks
- Expressed lack of control over self-care, current situation, and outcome
- Expressed self-doubt
- Failure to monitor progress
- Failure to seek information about care

- Irritability because of dependence on others
- Passivity
- Reluctance to express true feelings because of fear of alienating caregivers
- Reluctance to participate in decisions about health
- Resentment, anger, and guilt
- Uncertainty about fluctuating energy levels

Expected outcomes
- Patient will acknowledge fears, feelings, and concerns about current situation.
- Patient will make decisions regarding course of treatment.
- Patient will decrease level of anxiety by changing response to stressors.
- Patient will participate in self-care activities (specify).
- Patient will express feeling of regained control.
- Patient will accept and adapt to lifestyle changes.

Suggested NOC outcomes

Depression Self-Control; Family Participation in Professional Care; Health Beliefs; Health Beliefs: Perceived Ability to Perform; Participation in Health Care Decisions

Interventions and rationales
- Encourage patient to express his feelings and concerns. Set aside time for discussions with patient about daily events. *This helps patient bring vaguely understood emotions into focus.*
- Accept patient's feelings of powerlessness as normal. *This indicates respect for patient and enhances patient's feelings of self-worth.*
- Try to be present during situations where feelings of powerlessness are likely to be greatest *to help patient cope.*
- Identify and develop patient's coping mechanisms, strengths, and resources for support. *By making use of coping skills, patient can reduce anxiety and fears and successfully undergo grieving necessary to come to terms with chronic illness.*
- Discuss situations that provoke feelings of anger, anxiety, and powerlessness *to identify areas patient can control and to prevent anger from being inappropriately directed at self or others.*
- Encourage participation in self-care. Provide positive reinforcement for patient's activities. Encourage patient to take an active role as a member of the health care team. *This enhances patient's sense of control and reduces passive and dependent behavior.*
- Provide as many opportunities as possible for patient to make decisions about self-care (for instance, positioning, choosing an injection site, and visiting) *to communicate respect for patient and enhance feelings of independence.*
- Help patient learn about the health condition, treatment, and prognosis *to help patient feel in control.*
- Modify the environment when possible to meet patient's self-care needs *to promote patient's sense of control over his environment.*
- Decrease unpredictable events by discussing rules, policies, procedures, and schedules with patient. *Fear of the unknown interferes with patient's ability to cope.*

■ Encourage family members to support patient without taking control *to increase patient's feelings of self-worth.*

■ Reinforce patient's rights as stated in Patient's Bill of Rights *to protect patient's right to make decisions about health care treatment.*

■ Identify and arrange to accommodate patient's spiritual needs. *Spirituality enables patient to gain courage and resist despair.*

■ Respect and show your acceptance of patient's cultural beliefs about health. *The belief that each patient has the personal authority and responsibility to try to reach optimal well-being is a Western value not shared by all cultures.*

Suggested NIC interventions

Cognitive Restructuring; Decision-Making Support; Emotional Support; Health Education; Mood Management; Presence; Self- Care Assistance; Self-Responsibility Facilitation; Values Clarification

Evaluations for expected outcomes

■ Patient verbalizes positive and negative feelings about current situation.

■ Patient demonstrates increased control by participating in decisions related to health care.

■ Patient describes strategies for decreasing anxiety.

■ Patient actively participates in planning and executing aspects of care.

■ Patient communicates renewed sense of power and control of current situation.

■ Patient demonstrates ability to adapt to and accept lifestyle changes.

Documentation

■ Observations and interactions related to disease process and health care environment

■ Patient's responses to opportunities to participate in own care

■ Patient's feelings about chronic illness and situations that can't be changed

■ Teaching and counseling to enhance patient's decision-making ability

■ Interventions to help patient gain sense of control

■ Patient's response to nursing interventions

■ Evaluations for expected outcomes

Reference

Kylma, J. "Dynamics of Hope in Adults Living with HIV/AIDS: A Substantive Theory," *Journal of Advanced Nursing* 52(6):620-30, December 2005.

Ineffective
PROTECTION
related to myelosuppression and immunosuppression

Definition

A decrease in the ability to guard self from internal or external threats such as illness or injury

Assessment

- Vital signs
- Health maintenance, including high-risk behaviors and health-promoting activities
- Patient's knowledge of present condition, including diagnosis, treatment, prevention of complications, and management of adverse effects
- Coping skills, including physical, psychosocial, and spiritual strengths
- Mobility status
- Comfort level, including symptom management
- Activities of daily living, including rest, sleep, and exercise
- Cardiovascular status, including heart rate, rhythm, heart sounds, blood pressure, peripheral pulses, and electrocardiogram results
- Neurologic status, including sensory perception, decision-making abilities, and thought processes
- Respiratory status, including gas exchange and breathing patterns
- Nutritional status, including food preferences, modifications in diet, and weight changes
- Bowel and bladder elimination patterns
- Protective mechanisms, including immune, hematopoietic, integumentary, and sensorimotor systems
- Laboratory studies, including white blood cell count and differential, erythrocyte sedimentation rate, immunoelectrophoresis, enzyme-linked immunosorbent assay, and cultures of blood, body fluid, sputum, urine, and wound exudate
- Sexuality patterns

Defining characteristics

- Altered clotting
- Deficient immunity
- Dyspnea
- Immobility
- Impaired healing
- Insomnia
- Itching
- Maladaptive stress response
- Neurosensory alteration
- Perspiring
- Pressure ulcers
- Restlessness
- Weakness

Expected outcomes

- Patient won't experience chills, fever, or other signs and symptoms of illness.
- Patient will demonstrate use of protective measures, including conservation of energy, maintenance of balanced diet, and attainment of adequate rest.
- Patient will demonstrate effective coping skills.
- Patient will demonstrate personal cleanliness and will maintain clean environment.

■ Patient will maintain safe environment.
■ Patient will demonstrate increased strength and resistance.
■ Patient's immune system response will improve.

Suggested NOC outcomes

Abuse Protection; Immune Status; Immunization Behavior; Knowledge: Infection Control; Knowledge: Personal Safety

Interventions and rationales

■ Spend as much time as possible with patient *to provide comfort and support.*
■ Promote personal and environmental cleanliness *to decrease threat from microorganisms.*
■ Monitor vital signs. *This allows for early detection of complications.*
■ Institute safety precautions *to reduce risk of falls, cuts, or other injuries and subsequent infection, bleeding, and impaired healing.*
■ Teach protective measures, including the need to conserve energy, obtain adequate rest, and eat a balanced diet. Adequate sleep and nutrition enhance immune function. *Energy conservation can help decrease the weakness caused by anemia.*
■ Provide relief for symptoms (fever, chills, myalgia, weakness). *Discomfort interferes with rest, disturbs nutritional intake, and places added stress on patient.*
■ Teach patient coping strategies, including stress management and relaxation techniques. *Relaxation and decreased stress can increase immune function, thereby improving strength and resistance.*

Suggested NIC interventions

Coping Enhancement; Environmental Management: Safety; Infection Control; Infection Protection; Nutritional Counseling; Positioning; Risk Identification

Evaluations for expected outcomes

■ Patient doesn't develop petechiae, epistaxis, melena, hematuria, fever, cough, redness, drainage, pallor, headache, weakness, or dizziness. Vital signs remain within normal limits.
■ Patient demonstrates a normal pattern of rest, activity, and sleep. He consumes an adequate diet.
■ Patient reports being able to cope effectively.
■ Patient demonstrates personal cleanliness and maintains clean environment.
■ Patient uses safety precautions to avoid falls and other injuries.
■ Patient demonstrates increased strength and resistance.
■ Patient's immune system response improves.

Documentation

■ Patient's understanding of abnormal blood profiles
■ Patient's description of measures to prevent or manage complications
■ Observations of patient's behavior, including health-promoting and high-risk activities

■ Signs and symptoms of decreased immune resistance in body systems assessed (cardiopulmonary, neurologic, GI, genitourinary, and integumentary)
■ Observations of infection or bleeding
■ Interventions to assist with coping strategies and health maintenance and promotion
■ Patient's response to interventions
■ Evaluations for expected outcomes

Reference

Marrs, J.A. "Care of Patients with Neutropenia," *Clinical Journal of Oncology Nursing* 10(2):164-66, April 2006.

Readiness for enhanced
RELIGIOSITY
related to illness and hospitalization

Definition
Ability to increase reliance on religious beliefs or participation in rituals of a particular faith

Assessment
■ Age, gender, marital status
■ Health history
■ Support systems (family, clergy)
■ Communication skills
■ Cultural factors
■ Religious affiliation
■ Spiritual beliefs and practices that are important to patient
■ Perceptions of faith, life, death, and suffering

Defining characteristics
■ Desire to strengthen religious belief customs that had provided comfort
■ Need for increased participation in prescribed religious beliefs through:
– religious ceremonies, worship and religious services
– dietary regulations, clothing
– private religious behaviors, prayer
– holiday observances
■ Verbal expression of request to expand religious options, to meet with religious leaders, and to obtain religious material

Expected outcomes
■ Patient will articulate what gives him strength and hope.
■ Patient will discuss aspects of religion that are important to him.
■ Patient will list how staff can facilitate his participation in religious practices.

■ Patient will request or agree to talk to a spiritual professional.

■ Patient will express a feeling of peace with provided religious opportunities.

Suggested NOC outcomes

Health Beliefs; Health-promoting Behavior; Hope; Motivation; Quality of Life; Spiritual Health

Interventions and rationales

■ Perform a thorough spiritual assessment *to develop a holistic home care plan.*

■ Help patient list the religious practices most important to him *to determine what's possible to provide in the home.*

■ Acquire simple-to-obtain items, such as a Bible, *to comfort patient while planning more complex support.*

■ Suggest a referral to clergy *so patient may discuss deeper spiritual issues.*

■ Consider having a congregational nurse or faith community nurse visit weekly *to provide ongoing spiritual care.*

■ Confirm that patient's spiritual needs are being satisfied *if modifications are made to the plan.*

Suggested NIC interventions

Presence; Religious Ritual Enhancement; Spiritual Growth Facilitation; Spiritual Support; Values Clarification

Evaluations for expected outcomes

■ Patient describes what gives him strength and hope.

■ Patient discusses aspects of religion that are important to him.

■ Patient receives the assistance needed to participate in religious practices.

■ Patient talks to a spiritual professional.

■ Patient expresses peace with the ongoing attention to his spiritual needs.

Documentation

■ Assessment of spiritual needs

■ Religious practices to enjoy at home

■ Efforts to obtain resources to satisfy patient's needs

■ Visits by spiritual professional

■ Patient's responses to interventions

■ Evaluations for expected outcomes

Reference

Mattison, P. "Assessing Spiritual Health," *Health Ministry Journal* 2(2):5-13, Spring 2006.

Risk for impaired
RELIGIOSITY

Definition

At risk for an impaired ability to exercise reliance in belief or participate in rituals of a particular faith tradition

Assessment

- Age, gender
- Religious affiliation, beliefs, practices; importance of religion in daily life
- Environmental assessment of present living circumstances
- Support systems (family, clergy)

Risk factors

- Cultural or environmental barriers
- Illness or hospitalization
- Ineffective support/coping systems
- Lack of social interaction
- Lack of transportation
- Life transitions

Expected outcomes

- Patient will articulate those religious practices that are important to him.
- Patient will decide what changes to his practices are realistic and acceptable.
- Patient will cope with the limitations placed on him by current circumstances.
- Patient will make use of the available spiritual resources.
- Patient will express satisfaction with ability to practice his religion.

Suggested NOC outcomes

Health Beliefs; Health-promoting Behavior; Hope; Motivation; Quality of Life; Spiritual Health

Interventions and rationales

- Have patient talk about the religious practices that are important to him *to provide focus for interventions.*
- Help patient explore modifications to his activities without compromising spiritual comfort. *Decision making promotes feelings of independence, control.*
- Explain available resources *to prepare for developing a realistic plan.*
- Have patient list options for participation in religious activities *to promote optimism or acceptance in present situation.*
- Check daily, then weekly, *to assess patient's level of satisfaction with the plan.*
- Work with family, friends, or clergy *to provide appropriate spiritual support.*

Suggested NIC interventions

Active Listening; Emotional Support; Hope Instillation; Presence; Religious Addiction Prevention; Religious Ritual Enhancement; Spiritual Growth Facilitation; Spiritual Support; Values Clarification

Evaluations for expected outcomes

■ Patient expresses satisfaction with the religious activities that are provided.
■ Patient participates in practicing those religious activities that are available.
■ Patient asks to modify plan as needed.
■ Family and clergy visit and support.
■ Patient expresses feelings of health and wholeness.

Documentation

■ Thorough spiritual assessment
■ Religious practices that are meaningful to patient
■ Religious practices that can be provided in the present situation
■ Patient's satisfaction with options
■ Patient's participation in religious and other kinds of activities
■ Evaluations for expected outcomes

Reference

Elipoulos, E. "Belief as the Foundation for Health," *Health Ministry Journal* 1(3):5-13, Fall 2005.

RELOCATION STRESS SYNDROME

related to inadequate preparation for admission, transfer, or discharge

Definition

Physiologic or psychosocial disturbances caused by change in health care environment

Assessment

■ Reason for transfer or relocation
■ Nature of relocation
■ Physical and mental status of patient, including health condition, cognitive functioning, and functional abilities
■ Financial resources
■ Support systems, including family, friends, and health care workers
■ Resources available to help prepare for relocation
■ Conditions in original environment versus conditions in new environment
■ Coping and problem-solving abilities, including educational level, past experiences with relocation, and participation in recreational activities or hobbies

Defining characteristics

■ Anxiety
■ Apprehension

- Change in eating habits
- Change in environment
- Dependency
- Depression
- Expressed concern or anxiety about transfer
- Expressed unwillingness to relocate
- GI disturbances
- Increased confusion
- Increased expression of needs
- Insecurity
- Lack of trust
- Loneliness
- Restlessness
- Sad affect
- Sleep disturbance
- Unfavorable comparison of original and new staff or environment
- Vigilance
- Weight change
- Withdrawal

Expected outcomes

- Patient will request information about new environment.
- Patient will communicate understanding of relocation.
- Patient and family members will take steps to prepare for relocation.
- Patient will use available resources.
- Patient will express satisfaction with adjustment to new environment.

Suggested NOC outcomes

Anxiety Self-Control; Coping; Depression Level; Depression Self-Control; Loneliness Severity; Psychosocial Adjustment: Life Change; Quality of Life; Stress Level

Interventions and rationales

- Assign a primary nurse to patient *to provide a consistent, caring, and accepting environment that enhances patient's adjustment and well-being.*
- Help patient and family members prepare for relocation. Conduct group discussions, provide pictures of the new setting, and communicate any additional information that will ease transition *to help patient cope with a new environment.*
- If possible, allow patient and family members to visit the new location and provide introductions to the new staff. *The more familiar the environment, the less stress patient will experience during relocation.*
- Assess patient's needs for additional health care services before relocation *to ensure that patient receives appropriate care in the new environment.*
- Communicate all aspects of patient's discharge plan to appropriate staff members at the new location *to ensure continuity of care.*
- Educate family members about relocation stress syndrome and its potential effects *to encourage family members to provide needed emotional support throughout the transition period.*

■ Encourage patient to express emotions associated with relocation *to provide opportunity to correct misconceptions, answer questions, and reduce anxiety.*

■ Reassure patient that family members and friends know his new location and will continue to visit *to reduce feelings of abandonment and anxiety.*

Suggested NIC interventions

Active Listening; Coping Enhancement; Counseling; Hope Instillation; Mood Management; Presence; Sleep Enhancement; Self-Responsibility Facilitation; Spiritual Support

Evaluations for expected outcomes

■ Patient requests information about new environment.

■ Patient expresses understanding of relocation process.

■ Patient and family members complete preparations for relocation.

■ Patient makes use of available resources to smooth transition to new environment.

■ Patient expresses feelings associated with adjustment to new environment.

Documentation

■ Evidence of patient's emotional distress over relocation

■ Patient's needs in preparing for relocation

■ Available resources and support systems

■ Intervention to prepare patient and family members for relocation and patient's and family members' responses

■ Discharge plan instructions communicated to new staff

■ Evaluations for expected outcomes

Reference

Beard, H. "Does Intermediate Care Minimize Relocation Stress for Patients Leaving the ICU?" *Nursing in Critical Care* 10(6):272-78, November-December 2005.

Ineffective
ROLE PERFORMANCE
related to physical illness

Definition

Patterns of behavior and self-expression that don't match the environment context, norms, and exceptions

Assessment

■ Health history, including medical diagnosis, course and severity of illness, and reason for hospitalization

■ Patient's perception of illness and its effect on social, cultural, and vocational roles

■ Psychosocial status, including current stressors, support systems, hobbies, interests, work history, educational background, and changes in role function
■ Family status, including roles of family members, effect of illness on patient's family, and family's understanding of patient's illness

Defining characteristics

■ Ambivalence, denial, or confusion about role or responsibility
■ Anxiety, depression, dissatisfaction, pessimism, or uncertainty
■ Change in capacity to resume role
■ Change in perception of role (by self and others)
■ Change in usual responsibilities
■ Conflict among vocational, family, cultural, and social roles
■ Discrimination
■ Domestic violence or harassment
■ Inadequate adaptation to change or transition
■ Inadequate self-management, motivation, confidence, competence, or coping skills for fulfilling role
■ Inappropriate developmental expectations
■ Lack of external support for enacting role
■ Lack of knowledge about roles and responsibilities
■ Lack of opportunities for enacting role
■ Powerlessness
■ Role overload or strain

Expected outcomes

■ Patient will express feelings about diminished ability to perform usual roles.
■ Patient and family members will recognize and state feelings about limitations imposed by illness.
■ Patient will make decisions about course of treatment and management of illness.
■ Patient will continue to function in usual roles as much as possible.
■ Patient will express feelings of making productive contribution to self-care, to others, or to environment.

Suggested NOC outcomes

Caregiver Lifestyle Disruption; Coping; Depression Level; Psychomotor Energy; Psychosocial Adjustment: Life Change; Role Performance

Interventions and rationales

■ If possible, assign the same nurse to patient each shift *to establish rapport and foster development of a therapeutic relationship.*
■ Spend ample time with patient each shift *to foster a sense of safety and decrease loneliness.*
■ Provide opportunities for patient to express thoughts and feelings *to help patient identify how his altered role performance has affected his life.*
■ Convey a belief in patient's ability to develop the necessary coping skills. *By projecting a positive attitude, you can help patient gain confidence.*

■ Be aware of patient's emotional vulnerability, and allow open expression of all emotions. *An accepting attitude will help patient deal with the effects of chronic illness and loss of functioning.*

■ Provide opportunities for patient to make decisions, and encourage patient to maintain personal responsibilities. *Showing respect for patient's decision-making ability enhances feelings of independence.*

■ Encourage patient to participate in self-care activities, keeping in mind his physical and emotional limitations. *Involvement in self-care promotes optimal functioning.*

■ Assess patient's knowledge of illness, and educate patient about his condition, treatment, and prognosis. *Education helps patient cope with effects of illness more effectively.*

■ Encourage patient to recognize his personal strengths and to use them. *This will help maintain optimal functioning and foster a healthier self-image.*

■ Encourage patient to continue to fulfill life roles within the constraints posed by illness. *This will help patient maintain a sense of purpose and preserve connections with other people.*

■ Encourage patient to participate in his care as an active member of the health care team. *This will help establish mutually accepted goals between patient and his caregivers. Patient who participates in care is more likely to take an active role in other aspects of life.*

■ Help family members identify their feelings about patient's decreased role functioning. Encourage participation in a support group. *Relatives of patient may need social support, information, and an outlet for ventilating feelings.*

■ Offer patient and family members a realistic assessment of patient's illness, and communicate hope for the immediate future. *Education helps promote patient safety and security and helps family members plan for future health care requirements.*

■ Educate patient and family members about managing illness, controlling environmental factors that affect patient's health, and redefining roles *to promote optimal functioning. Through education, family members may become resources in patient's care.*

Suggested NIC interventions
Anticipatory Guidance; Caregiver Support; Coping Enhancement; Family Process Maintenance; Role Enhancement

Evaluations for expected outcomes
■ Patient shares feelings about illness and altered role performance in constructive manner.

■ Patient and family members understand role changes that are occurring because of chronic illness and express their feelings about these limitations.

■ Patient demonstrates increased functioning by making decisions about health care and participating in planning and implementing aspects of personal care.

■ Patient demonstrates ability to perceive options and uses options to function in usual roles as much as possible.

■ Patient expresses feelings of having made productive contribution to self-care, to others, or to the environment.

Documentation
- Observations of patient's physical, emotional, and mental status
- Patient's thoughts and feelings about illness and diminished role capacity
- Nursing interventions performed to help patient understand change in role functioning
- Patient's response to nursing interventions
- Health teaching, counseling, and precautions taken to maintain or enhance patient's level of functioning
- Referrals to sources of support for patient and family members
- Evaluations for expected outcomes

Reference
Emslie, C. "Women, Men and Coronary Heart Disease: A Review of the Qualitative Literature," *Journal of Advanced Nursing* 51(4):382-95, August 2005.

Bathing or hygiene
SELF-CARE DEFICIT
related to musculoskeletal impairment

Definition
Inability to carry out activities associated with bathing and hygiene

Assessment
- History of injury or disease associated with musculoskeletal impairment
- Self-care abilities, including knowledge and use of adaptive equipment, preparation of equipment and supplies, and technical or mechanical skills
- Musculoskeletal status, including coordination; functional ability; gait; mechanical restriction (such as cast, splint, and traction); muscle tone, size, and strength; range of motion; and tremors
- Psychosocial status, including coping mechanisms, family members, lifestyle, patient's perceptions of health problem and self, and personality

Defining characteristics
- Inability to dry body
- Inability to get into and out of bathroom
- Inability to obtain bath supplies
- Inability to obtain or get to water source
- Inability to regulate water temperature or flow
- Inability to wash body or body parts

Expected outcomes
- Patient will have his self-care needs met.
- Patient will have few if any complications.
- Patient will communicate feelings about limitations.
- Patient and family members will demonstrate correct use of assistive devices.

■ Patient and family members will carry out bathing and hygiene program daily.

Suggested NOC outcomes

Adaptation to Physical Disability; Energy Conservation; Pain Level; Self-Care: Activities of Daily Living (ADL); Self-Care: Bathing; Self-Care: Hygiene; Self-Care: Oral Hygiene

Interventions and rationales

■ Observe patient's functional level every shift; document and report any changes. *Careful observation helps you adjust nursing actions to meet patient's needs.*

■ Perform the prescribed treatment for underlying musculoskeletal impairment. Monitor patient's progress, reporting favorable and adverse responses to treatment. *Applying therapy consistently aids patient's independence.*

■ Encourage patient to voice feelings and concerns about self-care deficits *to help patient achieve the highest functional level possible.*

■ Monitor the completion of bathing and hygiene daily. Praise patient's accomplishments. *Reinforcement and rewards may encourage renewed effort.*

■ Provide assistive devices, such as a long-handled toothbrush, for bathing and hygiene; instruct patient on use. *Appropriate assistive devices encourage independence.*

■ Assist with or perform bathing and hygiene daily. Assist only when patient has difficulty *to promote feeling of independence.*

■ Instruct patient and family members in bathing and hygiene techniques (you can give family members written instructions). Have patient and family members demonstrate bathing and hygiene under supervision. *Return demonstration identifies problem areas and increases patients' and family members' self-confidence.*

■ As needed, refer patient to a psychiatric liaison nurse, support group, or home health care agency. *These extra resources will reinforce activities planned to meet patient's needs.*

Suggested NIC interventions

Bathing; Behavior Modification; Discharge Planning; Ear Care; Foot Care; Hair Care; Nail Care; Self-Care Assistance; Teaching: Individual

Evaluations for expected outcomes

■ Patient meets self-care needs with help of staff.

■ Patient participates in activities that minimize risk of such complications as infection and skin integrity alteration.

■ Patient expresses feelings about self-care deficit. If unable to meet his own needs, patient seeks assistance from a family member or the staff within 24 hours.

■ Patient or family members demonstrate appropriate use of assistive devices.

■ Patient follows daily bathing and hygiene program. Family members assist, as needed.

Documentation

- Patient's expression of feelings and concerns about self-care limitations and their impact on body image and lifestyle
- Patient's willingness to participate in bathing and hygiene routine
- Observations of patient's impaired ability to perform self-care
- Patient's response to treatment of underlying condition
- Interventions to provide supportive care
- Patient's response to nursing interventions
- Instructions to patient and family members and their understanding of instructions and demonstrated skill in carrying out self-care functions
- Evaluations for expected outcomes

Reference

Polzien, G. "Care After Hip Replacement," *Home Healthcare Nurse* 24(7):420-22, July-August 2006.

Bathing or hygiene
SELF-CARE DEFICIT
related to perceptual or cognitive impairment

Definition

Inability to carry out activities associated with bathing and hygiene

Assessment

- History of neurologic, sensory, or psychological impairment
- Age
- Self-care abilities, including knowledge and use of adaptive equipment, preparation of equipment and supplies, and technical and mechanical skills
- Neurologic status, including cognition, communication ability, insight or judgment, level of consciousness, memory, sensory and motor ability, and orientation
- Psychosocial status, including coping mechanisms, family members, lifestyle, patient's perceptions of self, and personality

Defining characteristics

- Inability to dry body
- Inability to get into and out of bathroom
- Inability to obtain bath supplies
- Inability to obtain or get to water source
- Inability to regulate water temperature or flow
- Inability to wash body or body parts

Expected outcomes

- Patient will have his self-care needs met.
- Patient will have few if any complications.
- Patient and family members will carry out self-care program daily.

■ Patient and family members will communicate feelings and concerns.
■ Patient and family members will identify resources to help cope with problems after discharge.

Suggested NOC outcomes

Self-Care: Activities of Daily Living (ADL); Self-Care: Bathing; Self-Care: Hygiene

Interventions and rationales

■ Observe, document, and report patient's functional and perceptual or cognitive ability daily. *Careful observation helps you adjust nursing actions to meet patient's needs.*
■ Perform the prescribed treatment for the underlying condition. Monitor patient's progress and report favorable and adverse responses. *Applying therapy consistently aids patient's independence.*
■ Allow patient to express frustration, anger, or feelings of inadequacy. Provide emotional support *to help patient achieve the highest functional level.*
■ Provide privacy *to enhance patient's self-esteem.*
■ Monitor the completion of bathing and hygiene daily. Remind patient of what he needs to accomplish. Offer praise. *Reinforcement and rewards may encourage daily activities.*
■ Allow ample time for patient to perform bathing and hygiene. *Rushing creates unnecessary stress and promotes failure.*
■ Direct patient in bathing and hygiene measures, giving simple instructions one at a time, *to aid comprehension.*
■ Assist with bathing and hygiene daily only when patient has difficulty *to encourage independence and self-reliance.*
■ Give written instructions to family members in bathing and hygiene techniques and supervise return demonstration. *Return demonstration identifies problem areas and increases family members' self-confidence.*
■ Discuss the normal aspects of bathing. Reassure patient with such statements as "You're in the tub" and "The water is only 3 inches deep" *to guard against a panic reaction caused by the fear of being drowned.*
■ Refer patient to a psychiatric liaison nurse, support group, or home health care agency, as needed. *These extra resources will reinforce activities planned to meet patient's needs.*

Suggested NIC interventions

Energy Management; Oral Health Maintenance; Perineal Care; Self-Care Assistance: Bathing/Hygiene

Evaluations for expected outcomes

■ Patient meets self-care needs with help of staff.
■ Patient doesn't experience infection, skin integrity alteration, or other complications of altered self-care.
■ Patient and family members become more active in carrying out self-care program; need for staff assistance decreases.

■ Patient and family members express feelings about patient's self-care deficit. If unable to meet own needs, patient seeks help from family members or staff within 24 hours.

■ Patient and family members identify and contact support resources, as needed.

Documentation

■ Patient's and family members' expression of feelings and concern about self-care deficits

■ Observations of patient's impaired ability to perform bathing and hygiene

■ Patient's response to treatment of underlying condition

■ Interventions to provide supportive care

■ Instructions to patient (if capable) and family members, their understanding of instructions, and their demonstrated skill in carrying out self-care functions

■ Patient's response to nursing interventions

■ Evaluations for expected outcomes

Reference

Hoeffer, B., et al. "Assisting Cognitively Impaired Nursing Home Residents with Bathing: Effects of Two Bathing Interventions on Caregiving," *The Gerontologist* 46(4):524-32, August 2006.

Dressing or grooming
SELF-CARE DEFICIT
related to musculoskeletal impairment

Definition
Inability to perform activities associated with dressing and grooming

Assessment

■ History of injury or disease associated with musculoskeletal impairment

■ Self-care abilities, including knowledge and use of adaptive equipment, preparation of equipment and supplies, and technical or mechanical skills

■ Musculoskeletal status, including coordination; functional ability; gait; mechanical restriction (such as cast, splint, and traction); muscle tone, size, and strength; range of motion; and tremors

■ Psychosocial status, including coping mechanisms, family members, lifestyle, patient's perceptions of health problem and self, and personality

Defining characteristics

■ Impaired ability to clothe part or all of body

■ Impaired ability to fasten clothing (such as inability to use zippers)

■ Impaired ability to obtain or replace items of clothing

■ Impaired ability to put on or take off specific articles of clothing (such as socks and shoes)

■ Inability to choose clothing

- Inability to maintain appearance at satisfactory level
- Inability to pick up clothing
- Inability to use assistive devices

Expected outcomes
- Patient will have his self-care needs met.
- Patient will have few if any complications.
- Patient will communicate feelings about limitations.
- Patient and family members will demonstrate correct use of assistive devices.
- Patient and family members will carry out dressing and grooming program daily.

Suggested NOC outcomes

Adaptation to Physical Disability; Coordinated Movement; Energy Conservation; Mobility; Motivation; Self-Care: Activities of Daily Living (ADL); Self-Care: Dressing

Interventions and rationales
- Observe patient's functional level every shift; document and report any changes. *Careful observation helps you adjust nursing actions to meet patient's needs.*
- Perform the prescribed treatment for the underlying musculoskeletal impairment. Monitor patient's progress, reporting favorable and adverse responses to treatment. *Applying therapy consistently aids patient's independence.*
- Encourage patient to voice feelings and concerns about self-care deficits *to help patient achieve the highest functional level.*
- Provide enough time for patient to perform dressing and grooming. *Rushing creates unnecessary stress and promotes failure.*
- Monitor patient's abilities to dress and groom daily. *This identifies problem areas before they become sources of frustration.*
- Encourage family members to provide clothing patient can easily manage. Patient may benefit from clothing slightly larger than regular size and Velcro straps. *Such clothing makes independent dressing easier.*
- Provide necessary assistive devices, such as a long-handled shoehorn and zipper pull, as needed. Instruct patient on use. *Appropriate assistive devices encourage independence.*
- Assist with or perform dressing and grooming: fasten clothes, comb hair, and clean nails. Provide help only when patient has difficulty *to promote feeling of independence.*
- Instruct patient and family members in dressing and grooming techniques (you can give family members written instructions). Have patient and family members demonstrate dressing and grooming techniques under supervision. *Return demonstration reveals problem areas and increases self-confidence.*
- As needed, refer patient to a psychiatric liaison nurse, support group, or home health care agency. *Extra resources reinforce activities planned to meet patient's needs.*

Suggested NIC interventions

Body Image Enhancement; Energy Management; Exercise Promotion; Hair Care; Self-Care Assistance: Dressing/Grooming; Skin Surveillance

Evaluations for expected outcomes

■ Patient meets self-care needs with help of staff.
■ Patient participates in activities designed to minimize risk of complications, such as complying with treatment.
■ Patient expresses feelings about self-care limitations.
■ Patient and family members demonstrate appropriate use of assistive devices.
■ Patient follows daily dressing and grooming program. Family members assist, as needed.

Documentation

■ Patient's expression of feelings and concerns about self-care limitations and their impact on body image and lifestyle
■ Patient's willingness to participate in dressing and grooming
■ Observations of patient's impaired ability to perform dressing and grooming
■ Interventions to provide supportive care
■ Patient's response to nursing interventions
■ Instructions given to patient and family members, their understanding of instructions, and their demonstrated skill in carrying out self-care functions
■ Evaluations for expected outcomes

Reference

Suzuki, M., et al. "Predicting Recovery of Upper-body Dressing Ability After Stroke," *Archives of Physical Medicine and Rehabilitation* 87(11):1496-502, November 2006.

Dressing or grooming
SELF-CARE DEFICIT

related to perceptual or cognitive impairment

Definition
Inability to carry out activities associated with dressing and grooming

Assessment

■ History of neurologic, sensory, or psychological impairment
■ Age
■ Self-care abilities, including knowledge and use of adaptive equipment, preparation of equipment and supplies, and technical and mechanical skills
■ Neurologic status, including cognition, communication ability, insight or judgment, level of consciousness, memory, motor and sensory ability, and orientation
■ Psychosocial status, including coping mechanisms, family members, lifestyle, patient's perceptions of self, and personality

Defining characteristics

- Impaired ability to clothe part or all of body
- Impaired ability to fasten clothing (such as inability to use zippers)
- Impaired ability to obtain or replace items of clothing
- Impaired ability to put on or take off specific articles of clothing (such as socks and shoes)
- Inability to choose clothing
- Inability to maintain appearance at satisfactory level
- Inability to pick up clothing
- Inability to use assistive devices

Expected outcomes

- Patient will have his self-care needs met.
- Patient will have few if any complications.
- Patient and family members will carry out self-care program daily.
- Patient and family members will communicate feelings and concerns.
- Patient and family members will identify resources to help cope with problems and discharge.

Suggested NOC outcomes

Adaptation to Physical Disability; Anxiety Self-Control; Energy Conservation; Mobility; Motivation; Pain Level; Self-Care: Activities of Daily Living (ADL); Self-Care: Dressing

Interventions and rationales

- Observe, document, and report patient's functional and perceptual or cognitive ability daily. *Careful observation helps you adjust nursing actions to meet patient's needs.*
- Perform the prescribed treatment for the underlying condition. Monitor patient's progress, and report favorable and adverse responses. *Applying therapy consistently aids patient's independence.*
- Allow patient to express frustration, anger, or feelings of inadequacy. Provide emotional support *to help patient achieve the highest functional level.*
- Provide privacy *to enhance patient's self-esteem.*
- Monitor dressing and grooming daily. *This identifies problem areas before they become sources of frustration.*
- Provide assistive devices, as needed. *Appropriate assistive devices can encourage independence.*
- Don't rush patient. *Rushing creates unnecessary stress and promotes failure.*
- Remind patient of what he needs to accomplish while performing actual task. Praise accomplishments *to foster self-confidence.*
- Assist with dressing and grooming daily: fasten clothes, clean nails, and comb hair. Select clothes and hand garments to patient one at a time in appropriate order. Provide help only when patient has difficulty *to promote feeling of independence.*
- Direct patient in grooming measures, giving simple instructions one at a time, *to aid comprehension.*

■ Encourage patient to complete dressing and grooming measures. Provide positive feedback during task performance. *Reinforcement and rewards may encourage effort.*

■ Encourage family member to provide clothing patient can easily manage: Patient may benefit from clothing slightly larger than regular size and Velcro straps. *Such clothing makes independent dressing easier.*

■ Give written instructions to family member in dressing and grooming technique, and supervise return demonstration *to identify problem areas and increase family member's self-confidence.*

■ As needed, refer patient to a psychiatric liaison nurse, support group, or home health care agency. *These extra resources will reinforce activities planned to meet patient's needs.*

Suggested NIC interventions

Dressing; Fall Prevention; Foot Care; Hair Care; Nail Care; Oral Health Promotion

Evaluations for expected outcomes

■ Patient meets self-care needs with help of staff.

■ Patient doesn't experience infection, skin integrity alteration, or other complications of altered self-care.

■ Patient and family members become more active in carrying out self-care program; need for staff assistance decreases.

■ Patient and family members discuss feelings about patient's self-care deficit. If unable to meet own needs, patient seeks help from family member or staff within 24 hours.

■ Patient and family members identify and contact available support resources, as needed.

Documentation

■ Patient's and family members' expression of feelings and concern about self-care deficits

■ Observations of patient's impaired ability to perform dressing and grooming activities

■ Patient's response to underlying treatment

■ Interventions to provide supportive care

■ Instructions to patient (if capable) and family members, their understanding of instructions, and their demonstrated skill in carrying out self-care functions

■ Patient's response to nursing interventions

■ Evaluations for expected outcomes

Reference

Cohen-Mansfield, J., et al. "Dressing of Cognitively Impaired Nursing Home Residents: Description and Analysis," *The Gerontologist* 46(1):89-96, February 2006.

Feeding
SELF-CARE DEFICIT
related to musculoskeletal impairment

Definition
Inability to carry out the self-care activity of feeding

Assessment
- History of injury or disease associated with musculoskeletal impairment
- Self-care abilities, including knowledge and use of adaptive equipment, preparation of equipment and supplies, and technical and mechanical skills
- Musculoskeletal status, including coordination; functional ability; gait; mechanical restriction (such as cast, splint, and traction); muscle tone, size, and strength; range of motion; and tremors
- Psychosocial status, including coping mechanisms, family members, lifestyle, motivation, patient's perception of health problem and self, and personality

Defining characteristics
Inability to perform one or more of the following:
- Bring food from receptacle to mouth
- Chew food
- Complete meals
- Get food onto utensil
- Handle cup or glass
- Handle utensils
- Ingest food safely and in socially acceptable manner
- Ingest sufficient food
- Open containers
- Prepare food
- Swallow food
- Use assistive devices

Expected outcomes
- Patient will express feelings about feeding limitations.
- Patient will maintain weight at ___ lb.
- Patient won't have evidence of aspiration.
- Patient will consume ___ % of diet.
- Patient and family members will demonstrate correct use of assistive devices.
- Patient and family members will carry out feeding program daily.

Suggested NOC outcomes
Nutritional Status; Self-Care: Activities of Daily Living (ADL); Self-Care: Eating; Swallowing Status

Interventions and rationales

■ Observe patient's functional level every shift; document and report changes. *Careful observation helps you adjust nursing actions to meet patient's needs.*

■ Perform the prescribed treatment for the underlying musculoskeletal impairment. Monitor patient's progress and report responses. *Applying therapy consistently aids patient's independence.*

■ Weigh patient weekly and record his weight. Report a change of more than 1 lb/week *to ensure adequate nutrition and fluid balance.*

■ Monitor and record breath sounds every 4 hours *to check for aspiration of food.* Report crackles, wheezes, or rhonchi.

■ Encourage patient to express feelings and concerns about feeding deficits *to help patient achieve the highest functional level.*

■ Initiate an ordered feeding program:

– Determine the types of food best handled by patient *to encourage patient's feelings of independence.*

– Place patient in high Fowler's position to feed *to aid swallowing and digestion.* Support weakened extremities, and wash patient's face and hands before meals.

– Provide assistive devices; instruct patient on their use *to allow more independence.*

– Supervise or assist at each meal—for example, cut food into small pieces. *This aids chewing, swallowing, and digestion and reduces the risk of choking or aspiration.*

– Feed patient slowly. *Rushing causes stress, reducing digestive activity and causing intestinal spasms.*

– Keep suction equipment at the bedside *to remove aspirated foods, if necessary.*

– Instruct patient and family members in feeding techniques and equipment. *This aids understanding and encourages compliance.*

– Record the percentage of food consumed *to ensure adequate nutrition.*

■ Encourage patient to carry out the aspects of feeding according to his abilities. *This gives patient a sense of achievement and control.*

■ Refer patient to a psychiatric liaison nurse, support group, or such community agencies as Visiting Nurse Association and Meals On Wheels. *Additional resources reinforce activities planned to meet patient's needs.*

Suggested NIC interventions

Fluid Management; Nutrition Management; Nutritional Monitoring; Self-Care Assistance: Feeding; Swallowing Therapy

Evaluations for expected outcomes

■ Patient expresses frustration with feeding limitations.

■ Patient obtains adequate fluid and nutritional intake and maintains weight at or above established limit.

■ Patient doesn't experience aspiration.

■ Patient consumes established percentage of diet.

■ Patient and family members demonstrate proper use of assistive devices.

■ Patient follows daily self-care feeding program. Family members provide assistance, as needed.

Documentation
- Patient's expression of feelings and concerns about inability to feed self
- Observations of patient's impaired ability to perform self-care
- Patient's response to treatment
- Patient's weight
- Patient's intake
- Interventions to provide supportive care
- Instructions given to patient and family members, their understanding of instructions, and their demonstrated skill in carrying out self-care functions
- Patient's response to interventions
- Evaluations for expected outcomes

Reference
Westergren, A. "Detection of Eating Difficulties After Stroke: A Systematic Review," *International Nursing Review* 53(2):143-49, June 2006.

Feeding
SELF-CARE DEFICIT
related to perceptual or cognitive impairment

Definition
Inability to feed self

Assessment
- History of neurologic, sensory, or psychological impairment
- Age
- Self-care abilities, including knowledge and use of adaptive equipment, preparation of equipment and supplies, and technical and mechanical skills
- Neurologic status, including cognition, communication ability, insight or judgment, level of consciousness, memory, motor and sensory ability, and orientation
- Psychosocial status, including coping mechanisms, family members, lifestyle, patient's perceptions of self, and personality

Defining characteristics
Inability to perform one or more of the following:
- Bring food from receptacle to mouth
- Chew food
- Complete meals
- Get food onto utensil
- Handle cup or glass
- Handle utensils
- Ingest food safely and in socially acceptable manner
- Ingest sufficient food
- Open containers
- Prepare food

- Swallow food
- Use assistive devices

Expected outcomes

- Patient will have his self-care needs met.
- Patient will have few if any complications.
- Patient and family members will carry out feeding program daily.
- Patient will maintain weight.
- Patient and family members will communicate feelings and concerns.
- Patient and family members will identify resources to help cope with problems and discharge.

Suggested NOC outcomes

Nutritional Status; Nutritional Status: Food & Fluid Intake; Self-Care: Eating; Swallowing Status

Interventions and rationales

- Observe, document, and report patient's functional and perceptual or cognitive ability daily. *Careful observation helps you adjust nursing actions to meet patient's needs.*
- Weigh patient weekly and record the results. Report a loss of 2 lb or more *to ensure adequate nutrition and fluid balance.*
- Perform the prescribed treatment for the underlying condition. Monitor patient's progress and report favorable and adverse responses. *Applying therapy consistently aids patient's independence.*
- Allow patient to express frustration, anger, or feelings of inadequacy. Provide emotional support *to help patient come to terms with his self-care deficit and achieve the highest functional level.*
- Determine the types of food best handled by patient — for example, finger foods or soft or liquid diet. *Easily handled foods encourage patient's feelings of independence.*
- Provide assistive devices at each meal, as needed. *These allow patient to do as much as possible for self.*
- Place patient in high Fowler's position *to reduce swallowing difficulty and aid digestion.*
- Supervise or assist at each meal; for example, cut food into small pieces. *Cutting food into small bites aids chewing, swallowing, and digestion and reduces the risk of choking or aspiration.*
- Feed patient slowly. Don't rush. *Rushing causes stress, reducing digestive activity and causing intestinal spasms.*
- Encourage patient to do as much for self as possible, giving simple instructions one at a time, *to aid comprehension.*
- Keep suction equipment at the bedside *to remove aspirated foods, if necessary.*
- Instruct patient and family members in feeding techniques and use of equipment. Have patient and family members give a return demonstration of feeding and equipment use under supervision. *This aids understanding and encourages compliance.*

■ As needed, refer patient to a psychiatric liaison nurse, support group, or home health care agency. *These extra resources will reinforce activities planned to meet patient's needs.*

Suggested NIC interventions

Aspiration Precautions; Family Involvement Promotion; Feeding; Fluid Management; Nutritional Monitoring; Swallowing Therapy

Evaluations for expected outcomes

■ Patient meets self-care needs with help of staff.
■ Patient doesn't experience infection, skin integrity alteration, weight loss, or other complications of altered self-care.
■ Patient and family members become more active in carrying out self-care program; need for staff assistance decreases.
■ Patient maintains weight at designated level.
■ Patient and family members express feelings about patient's self-care deficit. If unable to meet own needs, patient seeks help from family member or staff within 24 hours.
■ Patient and family members identify and contact available support resources, as needed.

Documentation

■ Patient's and family members' expression of feelings and concerns about difficulty with feeding
■ Observations of patient's impaired ability to feed self
■ Weight
■ Patient's response to treatment
■ Interventions to provide supportive care
■ Instructions to patient (if capable) and family members, their understanding of instructions, and their demonstrated skill in carrying out instructions
■ Patient's response to nursing interventions
■ Evaluations for expected outcomes

Reference

DiBartolo, M.C. "Careful Hand Feeding: A Reasonable Alternative to PEG Tube Placement in Individuals with Dementia," *Journal of Gerontological Nursing* 32(5):25-33, May 2006.

Toileting
SELF-CARE DEFICIT
related to musculoskeletal impairment

Definition

Inability to carry out toileting routine

Assessment

■ History of injury or disease associated with musculoskeletal impairment
■ Self-care abilities, including knowledge and use of adaptive equipment, preparation of equipment and supplies, and technical or mechanical skills
■ Musculoskeletal status, including coordination; functional ability; gait; mechanical restriction (such as cast, splint, and traction); muscle tone, size, and strength; range of motion; and tremors
■ Psychosocial status, including coping mechanisms, family members, lifestyle, patient's perceptions of health problem and self, and personality

Defining characteristics

■ Inability to carry out proper toilet hygiene
■ Inability to flush toilet or empty commode
■ Inability to get to toilet or commode
■ Inability to manipulate clothing for toileting
■ Inability to sit on or rise from toilet or commode

Expected outcomes

■ Patient will have his self-care needs met.
■ Patient will have few if any complications.
■ Patient will communicate feelings about limitations.
■ Patient will maintain continence.
■ Patient and family members will demonstrate correct use of assistive devices.
■ Patient and family members will carry out toileting program daily.

Suggested NOC outcomes

Self-Care: Activities of Daily Living (ADL); Self-Care: Hygiene; Self-Care: Toileting

Interventions and rationales

■ Observe patient's functional level every shift; document and report any changes. *Careful observation helps you adjust nursing actions to meet patient's needs.*
■ Perform the prescribed treatment for the underlying musculoskeletal impairment. Monitor patient's progress, reporting favorable and adverse responses to treatment. *Applying therapy consistently aids patient's independence.*
■ Encourage patient to voice feelings and concerns about his self-care deficits *to help patient achieve the highest functional level possible.*
■ Monitor intake and output and skin condition; record episodes of incontinence. *Accurate intake and output records can identify potential imbalances.*
■ Use assistive devices, as needed, such as an external catheter at night, a bedpan or urinal every 2 hours during the day, and adaptive equipment for bowel care. Instruct on use. As control improves, reduce the use of assistive devices. *Assisting at an appropriate level helps maintain patient's self-esteem.*
■ Assist with toileting, only if needed. Allow patient to perform independently as much as possible *to promote independence.*

■ Perform urinary and bowel care, if needed. Follow urinary or bowel elimination plans. *Monitoring success or failure of toileting plans helps identify and resolve problem areas.*

■ Instruct patient and family members in toileting routine (you can give family members written instructions). Have patient and family members demonstrate toileting routine under supervision. *Return demonstration identifies problem areas and increases patient's self-confidence.*

■ As needed, refer patient to a psychiatric liaison nurse, support group, or home health care agency. *Extra resources reinforce activities planned to meet patient's needs.*

Suggested NIC interventions

Bowel Training; Self-Care Assistance: Toileting; Urinary Elimination Management

Evaluations for expected outcomes

■ Patient meets self-care needs with help of staff.

■ Patient doesn't experience constipation, infection, skin integrity alteration, weight loss, or other complications of altered self-care.

■ Patient expresses feelings about self-care deficit. If unable to meet own needs, patient seeks assistance from family member or staff within 24 hours.

■ Patient maintains continence.

■ Patient and family members demonstrate appropriate use of assistive devices.

■ Patient follows toileting program daily. Family members assist, as needed.

Documentation

■ Patient's expression of feelings and concerns about self-care limitations and their impact on body image and lifestyle

■ Patient's willingness to participate in self-care

■ Observations of patient's impaired ability to perform toileting routine and patient's response to treatment

■ Patient's intake and output

■ Interventions to provide supportive care

■ Instructions given to patient and family members, their understanding of instructions, and their demonstrated skill in carrying out self-care functions

■ Patient's response to nursing interventions

■ Evaluations for expected outcomes

Reference

Polzien, G. "Care After Hip Replacement," *Home Healthcare Nurse* 24(7):420-22, July-August 2006.

Toileting
SELF-CARE DEFICIT

related to perceptual or cognitive impairment

Definition
Inability to carry out toileting routine

Assessment
■ History of neurologic, sensory, or psychological impairment
■ Age
■ Self-care abilities, including knowledge and use of adaptive equipment, preparation of equipment and supplies, and technical or mechanical skills
■ Neurologic status, including cognition, communication ability, insight or judgment, level of consciousness, memory, motor and sensory ability, and orientation
■ Psychosocial status, including coping mechanisms, family members, lifestyle, patient's perceptions of self, and personality

Defining characteristics
■ Inability to carry out proper toilet hygiene
■ Inability to flush toilet or empty commode
■ Inability to get to toilet or commode
■ Inability to manipulate clothing for toileting
■ Inability to sit on or rise from toilet or commode

Expected outcomes
■ Patient will have his self-care needs met.
■ Patient will have few if any complications.
■ Patient and family members will carry out toileting program daily.
■ Patient will maintain continence.
■ Patient and family members will communicate feelings and concerns.
■ Patient and family members will identify resources to help cope with problems and discharge from facility.

Suggested NOC outcomes
Self-Care: Activities of Daily Living (ADL); Self-Care: Hygiene; Self-Care: Toileting

Interventions and rationales
■ Observe, document, and report patient's functional and perceptual or cognitive ability daily. *Careful observation helps you adjust nursing actions to meet patient's needs.*
■ Perform the prescribed treatment for the underlying condition. Monitor patient's progress and report favorable and adverse responses. *Applying therapy consistently aids patient's independence.*
■ Allow patient to express frustration, anger, and feelings of inadequacy. Provide emotional support *to help patient achieve the highest functional level.*

■ Monitor intake and output; record episodes of incontinence. *Accurate intake and output records can identify potential imbalances.*

■ Use assistive devices, as needed, such as an external catheter at night, a bedpan or urinal every 2 hours during the day, and adaptive equipment for bowel care. As control improves, reduce the use of assistive devices. *Assisting at an appropriate level helps maintain patient's self-esteem.*

■ Assist with toileting, if needed, using visual and auditory cues to stimulate urination. *This allows patient to perform independently as much as possible.*

■ Allow ample time for patient to perform toileting routine. *Rushing creates unnecessary stress and promotes failure.*

■ Provide positive, constructive feedback when assisting with toileting. *Reinforcement and rewards may enhance self-esteem.*

■ Assist with toileting, giving simple instructions one at a time, *to aid comprehension.*

■ Complete urinary and bowel care if patient can't do so. Follow urinary and bowel elimination plans. *Monitoring success or failure of toileting plans helps identify and resolve problem areas.*

■ Give written instructions about the toileting routine to family members, and supervise a return demonstration. *A return demonstration identifies problem areas and increases family members' self-confidence.*

■ Refer patient to a psychiatric liaison nurse, support group, or community agency, as needed. *These extra resources will reinforce activities planned to meet patient's needs.*

Suggested NIC interventions

Bowel Incontinence Care; Self-Care Assistance: Toileting; Urinary Elimination Management

Evaluations for expected outcomes

■ Patient meets self-care needs with help of staff.

■ Patient doesn't experience constipation, infection, skin integrity alteration, weight loss, or other complications of altered self-care.

■ Patient and family members become more active in carrying out toileting program; need for staff assistance decreases.

■ Patient maintains continence.

■ Patient and family members express feelings about patient's self-care deficit. If unable to meet own needs, patient seeks help from family member or staff within 24 hours.

■ Patient and family members identify and contact available support resources, as needed.

Documentation

■ Patient's and family members' expressions of feelings and concerns about self-care deficits

■ Observations of patient's impaired ability to perform toileting routine

■ Patient's intake and output

■ Patient's response to treatment of underlying condition

■ Interventions to provide supportive care

■ Instructions given to patient (if capable) and family members, their understanding of instructions, and their demonstrated skill in carrying out self-care functions
■ Patient's response to nursing interventions
■ Evaluations for expected outcomes

Reference

Forbat, L. "Listening to Carers Talking about Subjects of Continence and Toileting," *Nursing Times* 100(2):46-49, January 2004.

Chronic low
SELF-ESTEEM

Definition

Long-standing negative self-evaluation or feelings about self or capabilities

Assessment

■ Reason for hospitalization or outpatient treatment
■ Age
■ Gender
■ Developmental stage
■ Family system, including marital status, role in family, and sibling position
■ Perception of health problem
■ Past experience with health care system
■ Mental status, including abstract thinking, affect, communication, general appearance, judgment or insight, memory, mood, orientation, perception, and thinking process
■ Belief system, including norms, religion, and values
■ Social interaction pattern
■ Social and occupational history
■ Perception of self (past and present), including body image, coping mechanisms, problem-solving ability, and self-worth
■ Past experience with crisis
■ Past history of treatment for psychosocial disturbance, including hospitalization, medication, psychotherapy, and suicidal ideation, plans, and attempts
■ Neurovegetative signs, including ability to experience pleasure, appetite, energy level, and sleep

Defining characteristics

■ Expressions of self-negating thoughts
■ Expressions of shame or guilt
■ Extreme conformity or dependency on others' opinions
■ Hesitation to try new things or situations
■ Indecisiveness

- Need for excessive reassurance
- Nonassertive or passive tendencies
- Perception of self as unable to deal with events
- Poor eye contact
- Rejection of positive feedback and exaggeration of negative feedback
- Repeated experience of failure in career or other aspects of life

Expected outcomes

- Patient will voice feelings related to self-esteem.
- Patient will report feeling safe in facility environment.
- Patient will make verbal contract not to harm self while in facility.
- Patient will gradually join in self-care and decision-making process.
- Patient will engage in social interaction with others.
- Patient will demonstrate verbal and behavioral decrease in negative self-evaluation.
- Patient will voice acceptance of positive and negative feedback without exaggeration.

Suggested NOC outcomes

Body Image; Depression Level; Mood Equilibrium; Motivation; Personal Autonomy; Quality of Life; Self-Esteem

Interventions and rationales

- Provide for a specific amount of uninterrupted non-care–related time to engage patient in conversation. *This gives patient time for self-exploration.*
- Listen to patient with understanding, responding with nonjudgmental acceptance, genuine interest, and sincerity. *This expands patient's self-awareness and reduces the element of threat.*
- Assess patient's mental status through interview and observation at least once per week. *High anxiety from self-rejection may cause cognitive, sensory, and perceptual disturbances.*
- Assess suicide risk and lethal potential, as indicated. *Extremely low levels of self-esteem may lead to suicide.*
- Institute suicidal precautions according to protocol. Patient needs supervision until he demonstrates adequate self-control *to ensure his own safety.*
- Provide patient with a simple, structured daily routine. *Structured activity limits patient's anxious behaviors.*
- Encourage patient to care for self to the extent possible. *Patient may neglect or reject aspects of self-care because of feelings of self-hate.*
- Involve patient in decisions about care on a gradual basis *to reduce feelings of ambivalence, prevent procrastination, and promote confidence in decision making.*
- Arrange situations to encourage social interaction between patient and others. *Disturbed interpersonal relationships are a direct expression of self-hate.*
- Provide patient with positive feedback for verbal reports and behaviors that indicate improved self-esteem. *This encourages future adaptive coping behaviors.*
- Help patient mobilize resources for assistance when discharged *to help patient replace maladaptive coping behaviors with more adaptive ones.*

■ Refer patient to a mental health professional, as indicated. *Severity of symptoms accompanying chronic low self-esteem may require long-term psychotherapy.*

Suggested NIC interventions
Active Listening; Body Image Enhancement; Coping Enhancement; Decision-Making Support; Hope Instillation; Self-Esteem Enhancement; Spiritual Support; Support Group

Evaluations for expected outcomes
■ Patient expresses feelings about self-esteem.
■ Patient doesn't feel threatened by facility environment.
■ At least once daily, patient reiterates commitment not to harm self.
■ Patient participates in at least one aspect of self-care daily.
■ Patient converses with others on daily basis.
■ Patient states at least two positive aspects about self.
■ Patient accepts positive feedback and constructive criticism.

Documentation
■ Patient's verbal expressions and behaviors that indicate low self-esteem
■ Mental status examination (baseline and ongoing)
■ Suicide assessment, interventions, and patient's response
■ Nursing interventions implemented to promote self-esteem
■ Patient's response to interventions
■ Evaluations for expected outcomes

Reference
Captain, C. "Is Your Patient a Suicide Risk?" *Nursing* 36(8):43-47, August 2006.

Situational low
SELF-ESTEEM
related to an unexpected change in health status

Definition
Development of a negative perception of self-worth in response to a current situation

Assessment
■ Age
■ Gender
■ Developmental stage
■ Family system, including marital status, role in family, and sibling position
■ Reason for health care visit
■ Mental status, including affect, general appearance, and mood
■ Cognitive ability
■ Behavior

■ Perception of self (past and present), including body image, coping mechanisms, and self-worth

Defining characteristics
■ Difficulty making decisions
■ Evaluation of self as unable to handle life events
■ Expression of negative feelings about self (such as helplessness and uselessness)
■ Expressions of self-negating thoughts
■ Expressions of shame or guilt
■ Negative self-appraisal in response to life events in a patient who previously exhibited positive self-evaluation

Expected outcomes
■ Patient will voice feelings related to current situation and its effect on self-esteem.
■ Patient will verbally appraise self before and during current health problem.
■ Patient will participate in decisions related to care and therapies.
■ Patient will report sense of control over life events.
■ Patient will articulate return to previous positive feelings about self.

Suggested NOC outcomes
Decision-Making; Grief Resolution; Psychosocial Adjustment: Life Change; Self-Esteem

Interventions and rationales
■ Encourage patient to express feelings about self (past and present). *Self-exploration encourages patient to consider future change.*
■ Provide a specific amount of uninterrupted non-care–related time to engage patient in conversation. *Such discussions help patient assume ultimate responsibility for coping responses.*
■ Assess patient's mental status through interview and observation at least once per day. *If anxiety resulting from self-rejection becomes severe, patient may experience disorientation and psychotic symptoms.*
■ Involve patient in the decision-making process. *Making such decisions can help combat ambivalence and procrastination associated with low self-esteem.*
■ Provide patient with positive feedback for verbal reports or behaviors that indicate a return to positive self-appraisal. *This gives patient feelings of significance, approval, and competence, which can help him cope effectively with stressful situations.*

Suggested NIC interventions
Anticipatory Guidance; Decision-Making Support; Grief Work Facilitation; Self-Esteem Enhancement

Evaluations for expected outcomes
■ Patient expresses feelings about self in relation to recent stressful events.

■ Patient describes how feelings about self have changed since current health problem began.
■ Patient makes decisions related to care daily.
■ Patient reports feeling more self-confident and in control of current situation.
■ Patient states at least two positive feelings about self.

Documentation

■ Patient's expressions of lowered self-esteem
■ Mental status assessment (baseline and ongoing)
■ Nursing interventions directed toward return to previous positive self-esteem
■ Patient's response to interventions
■ Evaluations for expected outcomes

Reference

Raty, L., and Gustafsson, B. "Emotions in Relation to Healthcare Encounters Affecting Self-esteem," *The Journal of Neuroscience Nursing* 38(1):42-50, February 2006.

Disturbed
SENSORY PERCEPTION

related to altered sensory perception

Definition

Change in the amount or patterning of incoming stimuli accompanied by a diminished, exaggerated, distorted, or impaired response to such stimuli

Assessment

■ Nature of medical diagnosis
■ Mobility
■ Neurologic status, including cognition (insight or judgment and recent and remote memory), level of consciousness, orientation, and sensory function
■ Diagnostic tests, including EEG and computed tomography scan
■ Communication status, including adaptive responses (such as gestures, lipreading, and signing), level of comprehension and expression, and speech pattern
■ Environmental status, including equipment and supplies, lighting, location of patient's personal belongings, noise, privacy, and space
■ Psychosocial status, including alcohol and drug use, behavior and personality, coping mechanisms, history of depression, and support systems

Defining characteristics

■ Altered communication pattern
■ Auditory distortions
■ Change in behavior pattern
■ Change in problem-solving abilities
■ Change in usual response to stimuli

- Disorientation
- Hallucinations
- Irritability
- Poor concentration
- Reported or measured change in sensory acuity
- Restlessness
- Visual distortions

Expected outcomes

- Patient will use adaptive equipment (such as glasses and hearing aid), as needed.
- Patient will remain oriented to time, place, and person.
- Patient will remain safe in environment.
- Patient will respond to environmental stimuli.
- Patient or family members will communicate understanding of sensory stimulation exercises.
- Patient or family members will take active role in preventing sensory deprivation and isolation.

Suggested NOC outcomes

Communication: Receptive; Hearing Compensation Behavior; Sensory Function: Taste & Smell

Interventions and rationales

- Assist or encourage patient to use glasses, a hearing aid, or other adaptive devices *to help reduce sensory deprivation.*
- Reorient patient to reality:
- Call patient by name.
- Tell patient your name.
- Give background information (time, place, and date) frequently throughout day.
- Orient to the environment, including sights and sounds.
- Use large signs as visual cues.
- Post a photo of patient on the door if patient is ambulatory and disoriented.
- Provide visual contrast in the environment.
These measures help reduce patient's sensory deprivation.
- Arrange the environment to offset deficit:
- Place patient in a room that allows him a full view of his environment.
- Encourage family to bring in personal articles, such as books, cards, and photos.
- Keep articles in the same place to promote a sense of identity.
- Use such safety precautions as a nightlight, when needed.
These measures reduce sensory deprivation.
- Communicate patient's response level to family members and staff; record on the care plan and update, as needed. *Patient's response to stimuli allows evaluation of his sensory deprivation level.*

■ Talk to patient while providing care; encourage family members to discuss past and present events with patient. *Verbal stimuli can improve patient's reality orientation.*

■ Arrange to be with patient at predetermined times during the day *to avoid isolation.*

■ Turn on the television and radio for short periods of time based on patient's interests *to help orient patient to reality.*

■ Hold patient's hand when talking. Discuss interests with patient and family members. Obtain needed items such as talking books. *Sensory stimuli help reduce patient's sensory deprivation.*

■ Assist patient and family members in planning short trips outside the facility or health care environment. Educate about mobility, toileting, feeding, suctioning, and other requirements. *Trips help reduce patient's sensory deprivation.*

Suggested NIC interventions

Cognitive Stimulation; Environmental Management; Fluid Management; Nutrition Management

Evaluations for expected outcomes

■ Patient uses adaptive equipment to alleviate sensory deprivation.

■ Patient demonstrates ability to correctly identify time, places, and people and to recall past events.

■ Patient uses safety precautions to remain free from injury.

■ Patient responds to environmental stimuli.

■ Patient or family members communicate understanding of sensory stimulation exercises.

■ Patient or family members identify and use techniques to prevent sensory deprivation.

Documentation

■ Patient's or family members' expressions of concern about sensory deprivation

■ Observations of patient's orientation, response to environmental stimuli, and safety

■ Patient's or family members' response to nursing interventions

■ Instructions and demonstration of skill in providing sensory stimuli

■ Evaluations for expected outcomes

Reference

Mauk, K.L. "Reaching and Teaching Older Adults," *Nursing* 36(2):17, February 2006.

Disturbed
SENSORY PERCEPTION
related to hallucinations

Definition
Change in the amount or patterning of incoming stimuli accompanied by a diminished, exaggerated, distorted, or impaired response to such stimuli

Assessment
- Age
- Gender
- Reason for hospitalization or outpatient visit, including patient's perception of problem, recent stressors, changes in somatic functioning, circumstances surrounding onset of hallucinations, duration and diurnal nature of experiences, and delusional beliefs
- Mental status, including insight about current situation, judgment, abstract thinking, general information, mood, affect, recent and remote memory, thought processes, thought content, and orientation to time, place, and person
- Physical characteristics, including manner of dress, personal hygiene, posture, and gait
- Communication skills, including attitude toward interviewer, body language, and facial expressions
- Psychosocial assessment, including coping mechanisms, support systems, willingness to cooperate with treatment, ability to perform activities of daily living, and social interactions
- Health history, including medication history (response, effectiveness, and adverse reactions), substance abuse history (type and effect on mental status), sleep habits, and dietary and nutritional status
- Laboratory studies, including blood chemistry and toxicology screening
- Diagnostic tests, including computed tomography scan and EEG

Defining characteristics
- Acting out of hallucinatory experience (command hallucinations)
- Perception of images that occur in absence of external stimuli (visual hallucinations)
- Perception of odors of specific or unknown origin (olfactory hallucinations)
- Perception of taste sensations with no basis in reality (gustatory hallucinations)
- Perception of voices or sounds not heard by others and unrelated to objective reality (auditory hallucinations)
- Preoccupation and lack of awareness of surroundings
- Strange body sensations, including misperceptions about body parts (tactile hallucinations)
- Talking to self
- Watchfulness and listening in absence of external stimuli

Expected outcomes
■ Patient will report decrease in number of hallucinatory experiences.
■ Patient will report decrease in anxiety levels that lead to hallucinations.
■ Patient will demonstrate increased ability to test reality at onset of hallucinations.
■ Patient will meet interpersonal needs in realistic ways.

Suggested NOC outcomes
Cognitive Orientation; Distorted Thought Self-Control; Risk Control

Interventions and rationales
■ Provide a safe and structured environment. Identify and reduce as many stressors as possible. Be honest and consistent in all interactions with patient. *These measures will help decrease patient's anxiety.*
■ Encourage patient to identify and initiate anxiety-reducing measures *to give patient a sense of control.*
■ In organic hallucinations, use reality orientation and factual information to help patient cope. Tell patient that the hallucination results from organic causes and can be reversed. *This will reduce anxiety.* In nonorganic hallucinations, don't attempt to reason with patient or challenge the hallucination. Instead, provide comfort and support. *Attempts at reasoning only increase anxiety, which exacerbates hallucinations.*
■ When speaking to patient, use directive statements such as "Look at me and listen; try not to pay attention to the voices right now." *Reacting verbally forces patient to focus on you rather than on internal stimuli.*
■ Provide regular physical activity that requires use of concentration and large muscles *to distract patient from internal stimuli.*
■ Help patient to identify situations that evoke hallucinatory experiences *to enable patient to anticipate hallucinations and possibly prevent their onset.*
■ Teach patient to intervene in a hallucinatory experience. Encourage patient to speak out against the hallucination, using such statements as "Go away; you aren't real." *Such responses foster a sense of control and help distract patient, thereby reducing frequency and duration of hallucinations.*
■ Teach patient to use consensual validation of perceptual experiences to test reality. *Having other people validate experiences will increase patient's orientation to reality.*
■ As patient's anxiety level decreases, encourage participation in group-oriented activities and involvement in the community *to increase patient's level of functioning.*
■ Refer patient to a psychiatric liaison nurse, social service, or support group, as appropriate, *to provide additional support for patient and family members.*

Suggested NIC interventions
Anxiety Reduction; Delusion Management; Hallucination Management; Reality Orientation

Evaluations for expected outcomes
- Within 2 weeks, patient states that hallucinatory experiences have decreased in intensity and frequency.
- Patient reports reduced anxiety levels that lead to hallucination.
- Patient employs self-control measures to reduce hallucinations.
- Patient demonstrates improved social skills.

Documentation
- Patient's statements about type, frequency, and intensity of hallucinations
- Observations about environmental factors that precipitate hallucinatory experiences
- Patient's anxiety level
- Interventions to help patient cope
- Patient's response to nursing interventions
- Referrals
- Evaluations for expected outcomes

Reference
Marco, C.A., and Vaughan, J. "Emergency Management of Agitation in Schizophrenia," *The American Journal of Emergency Medicine* 23(6):767-76, October 2005.

Disturbed
SENSORY PERCEPTION
related to sensory overload

Definition
Change in the amount or patterning of incoming stimuli accompanied by a diminished, exaggerated, distorted, or impaired response to such stimuli

Assessment
- History of major trauma or surgery, seizures, alcoholism, or psychiatric disorders
- Mobility status
- Neurologic status, including cognition (recent and remote memory and insight or judgment), level of consciousness, orientation, and sensory function
- Sleep-wake status
- Communication status, including adaptive responses (such as gestures, lipreading, and signing), level of comprehension and expression, and speech pattern
- Environmental status, including equipment and supplies, lighting, location of patient's personal belongings, noise, privacy, and space
- Psychosocial status, including alcohol and drug use, behavior and personality, coping mechanisms, history of depression, and support systems

Defining characteristics

- Altered communication pattern
- Auditory distortions
- Change in behavior pattern
- Change in problem-solving abilities
- Change in usual response to stimuli
- Disorientation
- Hallucinations
- Irritability
- Poor concentration
- Reported or measured change in sensory acuity
- Restlessness
- Visual distortions

Expected outcomes

- Patient will remain oriented to time, place, and person.
- Patient will voice decreased anxiety and irritability.
- Patient will communicate in a lucid manner.
- Patient will recognize when sensory stimuli are excessive.
- Patient will reestablish usual sleep-wake cycle.
- Patient will state measures to reduce sensory overload.
- Patient will demonstrate positive coping behavior when sensory overload situation arises.

Suggested NOC outcomes

Cognitive Orientation; Distorted Thought Self-Control

Interventions and rationales

- Reorient patient to reality: call patient by name, tell patient your name, give background information (time, place, and date) frequently, and orient to the environment, including sights, sounds, and smells. *These measures will reduce susceptibility to sensory overload.*
- Provide a nonthreatening environment, reduce excessive noise and lights, and keep the environment uncluttered *to reduce sensory overload.*
- Accept patient's perception of stimuli. Don't challenge hallucinations or delusions; don't ridicule or tease. *Challenging patient's perceptions doesn't reduce sensory overload.*
- Help patient interpret the environment (for example, "This is the hospital," "I am a nurse," "You're hearing the food cart go down the hall"). *This helps reduce anxiety.*
- Simulate a "normal" environment: keep lights off (or dim) at night, let in light during day, provide a clock and calendar, and place family photos at the bedside. *This reduces sensory overload.*
- Explain procedures, tests, special equipment, and unusual sounds (such as alarms). Prepare patient for procedures in advance. *Increased knowledge reduces sensory overload.*

■ Cluster procedures and treatments. Avoid disturbing patient unnecessarily. Always approach in a calm, gentle manner to avoid startling patient. *Approaching patient in a compassionate manner helps reduce sensory overload.*

■ Help patient use coping strategies such as talking to someone when sensory overload occurs. *This provides a sense of control.*

■ Teach patient how to limit sensory overload—for example, turning off the television and removing self from a stimulating environment. *Knowledgeable patient is better able to reduce sensory overload.*

■ Encourage regular sleep pattern and routines, possibly including milk or a warm bath before bedtime. *Sufficient rest improves tolerance of stimuli.*

■ Encourage family members to visit frequently; provide reassurance and explanations to aid understanding of patient's condition. *Orientation to reality through family visits helps to promote relaxation.*

Suggested NIC interventions

Cognitive Stimulation; Delusion Management; Medication Management; Reality Orientation

Evaluations for expected outcomes

■ Patient demonstrates ability to correctly identify time, places, and people and to recall past events.

■ Patient reports feeling less irritable and anxious.

■ Patient communicates clearly.

■ Patient recognizes when sensory stimuli are becoming excessive.

■ Patient states that he feels rested.

■ Patient identifies measures to avoid sensory overload.

■ Patient demonstrates positive coping behavior to handle sensory overload.

Documentation

■ Patient's and family members' expressions of concern about sensory overload

■ Observations of orientation, response to environment, anxiety level, and sleep pattern

■ Patient's or family members' responses to nursing interventions

■ Instructions and demonstration of skill in managing sensory overload

■ Evaluations for expected outcomes

Reference

Wheeler, S.L., and Houston, K. "The Role of Diversional Activities in the General Medical Hospital Setting," *Holistic Nursing Practice* 19(2):87-89, March-April 2005.

Disturbed
SENSORY PERCEPTION (AUDITORY)
related to altered sensory reception, transmission, or integration

Definition
Change in the amount or patterning of incoming stimuli accompanied by a diminished exaggerated, distorted, or impaired response to such stimuli

Assessment
- History of ear disorders, trauma, or surgery
- Age
- Auditory status, including ear position, size, and symmetry; skin color and texture; tympanic membrane (cerumen, color of canal, deformities, discharge, intactness or tension, and landmarks); and hearing aid use
- Rinne test
- Weber's test
- Communication status, including adaptive responses (such as gestures, lipreading, and signing), level of comprehension and expression, and speech pattern
- Environmental factors such as factory noise
- Activities of daily living
- Behavioral assessment, including coping mechanisms and willingness to cooperate with treatment

Defining characteristics
- Altered communication pattern
- Auditory distortions
- Change in behavior pattern
- Change in problem-solving abilities
- Change in usual response to auditory stimuli
- Disorientation
- Hallucinations
- Irritability
- Poor concentration
- Reported or measured change in auditory acuity
- Restlessness

Expected outcomes
- Patient will discuss impact of hearing loss on lifestyle.
- Patient will remain oriented to time, place, and person.
- Patient will express feeling of comfort and security.
- Patient will show interest in external environment.
- Patient will compensate for auditory loss by using signing, gestures, lip-reading, hearing aid, or other measures.
- Patient will plan to use community resources to assist with auditory deficit.

Suggested NOC outcomes

Cognitive Orientation; Communication: Receptive; Hearing Compensation Behavior

Interventions and rationales

■ Allow patient to express feelings about hearing loss. Convey willingness to listen, but don't pressure patient to talk. *Giving patient a chance to talk about hearing loss enhances acceptance of loss.*

■ Determine how to communicate effectively with patient, using gestures, written words, signing, or lip-reading. If patient has a hearing aid, encourage its use. *Planned communication with patient improves care delivery.*

■ Give patient clear, concise explanations of treatments and procedures, avoiding information overload. Face patient when speaking; enunciate words clearly, slowly, and in a normal speaking voice; and avoid putting your hands to your mouth when speaking. *Patient will be better able to join in his care with a better understanding of the treatment plan.*

■ Provide sensory stimulation by using tactile and visual stimuli to help compensate for hearing loss. Encourage family members to bring familiar objects from home. *Sensory stimulation of patient's other senses helps compensate for hearing loss.*

■ Provide reality orientation if patient is confused or disoriented *to permit more effective patient-staff interaction.*

■ Make sure other staff members are aware of patient's hearing deficit. Record information on patient's care plan and chart cover *to ensure effective nursing care delivery by all staff members.*

■ Respond to the call bell by going to patient's room as soon as possible. If feasible, assign the same staff members to care for patient. *These measures provide continuity of care and reduce patient's fears.*

■ Teach patient alternative ways to cope with hearing loss; care of hearing aid, if prescribed; and safety and protective measures to avoid harm or injury (such as an amplifier or signal devices on telephone and visual cues in environment). *A knowledgeable patient can better cope with hearing loss.*

■ Refer patient to appropriate community resources, such as Self-help for Hard of Hearing People, to help patient adapt to loss. Involve family members in planning, and encourage their participation. *These measures help patient and family cope better with hearing loss.*

Suggested NIC interventions

Cognitive Stimulation; Communication Enhancement: Hearing Deficit; Environmental Management

Evaluations for expected outcomes

■ Patient discusses impact of hearing loss on lifestyle.

■ Patient demonstrates ability to correctly identify time, places, and people and to recall past events.

■ Because of reduction in environmental risk factors, patient expresses comfort in surroundings.

■ Patient expresses interest in interacting with others.

■ Patient identifies and uses alternative methods of communication.

■ Patient recognizes need for support during transition from facility to outside environment and states plans to use community resources to help him cope with auditory deficit.

Documentation

■ Patient's statements of feelings about auditory loss

■ Observations of patient's behavior or response to auditory loss and use of adaptive aids

■ Instructions about safety and protective measures and patient's intent to use appropriate resources

■ Patient's response to nursing interventions

■ Evaluations for expected outcomes

Reference

Wallhagen, M.I., et al. "Sensory Impairment in Older Adults: Part 1: Hearing Loss," *AJN* 106(10):40-48, October 2006.

Disturbed
SENSORY PERCEPTION (GUSTATORY)

Definition

Change in the amount or patterning of incoming stimuli accompanied by a diminished exaggerated, distorted, or impaired response to such stimuli

Assessment

■ Taste sensation, including change from baseline and ability to differentiate sweet, salty, sour, and bitter tastes

■ Health history, including trauma, infection, vitamin or mineral deficiency, neurologic or oral disorders, and chemotherapy or radiation therapy

■ Medication history, including use of certain antidepressants (such as clomipramine), antineoplastics, captopril, interferon alfa-2a, levamisole, lithium, penicillamine, or zidovudine

■ Evidence of loss of appetite

■ Weight change from baseline

■ Mouth dryness

■ Smoking history

■ Sense of smell

Defining characteristics

■ Altered taste sense:

– Complete loss of taste (ageusia)

– Distorted sense of taste (dysgeusia)

– Partial loss of taste (hypogeusia)

- Loss of appetite
- Reported or measured change in sensory acuity
- Weight loss

Expected outcomes
- Patient will report changes in sense of taste.
- Patient will identify ways to enhance enjoyment of food.
- Patient will consume ___ % of diet.
- Patient will maintain weight.

Suggested NOC outcomes

Appetite; Cognitive Orientation; Nutritional Status: Food & Fluid Intake; Sensory Function: Taste & Smell; Stress Level

Interventions and rationales
- Assess changes in sense of taste *to establish baseline.*
- Gently raise patient's tongue slightly with a gauze sponge. Use moistened applicator to place a few crystals of salt or sugar on one side of the tongue. Wipe the tongue clean and ask patient to identify the taste sensation *to test sweet and salt taste sensation.*
- Apply a tiny amount of quinine to the base of the tongue *to test bitter taste sensation.*
- Place a small piece of sour pickle on patient's tongue *to test sour taste sensation.*
- Pinch off one nostril and ask patient to close his eyes and sniff through the open nostril to identify nonirritating odors, such as coffee, lime, and wintergreen, *to evaluate sense of smell; much of what constitutes taste is actually smell.* Repeat the test on the opposite nostril.
- Monitor and record patient's weight each week *to detect signs of weight loss.*
- Modify patient's diet *so he can distinguish and enjoy as many tastes as possible.* Identify ways to emphasize smell and enhance the flavor of food, such as using herbs and spices, *to compensate for loss of taste.*
- Serve food in attractive surroundings. Prepare meals in an inviting manner, using various different-colored foods, *to appeal to patient's visual sense.*

Suggested NIC interventions

Electrolyte Management; Environmental Management; Feeding; Fluid Management; Neurologic Monitoring; Nutritional Monitoring; Reality Orientation

Evaluations for expected outcomes
- Patient reports changes in sense of taste.
- Patient identifies ways to make meals more appealing.
- Patient consumes ___ % of diet.
- Patient maintains weight.

Documentation
- Evidence of changes in patient's sense of taste

- Patient's weight
- Techniques used to modify patient's diet
- Evaluations for expected outcomes

Reference

Ravasco, P. "Aspects of Taste and Compliance in Patients with Cancer," *European Journal of Oncology Nursing* 9(Suppl 2):S84-S91, 2005.

Disturbed
SENSORY PERCEPTION (KINESTHETIC)

Definition

Change in the amount or patterning of incoming stimuli accompanied by a diminished exaggerated, distorted, or impaired response to such stimuli

Assessment

- Health history, including presence of neurologic or musculoskeletal conditions
- Musculoskeletal status, including motor coordination and muscular weakness
- Use of safety devices
- Presence of other sensory impairments
- Neurologic status, including cognition (insight, judgment, and memory), level of consciousness, and orientation
- Coping behaviors
- Emotional response to illness
- Self-concept, including self-esteem and body image

Defining characteristics

- Diminished motor coordination
- Inability to identify position or location of body parts
- Inability to perceive changes in angles of joints
- Muscular weakness, flaccidity, rigidity, or atrophy
- Paralysis

Expected outcomes

- Patient will express feelings associated with changes in kinesthetic perception.
- Patient will implement safety precautions.
- Patient won't experience skin breakdown, especially in areas around vulnerable joints.
- Patient will participate in self-care activities to maximum ability.
- Patient will participate in appropriate exercise program.
- Patient won't experience injury.

Suggested NOC outcomes

Balance; Body Positioning: Self-Initiated; Sensory Function: Propriocep-
tion

Interventions and rationales

■ Encourage patient to express feelings related to diminished kinesthetic perception *to promote acceptance of perceptual impairment.*

■ Assess changes in motor coordination, paralysis, or muscular weakness and report observations to health care team *to ensure appropriate care.*

■ Implement appropriate safety measures, such as installing padded bed rails,
maintaining bed in low position, and using wheelchair lapboard, *to avoid patient
injury.*

■ Remind patient to regularly check placement of his hands and feet *to avoid
injury.*

■ Teach staff members to remind patient of the need to check the positioning of
hands and feet *to ensure safety and avoid injury.* Emphasize importance of communicating a supportive and accepting attitude *to enhance patient's emotional
well-being.*

■ Inspect patient's skin daily, especially areas around vulnerable joints, *to detect
signs of skin breakdown.*

■ Encourage use of a letter board, electric wheelchair, and feeding and dressing
devices *to promote independence.*

■ Provide patient with an exercise program that includes active and passive
range-of-motion (ROM) routines *to maintain ROM and prevent musculoskeletal
degeneration.*

Suggested NIC interventions

*Energy Management; Exercise Promotion: Strength Training; Exercise
Therapy: Balance; Progressive Muscle Relaxation*

Evaluations for expected outcomes

■ Patient describes feelings brought on by changes in kinesthetic perception.
■ Patient implements safety precautions.
■ Patient doesn't exhibit signs of skin breakdown.
■ Patient participates in self-care activities to maximum ability.
■ Patient participates in selected exercise program.
■ Patient doesn't experience injury.

Documentation

■ Observations of diminished kinesthetic perception
■ Evidence of patient's understanding of instructions about safety and protective
measures and intent to use appropriate safety devices
■ Patient's response to nursing interventions
■ Evaluations for expected outcomes

Reference

Bunting-Perry, L.K. "Palliative Care in Parkinson's Disease: Implications for Neuroscience Nursing," *Journal of Neuroscience Nursing* 38(2):106-13, April 2006.

Disturbed
SENSORY PERCEPTION (OLFACTORY)

Definition

Change in the amount or patterning of incoming stimuli accompanied by a diminished exaggerated, distorted, or impaired response to such stimuli

Assessment

■ Alterations in olfactory sense and related symptoms, including nosebleeds, foul taste in mouth, sneezing, postnasal drip, dry or sore mouth or throat, loss of sense of taste or appetite, excessive tearing, and facial or eye pain
■ Nutritional status, including weight, usual dietary intake, and nausea
■ Medication history, including use of phenothiazines, estrogen, metronidazole, or antineoplastics and prolonged use of nasal decongestants or topical anesthetics
■ History of intranasal drug abuse, such as cocaine and amphetamines
■ Respiratory status, including nasal drainage, sputum characteristics, and history of colds, hay fever, or polyps
■ Health status, including presence of any condition that causes irritation and swelling of nasal mucosa and obstruction of the olfactory area (such as nasal disease and allergies) and any condition that may cause a lesion in the olfactory nerve pathway (such as head trauma)
■ Smoking history
■ Inhalation of irritants such as chlorine fumes
■ Physical examination, including inspection and palpation of nasal structures, contour and color of nasal mucosa, size and color of turbinates, presence of polyps, source and character of nasal discharge, and olfactory nerve (cranial nerve I) function
■ Home environment, including presence of gas or propane heating systems, smoke detectors, and chemical substances

Defining characteristics

■ Altered sense of smell: diminished (hyposmia) or absent (anosmia)
■ Diminished sense of taste and loss of appetite
■ Weight changes

Expected outcomes

■ Patient will express understanding that decreased olfactory perception is temporary.
■ Patient will report improvements in olfactory perception.
■ Patient will maintain weight.

■ Patient will describe how to identify noxious odors and maintain safe home environment.

Suggested NOC outcomes

Cognitive Orientation; Nutritional Status: Food & Fluid Intake; Sensory Function: Taste & Smell

Interventions and rationales

■ Assess patient's ability to smell and document findings *to establish baseline.*

■ Prepare foods the patient likes and serve them in an inviting manner *to stimulate patient's appetite.* Use various different-colored foods with each meal *to appeal to patient's visual sense.*

■ Weigh patient weekly *to detect weight loss and monitor for possible malnutrition.*

■ If altered olfactory perception results from nasal congestion, follow these steps:

– Reassure patient that the condition is temporary and his sense of smell should return *to diminish anxiety.*

– Tell patient with nasal packing that his sense of smell will return after packing is removed and swelling decreases *to provide reassurance.*

– Administer prescribed medications, such as antihistamines and nose drops or sprays, *to relieve nasal congestion.*

– Monitor laboratory values and vital signs *to detect signs of infection.*

– Record nasal drainage characteristics, including amount, color, consistency, and odor, *to assess for changes in olfactory condition.*

– Ensure adequate hydration, and provide for humidification in patient's room *to prevent drying of mucous membranes.*

■ If altered olfactory perception doesn't result from simple nasal congestion, prepare patient for diagnostic tests, such as sinus transillumination, skull X-ray, and computed tomography scan, as ordered, *to guide further treatment.*

■ Provide home care instructions, as necessary. Teach patient to:

– contact utility company *to implement measures for protecting against possible gas leaks*

– place smoke detectors throughout his home *to signal danger of fire*

– discard food according to dates on packages rather than relying on his sense of smell *to avoid eating spoiled food.*

Suggested NIC interventions

Cognitive Stimulation; Environmental Management; Nutrition Management

Evaluations for expected outcomes

■ Patient expresses understanding that change in olfactory perception is temporary.

■ Patient reports improvement in olfactory perception.

■ Patient's weight stabilizes.

■ Patient demonstrates the ability to identify noxious odors and maintain a safe home environment.

Documentation
- Evidence of changes in patient's olfactory perception
- Nursing interventions performed and patient's response
- Patient's dietary preferences
- Patient's weight
- Instructions for home care and patient's or caregiver's response
- Evaluations for expected outcomes

Reference
Vance, D., and Burrage, J. "Chemosensory Declines in Older Adults with HIV: Identifying Interventions," *Journal of Gerontological Nursing* 32(7):42-48, July 2006.

Disturbed
SENSORY PERCEPTION (TACTILE)

Definition
Change in the amount or patterning of incoming stimuli accompanied by a diminished exaggerated, distorted, or impaired response to such stimuli

Assessment
- Vital signs
- Evidence of impaired tactile perception, including complaints of tingling, pain, or numbness; response to sharp and dull stimuli; and signs of bruises, cuts, scrapes, or other injury
- Neurologic status, including level of consciousness, cranial nerve function, muscle strength, deep tendon reflexes, and light touch, pain, temperature, vibration, and position sensation
- Skin color and temperature
- History of chemotherapy treatment
- History of alcohol abuse
- Medication history, including use of amiodarone, anistreplase, ceftizoxime, clomipramine, dichlorphenamide, guanadrel, interferon alfa-2b, or zidovudine

Defining characteristics
- Altered sense of touch:
- Abnormal sensation, such as numbness, prickling, and tingling (paresthesia)
- Decreased sensitivity to stimulation (hypoesthesia)
- Diminished sensitivity to pain (hypalgesia)
- Impaired sense of touch (dysesthesia)

Expected outcomes
- Patient will express feelings about changes in tactile perception.
- Patient won't experience falls or injury.

- Patient won't experience skin breakdown.
- Patient will describe safety measures to avoid injury.
- Family member or caregiver will describe a program to provide patient with increased tactile stimulation.

Suggested NOC outcomes

Ambulation; Balance; Body Mechanics Performance; Body Positioning: Self-Initiated; Coordinated Movement; Neurological Status: Spinal Sensory/Motor Function; Sensory Function: Cutaneous

Interventions and rationales

- Allow patient to express feelings associated with altered tactile perception. Be willing to listen, but don't pressure patient to talk. *Providing a chance to talk will help patient cope with sensory deficits.*
- Teach patient to regularly check placement of his hands and feet *to avoid injury.*
- Inspect patient's skin daily, especially on his feet, *to detect signs of skin breakdown.*
- Use padded side rails or a lapboard on the wheelchair, if appropriate. Make any other environmental modifications, as needed, *to promote safe tactile experiences and prevent accidental injury.*
- Teach patient safety measures, such as testing bath water with a thermometer, *to prevent injury.*
- Teach family members or caregiver to touch patient in areas with preserved sensation, using various textures, *to promote sensory input.* For example, suggest family members provide a satin pillowcase, wrap a soft scarf around patient's neck, or give a gentle massage with scented lotion.

Suggested NIC interventions

Activity Therapy; Environmental Management: Safety; Fluid Management; Fluid Monitoring; Neurologic Monitoring; Nutrition Management; Peripheral Sensation Management; Pressure Management; Skin Surveillance

Evaluations for expected outcomes

- Patient expresses feelings associated with changes in tactile perception.
- Patient doesn't experience falls or injury.
- Patient's skin remains intact.
- Patient lists ways to protect against risk of injury caused by diminished tactile sensation.
- Family member or caregiver describes program to provide patient with increased tactile sensation.

Documentation

- Evidence of diminished tactile sensation
- Patient's expression of feelings about diminished tactile perception
- Instructions about safety and protective measures
- Patient's response to nursing interventions

■ Evaluations for expected outcomes

Reference
Crimlisk, J.T., and Grande, M.M. "Neurologic Assessment Skills for the Acute Medical Surgical Nurse," *Orthopedic Nursing* 23(1):3-9, January-February 2004.

Disturbed
SENSORY PERCEPTION (VISUAL)
related to altered sensory reception, transmission, or integration

---

Definition
Change in the amount or patterning of incoming stimuli accompanied by a diminished exaggerated, distorted, or impaired response to such stimuli

Assessment
■ History of eye disorders, trauma, or surgery
■ Age
■ Visual status, including corneal reflex, extraocular movement, inspection of lid and eyeball, ophthalmoscopy, palpation of lid and eyeball, pupil size and accommodation, tonometry, use of glasses or contact lenses, visual acuity (near and distant), and visual fields
■ Environmental and occupational factors
■ Activities of daily living
■ Behavioral assessment, including coping mechanisms, support system, and willingness to cooperate with treatment

Defining characteristics
■ Altered communication pattern
■ Change in behavior pattern
■ Change in problem-solving abilities
■ Change in usual response to stimuli
■ Disorientation
■ Hallucinations
■ Irritability
■ Poor concentration
■ Reported or measured change in visual acuity
■ Restlessness
■ Visual distortions

Expected outcomes
■ Patient will discuss impact of vision loss on lifestyle.
■ Patient will express feelings of safety, comfort, and security.
■ Patient will maintain orientation to time, place, and person.
■ Patient will show interest in external environment.

- Patient will regain visual functioning and will come to terms with any vision loss.
- Patient will compensate for vision loss by use of adaptive devices.
- Patient will plan to use appropriate resources.

Suggested NOC outcomes

Body Image; Distorted Thought Self-Control; Risk Control; Sensory Function: Vision; Vision Compensation Behavior

Interventions and rationales

- Allow patient to express feelings about vision loss such as its impact on his lifestyle. Convey willingness to listen, but don't pressure patient to talk. *Allowing patient to voice fears aids acceptance of vision loss.*
- Provide a safe environment by removing excess furniture or equipment from patient's room. Orient patient to the room. Show patient how to use the call bell. Don't move furniture or leave objects in the hallway. *Orienting patient to his surroundings reduces the risk of injury.*
- If patient is blind on admission, allow patient to direct arrangement of the room; walk with patient to the bathroom and other key areas until he becomes familiar with his environment. If patient has a seeing-eye dog, make arrangements for the dog's needs. *Maintaining patient's optimal level of independence fosters a sense of control.*
- Modify the environment to maximize any vision patient may have. For example, with hemianopia, place patient in the room to maximize his visual field, approach patient from the best visual angle, remind patient to scan the environment to pick up visual cues, and place objects within his visual field. *Modifying the environment helps patient meet self-care needs.*
- If patient has diplopia, patch one eye *to ameliorate double vision.*
- Always introduce yourself or announce your presence upon entering patient's room; let patient know when you're leaving. *Familiarizing patient with the caregiver aids reality orientation and conveys respect.*
- Provide sensory stimulation by using tactile, auditory, and gustatory stimuli to help compensate for vision loss. Obtain large-print books, talking books, audiotapes, or radio, as preferred by patient. *Nonvisual sensory stimulation helps patient adjust to vision loss.*
- Provide reality orientation if patient is confused or disoriented *to allow for more effective patient-staff interaction.*
- Give patient clear, concise explanations of treatments and procedures, avoiding information overload. When speaking to patient, enunciate words clearly, slowly, and in a normal speaking voice. *A knowledgeable patient will be better able to participate in the treatment plan.*
- Encourage family and friends to visit patient and bring familiar objects to leave in patient's room. *Presence of familiar objects aids reality orientation.*
- Make sure that health care personnel are aware of patient's vision loss. Record information on patient's care plan and chart cover or post in patient's room. *Nursing care is improved if staff is aware of patient's vision loss.*

■ Respond to the call bell as soon as possible. Assign the same staff members to care for patient if possible. *These measures help reduce patient's fears and provide continuity of care.*

■ If patient has had eye surgery, provide appropriate care, as indicated. Be aware of and take steps to limit activities that increase intraocular pressure, such as bending, stooping, getting on and off the bedpan, coughing, and vomiting. *Avoiding postoperative activities that increase intraocular pressure helps reduce complications.*

■ Administer and monitor the effectiveness of medications. Report any adverse effects. *Medications help reduce pain and may control the disease process.*

■ Educate patient in alternative ways of coping with vision loss; care of such adaptive devices as eyeglasses, magnifying glass, contact lenses, and artificial eye; and administration of eyedrops, including name, dosage, and therapeutic and adverse effects. *A knowledgeable patient will be better able to cope with vision loss.*

■ Refer patient and his family to appropriate community resources; for example, the American Foundation for the Blind or other community agencies or support groups. *Postdischarge support will help patient and family cope better with patient's vision loss.*

Suggested NIC interventions

Activity Therapy; Cognitive Stimulation; Communication Enhancement: Visual Deficit; Emotional Support; Environmental Management; Exercise Therapy: Balance; Fall Prevention; Medication Administration; Self-Esteem Enhancement; Surveillance: Safety

Evaluations for expected outcomes

■ Patient discusses effects of vision loss on lifestyle.

■ Because of reduction in environmental risk factors, patient reports comfort in surroundings.

■ Patient maintains ability to correctly identify time, places, and people and to recall past events.

■ Patient expresses interest in interacting with others.

■ Patient regains visual functioning to the extent possible and begins to come to terms with any permanent vision loss.

■ Patient uses adaptive devices to compensate for vision loss.

■ Patient recognizes need for support during transition from facility to outside environment and plans to use appropriate resources, as needed.

Documentation

■ Patient's feelings about visual deficits

■ Observations of patient's behavior and response to visual deficit and use of adaptive equipment or devices

■ Instructions about safety and protective measures, coping strategies, and postoperative management

■ Patient's and family members' intent to use appropriate resources

■ Patient's response to nursing interventions

■ Evaluations for expected outcomes

Reference

Whiteside, M.M., et al. "Sensory Impairment in Older Adults: Part 2: Vision Loss," *AJN* 106(11):52-61, November 2006.

SEXUAL DYSFUNCTION

related to altered body structure or function

Definition

Change in sexual function that's viewed as unsatisfying, unrewarding, and inadequate

Assessment

- History of problem that caused change in structure or function
- Patient's perception of change's effect
- Marital status and attitude of spouse or significant other
- Living arrangement
- Usual sexual patterns
- Sexual problems before current health problem
- Patient's attitude toward modifying sexual patterns
- Patient's present knowledge about appropriate options available

Defining characteristics

- Actual or perceived limitation imposed by disease or therapy
- Change in achieving perceived sex role
- Change in relationship with spouse or significant other
- Change of interest in self and others
- Conflicts involving values
- Inability or change in ability to achieve sexual satisfaction
- Need for confirmation of sexual desirability
- Verbal expression of problem

Expected outcomes

- Patient will acknowledge problem or potential problem in sexual function.
- Patient will voice feelings about changes in sexual identity.
- Patient will explain reason for sexual dysfunction.
- Patient will express willingness to obtain counseling.
- Patient will reestablish sexual activity at pre-illness level.

Suggested NOC outcomes

Adaptation to Physical Disability; Body Image; Fear Level; Physical Aging; Role Performance; Sexual Functioning; Sexual Identity; Stress Level

Interventions and rationales

■ Provide a nonthreatening atmosphere and encourage patient to ask questions about personal sexuality. *A nonthreatening atmosphere encourages patient to ask questions specifically related to the current situation.*

■ Allow patient to express feelings openly in a nonjudgmental atmosphere *to enhance communication and understanding between patient and caregiver.*

■ Provide answers to specific questions *to help patient focus on specific issues, clarify misconceptions, and build trust in the caregiver.*

■ Provide time for privacy *to demonstrate respect for patient, allow time for introspection, and give patient control over time spent interacting with others.*

■ Suggest that patient discuss concerns with partner. *Open discussion fosters sharing of concerns and strengthens relationships.*

■ Provide support for the partner. *Supportive interventions such as active listening communicate concern, interest, and acceptance.*

■ Educate patient and partner about limitations imposed by patient's current physical condition. *Education about limitations imposed on sexual activity by illness helps patient avoid complications or injury.*

■ Suggest referral to a sex counselor or other appropriate professional for future guidance *to provide patient with a resource for postdischarge support.*

Suggested NIC interventions

Anxiety Reduction; Emotional Support; Mutual Goal Setting; Role Enhancement; Self-Awareness Enhancement; Self-Esteem Enhancement; Sexual Counseling; Teaching: Individual; Values Clarification

Evaluations for expected outcomes

■ Patient acknowledges existence of problem or potential problem in sexual function.

■ Patient expresses anxiety, anger, depression, or frustration over changes in sexual function.

■ Patient explains relationship between illness or treatment and sexual dysfunction.

■ Patient expresses willingness to obtain counseling.

■ Patient resumes usual level of sexual activity.

Documentation

■ Patient's perception of problem

■ Subtle comments made by patient about inability to cope with change in structure or function

■ Observations of patient's behavior

■ Interventions performed to assist patient and spouse or significant other; response to interventions

■ Evaluations for expected outcomes

Reference
Bakewell, R.T., and Volker, D.L. "Sexual Dysfunction Related to the Treatment of Young Women with Breast Cancer," *Clinical Journal of Oncology Nursing* 9(6):697-702, December 2005.

SEXUAL DYSFUNCTION
related to biopsychosocial alteration of sexuality

Definition
Change in sexual function that's viewed as unsatisfying, unrewarding, and inadequate

Assessment
- Age
- History of impotence
- Organic (anatomic or central nervous system defect)
- Functional (physiologic alterations in nervous and cardiovascular systems)
- Psychogenic (inhibition by emotions of neural transmission from brain to sexual organs)
- Primary (failure to ever achieve satisfactory erection for coitus)
- Secondary (at least one successful coitus)
- History of organic impotence or physiologic disorders that interfere with erection
- Anatomic anomalies of penis
- Psychological variables, including patient's perception of sexual performance, relationships, desire for erection, guilt, shame, relationship with parents (presence of overbearing mother), and family or social pressures
- Physiologic status, including medication history (response, effectiveness, and adverse reactions) and history of substance abuse (type and effect on mental status)
- Sociocultural factors, including educational level, socioeconomic status, ethnic group, and religious beliefs and practices
- Sexual history, including sexual drive, sexual preference, frequency of impotence, premature ejaculation, spontaneous morning erections, positive coital experiences, types of erotic stimulation used, past professional counseling or sex therapy, homosexual experiences, affairs (other partners or prostitutes), and feelings of anger, hostility, or disgust toward partner

Defining characteristics
- Actual or perceived limitation imposed by disease or therapy
- Change in achieving perceived sex role
- Change in relationship with spouse or significant other
- Change of interest in self and others
- Conflicts involving values
- Inability or change in ability to achieve sexual satisfaction

■ Need for confirmation of sexual desirability
■ Verbal expression of problem

Expected outcomes

■ Patient will acknowledge problem in sexual function.
■ Patient will voluntarily discuss his problem.
■ Patient and partner will discuss their feelings and perceptions about changes in sexual performance.
■ Patient will learn methods to enhance sexual pleasure for himself and his partner and incorporate them into his sexual activities.
■ Patient will continue to communicate with partner about sexual issues and needs.
■ Patient will agree to obtain sexual evaluation and therapy, if needed.
■ Patient will develop and maintain positive attitude toward his sexuality and sexual performance.

Suggested NOC outcomes

Body Image; Fear Level; Physical Aging; Role Performance; Sexual Functioning; Sexual Identity; Social Interaction Skills; Stress Level

Interventions and rationales

■ Establish a therapeutic relationship with patient *to provide a safe, comfortable atmosphere for discussing sexual concerns.*
■ Encourage patient to discuss feelings and perceptions about his sexual dysfunction *to help him validate perceptions and reduce emotional distress through catharsis.*
■ Encourage partner to discuss feelings and perceptions *to help the couple clarify issues about their relationship and improve communication.*
■ Educate patient and partner about alternative methods of lovemaking and expressing affection. *Alternative expressions of love and intimacy can raise patient's self-esteem until impotence is evaluated and treated.*
■ Encourage use of sexual fantasies and erotica to promote sexual stimulation and erection. *This helps patient and partner achieve sexual satisfaction and decreases "spectatoring" (watching oneself during sexual activity with partner), which can inhibit performance.*
■ Encourage patient to seek professional evaluation and therapy *to obtain proper diagnosis and treatment.*

Suggested NIC interventions

Active Listening; Anxiety Reduction; Behavior Management: Sexual; Counseling; Role Enhancement; Self-Awareness Enhancement; Self-Esteem Enhancement; Sexual Counseling; Teaching: Sexuality

Evaluations for expected outcomes

■ Patient states that he has problem in sexual function.
■ Patient states that he feels comfortable discussing his sexual concerns.

- Patient and partner communicate with each other about their sexual relationship.
- Patient states specific ways in which he'll enhance sexual pleasure with his partner.
- Patient continues to communicate with his partner about sexual issues and needs.
- Patient participates in sexual evaluation and sex therapy, if needed.
- Patient makes positive comments about self, sexuality, and sexual performance.

Documentation
- Patient's perception of sexual problem
- Overt and covert remarks made by patient that indicate his difficulty dealing with impotence
- Observations of patient's behavior in response to his inability to perform
- Interventions performed to assist patient and his partner
- Response to nursing interventions
- Evaluations for expected outcomes

Reference
Rice, D., and Jack, L. "Use of an Assessment Tool to Enhance Diabetes Educators' Ability to Identify Erectile Dysfunction," *The Diabetes Educator* 32(3):373-80, May-June 2006.

Ineffective
SEXUALITY PATTERNS

related to impaired relationship with significant other

Definition
State in which an individual expresses concern about personal sexuality

Assessment
- Reason for hospitalization
- Current and anticipated length of stay
- Marital status and family members
- Living arrangement
- Patient's perception of sexual identity and role
- Usual sexual activity pattern
- Patient's perception of limitation on sexual activity resulting from hospitalization
- Significance of sexual relationship to patient and his partner
- Emotional reactions (affect and mood)
- Behavioral reactions (specify)

Defining characteristics
- Reported difficulties, limitations, or changes in sexual activity

Expected outcomes

■ Patient will voice feelings about changes in usual sexual activity.
■ Patient and his partner will discuss possible realistic alternatives for intimacy within hospital setting.
■ Patient and his partner will use available counseling referrals.

Suggested NOC outcomes

Anxiety Level; Body Image; Role Performance; Self-Esteem; Sexual Identity; Stress Level

Interventions and rationales

■ Allow a specific amount of uninterrupted, non-care-related time to talk with patient *to demonstrate your comfort with sexuality issues and reassure patient that his concerns are acceptable for discussion.*
■ Display an accepting, nonjudgmental manner *to encourage patient to discuss concerns about sexuality.* Approach the partner in the same manner and include the partner in discussions with patient, if agreeable to both. *A nonjudgmental approach demonstrates unconditional positive regard for both patient and his partner.*
■ Include patient in a plan for setting limits on inappropriate behavior, if indicated by behavioral assessment.
– Explain aspects of patient's behavior that are inappropriate.
– Share the proposed care plan with patient, including expectations, goals, and approaches for reducing bothersome behavior.
– Request patient's cooperation, but be willing to compromise if he offers acceptable alternatives.
Working together to set limits allows patient to take part in planning to reduce undesirable behaviors.
■ Discuss with patient and his partner realistic, acceptable alternatives for intimacy needs. *Discussion encourages open communication between them as sexual partners.*
■ Explain to patient and his partner the limitations related to illness and facility environment *to establish a standard for realistic and acceptable behavior.*
■ Provide time for privacy to allow patient and his partner *to discuss feelings about sexuality and to engage in alternatives for intimacy while patient is hospitalized.*
■ Offer referral for counseling, such as a mental health professional and sex counselor, if indicated. *Referrals provide opportunities for additional ongoing therapy during hospitalization and after discharge.*

Suggested NIC interventions

Anticipatory guidance; Anxiety Reduction; Coping Enhancement; Role Enhancement; Self-Esteem Enhancement; Sexual Counseling; Teaching: Sexuality

Evaluations for expected outcomes

■ Patient describes usual sexual activity pattern and expresses feelings resulting from changes in pattern.

■ Patient and his partner request privacy and seek permission to use acceptable alternatives for intimacy, such as holding and kissing.

■ Patient and his partner seek counseling.

Documentation

■ Patient's verbal and nonverbal behaviors

■ Patient's and his partner's perception of current situation

■ Specific nursing interventions to reduce emotional and behavioral reactions, such as active listening, limit setting, and counseling referrals

■ Patient's and his partner's response to nursing interventions

■ Evaluations for expected outcomes

Reference

Magnan, M.A., et al. "Barriers to Addressing Patient Sexuality in Nursing Practice," *Medsurg Nursing* 14(5):282-89, October 2005.

Ineffective
SEXUALITY PATTERNS

related to skill deficit about alternative responses to health related transitions

Definition

State in which an individual expresses concern about personal sexuality

Assessment

■ History of current illness

■ Current treatment regimen (medications and therapies)

■ Marital status and family members

■ Patient's perception of sexual identity and role

■ Usual sexual activity pattern

■ Patient's perception of changes in sexual activity resulting from illness or treatment

■ Significance of sexual relationship to patient and partner

■ Emotional reactions (affect and mood)

■ Behavioral reactions (specify)

Defining characteristics

■ Reported difficulties, limitations, or changes in sexual activity

Expected outcomes

■ Patient will voice feelings about potential or actual changes in sexual activity.

■ Patient will express concern about self-concept, self-esteem, and body image.

■ Patient will state at least one effect of illness or treatment on sexual behavior.

■ Patient and his partner will resume effective communication patterns.

■ Patient and his partner will use available counseling referrals or support groups.

Suggested NOC outcomes

Anxiety Level; Body Image; Role Performance; Self-Esteem; Sexual Identity; Stress Level

Interventions and rationales

■ Allow for a specific amount of uninterrupted time to talk with patient *to demonstrate your comfort with sexuality issues and reassure patient that his concerns are acceptable for discussion.*

■ Provide a nonthreatening, nonjudgmental atmosphere for patient to verbalize feelings about perceived changes in sexual identity and behaviors *to demonstrate unconditional positive regard for patient and his concerns about sexuality patterns.*

■ Provide patient and his partner with information about the illness and treatment. Answer any questions and clarify any misconceptions they may have *to help them focus on specific concerns, encourage questions, and avoid misunderstandings.*

■ Provide time for privacy *to demonstrate respect for patient, allow time for introspection, and give patient control over time spent interacting with others.*

■ Encourage social interaction and communication between patient and his partner *to foster sharing of concerns and strengthen relationship.*

■ Offer referral to counselors or support persons, such as a mental health professional, sex counselor, and illness-related support groups, such as "I Can Cope," Reach for Recovery, and the Ostomy Association, *to provide patient with resources for postdischarge support.*

Suggested NIC interventions

Anticipatory Guidance; Body Image Enhancement; Coping Enhancement; Counseling; Emotional Support; Self-Awareness Enhancement; Support Group; Support System Enhancement

Evaluations for expected outcomes

■ Patient expresses concerns and fears related to potential or actual changes in sexual activity.

■ Patient expresses feelings about change in self-image resulting from illness or medical treatment.

■ Patient identifies specific physical symptom that has negative effect on sexual behavior.

■ Patient and his partner communicate effectively.

■ Patient and his partner participate in therapy with appropriate counselor.

Documentation

■ Patient's perception of changes in sexual patterns
■ Patient's ability to interact with other people
■ Interventions to support and educate patient and his partner
■ Response to nursing interventions
■ Evaluations for expected outcomes

Reference

Christopherson, J.M., et al. "A Comparison of Written Materials vs. Materials and Counseling for Women with Sexual Dysfunction and Multiple Sclerosis," *Journal of Clinical Nursing* 15(6):742-50, June 2006.

Impaired
SKIN INTEGRITY

related to internal (somatic) factors

Definition
Altered epidermis and/or dermis

Assessment
- History of skin problems, trauma, chronic debilitating disease, or immobility
- Age
- Integumentary status, including color, elasticity, hygiene, lesions, moisture, texture, turgor, sensation, temperature, and quantity and distribution of hair
- Musculoskeletal status, including joint mobility, muscle strength and mass, paralysis, and range of motion
- Nutritional status, including appetite, dietary intake, hydration, current weight, and change from normal weight
- Hemoglobin and serum albumin levels and hematocrit
- Psychosocial status, including coping patterns, family members, mental status, occupation, self-concept, and body image
- Knowledge level, including patient's current understanding of his physical condition and physical, mental, and emotional readiness to learn

Defining characteristics
- Destruction of skin layers
- Disruption of skin surfaces
- Invasion of body structures

Expected outcomes
- Patient won't show evidence of skin breakdown.
- Patient will exhibit improved or healed lesions or wounds.
- Patient will report increased comfort.
- Patient will have few if any complications.
- Patient will correlate precipitating factors with appropriate skin care regimen.
- Patient will explain skin care regimen.
- Patient and family members will demonstrate skin care regimen.
- Patient will voice feelings about changed body image.

Suggested NOC outcomes
Immobility Consequences: Physiological; Tissue Integrity: Skin & Mucous Membranes; Wound Healing: Secondary Intention

Interventions and rationales

■ Inspect patient's skin every shift, describe and document skin condition, and report changes *to provide evidence of the effectiveness of skin care regimen.*

■ Perform prescribed treatment regimen for the skin condition involved; monitor progress. Report favorable and adverse responses to treatment regimen *to maintain or modify current therapies, as needed.*

■ Provide supportive measures, as indicated:

– Assist with general hygiene and comfort measures *to promote comfort and general sense of well-being.*

– Administer pain medications and monitor effectiveness. *Patient needs pain relief to maintain health.*

– Maintain proper environmental conditions, including room temperature and ventilation. *Providing a comfortable environment promotes sense of well-being.*

– Apply a bed cradle *to protect lesions from bed covers.*

– Remind patient not to scratch *to avoid skin injury.*

– Administer and monitor effectiveness of antipruritic medications. *Antipruritics reduce the itching sensation.*

– Explain dietary restrictions—for example, explain that certain foods may cause a skin allergy. *Avoiding foods that cause skin allergy helps prevent skin breakdown.*

■ Encourage patient to express his feelings about his skin condition *to enhance coping.*

■ Explain the therapy to patient and his family *to encourage compliance.*

■ Discuss precipitating factors, if known, and long-term effects of skin integrity interruption. *Knowledge of precipitating factors helps patient reduce their occurrence and severity.*

■ Instruct patient and his family in the skin care regimen *to ensure compliance.*

■ Supervise patient and his family in the skin care regimen. Provide feedback. *Practice helps improve skill in managing patient's skin care regimen.*

■ Encourage adherence to other aspects of health care management *to control or minimize effects on skin.*

■ Refer patient to a psychiatric liaison nurse, social service, or support group, as appropriate. *These resources provide additional support for patient and his family.*

Suggested NIC interventions

Infection Control; Nutrition Therapy; Positioning; Pressure Ulcer Prevention; Skin Surveillance

Evaluations for expected outcomes

■ Patient's skin remains intact.

■ Patient's wounds or lesions heal.

■ Patient reports feeling of comfort.

■ Patient doesn't experience further skin breakdown or other complications.

■ Patient lists factors precipitating skin breakdown.

■ Patient explains skin care regimen.

■ Patient and family members demonstrate skin care regimen.

■ Patient expresses feelings about changed body image.

Documentation
- Patient's concerns about his skin disorder and its impact on body image and lifestyle
- Patient's willingness to participate in care
- Observations of skin condition, healing, and response to treatment regimen
- Interventions to provide supportive care
- Instructions about treatment regimen
- Patient's or family members' understanding of and skill in carrying out instructions
- Patient's response to nursing interventions
- Evaluations for expected outcomes

Reference
Hoggarth, A., et al. "A Controlled, Three-part Trial to Investigate the Barrier Function and Skin Hydration Properties of Six Skin Protectants," *Ostomy/Wound Management* 51(12):30-42, December 2005.

Impaired
SKIN INTEGRITY
related to physical immobilization

Definition
Altered epidermis and/or dermis

Assessment
- History of skin problems, trauma, surgery, or immobility
- Age
- Integumentary status, including color, elasticity, hygiene, lesions, moisture, texture, turgor, sensation, temperature, and quantity and distribution of hair
- Musculoskeletal status, including joint mobility, muscle strength and mass, paralysis, and range of motion
- Nutritional status, including appetite, dietary intake, hydration, current weight, and change from normal weight
- Hemoglobin and serum albumin levels and hematocrit
- Psychosocial status, including coping skills, family members, mental status, self-concept, and body image
- Occupational hazards
- Knowledge level, including patient's current understanding of physical condition and physical, mental, and emotional readiness to learn

Defining characteristics
- Destruction of skin layers
- Disruption of skin surface
- Invasion of body structures

Expected outcomes

- Patient won't show evidence of skin breakdown.
- Patient will show normal skin turgor.
- Patient will regain skin integrity (specify) — for example, pressure ulcer will decrease in size.
- Patient's surgical wound will heal.
- Patient will communicate understanding of skin protection measures.
- Patient will demonstrate skill in care of wound, burn, or incision.
- Patient will demonstrate skin inspection technique.
- Patient will perform skin care routine.
- Patient will communicate feelings about change in body image.

Suggested NOC outcomes

Immobility Consequences: Physiological; Tissue Integrity: Skin & Mucous Membranes; Tissue Perfusion: Peripheral; Wound Healing: Primary Intention; Wound Healing: Secondary Intention

Interventions and rationales

- Inspect skin every shift, describe and document skin condition, and report changes *to provide evidence of the effectiveness of the skin care regimen.*
- Perform prescribed treatment regimen for the skin condition involved; monitor progress. Report responses to the treatment regimen *to maintain or modify current therapy.*
- Provide supportive measures, as indicated:
- Assist with general hygiene and comfort measures *to promote comfort and sense of well-being.*
- Administer pain medication and monitor its effectiveness. *Patient needs pain relief to maintain health.*
- Maintain proper environmental conditions *to promote patient's sense of well-being.*
- Use a foam mattress, bed cradle, or other devices *to minimize skin breakdown.*
- Warn against tampering with the wound or dressings *to reduce potential for infection.*
- Maintain infection control standards *to reduce the risk of spreading disease.*
- Position patient for comfort and minimal pressure on bony prominences. Change his position at least every 2 hours. Monitor frequency of turning and skin condition. *These measures reduce pressure, promote circulation, and minimize skin breakdown.*
- Explain the therapy to patient and family members *to encourage compliance.*
- Allow patient to express his feelings about skin problem. *Verbalization of feelings helps allay anxiety and develops coping skills.*
- Instruct patient and family members in a skin care regimen *to encourage compliance.*
- Supervise patient and family members in skin care management. Provide feedback *to improve skill in managing skin care.*
- Provide a referral to a psychiatric liaison nurse, social service, or support group, as appropriate *to provide additional support for patient and his family.*

Suggested NIC interventions

Fluid Management; Infection Protection; Positioning; Pressure Management; Pressure Ulcer Care; Pressure Ulcer Prevention; Skin Surveillance; Wound Care

Evaluations for expected outcomes

- Patient's skin remains intact.
- Patient's skin turgor remains normal.
- Patient's pressure ulcer heals, as evidenced by presence of granulation tissue and decreased size and depth of ulcer.
- Patient's surgical wound heals, as evidenced by clean suture line and absence of scar discoloration and skin breakdown.
- Patient understands necessity of avoiding prolonged pressure, obtaining adequate nutrition, and using protective devices.
- Patient demonstrates skill in care of wound, burn, or incision.
- Patient demonstrates skin inspection techniques.
- Patient performs skin care routine.
- Patient expresses feelings about changes in body image.

Documentation

- Patient's concerns about change in skin integrity, willingness to accept treatment, and participation in treatment regimen
- Observations of wound, pressure ulcer, and incision healing and response to treatment regimen
- Interventions to provide supportive care and prescribed treatment
- Patient's response to nursing interventions
- Patient's and family members' understanding and skill in performing skin care measures
- Evaluations for expected outcomes

Reference

Mackey, D. "Support Surfaces: Beds, Mattresses, Overlays-Oh My!" *The Nursing Clinics of North America* 40(2):251-65, June 2005.

Risk for impaired
SKIN INTEGRITY

Definition

At risk for skin being adversely altered

Assessment

- History of skin problems, trauma, chronic debilitating disease, or immobility
- Age

■ Integumentary status, including color, elasticity, hygiene, lesions, moisture, sensation, temperature, texture, turgor, and quantity and distribution of hair
■ Musculoskeletal status, including muscle strength and mass, joint mobility, paralysis, and range of motion (ROM)
■ Nutritional status, including appetite, dietary intake, hydration, current weight, and change from normal weight
■ Hemoglobin and serum albumin levels and hematocrit
■ Psychosocial status, including activities of daily living, mental status, occupation (sun exposure), and recreational activities

Risk factors

■ External factors, including pressure, friction and shearing, restraints, physical immobilization, humidity and moisture, chemical substances, radiation, excretions and secretions, hypothermia or hyperthermia, and extreme youth or age
■ Internal factors, including effects of medications, skeletal prominences, and altered nutritional status (obesity or emaciation), sensation, pigmentation, metabolic state, circulation, or skin turgor

Expected outcomes

■ Patient won't experience skin breakdown.
■ Patient will maintain muscle strength and joint ROM.
■ Patient will sustain adequate food and fluid intake.
■ Patient's mucous membranes will remain intact.
■ Patient will maintain adequate skin circulation.
■ Patient will communicate understanding of preventive skin care measures.
■ Patient and family members will demonstrate preventive skin care measures.
■ Patient and family members will correlate risk factors and preventive measures.

Suggested NOC outcomes

Immobility Consequences: Physiological; Nutritional Status; Physical Aging; Risk Control; Risk Detection; Tissue Integrity: Skin & Mucous Membranes

Interventions and rationales

■ Inspect patient's skin every shift; document skin condition and report status changes. *Early detection of changes prevents or minimizes skin breakdown.*
■ Change patient's position at least every 2 hours; follow turning schedule posted at bedside. Monitor frequency of turning. *These measures reduce pressure on tissues, promote circulation, and help prevent skin breakdown.*
■ Encourage ambulation or perform or assist with active ROM exercises at least every 4 hours while patient is awake. *Exercises prevent muscle atrophy and contracture; ambulation promotes circulation and relieves pressure.*
■ Use preventive skin care devices, as needed, such as a foam mattress, alternating pressure mattress, sheepskin, pillows, and padding, *to avoid discomfort and skin breakdown.*

■ Keep patient's skin clean and dry; lubricate, as needed. Don't use irritating soap, and rinse skin well. *These measures alleviate skin dryness, promote comfort, and reduce the risk of irritation and skin breakdown.*

■ Protect bony prominences with foam padding. *Prominences have little subcutaneous fat and are prone to breakdown; using foam padding may help promote skin integrity.*

■ Lift patient's body when moving him, using a lifting sheet, if needed. Avoid shearing force. *Shearing force results when tissues slide against each other; a lifting sheet reduces sliding.*

■ Keep linen dry, clean, and free from wrinkles or crumbs. Change wet bed linens and incontinence pads immediately. *Dry, smooth linens help prevent excoriation and skin breakdown.*

■ Monitor nutritional intake; maintain adequate hydration. *Anemia (less than 10 mg hemoglobin) and low serum albumin concentrations (less than 2 mg) are associated with the development of pressure ulcers. Hydration helps maintain skin integrity.*

■ Educate patient and his family in preventive skin care. Teach them how to maintain good personal hygiene; use nonirritating (nonalkaline) soap; pat rather than rub skin dry; inspect skin regularly; avoid prolonged exposure to water, sun, cold, and wind; avoid rubber rings; recognize the beginning of skin breakdown (redness, blisters, and discoloration); and report signs and symptoms. *These measures encourage compliance with patient's skin care regimen.*

■ Indicate the risk factor potential on patient's chart and care plan, and reevaluate weekly, using an accepted form such as the Braden Scale. *The risk factor score helps evaluate treatment progress.*

■ Explain the importance of practicing preventive skin care measures *to encourage compliance with skin care regimen.*

■ Supervise patient and his family in preventive skin care measures. Give constructive feedback. *Practice helps improve skill in managing the skin care regimen.*

Suggested NIC interventions
Circulatory Precautions; Infection Prevention; Positioning; Pressure Management; Pressure Ulcer Prevention; Skin Surveillance; Splinting

Evaluations for expected outcomes
■ Patient's skin remains intact.
■ Patient maintains muscle strength and joint ROM.
■ Patient's weight remains within established limits.
■ Patient's mucous membranes remain intact.
■ Patient maintains adequate skin circulation.
■ Patient lists preventive skin care measures.
■ Patient and family members demonstrate skin care measures.
■ Patient and family members understand need to avoid prolonged pressure, obtain adequate nutrition, prevent incontinence, and consistently perform skin care measures.

Documentation
■ Patient's and family members' expressions of concern about potential skin breakdown
■ Observations of risk factors and skin condition
■ Use of preventive skin care devices and their effectiveness
■ Instructions about preventive skin care; patient's and family members' understanding of instructions
■ Patient's and family members' demonstrated skill in carrying out preventive skin care measures
■ Results of Braden Scale
■ Patient's response to nursing interventions
■ Evaluations for expected outcomes

Reference
Lyder, C.H. "Assessing Risk and Preventing Pressure Ulcers in Patients with Cancer," *Seminars in Oncology Nursing* 22(3):178-84, August 2006.

SLEEP DEPRIVATION

Definition
Prolonged periods of time without sustained natural, periodic suspension of relative unconsciousness

Assessment
■ Number of hours of sleep patient usually needs to feel rested
■ Premorbid sleep patterns and current sleep patterns
■ Daytime activity and work patterns
■ Recent changes in health status or lifestyle
■ Sleep environment, including recent changes to environment
■ Activities that promote sleep
■ Quality of sleep, as described by patient
■ Dietary and drug history, including ingestion of caffeine or other stimulants, nicotine, alcohol, and sedative-hypnotics

Defining characteristics
■ Acute confusion
■ Agitation or combativeness
■ Daytime drowsiness
■ Decreased ability to function
■ Hallucination
■ Hand tremors
■ Heightened sensitivity to pain
■ Inability to concentrate
■ Irritability, lethargy, listlessness, restlessness, anxiety, malaise, apathy

- Mild, fleeting nystagmus
- Perceptual disorders (for example, disturbed body sensation, delusions, feeling afloat)
- Transient paranoia

Expected outcomes

- Patient will identify factors that prevent or disrupt sleep.
- Patient will sleep ___ (specify) hours without interruption.
- Patient will express feeling well rested.
- Patient will show no physical signs of sleep deprivation.
- Patient will not exhibit complications associated with sleep deprivation, such as sleep apnea and nocturnal hypoxic episodes.
- Patient will alter diet and habits to promote sleep — for example, by reducing caffeine intake and limiting alcohol intake.
- Patient will not exhibit such sleep-related behavioral symptoms as irritability, lethargy, listlessness, restlessness, anxiety, worry, or depression.
- Patient will perform relaxation exercises at bedtime.
- Health care providers will schedule nighttime treatments to allow for maximum restful sleep.

Suggested NOC outcomes

Concentration; Endurance; Energy Conservation; Mood Equilibrium; Rest; Sleep; Stress Level; Symptom Severity

Interventions and rationales

- Encourage patient to identify factors in the environment that make sleeping difficult. *A strange or new environment may affect rapid-eye-movement (REM) and non-rapid-eye-movement (NREM) sleep.*
- Ask patient what changes would help promote sleep *to encourage patient to play an active role in care.*
- Advise patient to avoid daytime naps *to promote restful nocturnal sleep.*
- Tell patient to avoid spending long periods in bed without sleep. *Activity produces healthy fatigue, which promotes restful sleep.*
- Make immediate changes to accommodate patient — for example, reduce noise; change catheterization, medication, or treatment schedule; change lighting; and close door. *These measures promote rest and sleep.*
- Develop a plan to allow patient to have ___ hours of uninterrupted sleep, if possible. *This provides consistent nursing care and provides patient with maximum hours of uninterrupted sleep.*
- Perform interventions to promote sleep, such as giving patient a bath or back rub, ensuring that patient is positioned properly, or providing pillows, food, or drink. *Personal hygiene routine precedes sleep for many individuals. Milk and some high-protein snacks, such as cheese or nuts, contain L-tryptophan, a sleep promoter.*
- Assess patient each morning to determine quality of sleep the night before *to help detect sleep-related behavioral symptoms.*
- Teach patient relaxation techniques, such as guided imagery, meditation, and progressive muscle relaxation. Practice them with patient at bedtime. *Purposeful relaxation efforts commonly promote sleep.*

■ Instruct patient to limit alcohol and caffeine intake and avoid foods that interfere with sleep (such as spicy foods). Foods and beverages with caffeine should be avoided for 4 to 5 hours before bedtime. *Dietary changes may help to promote restful sleep.*

■ Avoid quick, unanticipated movements when turning and positioning patients with neuromuscular dysfunction *to prevent spasticity, which may interrupt sleep.*

■ In stroke patients with muscle tone problems, plan to position patient on the affected side during the last turn of the night *to promote restful sleep and help normalize patient's muscle tone for morning activities.*

■ Refer patient experiencing sleep deprivation to a sleep disorder center especially if activities of daily living are affected or sleep apnea occurs. *A specialist may be required to assist in treatment.*

■ Assess the daytime schedule to ensure adequate time for rest. *Excessive fatigue can result in insomnia.*

■ Help patient with chronic illness or disability find resources for addressing psychosocial issues. *Fears and concerns about future prevent restful sleep.*

Suggested NIC interventions

Anxiety Reduction; Coping Enhancement; Energy Management; Environmental Management: Comfort; Progressive Muscle Relaxation; Sleep Enhancement

Evaluations for expected outcomes

■ Patient identifies factors that prevent or disrupt sleep.

■ Patient sleeps ___ (specify) hours without interruption.

■ Patient expresses feeling of being well rested.

■ Patient shows no physical signs of sleep deprivation.

■ Patient doesn't exhibit complications associated with sleep deprivation, such as sleep apnea and nocturnal hypoxic episodes.

■ Patient alters diet and habits to promote sleep — for example, by reducing caffeine intake and limiting alcohol intake.

■ Patient doesn't exhibit such sleep-related behavioral symptoms, such as irritability, lethargy, listlessness, restlessness, anxiety, worry, or depression.

■ Patient performs relaxation exercises at bedtime.

■ Health care providers schedule nighttime treatments to allow for maximum restful sleep.

Documentation

■ Patient's reports of sleep disturbances

■ Patient's expressions of feelings related to sleep deprivation

■ Observations of behaviors that indicate sleep deprivation

■ Nursing interventions to alleviate sleep deprivation

■ Patient's response to nursing interventions

■ Evaluations for expected outcomes

Reference

Frank, M.G. "The Mystery of Sleep Function: Current Perspectives and Future Directions," *Review in Neuroscience* 17:375-92, 2006.

Impaired
SOCIAL INTERACTION
related to altered thought processes

Definition

Insufficient quantity or ineffective quality of social exchange

Assessment

- Reason for hospitalization (physiologic or psychiatric)
- Usual pattern of social interaction (nonverbal behaviors and verbal communication)
- Neurologic functioning, including level of consciousness, orientation, and sensory and motor ability
- Mental status, including abstract ability, affect, concentration ability, insight and judgment, memory, mood, and thought content
- History of substance abuse
- Education and intelligence level
- Sociocultural background, including beliefs, norms, religion, and values
- Support systems, including clergy, family members, and friends

Defining characteristics

- Discomfort in social situations
- Family report of change in style of interaction
- Inability to receive or communicate satisfying sense of belonging, caring, interest, or shared history
- Use of unsuccessful or dysfunctional social interaction skills

Expected outcomes

- Patient will remain free from injury.
- Patient and family members will report concern about difficulties in social interaction.
- Patient will maintain orientation to time, place, and person.
- Patient's perceptions will be reality-based.
- Patient and family members will participate in care and prescribed therapies.
- Patient will express needs and will communicate whether needs are met.
- Patient will regain appropriate neurologic function to extent possible.
- Patient will demonstrate effective social interaction skills in one-on-one and group settings.
- Patient and family members will identify and mobilize resources for rehabilitation and discharge planning, as necessary.

Suggested NOC outcomes

Family Social Climate; Immobility Consequences: Psycho-Cognitive; Self-Esteem; Social Interaction Skills; Social Involvement;

Interventions and rationales

■ Follow the medical regimen to treat the underlying condition. *The nurse is responsible for following the medical regimen and working with the physician to plan appropriate care.*

■ Take precautions to ensure a safe and protected environment (provide side rails, help with out-of-bed activities, keep the room free from clutter, and use physical restraints, as necessary) *to reduce the potential for patient injury.*

■ Assess neurologic function and mental status every shift *to monitor changes in patient's status;* reorient patient as often as necessary:

– Call patient by name and say your name each time you interact with him.

– Tell patient the correct day, date, time, and place at least once per shift.

– Teach family members how to reorient patient, and help them do so.

– Ask family members to bring patient familiar objects from home, such as clock, radio, and photographs.

– Post a structured schedule of daily activities in patient's room within visual range.

– Explain the schedule to family members and other caregivers to provide consistency and continuity.

Reorienting patient and involving family members enhances patient's reality-testing ability and overall mental status. Scheduling a daily routine narrows patient's frame of reference, thereby decreasing the potential for increased confusion.

■ If delusions and hallucinations occur, don't focus on them; provide patient with reality-based information and reassure patient of his safety *to increase patient's ability to grasp reality and reduce fears associated with these disturbances.*

■ Provide specific, non-care-related time with patient each shift *to encourage social interaction.* Begin with one-on-one interaction and increase to group interaction as patient's skills indicate. *Gradually increasing social interaction reduces patient's feeling of being overwhelmed and eliminates sensory input that may renew a cognitive or perceptual disturbance.*

■ Give positive reinforcement for appropriate and effective interaction behaviors (verbal and nonverbal) *to help patient recognize progress and enhance feelings of self-worth.*

■ Assist patient and family members in progressive participation in care and therapies *to reduce feelings of helplessness and enhance patient's feeling of control and independence.*

■ Initiate or participate in multidisciplinary patient-centered conferences to evaluate progress and plan discharge. In addition to patient and family members, conferences may include physical, occupational, and speech therapists; a social worker; the attending physician; and other consultants, as necessary. *These conferences involve patient and his family in a cooperative effort to develop strategies for altering the care plan, as necessary.*

Suggested NIC interventions

Behavior Modification: Social Skills; Complex Relationship Building; Family Integrity Promotion; Family Therapy; Normalization Promotion; Support System Enhancement

Evaluations for expected outcomes
- Patient doesn't exhibit physical evidence of injury.
- Patient and family members express concern about patient's inability to interact normally.
- Patient remains oriented to time, place, and person.
- Patient's verbal responses and behavior don't indicate delusions or hallucinations.
- Patient and family members perform care-related procedures to extent possible.
- Patient uses words, gestures, or writing to communicate needs and whether needs are met.
- Patient maintains appropriate cognitive and perceptual functioning to extent possible.
- Patient communicates effectively in one-on-one and group settings.
- Patient and family members identify and contact available support resources, as needed.

Documentation
- Patient's verbal and nonverbal behaviors
- Neurologic and mental status assessment
- Observations of patient's social interaction skills
- Interventions to facilitate appropriate and effective social interaction
- Patient's responses to nursing interventions
- Evaluations for expected outcomes

Reference
Oliver, D.P., et al. "A Promising Technology to Reduce Social Isolation of Nursing Home Residents," *Journal of Nursing Care Quality* 21(4):302-305, October-December 2006.

Impaired
SOCIAL INTERACTION
related to sociocultural dissonance

Definition
Insufficient quantity or ineffective quality of social exchange

Assessment
- Reason for hospitalization (physiologic or psychiatric)
- Sociocultural background (beliefs, norms, rituals, and values)

■ Usual pattern of social interaction, including dominant language, group participation, level of comprehension, nonverbal communication skills (such as drawing and gestures), and speech pattern
■ Patient's position in family
■ Support systems, including clergy, family members, and friends
■ Education and intelligence level

Defining characteristics
■ Discomfort in social situations
■ Family report of change in style of interaction
■ Inability to receive or communicate satisfying sense of belonging, caring, interest, or shared history
■ Use of unsuccessful or dysfunctional social interaction skills

Expected outcomes
■ Patient will provide information concerning cultural background.
■ Patient will identify needs and will communicate (verbally or through behavior) whether needs are met.
■ Patient will express understanding of care-related instruction.
■ Patient and family members will participate in planning care.
■ Patient will identify effective coping techniques to deal with sociocultural differences.
■ Patient will express feelings of comfort and trust in interaction with caregivers.
■ Patient will use resources outside normal sociocultural group, as necessary.

Suggested NOC outcomes
Communication; Social Interaction Skills; Social Involvement; Stress Level

Interventions and rationales
■ Assign a primary nurse to patient if possible. *Primary nursing provides consistency, enhances trust, and decreases the potential for fragmented care.*
■ Provide a specific time (for example, 10 minutes each shift) to talk with patient and family members about sociocultural background. *In many cultural groups, trust develops slowly and may be hampered by lengthy interviews.*
■ Take care not to stereotype the patient into what the nurse knows about the patient's cultural background. *Stereotyping is destructive when providing individualized care to a patient. Keep in mind that not all persons in a particular culture fit a pattern.*
■ Explain care-related activities clearly and answer questions as accurately as possible *to enhance patient's understanding of care-related procedures and facility routine.*
■ Use an interpreter when necessary *to ensure effective communication for non-English-speaking patients. The primary reasons for using an interpreter to communicate with a patient are legal, financial, and to provide quality care.*
■ Involve patient and family members in planning care, and continually encourage patient's participation in self-care *to increase their sense of control and reduce feelings of helplessness and isolation.*

■ Help patient identify and use effective social-interaction behaviors, such as increased eye contact, calling people by name, and asking questions. *Teaching patient effective interpersonal communication helps him function more effectively in a social environment.*

■ Demonstrate respect for patient's privacy, personal belongings, cultural norms, and religious beliefs and practices *to provide sensitive care to patients from varied cultural backgrounds.*

■ Offer a referral to other support systems (such as social services, financial counseling, home health care, mental health care, and professional care), if indicated. *This ensures comprehensive approach to patient's care.*

Suggested NIC interventions

Active Listening; Anxiety Reduction; Coping Enhancement; Family Process Maintenance; Family Support; Mutual Goal Setting; Normalization Promotion

Evaluations for expected outcomes

■ Patient provides information about his culture, including values, attitudes, roles, and beliefs.

■ Patient reports needs and gratification of these needs, either verbally or through behavior.

■ Patient demonstrates care-related procedures.

■ Patient and family members help develop care plan.

■ Patient specifies positive ways to cope with cultural differences.

■ Patient communicates sense of security and demonstrates decrease in anxiety-related behaviors.

■ Patient uses appropriate resources outside his normal sociocultural group, as needed.

Documentation

■ Patient's and family members' perceptions of current situation

■ Interventions to promote effective social interaction

■ Patient's verbal and nonverbal responses to nursing interventions

■ Evaluations for expected outcomes

Reference

van Servellen, G., et al. "Continuity of Care and Quality Outcomes for People Experiencing Chronic Conditions: A Literature Review," *Nursing & Health Sciences* 8(3):185-95, September 2006.

SOCIAL ISOLATION
related to altered state of wellness

Definition
Aloneness that patient perceives negatively; may be self-imposed or be perceived as being imposed by others; alternatively, may result from environmental factors

Assessment
- Reason for hospitalization (physiologic or psychiatric)
- Support systems available, including clergy, family members, and friends
- Functional ability
- Diversional interests
- Attitudes of family or friends toward patient
- Financial resources
- Occupation
- Education level
- Coping and problem-solving ability
- Self-esteem

Defining characteristics
- Absence of supportive significant other
- Culturally unacceptable behavior
- Description of lifestyle as solitary or circumscribed by membership in subculture
- Evidence of physical or mental disability or altered state of wellness
- Expressed feelings of being different from others
- Expressed feelings of rejection or aloneness
- Expressed frustration over inability to meet expectations of others
- Inappropriate or immature interests or activities
- Insecurity in public
- Lack of family, friends, and social groups
- Lack of purpose in life
- Preoccupation with own thoughts
- Projection of hostility in voice and behavior
- Repetitive, meaningless actions
- Sad, dull affect
- Uncommunicative and withdrawn behavior, with poor eye contact

Expected outcomes
- Patient will express feelings associated with social isolation.
- Patient will identify causes of social isolation and participate in developing plan for increasing social activity.
- Patient will interact with family members or friends.
- Patient will interact with caregivers.
- Patient will perform self-care activities independently.
- Patient will participate daily in meaningful diversional activity (specify).

- Patient will indicate that social relationships have improved and negative feelings have diminished.
- Patient will achieve expected state of wellness.

Suggested NOC outcomes

Leisure Participation; Loneliness Severity; Personal Well-Being; Social Interaction Skills; Social Involvement; Social Support

Interventions and rationales

- Assign a primary nurse to patient, if possible, *to provide continuity, enhance trust, and decrease the potential for fragmented care.*
- Initiate a trusting nurse-patient relationship *to help gain patient's confidence.*
- Provide honest and immediate feedback about patient's behavior *to help patient become aware of the effects of behavior and to modify, verify, or correct patient's perceptions.*
- Help patient identify causes of social isolation *to identify patient's needs and guide planning of care.* Involve patient and his family or friends in setting goals and planning care *to individualize the care plan and decrease patient's feelings of helplessness and isolation.*
- Encourage patient to perform such self-care activities as bathing, grooming, dressing, eating, and ambulating *to reduce feelings of helplessness and foster independence.*
- Spend at least 15 minutes each shift sitting with patient and listening to him. *Listening communicates concern, interest, and acceptance and allows time for patient to collect thoughts and express feelings.*
- Arrange with patient for specific periods of appropriate planned diversional activity *to provide pleasure, increase feelings of self-worth, and decrease negative self-absorption.*
- Allow ample private time for patient to spend with his family or friends *to demonstrate respect for patient and for patient's relationships with others.*
- Identify appropriate social agencies and support groups for patient and provide referrals *to ensure ongoing opportunities for patient to increase social interaction.*
- Educate patient and his family about health care needs and treatment *to promote optimal health and well-being, thereby allowing for greater social activity.*

Suggested NIC interventions

Activity Therapy; Family Integrity Promotion; Mood Management; Mutual Goal Setting; Recreation Therapy; Socialization Enhancement; Support System Enhancement

Evaluations for expected outcomes

- Patient expresses sadness, frustration, anxiety, and other feelings associated with social isolation.
- Patient identifies causes of social isolation and helps develop plan for increasing social activity.
- Patient interacts with family members or friends.
- Patient interacts with caregivers.

■ Patient initiates self-care activities, such as bathing, dressing, eating, and grooming, to extent possible.

■ Patient identifies at least three activities that provide enjoyment and participates in one activity daily.

■ Patient reports decreased feelings of isolation and increased social interaction.

■ Patient reports regaining physical and psychological health. Assessment data and perceptions of physicians and other caregivers confirm patient's reports.

Documentation

■ Observations of patient's social interaction skills
■ Causes of social isolation identified by patient
■ Resources identified to help patient increase social interaction
■ Interventions to encourage social interaction and patient's response
■ Evaluations for expected outcomes

Reference

Arthur, H.M. "Depression, Isolation, Social Support, and Cardiovascular Disease in Older Adults," *The Journal of Cardiovascular Nursing* 21(5 Suppl 1):S2-S7, September-October 2006.

SPIRITUAL DISTRESS
related to situational crisis

Definition
Impaired ability to experience and integrate meaning and purpose in life through a person's connectedness with self, others, art, music, literature, nature, or a power greater than oneself

Assessment
■ General spiritual beliefs
■ Personal spiritual beliefs
■ Spiritual support systems
■ Religious affiliation
■ Impact of illness on spiritual beliefs

Defining characteristics
■ Anger toward God
■ Change in behavior and mood (anger, crying, withdrawal, anxiety)
■ Desire for spiritual assistance
■ Displaced anger toward religious representatives
■ Display of gallows humor
■ Expressed concern about meaning of life and death, belief systems, and relationship with deity
■ Expressed inner conflicts about beliefs
■ Questioning of meaning of own existence

- Questioning of meaning of suffering
- Questioning of moral and ethical implications of therapeutic regimen

Expected outcomes

- Patient will express feelings about his usual and current spiritual beliefs.
- Patient will identify areas of ambivalence and conflict resulting from current situation.
- Patient will state an understanding of grief process and its stages.
- Patient will use effective coping strategies to ease spiritual discomfort.
- Patient will seek appropriate support persons (family members, priest, minister, imam, or rabbi) for assistance.

Suggested NOC outcomes

Dignified Life Closure; Hope; Quality of Life; Spiritual Health

Interventions and rationales

- Approach patient in an accepting, nonjudgmental manner *to demonstrate unconditional positive regard for patient.*
- Acknowledge patient's spiritual concerns and encourage expression of feelings *to help build a therapeutic relationship.*
- Encourage patient to provide information about his spiritual or religious beliefs and practices. *Acquiring this initial database is the first step in the nursing process.*
- Instruct patient on stages of grieving and on emotions and behaviors common to each stage *to promote understanding and encourage feelings of normalcy.*
- Provide for the continuation of patient's spiritual or religious practices (allow for specific religious materials or clothing; respect dietary restrictions, if possible). *These measures demonstrate support and convey caring and acceptance to patient.*
- Facilitate visits from clergy and provide privacy during visits *to demonstrate respect for patient's relationship with clergy.*
- Encourage patient to discuss concerns with clergy, *thereby using expert spiritual care resources to help patient.*

Suggested NIC interventions

Active Listening; Anxiety Reduction; Coping Enhancement; Hope Instillation; Spiritual Growth Facilitation; Spiritual Support

Evaluations for expected outcomes

- Patient discusses feelings about his spiritual or religious beliefs.
- Patient specifies areas of spiritual conflict, such as anger toward God, questioning of his usual beliefs about an afterlife, and guilt related to loss of faith.
- Patient communicates understanding of grief process and its stages.
- Patient continues religious practices that ease spiritual distress.
- Patient makes use of available resources for spiritual assistance.

Documentation

- Patient's verbal and nonverbal communication of spiritual discomfort

- Stage of anticipatory grief, as indicated by behavior
- Interventions to promote spiritual comfort
- Patient's response to interventions
- Evaluations for expected outcomes

Reference
McClung, E. "Collaborating with Chaplains to Meet Spiritual Needs," *Medsurg Nursing* 15(3):147-56, June 2006.

SPIRITUAL DISTRESS
related to sociocultural deprivation

Definition
Impaired ability to experience and integrate meaning and purpose in life through a person's connectedness with self, others, art, music, literature, nature, or a power greater than oneself.

Assessment
- General spiritual beliefs
- Personal spiritual beliefs
- Spiritual support systems
- Religious affiliation
- Impact of illness on spiritual beliefs

Defining characteristics
- Change in behavior and mood (anger, crying, withdrawal, anxiety)
- Desire for spiritual assistance
- Displaced anger toward religious representatives
- Expressed concern about meaning of life and death, belief systems, and relationship with deity
- Expressed inner conflicts about beliefs
- Guilt
- Inability to participate in usual religious practices
- Inability to express previous state of creativity
- No interest in nature
- No interest in reading spiritual literature
- Poor coping
- Questioning of meaning of own existence
- Questioning of meaning of suffering
- Questioning of moral and ethical implications of therapeutic regimen

Expected outcomes
- Patient will communicate conflict about beliefs.
- Patient will identify source of spiritual conflict.
- Patient will specify whatever spiritual assistance he needs.

- Patient will discuss beliefs about religious practices.
- Patient will identify coping techniques to deal with spiritual discomfort.
- Patient will express feelings of spiritual comfort.

Suggested NOC outcomes

Hope; Personal Autonomy; Quality of Life; Spiritual Health; Will to Live

Interventions and rationales

- Listen for cues about patient's feelings. ("Why did God do this to me?" or "God is punishing me.") *Active listening demonstrates involvement with patient and allows you to hear important messages indicating spiritual distress.*
- Approach patient in a nonjudgmental way *to focus on patient's feelings without evaluating them as right or wrong, good or bad.*
- Acknowledge patient's spiritual concerns, and encourage expression of thoughts and feelings *to help build therapeutic relationship.*
- Help patient concretely define the problem causing inner conflict. *This is the first step in developing strategies for resolving conflicts.*
- For the patient whose spiritual comfort is derived from music, art, or nature, attempt to find such items (for example, CD's, posters, or picture books) that will provide spiritual nourishment. *Not everyone finds spiritual comfort in organized religion. Indeed, each person is entitled to find spiritual hope and consolation in whatever way meets their needs.*
- Arrange for visits by clergy, as appropriate, *thereby using spiritual care resources to help patient.*
- Encourage patient to continue religious practices during hospitalization; do whatever you must to facilitate this. For example:
– If patient is accustomed to reading Scripture and doesn't have a Bible, try to obtain one.
– If a Jewish male wears a yarmulke, allow him to continue wearing it, if possible.
– In cases in which patient's religious traditions prohibit or require certain foods, make every effort to communicate these needs to the dietary department and see that they're honored.
These measures demonstrate support and convey caring and acceptance to patient.
- Communicate and collaborate with patient's clergy person or with the hospital chaplain, as appropriate. *This ensures consistent care and provides a more complete database.*
- Arrange for patient to have bedside objects that provide spiritual comfort (such as a Bible, prayer shawl, pictures, statues, and rosary beads). *Items of spiritual significance may influence patient's ability to reduce conflict.*
- Provide privacy during patient's visits with a clergy person or chaplain *to demonstrate respect for patient's relationship with clergy.*

Suggested NIC interventions

Active Listening; Hope Instillation; Referral; Spiritual Growth Facilitation; Spiritual Support

Evaluations for expected outcomes

■ Patient expresses feelings of uncertainty or ambivalence related to spiritual beliefs.
■ Patient states specific causes of spiritual distress.
■ Patient requests spiritual assistance, if needed.
■ Patient discusses usual religious practices, including rituals, prayers, values, and beliefs.
■ Patient reports decreased spiritual discomfort.
■ Patient expresses desire to resume usual religious practices.

Documentation

■ Patient's expressions of concern about spiritual matters, whether direct or indirect
■ Observations about patient's spiritual distress or well-being
■ Interventions carried out to promote spiritual comfort
■ Observations about patient's responses to interventions
■ Evaluations for expected outcomes

Reference

Mohr, W.K. "Spiritual Issues in Psychiatric Care," *Perspectives in Psychiatric Care* 42(3):174-83, August 2006.

Risk for
SPIRITUAL DISTRESS

Definition

At risk for an impaired ability to experience and integrate meaning and purpose in life through a person's connectedness with self, others, art, music, literature, nature, or a power greater than oneself

Assessment

■ Health history, including debilitating disease (for example, rheumatoid arthritis); terminal illness; recurrent cancer; conditions that alter body image (for example, burns and scars); relapse or exacerbation of neurologic disease (for example, multiple sclerosis); alcoholism, depression, and drug abuse; and major traumatic injury
■ Impact of current illness, injury, or disability on lifestyle
■ Spiritual status, religious affiliation, beliefs, and practices; relationship with spiritual authority (such as priest, rabbi); beliefs about life, death, and suffering
■ Psychological status, including perception of self, body image, problem-solving ability, and coping mechanisms; sources of support (family, partner, friends, caregivers); perception of medical diagnosis or health problem (progression, severity, prognosis, treatment options); reaction to illness, injury, or disability; self-image, mood, behavior, motivation, and energy level; stressors (finances, job, marital or

partner discord, losses through death or separation); expressions of grief; and changes in sleep pattern
■ Family status, including socioeconomic status; quality of relationships; communication patterns; methods of conflict resolution; ability of family members to meet patient's physical, emotional, and social needs; and family goals

Risk factors
Physical
■ Physical illness, including chronic illness
■ Substance abuse, excessive drinking

Psychosocial
■ Low self-esteem
■ Depression, anxiety, stress
■ Poor relationships
■ Separation from support systems
■ Blocks to experiencing love
■ Inability to forgive
■ Loss
■ Racial or cultural conflict
■ Change in religious rituals, practices

Developmental
■ Life change
■ Developmental life changes

Environmental
■ Environmental changes
■ Natural disasters

Expected outcomes
■ Patient will discuss his current spiritual beliefs and concerns.
■ Patient will discuss effects of illness, injury, or disability on his beliefs and spiritual practices.
■ Patient will use healthy coping techniques to maintain his spiritual well-being.
■ Patient will express feelings of spiritual well-being.
■ Patient will be supported in efforts to pursue spirituality in coping with illness, injury, or disability.
■ Patient will reach out to family members, partner, priest, minister, imam, rabbi, or others for assistance.

Suggested NOC outcomes
Coping; Grief Resolution; Hope; Spiritual Health

Interventions and rationales

■ Assess the importance of spirituality in patient's life and in coping with illness. Note patient's participation in religious rituals and practices and his desire to discuss spiritual beliefs. Assess the impact of the illness, injury, or disability on patient's spiritual outlook. *Accurate assessment of the meaning of spirituality for patient is necessary before intervening.*

■ Assess patient's desire for help in coping with spiritual concerns *to determine the extent to which patient is motivated to address spiritual concerns and open to help from others.*

■ Express your willingness to discuss spirituality if patient desires *to reduce isolation and to bring spiritual issues into the open.*

■ Encourage patient to talk about spiritual or religious beliefs and practices. Listen actively to patient's discussion of spiritual concerns *to foster open discussion.*

■ Encourage patient to express feelings related to his recent life-threatening experience *to help him clarify and cope with his feelings.*

■ Communicate to patient that you accept his expression of spiritual concerns, even if his feelings are angry and negative *to reassure him that his feelings are valid.*

■ Show willingness to pray with patient, if he wishes, *to provide spiritual support.*

■ Maintain a nonjudgmental manner. Keep conversation focused on patient's spiritual values *to maintain the therapeutic value of your interaction with patient.*

■ Provide for continuation of patient's religious practices (for example, help patient obtain ritual items and respect dietary restrictions, if possible) *to demonstrate support and convey caring and acceptance to patient.*

■ Arrange for visits by clergy, as appropriate, *to provide patient with expert spiritual support.* Provide privacy during visits.

■ Collaborate with patient's clergyman or hospital chaplain to develop a plan to integrate spiritual interventions into patient's care *to ensure continuity of care.*

Suggested NIC interventions

Active Listening; Anticipatory Guidance; Anxiety Reduction; Caregiver Support; Emotional Support; Hope Instillation; Spiritual Growth Facilitation; Spiritual Support

Evaluations for expected outcomes

■ Patient discusses current spiritual or religious beliefs.
■ Patient discusses effects of illness, injury, or disability on beliefs and spiritual practices.
■ Patient uses healthy coping techniques to maintain spiritual well-being.
■ Patient expresses feelings of spiritual well-being.
■ Patient is supported in efforts to pursue spirituality in coping with illness, injury, or disability.
■ Patient reaches out to family members, partner, priest, minister, rabbi, imam, or others for assistance.

Documentation

■ Patient's statements regarding religious beliefs and practices
■ Patient's statements indicating effect of current crisis on spiritual outlook

■ Patient's statements indicating which rituals and practices help maintain spiritual well-being

■ Patient's statements indicating effectiveness of interventions to promote spiritual well-being

■ Visits with selected spiritual authority

■ Additional referrals to clergy or chaplain

■ Evaluations for expected outcomes

References

Bauer-Wu, S., and Farran, C.J. "Meaning in Life and Psycho-spiritual Functioning: A Comparison of Breast Cancer Survivors and Healthy Women," *Journal of Holistic Nursing* 23(2):172-90, June 2005.

Villagomeza, L.R. "Spiritual Distress in Adult Cancer Patients: Toward Conceptual Clarity," *Holistic Nursing Practice* 19(6):285-94, November-December 2005.

STRESS OVERLOAD

Definition

Excessive amounts and types of demands that require action; human response that's experienced as a problem and contributes to the development of other problems

Assessment

■ History or current presence of stress reactions in response to internal or external forces expressed by such physical findings as choking sensation, hyperventilation, dizziness, increased heart rate and/or blood pressure, perspiration, pupillary dilation, polyuria, and elevated blood glucose, cholesterol, and free fatty acid levels

■ History or current presence of stress reactions in response to internal or external forces expressed by such behavioral cues as insomnia, restlessness, "scattered" thoughts, disorganized speech, restlessness, irritability, and altered concentration

■ Physical stressors, including extreme heat or cold, malnutrition, disease, infection, and pain

■ Psychological stressors, including fear, sense of failure, move in company or home location, success, holiday, vacation, or promotion

■ Level of stress, positive coping mechanisms, realistic thought patterns, behaviors, or energy level

■ Medication history, including use of drugs, caffeine, tobacco, or alcohol that stimulate the sympathetic nervous system

■ Sleep patterns or changes in daily activities that could be perceived as stressful including too many or too few activities

■ Sociologic factors, including job satisfaction, presence of support systems, family coping mechanisms, or hobbies

Defining characteristics

■ Demonstrates excessive fear, worry, and hypervigilance

■ Demonstrates signs and symptoms of sympathetic stimulation, including increased heart rate or blood pressure, dilated pupils, increased respirations, and increased blood sugar

■ Exhibits dry mouth, tense muscles, or headaches

■ Expresses difficulty in functioning

■ Expresses feelings of pressure or tension

■ Expresses feelings of anger

■ Expresses feelings of guilt and failure or exhibits procrastination

■ Expresses feelings of impatience

■ Expresses problems with decision-making

■ Increase in tense expression, restlessness, or tearful outbursts

■ Increased number of deadlines and difficulty saying "No" to requests for added job or relationship responsibilities

■ Insomnia or tiredness/weariness

■ Lack of organized exercise plan or recreation efforts

■ Multiple lifestyle changes, including moves, job change, relationship changes, and losses

■ Overuse of alcohol, nicotine, caffeine, and carbohydrates

■ Reports decreased concentration and disorganized thought patterns

■ Reports negative physical and psychological impact from stress such as "feeling of being sick or going to get sick"

■ Reports situational stress as a 7 or above on a 10-point scale

Expected outcomes

■ Patient will experience reduced signs of stress overload as evidenced by subjective report and observations of reduced stress, such as less facial tension and less restlessness.

■ Patient will connect environmental stressors with manifestations of stress such as insomnia, tearful outbursts, irritability, or headache.

■ Patients will set limits on activities assumed by saying no without expressions of guilt.

■ Patient will develop more effective coping strategies to manage stress, such as guided imagery, exercise, healthy diet, and recreation and leisure activities.

■ Patient will develop strategies to reframe distorted thinking patterns relating to internal and environmental demands, such as talking about feelings and asking for help.

Suggested NOC outcomes

Abusive Behavior; Aggression Self-Control; Anxiety Self-Control; Coping; Self-Restraint; Stress Level

Interventions and rationales

■ Establish and promote a trusting relationship before asking patient to make any changes. *A trusting relationship can facilitate patient's attempts to make changes; whereas too many demands early in relationship can foster resistance.*

■ Teach prioritization of responsibilities and deadlines to facilitate patient's sense of control over stressors. *Stressors may seem overwhelming, and nurse can promote increased self-esteem when a plan is made cooperatively with nurse and patient as partners.*

■ Teach patient about positive self-talk. *Positive self-talk helps change and, ultimately, reverse negative emotions of guilt, fear, and worry.*

■ Teach coping strategies, such as reframing thoughts or using music, guided imagery, yoga, deep-breathing exercises, progressive neuromuscular relaxation, or pet therapy. *Strategies that reduce tense muscles and feelings can promote deeper relaxation and reduce heart rate, respirations, and blood pressure by promoting the parasympathetic response.*

■ Teach assertiveness training techniques with role-play exercises. *Assertiveness training can provide a concrete way to manage stressors and enhance feeling of being empowered, such as in communicating with demanding individuals.*

■ Explore support systems with patient, such as appropriate Internet chat rooms, support groups, or hobbies and outings with partner or family and friends. *Often patient is caretaker who perceives there is little time for self and is at risk for caregiver burden. Promoting verbalization of feelings with support persons can reduce feeling of stress overload.*

■ Explore role of food, lack of exercise, and excessive intake of caffeine, alcohol, nicotine, and carbohydrates during periods of stress overload and adoption of healthier alternatives. *Inappropriate food choices, inactivity, and substance abuse can occur when patient feels stress overload.*

■ Provide opportunities for patient to ventilate feelings about stressors. *Promoting a time to talk can help the patient share his feelings of mounting stress before irritability and tension worsen.*

Suggested NIC interventions

Anger Control Assistance; Assertiveness Training; Behavior Management; Behavior Modification; Calming Techniques; Cognitive Restructuring; Coping Enhancement; Impulse Control Training; Stress Management Assistance

Evaluations for expected outcomes

■ Patient experiences reduced signs of stress overload as evidenced by subjective report and observations of reduced stress, such as less facial tension and less restlessness.

■ Patient connects environmental stressors with manifestations of stress, such as insomnia, tearful outbursts, irritability, or headache.

■ Patient sets limits on activities assumed by saying no without expressions of guilt.

■ Patient addresses usual coping mechanisms for dealing with stress overload, such as increased use of alcohol, caffeine, tobacco, or carbohydrates, and adopts more effective coping strategies, such as guided imagery, exercise, healthy diet, and recreation and leisure activities.

■ Patient develops strategies to reframe distorted thinking patterns relating to internal and environmental demands, such as talking about feelings and asking for help.

Documentation
- Observations of subjective and objective data
- Documentation of interventions such as yoga, guided imagery, deep-breathing exercises, talking about feelings
- Patient's response to interventions
- Evaluations for expected outcomes

Reference
Learn Well Resources. "Managing Stress: Living without Stress Overload," Course Number LWH102, January 2006.

Risk for
SUFFOCATION
related to external factors

Definition
Accentuated risk of accidental suffocation (inadequate air available for inhalation)

Assessment
- Health history, including accidents, allergies, exposure to pollutants, falls, hyperthermia, hypothermia, poisoning, seizures, sensory or perceptual changes (auditory, gustatory, kinesthetic, olfactory, tactile, or visual), and trauma
- Circumstances of current situation that might lead to injury
- Neurologic status, including level of consciousness, mental status, and orientation
- Laboratory studies, including clotting factors, hemoglobin level, hematocrit, platelet count, and white blood cell count

Risk factors
- Access to unattended bathtub or pool (children)
- Consumption of large mouthfuls of food
- Discarded refrigerators or freezers with doors still in place
- Fuel-burning heater used in area without ventilation
- Habit of smoking in bed
- Household gas leaks
- Low-strung clotheslines
- Pacifier hung around neck (infant)
- Plastic bags or small objects within reach of children
- Propped bottle or pillow in infant's crib
- Vehicle left running in closed garage

Expected outcomes
- Patient's airway will remain patent at all times.
- Patient's vital signs will remain within normal parameters.

■ Patient and family members will demonstrate knowledge of safety measures to prevent suffocation.

Suggested NOC outcomes

Aspiration Prevention; Personal Safety Behavior; Respiratory Status: Ventilation; Risk Control; Risk Detection

Interventions and rationales

■ Monitor and record patient's respiratory status. *Changes in parameters (such as respiratory rate, cough, sputum production, and skin color) may indicate airway obstruction.*

■ Monitor and record patient's neurologic status. *Headache, depression, apathy, memory loss, poor muscle coordination, fatigue, stupor, and loss of consciousness may indicate hypoxia.*

■ Monitor patient's vital signs and report changes. *Tachycardia and a slight rise in blood pressure may indicate hypoxia. Reduced heart rate and loss of consciousness indicate advanced hypoxia.*

■ Position patient on his side or position his head and neck to prevent relaxed neck muscles from obstructing airway *to allow maximal chest expansion and prevent aspiration and airway obstruction.*

■ Check all ventilator connections every 30 minutes if patient is on mechanical ventilation *to ensure patient receives proper amount of oxygen at appropriate volume and rate.*

■ Check ventilator alarms every 30 minutes and after suctioning *to ensure proper alarm function.*

■ Suction airway, as needed, *to prevent secretion accumulation.* Do this only as needed *to prevent tracheal irritation.*

■ Provide patient and family members with information about safety practices *to enable patient and family members to take an active role in patient's care and ensure performance of safety measures.*

Suggested NIC interventions

Airway Management; Aspiration Precautions; Energy Management; Respiratory Monitoring; Security Enhancement; Surveillance; Vital Signs Monitoring

Evaluations for expected outcomes

■ Patient's airway remains free from obstruction.
■ Patient's vital signs remain within normal parameters.
■ Patient and family members demonstrate safety measures to prevent suffocation.

Documentation

■ Patient's statements that indicate potential for injury
■ Physical findings
■ Observations or knowledge of unsafe practices
■ Interventions performed to prevent injury

- Patient's response to nursing interventions
- Evaluations for expected outcomes

Reference
Rosenthal, L.D. "Carbon Monoxide Poisoning. Immediate Diagnosis and Treatment are Crucial to Avoid Complications," *AJN* 106(3):40-46, March 2006.

Risk for
SUFFOCATION
related to internal factors

Definition
Accentuated risk of accidental suffocation (inadequate air available for inhalation)

Assessment
- Health history, including accidents, allergies, exposure to pollutants, falls, hyperthermia, hypothermia, poisoning, seizures, sensory or perceptual changes (auditory, gustatory, kinesthetic, olfactory, tactile, or visual), and trauma
- Circumstances of current situation that might lead to injury
- Neurologic status, including level of consciousness, mental status, and orientation
- Laboratory studies, including clotting factors, hemoglobin level, hematocrit, platelet count, and white blood cell count

Risk factors
- Cognitive or emotional difficulties
- Injury or disease process
- Lack of safety education
- Lack of safety precautions
- Reduced motor abilities
- Reduced olfactory sensation

Expected outcomes
- Patient will avoid accidental suffocation.
- Patient's vital signs will remain within normal parameters.
- Patient and family members will demonstrate knowledge of safety measures to prevent suffocation.

Suggested NOC outcomes
Aspiration Prevention; Neurological Status: Consciousness; Personal Safety Behavior; Respiratory Status: Ventilation; Risk Control; Risk Detection

Interventions and rationales
- Observe, record, and report falls, seizures, and unsafe practices *to ensure implementation of appropriate interventions.*

■ Monitor and record patient's respiratory status. *Changes in parameters (such as respiratory rate, cough, sputum production, and skin color) may indicate airway obstruction.*

■ Monitor and record patient's neurologic status. *Headache, depression, apathy, memory loss, poor muscle coordination, fatigue, stupor, and loss of consciousness may indicate hypoxia.*

■ Monitor patient's vital signs and report changes. *Tachycardia and a slight rise in blood pressure may indicate hypoxia. Reduced heart rate and loss of consciousness indicate advanced hypoxia.*

■ Position patient on his side or position his head and neck to prevent relaxed neck muscles from obstructing airway *to allow maximal chest expansion and prevent aspiration and airway obstruction.*

■ Obtain suction equipment, assemble, and keep at bedside *to assure equipment readiness in case of need.*

■ Suction, as needed, *to keep upper and lower airways clear and to stimulate cough reflex to enhance sputum removal.* Do this only as needed *to prevent tracheal irritation.*

■ Provide patient and family members with information about safety practices *to enable patient and family members to take an active role in patient's care and ensure performance of safety measures.*

Suggested NIC interventions

Airway Management; Aspiration Precautions; Surveillance: Safety; Vital Signs Monitoring

Evaluations for expected outcomes
■ Patient doesn't experience accidental suffocation.
■ Patient's vital signs remain within normal parameters.
■ Patient or caregiver demonstrates safety measures that prevent suffocation.

Documentation
■ Patient's statements about situation that indicate potential for injury
■ Physical findings
■ Record of falls, seizures, and unsafe practices
■ Interventions that reduce risk of injury
■ Patient's response to nursing interventions
■ Evaluations for expected outcomes

Reference
Westergren, A. "Detection of Eating Difficulties after Stroke: A Systematic Review," *International Nursing Review* 53(2):143-49, June 2006.

Delayed
SURGICAL RECOVERY

Definition
Extension of the number of postoperative days required to initiate and perform activities that maintain life, health, and well-being

Assessment
- Age
- Gender
- Reason for surgery
- Type and length of surgical procedure
- Current health status, including weight, vital signs, temperature, nutritional status, integumentary status, neurologic status, cardiovascular status, musculoskeletal status, and pain status
- Laboratory studies, including complete blood count, electrolyte studies, urinalysis, blood cultures, blood coagulation studies, immunologic and serologic tests, liver function tests, cardiac enzyme studies, and arterial blood gas levels
- Health history, including past surgical procedures, food or drug allergies, substance abuse, mental illness, and chronic metabolic or systemic disease (diabetes mellitus; cardiovascular, hepatic, renal, or immunologic disease; coagulation disorders; and splenic or bone marrow disorders)
- Mobility status
- Complications during surgical procedure, such as hemorrhage, drop in blood pressure, and cardiac arrhythmias
- Current medical treatments, including radiation therapy, chemotherapy, antibiotic or antifungal therapy, steroid treatment, anticoagulant or thrombolytic therapy, and immunosuppressive therapy
- Social support, including family status and presence of caregiver and health care provider

Defining characteristics
- Difficulty in moving about
- Evidence of interrupted healing of surgical area
- Fatigue
- Loss of appetite with or without nausea
- Perception that more time is needed to recover
- Postpones resumption of work or employment activities
- Report of pain
- Requires help to complete self-care

Expected outcomes
- Patient's vital signs and laboratory values will return to normal limits.
- Patient's wound will begin to heal; incision site will appear free from signs and symptoms of infection.

- Patient will exhibit improved nutritional status.
- Patient's postoperative complications will be resolved.
- Patient will resume normal mobility status.
- Patient will seek and obtain emotional support from family and friends.
- Patient will resume normal eating, bowel, and bladder habits.
- Patient and family members will use community resources that are available to assist after discharge.

Suggested NOC outcomes

Ambulation; Endurance; Health Beliefs; Immobility Consequences: Physiological; Nutritional Status; Pain Level; Wound Healing: Primary Intention

Interventions and rationales

- Assess for factors that may be related to a delay in recovery, such as respiratory complications and infection. Document and report assessment findings *to facilitate the development of an individualized care plan.*
- Monitor wound healing. Assess the surgical site for signs of infection, such as erythema, edema, pain, drainage, odor, incision approximation, and intact sutures. *Infection may delay surgical recovery.*
- Monitor nutritional status by evaluating intake, output, and integumentary status. Consult a dietitian regarding changes to diet *to promote optimal nutritional status. Optimal nutritional status promotes wound healing and provides energy for recovery.*
- Assess all body systems *to detect signs and symptoms of postoperative complications that can delay surgical recovery.*
- Follow the proper pulmonary regimen *to facilitate resolution of respiratory complications, if present. Respiratory complications can lead to decreased oxygen levels, which can slow wound healing and delay mobility.*
- Following postoperative bleeding, monitor hemoglobin level and hematocrit. *Bleeding can lead to a low hemoglobin level and hematocrit, reducing the ability of red blood cells to carry oxygen, which can hinder wound healing and diminish patient's energy level.*
- If patient is suffering from psychosis, continue to reorient him during the postoperative recovery period. Report any psychological reaction, such as development of depression-like symptoms. *Psychosis or depression may delay recovery.*
- Administer pain medication, as prescribed. *A patient in pain won't move, cough, and deep-breathe as needed for timely recovery from surgery.*
- As appropriate, make sure someone is available to walk with patient or that such devices as walkers or canes are available. Don't allow patient to ambulate alone until steady. *Assistance (from staff or with devices) enhances safety and encourages patient to improve mobility without fear of falling. Mobility will facilitate improved strength, help prevent such complications as deep vein thrombosis and, ultimately, enhance recovery.*
- Make sure patient wears support stockings or a sequential compression device *to facilitate venous return and prevent deep vein thrombosis.*
- Monitor bowel and bladder activity. Report urine retention and absent or decreased bowel sounds. *Abnormal bowel and bladder patterns slow surgical recovery. Continual assessment ensures prompt treatment and enhances recovery.*

■ Initiate a multidisciplinary care conference for patient with care providers from all disciplines as well as the patient and family. Facilitating this type of communication will help *to develop a plan that will put the patient on a faster track to recovery.*

■ Make sure patient and family members have access to community resources to assist with recovery when patient returns home *to ensure ongoing recovery.*

■ Educate patient and family members regarding appropriate care after discharge *to help them carry out medication and treatment regimens.*

Suggested NIC interventions

Bed Rest Care; Case Management; Discharge Planning; Energy Management; Exercise Therapy: Ambulation; Incision Site Care; Multidisciplinary Care Conference; Nutrition Management; Pain Management; Sleep Enhancement

Evaluations for expected outcomes

■ Patient's vital signs and laboratory values return to normal limits.

■ Patient's wound begins to heal; incision site appears free from signs and symptoms of infection.

■ Patient exhibits improved nutritional status.

■ Patient's postoperative complications are resolved.

■ Patient resumes normal mobility status.

■ Patient seeks and obtains emotional support from family and friends.

■ Patient resumes normal eating, bowel, and bladder habits.

■ Patient and family members use community resources that are available to assist after discharge.

Documentation

■ Assessment findings

■ Type and length of operation

■ Type of anesthesia

■ Intraoperative complications

■ Postoperative complications (as they occur)

■ Results of ongoing multisystem assessment

■ Treatment regimen (for normal recovery and complications)

■ Patient's and family members' progress in following treatment regimen

■ Teaching provided to patient and family members

■ Discharge plans

■ Evaluations for expected outcomes

Reference

Bedard, D., et al. "The Pain Experience of Post-surgical Patients Following Implementation of an Evidence-based Approach," *Pain Management Nursing* 7(3):80-92, September 2006.

Impaired
SWALLOWING

related to neuromuscular impairment

Definition
Abnormal functioning of the swallowing mechanism associated with deficits in oral, pharyngeal, or esophageal structure or function

Assessment
- History of neuromuscular, cerebral, or respiratory disease
- Age
- Gender
- Nutritional status, including appetite, dietary intake, hydration, current weight, and change from normal weight
- Neurologic status, including barium swallow; chest X-ray; cognition; esophageal video fluoroscopy; gag reflex; level of consciousness; memory; motor ability; orientation; symmetry of face, mouth, and neck; sensory function; and tongue movement

Defining characteristics
- Evidence of aspiration, nasal reflux, heartburn, or epigastric pain
- Observed evidence of difficulty in swallowing, including choking, coughing, vomiting, decreased gag reflex, and stasis of food in oral cavity
- Stroke

Expected outcomes
- Patient won't show evidence of aspiration pneumonia.
- Patient will achieve adequate nutritional intake.
- Patient will maintain weight.
- Patient will maintain oral hygiene.
- Patient and caregiver will demonstrate correct feeding techniques to maximize swallowing.
- Patient and caregiver will list strategies to prevent aspiration.

Suggested NOC outcomes
Appetite; Aspiration Prevention; Cognition; Nutritional Status: Food & Fluid Intake; Swallowing Status; Swallowing Status: Esophageal Phase; Swallowing Status: Oral Phase; Swallowing Status: Pharyngeal Phase

Interventions and rationales
- Elevate the head of the bed 90 degrees during mealtimes and for 30 minutes after the completion of a meal *to decrease the risk of aspiration.*
- Position patient on his side when recumbent *to decrease the risk of aspiration.*
- Keep suction apparatus at the bedside; observe and report instances of cyanosis, dyspnea, or choking. *Symptoms indicate the presence of material in the lungs.*

■ Monitor intake and output and weight daily until stabilized. Establish an intake goal — for example, "Patient consumes ____ ml of fluid and ____% of solid food." Record and report any deviation from this. *Evaluating calorie and protein intake daily allows any necessary modifications to begin quickly.*

■ Consult with a dietitian to modify patient's diet, and conduct a calorie count, as needed, *to establish nutritional requirements.*

■ Consult with a dysphagia rehabilitation team, if available, *to obtain expert advice.*

■ Provide mouth care three times daily *to promote comfort and enhance appetite.*

■ Keep the oral mucous membrane moist by frequent rinses; use a bulb syringe or suction, if necessary, *to promote comfort.*

■ Lubricate patient's lips *to prevent cracking and blisters.*

■ Encourage patient to wear properly fitted dentures *to enhance chewing ability.*

■ Serve food in attractive surroundings; encourage patient to smell and look at food. Remove soiled equipment, control smells, and provide a quiet atmosphere for eating. *A pleasant atmosphere stimulates appetite; food aroma stimulates salivation.*

■ Teach patient and his family about positioning, dietary requirements, and specific feeding techniques, including facial exercises (such as whistling), using a short straw to provide sensory stimulation to his lips, tipping his head forward to decrease aspiration, applying pressure above the lip to stimulate mouth closure and the swallowing reflex, and checking the oral cavity frequently for food particles (remove if present). *These measures allow patient to take an active role in maintaining health.*

Suggested NIC interventions

Airway Suctioning; Aspiration Precautions; Feeding; Positioning; Referral; Risk Identification; Swallowing Therapy

Evaluations for expected outcomes

■ Patient shows no evidence of aspiration pneumonia. Breath sounds remain bilaterally clear; fever, chills, purulent sputum, and rapid shallow respirations are absent.

■ Patient's fluid and dietary intake remains within established daily limits.

■ Patient's weight remains stable.

■ Patient demonstrates appropriate oral hygiene practices.

■ Patient and caregiver demonstrate feeding techniques to maximize swallowing and minimize risk of complications.

■ Patient and caregiver list strategies to prevent aspiration.

Documentation

■ Patient's expressions of feelings about current situation

■ Observations of weight, swallowing ability, intake and output, and oral hygiene

■ Patient's response to nursing interventions

■ Instructions about diet monitoring and feeding techniques

■ Evaluations for expected outcomes

Reference
Lorefalt, B., et al. "Avoidance of Solid Food in Weight Losing Older Patients with Parkinson's Disease," *Journal of Clinical Nursing* 15(11):1404-12, November 2006.

Effective
THERAPEUTIC REGIMEN MANAGEMENT

Definition
An effective pattern of regulating and integrating into daily life a program for treating illness and its sequelae that's satisfactory for meeting specific health goals

Assessment
- Family status, including marital status and family composition
- Psychological status, including changes in appetite, behavior, energy level, mood, motivation, self-image, and sleep; alcohol and drug use; life changes; psychiatric history; and blood and urine toxicology
- Self-care status, including ability to carry out voluntary activities, use of adaptive devices, and neurologic, sensory, and psychological impairment
- Social status, including communication skills, size of social network, quality of relationships, degree of trust in others, and ability to function in social and occupational roles
- Spiritual status, including religious or church affiliation, religious practices, and support network (family, clergy, and friends)

Defining characteristics
- Verbalizes appropriate choices for meeting the goals of a treatment or prevention program
- Manages illness symptoms within a normal range of expectation
- Verbalizes desire to manage the treatment of illness and prevention of sequelae
- Verbalizes intent to reduce risk factors for progression of illness and sequelae

Expected outcomes
- Patient will recognize potential problems and identify needs.
- Patient will work toward establishing specific objectives to meet needs.
- Patient will make plans to ensure meeting future needs.

Suggested NOC outcomes
Adherence Behavior; Compliance Behavior; Family Participation in Professional Care; Knowledge: Treatment Regimen; Participation in Health Care Decisions; Risk Control; Symptom Control

Interventions and rationales
- Help patient identify needs, potential problems, and sources of stress *to maintain highest level of well-being.*

■ Help patient identify resources necessary to meet needs and develop strategies for using these resources *to solve problems.*

■ Assist patient in identifying major stressors in his life and what needs demand immediate attention. Help to establish priorities for addressing problems *to focus energy on important issues.*

■ Encourage patient to contact appropriate agencies *so that they can give preventive care, reduce stress, and enhance patient's well-being.*

■ Continue to monitor patient's progress in identifying needs, problems, and stressors *to reinforce patient's efforts to obtain maximum well-being.*

■ Support patient's plans for meeting future needs *to foster independence.*

Suggested NIC interventions

Anticipatory Guidance; Behavior Modification; Health Education; Mutual Goal Setting; Patient Contracting; Self-Responsibility Facilitation

Evaluations for expected outcomes

■ Patient describes potential problems and establishes plan to meet therapeutic needs.

■ Patient includes specific objectives in plan to meet needs.

■ Patient makes changes to plan that allow him to meet needs and solve problems after discharge.

Documentation

■ Patient's description of problems and needs

■ Patient's plan to resolve current issues, including resources required, priorities, and strategies

■ Patient's progress toward meeting goals

■ Evaluations for expected outcomes

Reference

Arvidsson, S.B., et al. "A Nurse-Led Rheumatology Clinic's Impact on Empowering Patients with Rheumatoid Arthritis: A Qualitative Study," *Nursing & Health Sciences* 8(3):133-39, September 2006.

Ineffective
THERAPEUTIC REGIMEN MANAGEMENT
related to health beliefs

Definition

Pattern of regulating or integrating into daily living a program of treatment for illness and the sequelae of illness that's unsatisfactory for meeting specific health needs

Assessment

■ Medical history

■ Physical examination

■ Prescriptions for treatment, including medications, activity, diet, and other treatments

■ Current medication schedule, including medications used at home (prescribed and over-the-counter)

■ Activities of daily living and exercise pattern

■ Nutrition pattern, including 3-day diet history or 1-day diet recall

■ Weight

■ Patient's and family members' health-related goals

■ Self-care abilities and resources, including presence of family members or others

■ Health beliefs, including perception of susceptibility to illness, seriousness of illness, effectiveness of treatment, and barriers to managing regimen

■ Other influences on health-related behavior, including age, sex, knowledge, and social pressures

Defining characteristics

■ Verbalizes choices of daily living that are ineffective for meeting the goals of a treatment program

■ Verbalizes, but doesn't take action to reduce risk factors for progression of illness and sequelae

■ Verbalizes desire to manage the treatment of illness and prevention of sequelae

■ Verbalizes difficulty with regulation and integration of one or more prescribed regimens for prevention of complications and the treatment of illness or its effects

■ Verbalizes, but doesn't take action to include treatment regimens in daily routines

Expected outcomes

■ Patient will express personal beliefs about illness and its management.

■ Patient and family members will develop plan for integrating components of therapeutic regimen, such as medications, activity, and diet, into pattern of daily living.

■ Patient will select daily activities to meet goals of treatment or prevention program.

■ Patient will express intent to reduce risk factors for progression of illness.

■ Patient and family members will use available support services.

Suggested NOC outcomes

Compliance Behavior; Knowledge: Treatment Regimen; Participation in Health Care Decisions; Treatment Behavior: Illness or Injury

Interventions and rationales

■ Discuss patient's personal beliefs about illness and review relevant information *to establish a common understanding for developing a plan to improve management of the therapeutic regimen.*

■ Educate patient about the pathophysiology of the illness, and explain the relationship between the pathophysiology and the therapeutic regimen. *A patient who knows the reasons for specific behaviors may be more willing to adjust his lifestyle.*

■ Help patient and family members clarify values associated with their lifestyle *to enhance understanding of conflicts between lifestyle and demands of the therapeutic regimen.*

■ Work with patient and family members to develop a daily routine for managing the therapeutic regimen that fits with their lifestyle. *Collaboration with patient and family members makes it possible to combine scientific knowledge of the illness with lifestyle factors such as culture, family dynamics, and finances.*

■ Correct patient's misconceptions about susceptibility to and seriousness of the illness. *Misconceptions may undermine treatment.*

■ Assist patient and family members in modifying factors (such as social pressures, lack of family support, and previous behavior patterns) that interfere with treatment management *to enhance level of care.*

■ Provide verbal reminders to reinforce health-promoting behaviors. For example, remind patient with heart disease to stop smoking. *Verbal cues may stimulate patient to take action; if not immediately, then at a later time.*

■ Provide clearly written literature about the treatment regimen *to reinforce patient's knowledge.*

■ Assist patient and family members in selecting appropriate options for managing the therapeutic regimen *to help patient and family members integrate potentially complicated and disruptive therapeutic interventions into their lifestyle.*

■ Refer patient or family members to support groups or self-help organizations *to empower patient and family members to continue effective management of the therapeutic regimen.*

■ Help patient and family members plan for a future course of the illness. For example, patient or family members may need to make structural changes at home to accommodate a wheelchair or hospital bed. *Planning enhances patient's and family members' abilities to develop appropriate management strategies.*

Suggested NIC interventions

Behavior Modification; Decision-Making Support; Mutual Goal Setting; Patient Contracting; Teaching: Procedure/Treatment

Evaluations for expected outcomes

■ Patient expresses personal beliefs about illness and therapeutic regimen.

■ Patient and family members successfully incorporate components of therapeutic regimen into daily activities.

■ Patient describes daily activities that will help him achieve goals of treatment or prevention program and carries out therapeutic regimen.

■ Patient states intent to reduce risk factors for illness.

■ Patient and family members contact appropriate support services.

Documentation

■ Patient's knowledge and beliefs about illness and therapeutic regimen

■ Patient's explanation of values and lifestyle

■ Information provided to clarify misconceptions

■ Actions taken to modify patient's environment or behavior

■ Written materials given to patient

■ Referrals to support services

■ Evaluations for expected outcomes

Reference
Giger, J.N., et al. "Multi-cultural and Multi-ethnic Considerations and Advanced Directives: Developing Cultural Competency," *Journal of Cultural Diversity* 13(1):3-9, Spring 2006.

Ineffective family
THERAPEUTIC REGIMEN MANAGEMENT
related to family conflict, complex therapy, economic difficulties, or difficulty coping with the health care system

Definition
Pattern of regulating or integrating into daily living a program of treatment for illness and the sequelae of illness that's unsatisfactory for meeting specific health goals

Assessment
■ Family status, including marital status, family composition, communication patterns, coping skills, drug or alcohol abuse, psychiatric history, and beliefs and attitudes about health and illness
■ Health status, including chronic or terminal illness and severely disabling physical conditions
■ Socioeconomic factors, including financial status, insurance, accessibility of health care, availability of health care providers, and transportation system
■ Social status, including communication skills, size of social network, degree of trust in others, self-esteem, and ability to function in social and occupational roles
■ Spiritual status, including religious or church affiliation and description of faith and religious practices

Defining characteristics
■ Verbalizes choices of daily living that are ineffective for meeting the goals of a treatment program
■ Verbalizes, but doesn't take action to reduce risk factors for progression of illness and sequelae
■ Verbalizes desire to manage the treatment of illness and prevention of sequelae
■ Verbalizes difficulty with regulation and integration of one or more prescribed regimens for prevention of complications and the treatment of illness or its effects
■ Verbalizes, but doesn't take action to include treatment regimens in daily routines

Expected outcomes
■ Family members will identify behaviors that lead to conflict.
■ Family members will participate in family therapy sessions and openly express feelings about illness of family member.
■ Family members will express desire to have help in resolving conflicts.

■ Family members will describe coping mechanisms that help reduce conflicts.
■ Family members will cooperate in finding ways to incorporate therapeutic regimen into their lifestyle.
■ Family members will express desire to carry out therapeutic regimen.
■ Family members will plan for future course of illness.

Suggested NOC outcomes

Compliance Behavior; Family Coping; Family Functioning; Family Normalization; Family Participation in Professional Care; Knowledge: Treatment Regimen; Risk Control; Symptom Control

Interventions and rationales

■ Spend time with family, get to know each family member individually, and establish a trusting relationship with each family member *to help identify measures that will increase family cohesiveness.*
■ Encourage family members to attend and participate in family therapy sessions *to strengthen family unit and promote resolution of conflict.*
■ Help family members describe feelings associated with the illness of their relative to bring family conflict into the open. *Unresolved family conflicts may prevent family members from fully implementing therapeutic regimen.*
■ Elicit family members' personal beliefs about the illness and review relevant information *to establish their support for improving management of therapeutic regimen.*
■ Educate family members about the pathophysiology of illness, and explain the relationship between the pathophysiology and the therapeutic regimen. *If family members know reasons for specific behaviors, they may be more willing to adjust their lifestyle.*
■ Work with family members to identify behaviors that have contributed to family conflict, and help them identify alternative behaviors *to promote resolution of the conflict.*
■ Encourage family members to address individual needs assertively *to promote healthy interactions within family.*
■ Help family members clarify values associated with their lifestyle *to enhance understanding of conflicts between their lifestyle and demands of therapeutic regimen.*
■ Work with family members to develop a daily routine for managing the therapeutic regimen that fits with their lifestyle. *Collaboration with family members makes it possible to incorporate lifestyle factors, such as culture, family dynamics, and finances, into a plan for managing the illness.*
■ Assist family members in modifying factors (such as lack of supportive behaviors among family members) that interfere with treatment management *to enhance level of care.*
■ Work with the family in establishing goals for coping with conflicts *to focus their energy on achievable objectives and to foster hope.*
■ Refer the family members to appropriate agencies, if needed. *This can ensure continued family support and help reduce conflicts.*

- Help the family members plan for a future course of the illness. *Planning enhances family members' abilities to develop an appropriate strategy to manage the therapeutic regimen.*

Suggested NIC interventions

Case Management; Coping Enhancement; Decision-Making Support; Family Involvement Promotion; Family Process Maintenance; Family Therapy

Evaluations for expected outcomes
- Family members identify unresolved conflicts.
- Family members attend and participate in family therapy sessions.
- Family members express a desire to resolve conflicts.
- Family members describe coping mechanisms that can reduce conflicts.
- Family members successfully incorporate components of therapeutic regimen into daily activities.
- Family members carry out therapeutic regimen.
- Family members establish a plan for coping with future course of illness.

Documentation
- Description of each family member's understanding of patient's illness
- Family members' expressions of feelings regarding patient's illness
- Compliance with participation in family therapy sessions
- Evaluations for expected outcomes

Reference

Verhaeghe, S., et al. "Stress and Coping Among Families of Patients with Traumatic Brain Injury: A Review of the Literature," *Journal of Clinical Nursing* 14(8): 1004-1012, September 2005.

Ineffective
THERMOREGULATION
related to trauma or illness

Definition
Fluctuations in body temperature between hypothermia and hyperthermia

Assessment
- History of current illness
- Medication history
- Neurologic status, including level of consciousness (LOC), mental status, motor status, and sensory status
- Cardiovascular status, including blood pressure, capillary refill time, electrocardiogram, heart rate and rhythm, pulses (apical and peripheral), and temperature

■ Respiratory status, including arterial blood gas measurements, breath sounds, and rate, depth, and character of respirations
■ Integumentary status, including color, temperature, and turgor
■ Fluid and electrolyte status, including blood urea nitrogen level, intake and output, serum electrolyte levels, and urine specific gravity
■ Laboratory studies, including clotting factors, hemoglobin level, hematocrit, platelet count, and white blood cell count

Defining characteristics
■ Cyanotic nail beds
■ Fluctuations in body temperature above or below normal range
■ Flushed skin
■ Hypertension
■ Increased capillary refill time
■ Increased respiratory or heart rate
■ Mild shivering
■ Moderate pallor
■ Piloerection
■ Seizures
■ Warm or cool skin

Expected outcomes
■ Patient will maintain body temperature at normothermic levels.
■ Patient won't shiver.
■ Patient will express feelings of comfort.
■ Patient will have warm, dry skin.
■ Patient will maintain heart rate and blood pressure within normal range.
■ Patient won't exhibit signs of compromised neurologic status.
■ Patient and family members will voice an understanding of health problem.

Suggested NOC outcomes
Hydration; Thermoregulation; Vital Signs

Interventions and rationales
■ Monitor patient's body temperature every 4 hours, or more often if indicated. Record the temperature and route (keep in mind that the baseline depends on the route). *Monitoring determines the effectiveness of therapy or if intervention is required and allows accurate comparison of data.*
■ Monitor and record patient's neurologic status every 8 hours. Report any changes to the physician. *Changes in LOC can result from tissue hypoxia related to altered tissue perfusion. Hyperthermia increases cerebral edema and thus intracranial pressure (ICP); hypothermia depresses metabolic rate.*
■ Monitor and record patient's heart rate and rhythm, blood pressure, and respiratory rate every 4 hours. *Hyperthermia may create hypoxia by increasing oxygen demand, which results from increased tissue metabolism (metabolism increases 7% with each increase of 1° F [0.6° C]). This, in turn, results in faster breathing and a rising pulse rate.*

■ Administer analgesics, antipyretics, and medications that prevent shivering, as indicated. Monitor and record their effectiveness. *Antipyretics help reduce fever. Shivering tends to retard the lowering of body temperature.*

■ If patient develops excessive fever, take the following steps:

– Remove blankets; place a loincloth over patient.

– Apply ice bags to the axilla and groin.

– Initiate a tepid water sponge bath.

– Use a hypothermia blanket if temperature rises above ____. Cool patient to ____.

These measures help reduce excessive fever.

■ Maintain hydration.

– Monitor intake and output.

– Administer parenteral fluids, as ordered.

– Determine patient's fluid preference. Keep oral fluids at the bedside and encourage patient to drink.

These measures help maintain fluid balance. Keeping preferred fluids at the bedside allows patient to actively participate in the prescribed treatment.

■ Maintain the environmental temperature at a comfortable setting.

– Ensure that all metal and plastic surfaces that come into contact with patient's body are covered.

– Use warm blankets.

– Make sure that linens and clothing are clean and dry.

The temperature of the external environment affects ease of body temperature regulation.

■ Instruct patient and family members about:

– signs and symptoms of altered body temperature

– precautionary measures to avoid hypothermia or hyperthermia

– adherence to other aspects of health care management to help normalize patient's temperature (such as dietary habits and measures to prevent increased ICP)

– rationale for treatment.

These measures allow patient to take an active role in health maintenance.

Suggested NIC interventions

Bathing; Environmental Management; Fever Treatment; Fluid Management; Fluid Monitoring; Temperature Regulation; Vital Signs Monitoring

Evaluations for expected outcomes

■ Patient's temperature remains within normal parameters.

■ Patient doesn't shiver.

■ Patient indicates feelings of comfort, either verbally or through behavior.

■ Patient's skin remains warm and dry.

■ Patient's heart rate and blood pressure remain within normal range.

■ Patient doesn't exhibit signs of neurologic complications associated with extremes in temperature.

■ Patient and his family state understanding of health problem.

Documentation
- Patient's needs and perceptions of current problem
- Physical findings
- Intake and output
- Patient's response to nursing interventions
- Evaluations for expected outcomes

Reference
Lasater, M. "The Role of Thermoregulation in Cardiac Resuscitation," *Critical Care Nursing Clinics of North America* 17(1):97-102, March 2005.

Disturbed
THOUGHT PROCESSES

Definition
Disruption in cognitive operations and activities

Assessment
- Age
- Reason for hospitalization, including patient's perception of problem, recent stressors, and changes in somatic functioning
- Mental status, including insight about current situation, judgment (ask patient to solve a simple problem), abstract thinking (ask patient to interpret a proverb), general information (ask patient to name five states), mood, affect, recent and remote memory, thought processes, thought content, and orientation to time, place, and person
- Physical appearance, including manner of dress, personal hygiene, posture, and gait
- Communication status, including attitude toward interviewer, body language, and facial expressions
- Sleep habits
- Self-care status, including ability to perform activities of daily living and safety practices
- Physiologic status, including medication history (response, effectiveness, and adverse reactions) and history of substance abuse (type and effect on mental status)
- Dietary and nutritional status
- Laboratory studies, including toxicology screening and blood chemistry
- Diagnostic tests, including computed tomography scan and EEG

Defining characteristics
- Cognitive dissonance
- Distractibility
- Egocentricity

- Hypervigilance or hypovigilance
- Inaccurate interpretation of environment
- Inappropriate, fantasy-based thinking
- Memory impairment

Expected outcomes
- Patient will identify internal and external factors that trigger delusional episodes.
- Patient will identify and perform activities that decrease delusions.
- Patient will practice distraction techniques to reduce anxiety before the onset of delusion.
- Patient will interact with others without becoming delusional.
- Patient will consider alternative interpretation of situation without becoming unduly hostile or anxious.
- Patient will recognize how delusional system meets his interpersonal needs.
- Patient will recognize symptoms and comply with therapeutic regimen.

Suggested NOC outcomes
Cognition; Cognitive Orientation; Distorted Thought Self-Control; Identity; Information Processing

Interventions and rationales
- Project a nonjudgmental and trusting attitude toward patient through active listening. *Patient must trust you to talk openly about delusions and feelings.*
- Orient patient to reality, as needed.
- Call patient by name.
- Tell patient your name.
- Provide background information (place, time, and date) frequently throughout the day, verbally and visually, using a reality orientation board.
- Orient patient to his environment, including sights, sounds, and smells. *Reality orientation techniques foster patient's awareness of himself and his environment.*
- Explain to patient with organic delusions that distorted thinking is caused by temporary biochemical changes *to help decrease patient's anxiety level.*
- Don't argue, reason with, or challenge patient with nonorganic delusions; instead, provide comfort and support. *Attempts to correct delusional beliefs will increase anxiety.*
- Explore events that trigger delusions. Discuss anxiety associated with triggering events. *Exploring these topics will help you understand the dynamics of patient's delusional system.*
- Without arguing or agreeing, acknowledge plausible elements of delusion. Make such statements as "I don't doubt that your family brought you to the hospital. However, I have no reason to believe that they're cooperating with the CIA to kill you." *Delusions usually have some basis in reality. By conveying the acceptance of delusions but not a belief in them, you can better help patient.*
- When the dynamics of patient's delusions are understood, discourage repetitious talk about delusions and refocus the conversation on patient's underlying

feelings. *As patient begins to learn to cope with underlying feelings, delusions will become less necessary.*

■ Help patient find other means to meet the emotional needs that he attempts to fulfill through delusions. *Delusions usually decrease when needs are met in other ways.*

■ Educate patient and family members about the signs and symptoms of illness and the effects of medication. *Collaboration with family members promotes continuity of care.*

■ Refer family members to appropriate resources to plan for patient care after discharge. *Referrals help provide a comprehensive approach to postdischarge care.*

Suggested NIC interventions

Cognitive Restructuring; Cognitive Stimulation; Delusion Management; Emotional Support; Energy Management; Environmental Management: Safety; Reality Orientation

Evaluations for expected outcomes

■ Patient describes at least two situations that increase delusions.
■ Patient describes two self-initiated activities to decrease delusions.
■ Patient gives two concrete examples of anxiety-reducing techniques.
■ Patient interacts with primary nurse 30 minutes per day without delusional content.
■ Patient discusses two reality-based interpretations of events that are validated by others.
■ Patient communicates insight about his delusional system.
■ Patient and family members discuss delusional symptoms and adverse effects of medication.

Documentation

■ Patient's statements indicating type, number, and intensity of delusions
■ Observations about environmental factors that precipitate delusional behavior
■ Interventions that focus on helping patient maintain reality orientation
■ Patient's response to nursing interventions
■ Referrals
■ Evaluations for expected outcomes

Reference

Magarey, J.M., and McCutcheon, H.H. "Fishing with the Dead—Recall of Memories from ICU," *Intensive & Critical Care Nursing* 21(6):344-54, December 2005.

Disturbed
THOUGHT PROCESSES
related to loss of memory

Definition
Disruption in cognitive operations and activities

Assessment
- History of neurologic disorder, head injury, or psychiatric disorder
- Neurologic status, including cognition, insight and judgment, memory, motor ability, orientation, and sensory ability
- Self-care status, including ability to perform activities of daily living (ADLs) and safety practices
- Psychosocial status, including coping mechanisms, family members, occupation, personality, and stressors (finances, job, or marital discord)

Defining characteristics
- Cognitive dissonance
- Distractibility
- Egocentricity
- Hypervigilance or hypovigilance
- Inaccurate interpretation of environment
- Inappropriate, fantasy-based thinking
- Memory impairment

Expected outcomes
- Patient will maintain orientation to time, place, and person.
- Patient will sustain no harm or injury.
- Patient will maintain current health status.
- Patient and family members will voice feelings and concerns.
- Family members will communicate understanding of care required by patient.
- Family members will demonstrate appropriate coping skills.
- Family members will identify available health resources.

Suggested NOC outcomes
Cognition; Cognitive Orientation; Concentration; Decision-Making; Distorted Thought Self-Control; Fall Prevention Behavior; Identity; Information Processing; Memory; Safe Home Environment

Interventions and rationales
- Observe patient's thought processes every shift. Document and report any changes. *Changes may indicate progressive improvement or decline in the underlying condition.*
- Perform the prescribed treatment for the underlying condition; monitor progress. Report any favorable or adverse responses to treatment *to assess the effectiveness of treatment.*

■ Orient patient to reality, as needed.

– Call patient by name.

– Tell patient your name.

– Provide background information (place, time, and date) frequently throughout the day.

– Reinforce verbal reports with visual aids such as a reality orientation board.

– Orient patient to his environment, including sights, sounds, and smells.

– Use television or radio purposefully to augment orientation.

Reality orientation techniques foster patient's awareness of self and his environment.

■ Keep items in the same places. *A consistent, stable environment reduces confusion, decreases frustration, and aids successful completion of ADLs.*

■ Ask family members to provide patient with photos (labeled with name and relationship on back), favorite belongings, and cards. *Belongings promote a sense of continuity and memory and create a sense of security and comfort.*

■ Protect patient from sensory overload; allow frequent rest periods. *Sensory overload may increase confusion; frequent rest periods help avoid fatigue.*

■ Provide a structured environment for patient. List the daily routine and post in patient's room *to provide continuity of care.*

■ Communicate patient's skill level to all personnel *to preserve his level of independent functioning.*

■ Spend time daily with patient to encourage memories and discussion of past events. Encourage patient's participation in reminiscence groups. *Remote memory may be intact. Discussion of past events promotes a sense of continuity, aids memory, and promotes feelings of security. Joining in reminiscence groups provides a diversional activity and may increase socialization skills.*

■ Correct patient privately for inappropriate behavior; walk patient to his room or initiate another behavior *to help prevent feelings of embarrassment and frustration. Redirection and engagement in previously successful activities increase patient's sense of accomplishment and reinforce desirable behavior.*

■ Provide close supervision *to prevent patient from wandering off or incurring harm.* Instruct family members on how to maintain a safe home environment for patient. *Patient may be unable to consider his own safety needs or risks.* Place patient's photo or name on the door to his room *to aid memory and help patient find his room.*

■ Encourage patient to voice feelings and concerns about loss of memory. *Verbalization helps reduce anxiety and ventilate frustrations and promotes acceptance of the need for supervision and the treatment regimen.*

■ Help family members develop the necessary coping skills to deal with patient. *Family members need these skills to deal with patient's neurologic or psychiatric impairment and the potential for deterioration in patient's condition.*

■ Demonstrate reorientation techniques to family members, and provide time for supervised return demonstrations. *Informed family members are better prepared to cope with patient with altered thought processes.*

■ Help family members identify a community support group (such as a stroke club and Alzheimer's group) *to assist in coping with the effects of patient's illness.*

Suggested NIC interventions

Anxiety Reduction; Cognitive Stimulation; Decision-Making Support; Delusion Management; Dementia Management; Energy Management; Family Support; Reality Orientation; Surveillance: Safety

Evaluations for expected outcomes

■ Patient remains oriented to time, place, and person.
■ Patient doesn't show evidence of harm or injury.
■ Patient maintains current health status.
■ Patient and family members express concerns about loss of memory and effect on patient's lifestyle.
■ Family members report understanding of care required by patient.
■ Family members demonstrate appropriate interventions, reorientation techniques, and coping skills.
■ Family members identify and contact at least one support group to assist in coping with effects of illness.

Documentation

■ Patient's and family members' expressions of concern and feelings about patient's altered thought processes
■ Observations of patient's altered thought processes and response to treatment for underlying condition
■ Patient's response to nursing interventions
■ Instructions to family members and their understanding of instructions and demonstrated ability to care for patient
■ Referrals made for patient and family members
■ Evaluations for expected outcomes

Reference

Gilmour, J.A., and Huntington, A.D. "Finding the Balance: Living with Memory Loss," *International Journal of Nursing Practice* 11(3):118-24, June 2005.

Disturbed
THOUGHT PROCESSES
related to physiologic causes

Definition

Disruption in cognitive operations and activities

Assessment

■ Reason for hospitalization
■ Mental status, including abstract thinking (ask patient to interpret a proverb); general information (ask patient to name five states); insight concerning the present situation; judgment (ask patient to solve a simple problem); memory for recent and remote past; and orientation to time, place, and person

- Neurologic status, including level of consciousness, motor ability, and sensory ability
- Sleep habits
- Ability to perform activities of daily living (ADLs)
- Safety hazards
- Medication history
- Dietary and nutritional status
- History of alcohol consumption

Defining characteristics
- Cognitive dissonance
- Distractibility
- Egocentricity
- Hypervigilance or hypovigilance
- Inaccurate interpretation of environment
- Inappropriate, fantasy-based thinking
- Memory impairment

Expected outcomes
- Patient will remain safe and protected from injury.
- Patient will maintain awareness of need for assistance.
- Patient will maintain orientation to time, place, and person.
- Patient will perform ADLs with assistance.
- Patient's laboratory values will stay within normal range.
- Patient will receive treatment for physiologic causes of altered thought processes, resulting in restoration of thought processes.
- Family members will identify partial or complete confusion.
- Family members will make arrangements for home care.

Suggested NOC outcomes
Cognition; Cognitive Orientation; Concentration; Distorted Thought Self-Control; Information Processing; Safe Home Environment

Interventions and rationales
- Monitor and record patient's vital signs every 4 hours, neurologic status every shift, and laboratory values, as ordered (including blood glucose and alcohol, arterial blood gas, and electrolyte levels). *Vital signs allow assessment of patient for indications of infection or complication. Neurologic assessment and laboratory studies may reveal progressive improvement or decline of the underlying condition.*
- Carry out the medical regimen to treat the underlying causes of mental status deterioration. *The medical regimen aims to alleviate the causes of mental status deterioration.*
- Address patient by name and tell him your name. *Reality orientation techniques foster patient's awareness of himself and his environment.*
- Give short, simple explanations to patient each time you do something *to avoid confusion and aid successful task completion.*
- Schedule nursing care to provide quiet times. *Rest periods help prevent sensory overload.*

■ Mention time, place, and date frequently throughout the day. Have a clock and calendar where patient can easily see them; refer to these aids when orienting patient. *Reality orientation techniques foster patient's awareness of himself and his environment.*

■ Keep patient's things in the same places as much as possible. *A consistent, stable environment reduces confusion and frustration and aids successful completion of ADLs.*

■ Use appropriate safety measures to protect patient from injury. Avoid physical restraints if possible. *Patient may be unable to consider his own safety needs or risks. Restraints may agitate patient.*

■ Ask family members to bring photos (label with name and relationship on back), favorite articles, and cards. *Familiar items help create a more secure environment for patient.*

■ Plan patient's routine, and follow it as consistently as possible. *A consistent daily plan aids task completion and reduces confusion and frustration.*

■ Speak slowly and clearly. Allow ample time for patient to respond. *These measures reduce confusion and frustration and aid task completion.*

■ Encourage patient to perform ADLs. Be patient and specific in providing instructions. Allow time for patient to perform each task *to enhance patient's self-esteem and help prevent complications of inactivity.* Limit new skills or tasks to small, critical units *to aid learning.* If needed, provide extensive supervision and repetition *to allow patient to master new tasks.*

■ Encourage family members to share stories and discuss familiar things with patient. *Remote memory commonly remains intact. Sharing stories and familiar things promotes a sense of continuity, aids memory, and creates a sense of security and comfort.*

■ Support family members in their attempts to interact with patient. *Family members need positive reinforcement for visiting and attempting to interact with patient.*

■ Allow time before and after visits for family members to express feelings. *Expression of feelings in a supportive environment helps family members cope with patient's illness.*

■ Refer family members to appropriate resources to plan for patient care after discharge. *Referrals help provide a comprehensive approach to postdischarge care.*

Suggested NIC interventions

Calming Technique; Cognitive Stimulation; Decision-Making Support; Environmental Management: Safety; Family Support; Reality Orientation; Surveillance: Safety

Evaluations for expected outcomes

■ Patient remains free from injury.
■ Patient maintains awareness of need for assistance.
■ Patient maintains orientation to time, place, and person.
■ Patient performs ADLs with assistance.
■ Patient's laboratory values remain within set limits.
■ Patient receives treatment for physiologic causes of altered thought processes.

■ Family members identify partial or complete confusion as indicator of patient's changing physiologic state.

■ Family members contact appropriate resources to arrange for home care.

Documentation
■ Patient's verbal responses
■ Observations of patient's behavior indicating altered thought processes
■ Interventions that focus on helping patient maintain reality orientation
■ Patient's response to nursing interventions
■ Evaluations for expected outcomes

Reference
Hinkle, J.L. "Variables Explaining Functional Recovery Following Motor Stroke," *The Journal of Neuroscience Nursing* 38(1):6-12, February 2006.

Impaired
TISSUE INTEGRITY
related to altered circulation

Definition
Damage to mucous membranes or to corneal, integumentary, or subcutaneous tissue

Assessment
■ History of peripheral vascular disease or surgery
■ Age
■ Gender
■ Integumentary status, including color, skin care practices, temperature, tenderness, texture, turgor, and edema
■ Cardiovascular status, including blood pressure, cardiac output, patient and family history of cardiovascular disease, peripheral pulses, and smoking history
■ Nutritional status, including dietary patterns, laboratory tests, serum lipid level, serum protein level, and change from normal weight
■ Neurologic status, including motor function and sensory pattern

Defining characteristics
■ Damaged or destroyed tissue

Expected outcomes
■ Patient will attain relief from immediate signs and symptoms (pain, ulcers, color changes, and edema).
■ Patient will maintain collateral circulation.
■ Patient will voice intent to stop smoking.
■ Patient will voice intent to follow specific management routines after discharge.

Suggested NOC outcomes

Knowledge: Treatment Regimen; Self-Care Hygiene; Tissue Integrity: Skin & Mucous Membranes; Tissue Perfusion: Peripheral; Wound Healing: Secondary Intention

Interventions and rationales

▪ Provide scrupulous foot care. Administer and monitor treatments according to institutional protocols. *Foot care prevents fungal infections and ingrown toenails, stimulates circulation, and allows detection of signs and symptoms you should immediately report to the physician.*

▪ Instruct patient to avoid pressure on popliteal space. For example, say "Don't cross your legs or wear constrictive clothing," *to avoid reducing arterial blood supply and increasing venous congestion.*

▪ Encourage adherence to an exercise regimen, as tolerated. *Exercise improves arterial circulation and venous return by promoting muscle contraction and relaxation.*

▪ Educate patient about risk factors and prevention of injury. Refer patient to a smoking cessation program. *Teaching about factors influencing peripheral vascular disease and prevention of tissue damage helps prevent complications.*

▪ Maintain adequate hydration. Monitor intake and output and record daily weight. *Adequate hydration reduces blood viscosity and decreases the risk of clot formation.*

▪ If patient has venous insufficiency, apply antiembolism stockings or intermittent pneumatic compression stockings, removing them for 1 hour every 8 hours or according to institutional protocol. Elevate patient's feet when he's sitting and elevate foot of bed 6″ to 8″ (15 to 20.5 cm) when he's lying down. *These measures promote venous return and decrease venous congestion in lower extremities.*

▪ If patient has arterial insufficiency, elevate the head of the bed 6″ to 8″ when he's lying down *to increase arterial blood supply to extremities.*

Suggested NIC interventions

Circulatory Care: Arterial Insufficiency; Circulatory Precautions; Nutrition Management; Oral Health Maintenance; Positioning; Pressure Management; Pressure Ulcer Prevention; Skin Surveillance; Teaching: Foot Care

Evaluations for expected outcomes

▪ Patient attains relief from immediate symptoms.
– Patient's feet show no signs of infection, ingrown toenails, or impaired circulation.
– Patient maintains normal skin turgor.
– Patient's mucous membranes remain moist.
– Patient maintains balanced intake and output.
– Patient's weight remains stable.
– Patient's vital signs remain within normal parameters.
▪ Patient uses interventions (antiembolism stockings or intermittent pneumatic compression stockings, elevation of feet, and elevation of head of bed) to promote arterial and venous circulation.

■ Patient states rationale for quitting smoking and begins smoking-cessation program.

■ Patient describes plan to incorporate prescribed treatment program into post-discharge routine, including avoiding risk factors and activities that contribute to vascular compression (such as popliteal compression, leg crossing, and wearing constrictive clothing), following exercise program, and practicing foot care.

Documentation
■ Patient's expressions of feelings about current situation
■ Observations of skin color, turgor, temperature, and ulcer size
■ Patient's response to nursing interventions
■ Evaluations for expected outcomes

Reference
Bjellerup, M. "Determining Venous Incompetence: A Report from a Specialised Leg Ulcer Clinic," *Journal of Wound Care* 15(10):429-36, November 2006.

Impaired
TISSUE INTEGRITY
related to physical, chemical, or electrical hazards during surgery

Definition
Damage to mucous membranes or to corneal, integumentary, or subcutaneous tissue

Assessment
■ Reason for, type of, and anticipated length of surgery
■ Health status, including age, sex, weight, vital signs, and nutritional, integumentary, cardiovascular, neurologic, respiratory, and psychosocial status
■ Mobility status, including range of motion
■ Patient's description of pain, numbness, and tingling
■ Laboratory studies, including hematocrit, hemoglobin level, complete blood count, blood coagulation studies, immunologic and serologic tests, electrolyte levels, urinalysis, liver function tests, and serum protein levels
■ Wound classification (clean, clean-contaminated, contaminated, or dirty)
■ Allergies to medications, irrigation solutions, or cleaning solutions
■ Health history, including altered immunologic status, malnutrition, and chronic metabolic or systemic disease (diabetes mellitus; cancer; cardiovascular, renal, or hepatic diseases; coagulation disorders; blood dyscrasias; or hematopoietic diseases)
■ Current medical treatments, including chemotherapy and radiation, steroid, immunosuppressive, anticoagulant, thrombolytic, and antibiotic therapy
■ Presence of infection, draining wounds, bruises, shear ulcers, or pressure ulcers

Defining characteristics
■ Damaged or destroyed tissue

Expected outcomes

- Patient will express feelings of comfort.
- Patient will remain free from alteration in tissue integrity related to physical hazards.
- Patient will remain free from alteration in tissue integrity related to chemical hazards.
- Patient will remain free from alteration in tissue integrity related to electrical hazards.

Suggested NOC outcomes

Hydration; Infection Severity; Sensory Function: Cutaneous; Thermoregulation; Tissue Integrity: Skin & Mucous Membranes; Wound Healing: Secondary Intention

Interventions and rationales

- Document and report the results of the preoperative nursing assessment. Identify factors that predispose patient to impaired tissue integrity. *A complete nursing assessment allows the development of an individualized care plan.*
- Classify the surgical wound according to the degree of contamination of the wound and surrounding tissue. *Classifying the surgical wound facilitates the assessment of the risk of wound infection and subsequent tissue injury.*
- Use padding, special mattresses, and support devices during surgery. *These measures reduce undue pressure and decrease the risk of impaired tissue integrity.*
- Maintain the environmental temperature at a comfortable setting. Offer blankets, if needed. *A comfortable environment reduces shivering, muscle tension, and reactive pain. These metabolic stressors can affect the rate of cellular repair.*
- Monitor patient for signs of hypothermia (shivering, cool skin, pallor, piloerection, and increased heart rate) *to determine the need to implement warming measures.*
- Warm prepping and irrigation solutions *to prevent a reduction in patient's temperature.*
- For infants (age 1 year or younger), use a warming unit and head covering. *Infants have immature thermoregulatory mechanisms and don't retain adequate body heat.*
- When using pneumatic tourniquets, pad the skin, place the cuff so the skin is free from wrinkles, set to proper pressure, and monitor inflation time. *Improper tourniquet use can impair the circulatory status of the affected limb.*
- Check patient history for a sensitivity or allergy to prepping solution. Clean and prepare the skin incision site with nonirritating solutions. *Hypoallergenic, physiologic prepping and cleaning solutions reduce the risk of tissue reaction and injury.*
- To avoid the pooling of solutions, use towels or pads during prep. When using sprays, shield patient's face and eyes. *Pooled solutions can produce skin maceration. Sprays can damage the cornea and mucous membranes.*
- Ensure adequate aeration of items sterilized by ethylene oxide gas. *Residual gas is toxic to tissue.*

■ Rinse chemosterilized items adequately. *Residual chemosterilization solutions are toxic to tissue.*

■ Remove powder from gloves. *Glove powder can cause granulomas and other reactions.*

■ Perform sponge, sharp, and instrument counts according to protocol, account for other items (such as bulldogs, umbilical tapes, and vessel loops), and document results. *Retained objects can produce a foreign body reaction or injury to tissue.*

■ Follow the manufacturer's instructions for applying medications and chemical agents, such as glutaraldehyde and methylmethacrylate. *Agents can be toxic when applied directly to tissue.*

■ Use physiologic solutions or prescribed medications for irrigation or topical application. *Nonphysiologic solutions can cause interstitial edema and cellular injury or death.*

■ Check the label, route, dose, and expiration date of each medication with the scrub nurse *to reduce the risk of error.*

■ When administering medications, record the drug, dosage, and route. Document verbal orders and have the physician cosign. *Documentation helps reduce medication errors.*

■ Inspect all electrical, mechanical, and air-powered equipment before use. Operate equipment according to manufacturers' instruction *to reduce the chances of patient injury.*

■ Apply an electrosurgical dispersive pad to clean, dry skin near the operative site. Avoid bony prominences, hairy surfaces, scar tissue, and areas of poor circulation. *Proper placement reduces the risk of burn injury.*

■ When using a hypothermia or hyperthermia blanket, avoid creases, place a sheet between the skin and the blanket, and set and maintain the correct temperature. Pad the extremities during hypothermia therapy. *Proper use protects against tissue injury.*

Suggested NIC interventions

Hemorrhage Control; Incision Site Care; Infection Control: Intraoperative; Infection Protection; Medication Management; Positioning; Pressure Ulcer Prevention

Evaluations for expected outcomes

■ Patient has minimal or no shivering, muscle tension, or reactive pain.

■ Patient doesn't develop rash, edema, bruises, discoloration, redness, skin breakdown, or other signs of altered tissue integrity related to physical hazards.

■ Patient doesn't develop allergic or toxic reaction to sterilizing agents, glove powder, irrigating solutions, medications, or chemical agents and has little or no reaction to cleaning procedure.

■ Patient doesn't develop reddened or discolored areas at site of electrosurgical grounding pad or adjacent tissue or any other signs of postoperative alteration in tissue integrity related to electrical hazards.

Documentation

■ Results of preoperative nursing assessment

- Surgical procedure
- Type of anesthesia
- Preoperative and postoperative diagnosis
- Wound classification
- Preexisting conditions that increase risk of tissue injury
- Nursing interventions performed to protect tissue integrity
- Medications administered
- Patient's status on discharge to postanesthesia care unit (PACU)
- Skin condition on discharge to PACU
- Presence of lines, tubes, catheters, and drains
- Type of wound closure and dressing
- Evaluations for expected outcomes

Reference

Cunnington, J. "Facilitating Benefit, Minimising Risk: Responsibilities of the Surgical Practitioner During Electrosurgery," *Journal of Perioperative Practice* 16(4):195-202, April 2006.

Impaired
TISSUE INTEGRITY
related to radiation

Definition

Damage to mucous membranes or to corneal, integumentary, or subcutaneous tissue

Assessment

- History of radiation therapy or exposure
- Age
- Gender
- Integumentary status, including color, distribution of hair, mucous membranes, skin care practices, temperature, tenderness, texture, turgor, scars, lesions, and wounds
- Nutritional status, including dietary patterns and change from normal weight

Defining characteristics

- Damaged or destroyed tissue

Expected outcomes

- Patient will show no irritation or skin breakdown in irradiated areas.
- Patient's ulcerated areas will heal.
- Patient will maintain adequate fluid and nutritional intake.
- Patient and family members will communicate understanding of skin care regimen, medication use, and need for adequate fluid and nutritional intake.

Suggested NOC outcomes

Allergic Response: Localized; Knowledge: Treatment Regimen; Thermoregulation; Tissue Integrity: Skin & Mucous Membranes; Wound Healing: Primary Intention

Interventions and rationales

■ Keep patient's skin clean, dry, and exposed to air as much as possible *to promote healing of excoriated areas and prevent infection.*

■ Avoid constrictive clothing *to reduce the risk of friction and decreased blood flow.* Avoid exposure to the sun *to reduce the risk of sunburn and possible skin cancer.*

■ Avoid nonprescription ointments, creams, and warm packs *because they can increase skin irritation and possible radiation* (if they contain heavy metals).

■ Avoid extremes of hot and cold on affected skin areas *to prevent further irritation and skin breakdown.*

■ Avoid vigorous scrubbing of irradiated areas *to minimize skin breakdown.*

■ Use nonadhesive dressings *to avoid pulling on affected skin.*

■ Provide oral hygiene, as indicated, *to promote comfort and reduce the risk of infection.* Use a soft toothbrush *to reduce the risk of bleeding.*

■ Use cornstarch over unbroken areas *to decrease itching and friction.*

■ Provide a regular change of position, a bed cradle, or pressure-relieving devices, when indicated. *These measures reduce friction and the risk of skin breakdown on affected body parts.*

■ Inspect patient's skin every shift. Report areas of breakdown and signs of infection *to ensure early treatment.*

■ Follow facility protocol for treating infected lesions. Administer creams, antibiotic ointments, and irrigation solutions, as ordered, and monitor effectiveness. *Protocols are established to meet specific patient needs.*

■ Administer analgesics, as ordered, and monitor effectiveness. *Analgesics reduce pain resulting from skin problems.*

■ Consult a dietitian to assist with diet, emphasizing a diet high in protein, calories, vitamins, and minerals to promote tissue repair and prevent catabolism. *Positive nitrogen balance promotes wound healing.*

■ Administer antiemetics, as ordered, *to promote patient comfort and adequate nutrition.* Monitor their effectiveness.

■ Educate patient and his family in the skin care regimen, medication administration, and nutritional needs *to promote compliance and maintain tissue integrity.*

Suggested NIC interventions

Fluid Management; Infection Control; Medication Administration; Oral Health Maintenance; Positioning; Pressure Management; Radiation Therapy Management; Skin Surveillance; Wound Care

Evaluations for expected outcomes

■ Patient's irradiated areas don't show signs of cracking, oozing, sloughing, or infection.

■ Patient's ulcerated areas heal.

■ Patient maintains adequate fluid and nutritional intake.

■ Patient and family members demonstrate proper skin care and medication administration techniques and communicate understanding of importance of maintaining nutritional intake.

Documentation
■ Patient's expression of feelings
■ Physical findings
■ Interventions performed to prevent irritation or breakdown and to promote healing
■ Patient's response to nursing interventions
■ Patient's and family members' response to education
■ Evaluations for expected outcomes

Reference
McQuestion, M. "Evidence-based Skin Care Management in Radiation Therapy," *Seminars in Oncology Nursing* 22(3):163-73, August 2006.

Ineffective
TISSUE PERFUSION (CARDIOPULMONARY)
related to decreased cellular exchange

Definition
Decrease in oxygen resulting in the failure to nourish the tissues at the capillary level

Assessment
■ Health history, including presence of diabetes mellitus, high cholesterol, hypertension, obesity, smoking, stressful lifestyle, and family history of heart disease
■ Neurologic status, including level of consciousness, mental status, and orientation
■ Cardiovascular status, including blood pressure; heart rate and rhythm; heart sounds; peripheral pulses; skin color, temperature, and turgor; hepatojugular reflux; jugular vein distention; and history of congenital heart disease or valvular disorder
■ Diagnostic tests, including chest X-ray, regular and exercise electrocardiogram (ECG), echocardiogram, nuclear isotope studies, and cardiac angiography
■ Respiratory status, including arterial blood gas (ABG) levels, auscultation of breath sounds, and respiratory rate and depth
■ Renal status, including intake and output, serum electrolyte levels, urine specific gravity, and weight
■ Integumentary system, including cyanosis, pallor, and peripheral edema

Defining characteristics
■ Abnormal ABG levels
■ Arrhythmias
■ Bronchospasms

- Capillary refill time greater than 3 seconds
- Chest pain
- Chest retraction
- Dyspnea
- Nasal flaring
- Respiratory rate outside of acceptable parameters
- Sense of impending doom
- Use of accessory muscles

Expected outcomes

- Patient will attain hemodynamic stability, with pulse not less than _____ beats/minute and not greater than _____ beats/minute and blood pressure not less than _____ mm Hg and not greater than _____ mm Hg.
- Patient won't exhibit arrhythmias.
- Patient's skin will remain warm and dry.
- Patient's heart rate will remain within prescribed limits while he carries out activities of daily living (ADLs).
- Patient will maintain adequate cardiac output.
- Patient will modify lifestyle to minimize risk of decreased tissue perfusion.

Suggested NOC outcomes

Cardiac Pump Effectiveness; Circulation Status; Fluid Balance; Respiratory Status: Gas Exchange; Tissue Perfusion: Cardiac; Tissue Perfusion: Peripheral; Vital Signs

Interventions and rationales

- Monitor and document patient's vital signs (heart rate, blood pressure, and pulmonary artery pressure) every hour until stable, then every 2 hours. Report any findings outside prescribed limits. *Decreased heart rate and blood pressure may indicate increased arteriovenous exchange, which leads to decreased tissue perfusion.*
- Administer fluids, as needed, *to maintain preload.*
- Monitor skin color and temperature every 2 hours. Assess for signs of skin breakdown. *Cool, blanched, mottled skin and cyanosis may indicate decreased tissue perfusion.*
- Monitor respiratory rate and breath sounds. Document findings. *Increased respiratory rate may indicate that patient is compensating for tissue hypoxia.*
- Monitor ECG for changes in heart rate and rhythm. *Altered heart rate and rhythm can affect tissue perfusion and may indicate a life-threatening crisis.*
- Maintain oxygen therapy, as ordered, *to maximize oxygen exchange in the alveoli and at the cellular level.*
- Encourage patient to change position and participate in activity, as condition permits, *to enhance vital capacity and avoid lung congestion and skin breakdown.*
- Encourage frequent rest periods *to conserve energy and maximize tissue perfusion.*
- Monitor creatine kinase, lactate dehydrogenase, and ABG levels. *Abnormal findings may indicate tissue damage or decreased oxygen exchange in the lungs.*
- Inform patient about:
- risk factors for heart and lung disease

– proper use of nitroglycerin
– proper use of medications and possible adverse reactions
– benefits of a low-fat, low-cholesterol diet
– need to avoid straining with bowel movements
– benefits of quitting smoking.
Effective teaching encourages patient to take an active role in health maintenance.

Suggested NIC interventions

Acid-Base Management; Cardiac Care: Acute; Cardiac Precautions; Embolus Precautions; Fluid/Electrolyte Management; Hemodynamic Regulation; Respiratory Monitoring; Vital Signs Monitoring

Evaluations for expected outcomes

- Patient attains hemodynamic stability within specified parameters.
- Patient shows no signs of arrhythmias.
- Patient's skin remains warm, dry, and intact.
- Patient's heart rate remains within prescribed parameters while he carries out ADLs.
- Patient maintains adequate cardiac output.
- Patient describes plans to modify lifestyle to minimize cause of decreased tissue perfusion.

Documentation

- Observations of physical findings
- Observation of patient's response to activity
- Verbal statements and behavior indicating patient's perception of health problems and health needs
- Nursing interventions performed and patient's response
- Patient's demonstration of skills associated with maintaining diet, adhering to medication regimen, maintaining activity level, and managing stress
- Evaluations for expected outcomes

Reference

Klieman, L., et al. "Cardiovascular Disease Risk Reduction in Older Adults," *The Journal of Cardiovascular Nursing* 21(5):S27-S39, September-October 2006.

Ineffective
TISSUE PERFUSION (CARDIOPULMONARY)
related to hypovolemia

Definition

Decrease in oxygen resulting in the failure to nourish the tissues at the capillary level

Assessment

- History of trauma, surgery, or condition resulting in fluid volume depletion

■ Cardiovascular status, including blood pressure, capillary refill time, central venous pressure (CVP), electrocardiogram, heart rate and rhythm, heart sounds, hemoglobin (Hb) level and hematocrit (HCT), jugular filling, peripheral pulses, and tilt test
■ Respiratory status, including breath sounds and respiratory rate and rhythm
■ Renal status, including intake and output, urine specific gravity, and weight
■ Neurologic status, including level of consciousness (LOC), mental status, and orientation
■ Integumentary status, including color, moisture, and temperature

Defining characteristics

■ Alterations of cardiopulmonary, cerebral, GI, peripheral, or renal tissue perfusion

Expected outcomes

■ Patient will maintain hemodynamic stability: pulse greater than _____ and less than _____; systolic blood pressure greater than _____; CVP greater than _____; and mean arterial pressure greater than _____.
■ Patient will maintain fluid balance, with intake equal to output.
■ Patient will maintain urine specific gravity within normal parameters.
■ Patient will maintain respiratory rate within 5 breaths/minute of baseline.
■ Patient will maintain skin integrity.
■ Patient will remain oriented to time, place, and person.
■ Patient will have no crackles or rhonchi.
■ Patient will exhibit improved circulation.
■ Patient's Hb level, HCT, white blood cell (WBC) count, and coagulation studies will remain within normal parameters.
■ Patient will communicate understanding of medical regimen, diet, medications, and activity restrictions.

Suggested NOC outcomes

Cardiac Pump Effectiveness; Circulation Status; Fluid Balance; Tissue Perfusion: Cardiac; Vital Signs

Interventions and rationales

■ Monitor patient's heart rate and rhythm, CVP, and blood pressure every hour until stable, then every 2 hours; record and report any changes above or below established limits. Monitor skin color and temperature every 2 hours. *Decreased heart rate, CVP, and blood pressure can indicate hypovolemia, which leads to decreased tissue perfusion. Blanched or mottled, cool skin indicates decreased tissue perfusion.*
■ Monitor respiratory rate and depth every hour until stable, then every 2 to 4 hours. Record and report changes outside established limits. *Increased respiratory rate is a compensatory mechanism of tissue hypoxia that can result from decreased tissue perfusion.*
■ Measure and record urine output every hour until output exceeds 30 ml/hour, then every 2 to 4 hours. *If patient has no history of renal disease, urine output is a*

good indicator of tissue perfusion. Decreased or absent urine output usually indicates poor renal perfusion.

■ Perform appropriate measures to treat the underlying cause of hypovolemia. *Patient must receive treatment for the underlying cause to avoid continued or worsening hypovolemia.*

■ Administer fluid or blood, as ordered. Monitor for such adverse reactions as fluid overload and transfusion reactions. *Vigorous fluid or blood resuscitation can cause fluid overload and cardiac decompensation. Transfusion reactions can occur during blood administration and may further compromise patient's condition.*

■ Initiate measures to help improve perfusion.

– Keep patient warm, but don't overheat. *Warmth aids vasodilation, which improves tissue perfusion.*

– Relieve anxiety and pain. *Anxiety and pain can cause a sympathetic reaction that results in vasoconstriction and decreased tissue perfusion.*

– Elevate patient's lower extremities *to increase arterial blood supply and improve tissue perfusion.*

■ Perform pulmonary toilet, as ordered; follow facility policies. *Properly performed pulmonary toilet helps prevent pulmonary edema, respiratory complications, and possible respiratory failure.*

■ Test urine specific gravity every shift; record and report abnormalities. *Concentrated urine with increased specific gravity indicates hypovolemia.*

■ Weigh patient daily before breakfast and record weight. *Weighing patient daily helps predict total fluid status; weighing at regular times and using the same scale give a better indication of weight changes.*

■ Change patient's position regularly, follow turning schedule, inspect his skin every shift, and record and report any potential areas of breakdown. *These measures help prevent decreased tissue perfusion and reduce the risk of skin breakdown.*

■ Watch for signs of confusion and disorientation. Frequently reorient patient to reality: call him by name; tell him your name; and orient him to his surroundings (sounds, smells, and sights). *A change in LOC can result from decreased tissue perfusion. Reorientation helps patient recall time, place, and person and can also reduce fear and anxiety.*

■ Monitor Hb level, HCT, WBC count, and coagulation studies. Frequency depends on the severity of patient's problem. *Monitoring helps establish blood replacement requirements, fluid status, blood viscosity level, and anticoagulation therapy parameters and allows detection of infection.*

■ Educate patient in the medical regimen (diet, medications, and activity restrictions) *to allow patient to take an active role in health maintenance.*

Suggested NIC interventions

Circulatory Care: Arterial Insufficiency; Circulatory Care: Venous Insufficiency; Fluid Management; Hemodynamic Regulation; Intravenous (IV) Therapy; Shock Management

Evaluations for expected outcomes

■ Patient's hemodynamic measurements remain within established limits.

■ Patient's daily fluid intake equals output.

■ Patient's urine specific gravity remains within normal parameters.

■ Patient maintains respiratory rate within established limits.

■ Patient maintains normal skin color and doesn't exhibit redness or skin breakdown.

■ Patient can identify self and state time of day, date, and location.

■ Patient has clear lung fields on auscultation.

■ Patient exhibits improved circulation as evidenced by strong, palpable peripheral pulses; normal skin color and temperature; and normal blood pressure and other hemodynamic measurements.

■ Patient's Hb level, HCT, WBC count, and coagulation studies remain within normal parameters.

■ Patient communicates understanding of medical regimen, diet, medications, and activity restrictions.

Documentation

■ Patient's expression of concern about hemodynamic status

■ Observations of vital signs, intake and output, status of skin, and level of orientation

■ Patient's response to nursing interventions

■ Instructions about diet, monitoring, and medical regimen

■ Evaluations for expected outcomes

Reference

Cottingham, C.A. "Resuscitation of Traumatic Shock: A Hemodynamic Review," *AACN Advanced Critical Care* 17(3):317-26, July-September 2006.

Ineffective
TISSUE PERFUSION (CEREBRAL)

related to interruption of venous blood flow

Definition

Decrease in oxygen resulting in the failure to nourish the tissues at the capillary level

Assessment

■ Vital signs

■ History of the event, including presenting problem, history of development, chief complaint, associated vascular problems, and associated psychosocial problems (which may contribute to behavioral changes)

■ Neurologic status, including level of consciousness (LOC); Glasgow Coma Scale score (eye, motor, and verbal response); orientation; pupil size; response to light and accommodation; motor activity; strength, positioning, and appearance of all four extremities; presence of reflexes (corneal, gag, swallowing, and Babinski's); nuchal rigidity; weakness; numbness; headaches; dizziness; dysphagia; slurred speech; seizure activity; posturing; and Cushing's triad (increased systolic pressure, decreased diastolic pressure, and decreased heart rate)

■ Respiratory status, including shallow or irregular breathing pattern

Defining characteristics

- Altered mental status
- Behavioral changes
- Change in motor response
- Difficulty swallowing
- Pupillary changes
- Speech abnormalities
- Weakness or paralysis in extremity

Expected outcomes

- Patient will maintain or improve current LOC.
- Patient's intracranial pressure (ICP) will remain between ____ mm Hg and ____ mm Hg.
- Patient's blood pressure will remain high enough to maintain cerebral perfusion pressure but low enough to prevent increased bleeding or cerebral swelling.
- Patient won't develop hypercarbia.
- Patient will remain free from pain.
- Patient will stay in quiet environment.
- Patient will maintain balanced intake and output.
- Patient will perform activities of daily living (ADLs) with maximum level of mobility and independence.
- Patient's risk factors for altered cerebral perfusion and complications will be reduced as much as possible.

Suggested NOC outcomes

Circulation Status; Cognitive Orientation; Communication; Coordinated Movement; Information Processing; Neurological Status; Neurological Status: Consciousness; Seizure Control; Tissue Perfusion: Cerebral

Interventions and rationales

- Conduct a neurologic assessment every 1 to 2 hours initially, then every 4 hours after patient becomes stable *to screen for changes in LOC and neurologic status.*
- Take vital signs every 1 to 2 hours initially, then every 4 hours after patient becomes stable *to detect early signs of decreased cerebral perfusion pressure or ICP.*
- Take patient's temperature at least every 4 hours. *Hyperthermia causes increased ICP; hypothermia causes decreased cerebral perfusion pressure.*
- Elevate the head of patient's bed 30 degrees *to promote venous drainage, thereby reducing cerebral edema.*
- Keep patient's head in neutral alignment *to keep the carotid flow unobstructed, thereby promoting perfusion.*
- If patient scores less than 10 on the Glasgow Coma Scale, hyperventilate patient on a ventilator in accordance with facility policy *to increase oxygenation and prevent cerebral swelling and hypercarbia.*
- Monitor for Cushing's triad, *which indicates impending herniation.*
- Keep the environment and patient quiet. Space nursing activities over the shift. *These measures may help to avoid an increase in ICP.*

■ If patient has a potentially compromised airway, use antiemetics or nasogastric suction *to prevent nausea and vomiting, which may lead to increased ICP and aspiration.*

■ Institute physical and occupational rehabilitation *to increase patient's ability for independent functioning.*

■ Prepare patient's discharge plan *to make sure patient continues to receive necessary rehabilitative care after discharge.*

■ Maintain adequate nutrition *to promote tissue healing, oxygenation, and metabolism.*

■ Maintain routine bowel and bladder function and administer diuretics, such as mannitol, as ordered, *to prevent increased ICP.*

■ Monitor hematocrit and hemoglobin level and report abnormalities *to prevent ischemia.*

■ Take measures to ward off infection *to prevent increased metabolic and oxygen demands that can interfere with the brain's metabolic needs.*

■ Measure accurate intake and output *to prevent volume overload or deficit.*

■ Instruct patient and family members in ways to minimize risk factors for altered tissue perfusion *to increase the probability that healthy adaptation will continue.*

■ Administer histamine-2 receptor antagonists, as ordered, *to prevent the development of stress ulcers.*

Suggested NIC interventions

Acid-Base Management; Cerebral Perfusion Promotion; Fluid/Electrolyte Management; Hemodynamic Regulation; Intracranial Pressure (ICP) Monitoring; Intravenous (IV) Therapy Management; Invasive Hemodynamic Monitoring; Neurologic Monitoring; Oxygen Therapy; Seizure Management; Vital Signs Monitoring

Evaluations for expected outcomes

■ Patient regains sense of orientation.
■ Patient's ICP remains within prescribed limits.
■ Patient's blood pressure remains high enough to maintain cerebral perfusion pressure but low enough to prevent increased bleeding or cerebral swelling.
■ Patient doesn't develop hypercarbia.
■ Patient remains free from pain.
■ Patient's environment remains quiet.
■ Patient maintains balanced intake and output.
■ Patient performs ADLs with maximum level of mobility and independence.
■ Patient's risk factors are reduced as much as possible.

Documentation

■ Observations of vital signs and neurologic findings
■ Intake and output
■ Patient's response to treatment of underlying condition
■ Medications administered and patient's response
■ Nursing interventions performed and patient's response

■ Family members' response to education and nursing interventions
■ Patient's response to physical and occupational therapy
■ Evaluation of care plan
■ Evaluations for expected outcomes

Reference
Iocono, L.A., and Lyons, K.A. "Making GCS as Easy as 1, 2, 3, 4, 5, 6," *Trauma Nursing* 12(3):77-81, July-September 2005.

Ineffective
TISSUE PERFUSION (GI)
related to exchange problems

Definition
Decrease in oxygen resulting in the failure to nourish the tissues at the capillary level

Assessment
■ Vital signs
■ GI status, including abdominal distention; nausea and vomiting; usual bowel habits; change in bowel habits; stool characteristics (color and consistency); presence or absence of occult blood; history of GI problems, disease, or surgery; pain; inspection of abdomen; palpation for tenderness; auscultation of bowel sounds; and abdominal girth
■ Nutritional status, including dietary intake, change from normal diet, current weight, and change from normal weight
■ Laboratory studies, including complete blood count, serum electrolyte levels, and liver profile
■ Medications (especially those with vasoconstrictive properties)

Defining characteristics
■ Abdominal distention
■ Abdominal pain or tenderness
■ Hypoactive or absent bowel sounds
■ Nausea

Expected outcomes
■ Patient's intake and output will remain within normal limits.
■ Patient's normal bowel function will return.
■ Patient won't experience any more nausea and vomiting.
■ Patient and family members will express understanding of need to modify dietary habits.
■ Patient will discuss with the physician the possible need to alter medication regimen.
■ Patient will express understanding of benefits of regular exercise in maintaining routine bowel habits.

- Patient's abdominal pain will subside.
- Patient's laboratory values will return to normal.
- Patient's vital signs will remain stable.
- Patient will express understanding of need to check stools for occult blood.

Suggested NOC outcomes

Bowel Elimination; Electrolyte & Acid/Base Balance; Fluid Balance; Hydration; Nausea & Vomiting Severity; Nutritional Status; Pain Level; Tissue Perfusion: Abdominal Organs

Interventions and rationales

- Monitor intake and output every 4 hours *to prevent hypovolemia, which can cause poor perfusion and subsequent ischemia.*
- Monitor patient's vital signs, including temperature, every 4 hours *to detect possible hypovolemia and screen for infection.*
- Monitor for increased abdominal tenderness *to detect early signs of increased ischemia.*
- Monitor bowel sounds and report changes. *Changes in bowel sounds can signal impending obstruction or a return to normal bowel function.*
- Monitor complete blood count, serum electrolyte levels, and liver function daily, as ordered, *to detect ischemia caused by low hematocrit and hemoglobin level, monitor for improvement in organ function, and screen for infection.*
- Administer prescribed pain medications sparingly. *Many opioids decrease gastric motility.* Use pain distraction techniques, if possible, *to provide relief with nonpharmacologic methods.*
- Implement nasogastric suctioning *to eliminate nausea and vomiting, thereby reducing the risk of inflammation.*
- Establish a bowel regimen *to prevent constipation.*
- When appropriate, provide alternative methods of nutrition, such as total parenteral nutrition, *to allow bowel rest and recovery and to prevent ischemic episodes after meals.*
- Start enteral feedings slowly and increase them gradually *to allow the recovering bowel to adapt to increased tissue demands.*
- Teach patient and family members about dietary habits that may have contributed to poor perfusion *to prevent future episodes of altered GI tissue perfusion.*
- Encourage patient to eat small, frequent meals, to increase fluid intake, and to eat more high-fiber foods (such as cruciferous vegetables and whole grains) *to prevent constipation and potential obstruction.*
- Teach patient the importance of routine exercise. *Routine exercise stimulates peristalsis.*
- Instruct patient to limit alcohol and fat intake *to preserve adequate liver function.*
- Teach patient to check all stools for occult blood *to monitor for blood loss, which may indicate anemia.*
- Encourage patient to discuss with the physician the need to avoid medications that have vasoconstrictive properties or that decrease peristalsis. *Such medications can contribute to decreased perfusion.*

■ Teach patient to rest after meals *to allow adequate blood circulation, thereby ensuring an oxygen supply for increased metabolic demands.*

Suggested NIC interventions

Bowel Management; Fluid/Electrolyte Management; Medication Management; Nutrition Management; Total Parenteral Nutrition (TPN) Administration

Evaluations for expected outcomes

■ Patient's intake and output remain within normal limits.
■ Patient's normal bowel function returns.
■ Patient's nausea and vomiting cease.
■ Patient and family members recognize need to modify dietary habits.
■ Patient expresses understanding of need to alter medication regimen.
■ Patient recognizes benefits of regular exercise in maintaining bowel habits.
■ Patient's abdominal pain subsides.
■ Patient's laboratory values return to normal.
■ Patient's vital signs remain stable.
■ Patient recognizes need to check stool for occult blood.

Documentation

■ Observations of physical findings
■ Results of laboratory studies
■ Intake and output
■ Nursing interventions to treat altered tissue perfusion
■ Effectiveness of nursing interventions
■ Stool characteristics, including color, consistency, and presence of occult blood
■ Evaluations for expected outcomes

Reference

Mullady, D.K., and O'Keefe, S.J. "Treatment of Intestinal Failure: Home Parenteral Nutrition," *Nature Clinical Practice Gastroenterology & Hepatology* 3(9):492-504, September 2006.

Ineffective
TISSUE PERFUSION (PERIPHERAL)
related to reduced arterial blood flow

Definition

Decrease in oxygen resulting in the failure to nourish the tissues at the capillary level

Assessment

■ History of vascular problems and disease (self or family)
■ Age
■ Gender

■ Integumentary status, including color, condition of nails, distribution of hair, lesions, temperature, texture, and edema

■ Cardiovascular status, including blood pressure, capillary refill time, clotting profile, Doppler studies, exercise test, heart rate and rhythm, pulses (brachial, femoral, pedal, peripheral, popliteal, posterior tibial, and radial), serum cholesterol and triglyceride levels, and venogram or arteriogram

■ Neurovascular status, including activity tolerance, mobility, and sensation

■ Nutritional status, including dietary patterns and weight

■ Psychosocial status, including alcohol intake, family support, history of smoking, occupation, and stressors

Defining characteristics

■ Altered condition of hair and nails

■ Altered sensation

■ Blood pressure changes in extremities

■ Bruits

■ Claudication

■ Edema

■ Positive Homans' sign

■ Skin discoloration, temperature changes, and moisture

■ Weak or absent pulses

Expected outcomes

■ Patient will express feelings of comfort or absence of pain at rest.

■ Patient won't develop arrhythmias.

■ Patient's peripheral pulses will remain present and strong.

■ Patient's skin color and temperature will remain unchanged.

■ Patient's feet will remain clean and free from pressure areas.

■ Patient will perform Buerger-Allen exercises.

■ Patient will lose ___ lb/week.

■ Patient will have a prothrombin time of 35 to 60 seconds.

■ Patient will practice relaxation techniques at least once every 8 hours.

■ Patient's ulcerated areas will heal.

■ Patient will demonstrate ability to perform skills needed to follow prescribed care regimen.

■ Patient will identify risk factors that exacerbate problem.

■ Patient will maintain tissue perfusion and cellular oxygenation.

■ Patient will reduce metabolic needs.

Suggested NOC outcomes

Sensory Function: Cutaneous; Tissue Integrity: Skin & Mucous Membranes; Tissue Perfusion: Peripheral; Vital Signs

Interventions and rationales

■ Elevate the head of the bed 30 degrees or place the head of the bed on 6″ to 8″ (15 to 20.5 cm) blocks *to promote circulation to lower extremities.*

■ Change patient's position every 2 hours *to reduce risk of skin breakdown.*

■ Administer analgesics and monitor effectiveness *to help reduce ischemic pain. Recording effectiveness guides further analgesic administration.*

■ Monitor patient's vital signs and heart rhythm every 4 hours. Report the development of a rapid, irregular pulse. *Rapid, irregular pulse can cause decreased cardiac output, which results in decreased tissue perfusion.*

■ Check peripheral pulses every 4 hours. Document the presence or absence and intensity of each. Use an ultrasonic blood flow detector if one is available. *Palpable, strong peripheral pulses indicate good arterial flow. Documentation reveals changes from one assessment to the next.*

■ Assess patient's skin color, temperature, and texture at least every 4 hours. Note, record, and report the development of mottling or black-and-blue areas. *Decreased tissue perfusion causes mottling; skin also becomes cooler and skin texture changes.*

■ Don't apply direct heat to extremities. You can apply heat to the abdomen; this causes reflex dilation of arteries of the lower extremities. *Directly heating extremities causes increased tissue metabolism; if arteries don't dilate normally, tissue perfusion decreases and ischemia may occur.*

■ Use light cotton blankets to cover patient's legs. *These provide insulation from cold but don't exert pressure on extremities.*

■ Use a bed cradle when patient has ulcerations or gangrene *to help prevent heavy sheets and blankets from resting on affected extremities.*

■ Provide meticulous foot care daily: soak patient's feet in warm water; trim nails carefully; rub feet with lanolin-based lotion; dry feet thoroughly; apply heel protectors; and instruct patient to wear white cotton socks. *These measures prevent cracking of dry skin and other complications.*

■ Teach patient to perform Buerger-Allen exercises twice per day: Raise the affected extremity above heart level and hold for 2 minutes; then lower the extremity to the dependent position and hold for 3 minutes. Repeat. *These exercises aid collateral circulation to patient's legs.*

■ Encourage ambulation to the level of tolerance *to encourage circulation to extremities.*

■ Provide a diet low in saturated fat *to reduce the risk of atherosclerosis, which further decreases circulation and tissue perfusion.*

■ Reduce patient's caloric intake to promote weight reduction. *Extra weight can stress the heart and decrease circulation.*

■ Help patient set goals for weight reduction *to give patient a sense of control and provide motivation.*

■ Consult a dietitian *to help patient modify eating patterns and habits.*

■ Administer anticoagulants, as ordered, *to prevent thrombi. Thrombi and emboli can further reduce arterial circulation and decrease tissue perfusion.*

■ Monitor clotting data *to guide the administration of anticoagulants.*

■ Administer vasodilators, alpha-adrenergic blocking agents, and other medications, as ordered. Monitor effectiveness and document patient response. *These agents aid vessel dilation, which promotes increased circulation. They work only if vessels can dilate.*

■ Teach patient relaxation techniques *to help improve vasodilation and help prevent vasoconstriction caused by anxiety.*

■ For patients with leg ulcers, follow a prescribed regimen. *Collaborative practice enhances overall patient care.*

■ Educate patient about:

– foot care

– importance of exercise

– need for low-cholesterol, low-calorie diet

– need to avoid tight clothes, crossing legs, and keeping legs dependent

– need to avoid vasoconstrictors (such as cold, stress, and smoking)

– precautionary measures to prevent injury.

These measures enable patient and family members to join actively in care and allow patient to make more informed decisions about his health status.

Suggested NIC interventions

Circulatory Care: Arterial Insufficiency; Fluid & Electrolyte Management; Foot Care; Nutrition Management; Peripheral Sensation Management; Skin Surveillance

Evaluations for expected outcomes

■ Patient indicates feelings of comfort, either verbally or through behavior.

■ Patient doesn't display arrhythmias during monitoring or examination.

■ Patient's radial, brachial, pedal, and popliteal pulses are present and palpable.

■ Patient's skin remains warm and dry, with normal color.

■ Patient's feet remain clean and don't exhibit signs of redness or breakdown.

■ Patient performs Buerger-Allen exercises.

■ Patient's weight decreases by established amount weekly.

■ Patient's prothrombin time remains between 35 and 60 seconds.

■ Patient practices relaxation techniques at least once every 8 hours.

■ Patient's ulcerated areas heal and don't require dressings.

■ Patient demonstrates skills needed to follow self-care regimen.

■ Patient states risk factors that may exacerbate problem.

■ Patient maintains tissue perfusion and cellular oxygenation.

■ Patient reduces metabolic needs.

Documentation

■ Patient's expressions of symptoms, such as pain, numbness, and muscle weakness

■ Observations of physical findings

■ Nursing interventions performed for patient

■ Patient's response to nursing interventions

■ Patient's response to education

■ Evaluations for expected outcomes

Reference

Sieggreen, M. "A Contemporary Approach to Peripheral Arterial Disease," *The Nurse Practitioner* 31(7):14-18, 23-25, July 2006.

Ineffective
TISSUE PERFUSION (PERIPHERAL)
related to reduced venous blood flow

Definition
Decrease in oxygen resulting in the failure to nourish the tissues at the capillary level

Assessment
- History of vascular problems or disease (self or family)
- Age
- Gender
- Medication history
- Integumentary status, including color, condition of nails, distribution of hair, lesions, temperature, and texture
- Cardiovascular status, including capillary refill time, clotting profile, Doppler studies, exercise test, heart rate and rhythm, pulses (brachial, femoral, pedal, peripheral, popliteal, posterior tibial, and radial), serum cholesterol and triglyceride levels, and venogram or arteriogram
- Neurovascular status, including activity tolerance, mobility, and sensation
- Nutritional status, including dietary patterns and weight
- Psychosocial status, including alcohol intake, family support, history of smoking, occupation, and stressors

Defining characteristics
- Altered condition of hair and nails
- Altered sensation
- Edema
- Positive Homans' sign
- Skin discoloration, temperature changes, and moisture
- Weak or absent pulses

Expected outcomes
- Patient won't develop embolization of thrombi.
- Patient will have less inflammation and improved venous blood flow.
- Patient's clotting studies will remain within therapeutic range.
- Patient will explain reasons for measures used to prevent pooling of blood in lower extremities.
- Patient will defecate without straining.
- Patient will demonstrate ability to perform skills needed for prescribed care regimen.
- Patient will identify risk factors that exacerbate problem.

Suggested NOC outcomes
Circulation Status; Tissue Integrity: Skin & Mucous Membranes; Vital Signs

Interventions and rationales

■ Monitor and record patient's temperature, pulse, respiration, and blood pressure at least every 4 hours. *Accurate monitoring of vital signs allows the detection of increased respiratory rate, pulse rate, and blood pressure, which may indicate pulmonary embolus.*

■ Auscultate and record breath sounds every 4 hours. *Decreased, absent, or adventitious breath sounds may result from pulmonary embolus.*

■ Observe for the development of pulmonary emboli. Report immediately any increase in temperature, pulse, or respiratory rate; decrease in blood pressure; anxious, apprehensive behavior; complaints of dyspnea, cough, or hemoptysis; or development of crackles or red, frothy sputum. *Embolization of thrombi from deep veins (legs and pelvis) frequently causes pulmonary embolus.*

■ Monitor clotting profile, as ordered, *to guide anticoagulant therapy and indicate the potential for clot formation.*

■ Administer anticoagulant therapy, monitor effectiveness, and observe for bleeding (epistaxis, bleeding gums, and petechiae) *to reduce the risk of further thrombosis by preventing clot propagation.*

■ Measure and compare the size of patient's calves every 4 hours. *Venous pooling and stasis can cause fluid to move into interstitial space to cause edema.*

■ Apply antiembolism stockings or intermittent pneumatic compression stockings, as ordered. Remove stockings for 1 hour every 8 hours or according to policy. *Stockings can decrease venous stasis, but they can also cause edema from constriction. Monitor their use closely.*

■ Apply moist heat to the affected extremity, as ordered (may be contraindicated in chronic venous insufficiency). *Moist heat can aid vasodilation, reduce vasospasm, and enhance venous return.*

■ Elevate the affected extremity. Don't use a knee gatch or pillows under the knees, and explain the reasons for not using them to patient. *Elevation aids venous return; a knee gatch or pillows under the knees hinder venous return because they elevate the knees above the feet.*

■ Instruct patient not to cross his legs or lie in the fetal position. Explain the importance of remembering not to cross his legs. *Crossing legs constricts popliteal vessels, thus reducing venous return and promoting venous stasis.*

■ Increase patient's activity, as ordered. *This helps prevent venous pooling and stasis and promotes venous return.*

■ Urge patient to elevate his legs when sitting in a chair, supporting the entire length of his legs. *Elevating the legs aids venous return. Supporting the entire leg ensures blood flow.*

■ Encourage patient to walk. Discourage prolonged standing in one place. *Walking promotes venous blood flow by causing muscles to compress veins. Standing promotes venous stasis.*

■ Use stool softeners *to avoid constipation and straining during defecation. Valsalva's maneuver, used in straining during defecation, decreases venous blood return.*

■ Educate patient about anticoagulant therapy; the importance of having blood work done, as ordered; the need to report bleeding gums and blood in urine and secretions; and dietary precautions while on anticoagulant therapy, such as minimizing the intake of green, leafy vegetables if he's taking an oral agent. *Leafy vegetables contain vitamin K, which inhibits anticoagulants such as warfarin.*

■ Educate patient about the use of antiembolism stockings or intermittent pneumatic compression stockings; avoidance of crossing legs, wearing constrictive clothing, or standing in one place; and the importance of protecting extremities from injury. *Education allows patient and family members to take an active role in health maintenance.*

Suggested NIC interventions

Circulatory Care: Venous Insufficiency; Embolus Precautions; Exercise Therapy: Ambulation; Fluid Management; Neurologic Monitoring; Nutrition Management; Pain Management; Skin Surveillance

Evaluations for expected outcomes

■ Patient doesn't exhibit indications of embolization, such as increased respiratory rate, pulse rate, and blood pressure; decreased, absent, or adventitious breath sounds; and signs and symptoms of pulmonary embolus.

■ Patient's inflammation decreases and venous blood flow improves.

■ Patient's prothrombin time and partial thromboplastin time remain within established limits.

■ Patient explains reasons for measures used to prevent pooling of blood in lower extremities.

■ Patient defecates without straining.

■ Patient demonstrates ability to perform skills needed for prescribed care regimen.

■ Patient lists risk factors that exacerbate reduced venous blood flow or demonstrates understanding of risk factors through behavior.

Documentation

■ Patient's expression of feelings about hospitalization and current situation
■ Observations of physical findings
■ Clotting profile
■ Administration of anticoagulant therapy, including adverse effects
■ Nursing interventions performed to promote circulation to lower extremities
■ Patient's response to nursing interventions
■ Patient's response to education
■ Evaluations for expected outcomes

Reference

Sol, B.G., et al. "Vascular Risk Management Through Nurse-led Self-management Programs," *Journal of Vascular Nursing* 23(1):20-24, March 2005.

Ineffective
TISSUE PERFUSION (RENAL)
related to decreased cellular exchange

Definition
Decrease in oxygen resulting in the failure to nourish the tissues at the capillary level

Assessment
■ Health history, including surgery, any condition resulting in fluid volume depletion, and use of nephrotoxic drugs
■ Renal status, including color of urine, intake and output, presence of anuria or oliguria, urine specific gravity, and weight
■ Cardiovascular status, including blood pressure, central venous pressure, hemodynamic readings, jugular filling, and presence of dependent edema, fluid retention, or palpitations
■ Respiratory status, including auscultation of breath sounds, respiratory rate and rhythm, and shortness of breath
■ Neurologic status, including level of consciousness (LOC), mental status, orientation, decreased tolerance to activity, fatigue, and weakness
■ Integumentary status, including color, moisture, and presence of edema and secondary skin ulcerations from edema
■ Nutritional status, including thirst and signs of anorexia
■ Laboratory studies, including blood urea nitrogen (BUN) and creatinine levels, creatinine clearance, hemoglobin and serum electrolyte levels, and urine osmolality

Defining characteristics
■ Blood pressure readings outside acceptable parameters
■ Elevated BUN and creatinine levels
■ Hematuria
■ Oliguria or anuria

Expected outcomes
■ Patient will maintain fluid balance.
■ Patient will maintain urine specific gravity within normal limits (specify).
■ Patient's weight won't fluctuate.
■ Patient will report increased comfort.
■ Patient will maintain hemodynamic stability.
■ Patient will identify risk factors that exacerbate decreased tissue perfusion and will modify lifestyle appropriately.
■ Patient will communicate understanding of medical regimen, medications, diet, and activity restrictions.

Suggested NOC outcomes
Circulation Status; Electrolyte & Acid/Base Balance; Fluid Balance; Hydration; Tissue Perfusion: Abdominal Organs; Urinary Elimination

Interventions and rationales

■ Monitor and document intake and output every hour until output exceeds 30 ml/hour, then every 2 to 4 hours. *If patient has no history of renal disease, urine output is a good indicator of tissue perfusion. Decreased or absent urine output usually indicates poor renal perfusion.*

■ Document urine color and characteristics. Report changes. *Concentrated urine may indicate poor kidney function or dehydration.*

■ Weigh patient daily before breakfast and record weight. *Weighing patient daily helps predict total fluid status; weight gain may indicate fluid overload. Weighing at regular times gives a better indication of weight changes.*

■ Assess for dependent edema. *Dependent edema may indicate a lack of kidney function.*

■ Observe voiding patterns *to note deviations from normal.*

■ Monitor urine specific gravity and serum electrolyte, BUN, and creatinine levels. *Rising levels may indicate decreased kidney function.*

■ Monitor hemodynamic status and vital signs. Notify the physician of changes. *Increase from baseline may indicate fluid overload caused by a lack of kidney function.*

■ Explain the reasons for therapy and its intended effects to patient and his family *to encourage patient to take an active role in health maintenance.*

■ Allow for frequent rest periods *to enable patient to conserve energy.*

■ Refer patient to a dietitian for a special diet for renal impairment *to help patient avoid foods that place increased demands on the kidneys.*

■ Instruct patient to check with the physician before taking over-the-counter medications. *Some may be nephrotoxic.*

■ Provide patient and family members with psychological support if renal failure becomes chronic *to encourage healthy adaptation.*

Suggested NIC interventions

Acid-Base Management; Fluid Monitoring; Hemodynamic Regulation; Laboratory Data Interpretation; Medication Management; Nutrition Management

Evaluations for expected outcomes

■ Patient maintains fluid balance.

■ Patient maintains urine specific gravity within normal limits (specify).

■ Patient's weight doesn't fluctuate.

■ Patient reports increased comfort.

■ Patient maintains hemodynamic stability.

■ Patient recognizes risk factors that exacerbate problem and changes lifestyle appropriately.

■ Patient communicates understanding of medical regimen, medications, diet, and activity restrictions.

Documentation

■ Patient's expressions of concern over signs and symptoms of decreased tissue perfusion

■ Vital signs, intake and output, LOC, and other clinical findings
■ Nursing interventions performed to maintain fluid balance and hemodynamic stability
■ Patient's response to nursing interventions
■ Patient's response to education
■ Evaluations for expected outcomes

Reference
Chikotas, N., et al. "Uremic Syndrome and End-stage Renal Disease: Physical Manifestations and Beyond," *Journal of the American Academy of Nurse Practitioners* 18(5):195-202, May 2006.

Impaired
TRANSFER ABILITY
related to neuromuscular dysfunction

Definition
Limitation of independent movement between two nearby surfaces

Assessment
■ Age
■ Gender
■ Vital signs
■ Drug history
■ History of neuromuscular disorder or dysfunction
■ Musculoskeletal status, including coordination, muscle size and strength, muscle tone, range of motion (ROM), functional mobility as follows:
0 = completely independent
1 = requires use of equipment or device
2 = requires help, supervision, or teaching from another person
3 = requires help from another person and equipment or device
4 = dependent; doesn't participate in activity
■ Neurologic status, including level of consciousness, motor ability, and sensory ability
■ Endurance—for example, how long patient can remain sitting in wheelchair before becoming fatigued
■ Knowledge of wheelchair transfer techniques

Defining characteristics
■ Impaired ability to transfer:
– From bed to chair
– On or off a toilet or commode
– In and out of tub or shower
– Between uneven levels
– From chair to car or car to chair

– From chair to floor or floor to chair
– From standing to floor or floor to standing

Expected outcomes

■ Patient won't exhibit complications associated with impaired wheelchair transfer mobility, such as depression, altered health maintenance, and falls.
■ Patient will maintain or improve muscle strength and joint ROM.
■ Patient will achieve highest level of mobility possible (independence with regard to wheelchair transfer, ability to transfer to wheelchair with assistance, verbalization of needs regarding wheelchair transfer).
■ Patient will maintain safety during wheelchair transfer.
■ Patient will adapt to alteration in ability to perform wheelchair transfer.
■ Patient will demonstrate understanding of wheelchair transfer techniques.
■ Patient will participate in social and occupational activities to the greatest extent possible.

Suggested NOC outcomes

Balance; Body Positioning: Self-Initiated; Joint Movement: Hip, Knee, Spine; Knowledge: Body Mechanics; Mobility; Transfer Performance

Interventions and rationales

■ Perform ROM exercises to the joints of affected limbs, unless contraindicated, at least once per shift. Progress from passive to active ROM, as tolerated, *to prevent joint contractures and muscle atrophy.*
■ Identify patient's level of independence using the functional mobility scale. Report the findings to the staff *to provide continuity and preserve the documented level of independence.*
■ Monitor and record daily evidence of complications related to altered mobility or decreased ability to perform wheelchair transfer (contractures, venous stasis, skin breakdown, thrombus formation, depression, altered health maintenance, or self-care deficit). *Patients with neuromuscular dysfunction are at risk for complications.*
■ Teach patient wheelchair transfer techniques, such as performing a standing or sitting transfer, *to maintain muscle tone, prevent complications of immobility, and promote independence.* Adapt teaching to the limits imposed by his condition *to prevent injury.*
■ Refer patient to a physical therapist for the development of a wheelchair mobility program *to assist with rehabilitation of musculoskeletal deficits.*
■ Encourage patient to attend physical therapy. Request a written copy of wheelchair transfer instructions to use as a reference *to maintain continuity of care and foster safety.*
■ Assess patient's skin upon his return to bed and request a wheelchair cushion, if necessary, *to maintain skin integrity.*
■ As part of your teaching plan, demonstrate transfer techniques to family members and note the date. Have them perform a return demonstration *to ensure the use of proper technique and to promote continuity of care.*
■ Identify resources (stroke program, sports association for disabled, National Multiple Sclerosis Society) *to promote patient's reintegration into the community.*

Suggested NIC interventions

Body Mechanics Promotion; Energy Management; Exercise Promotion: Strength Training; Exercise Therapy: Balance; Fall Prevention; Self-Care Assistance: Transfer

Evaluations for expected outcomes

▪ Patient doesn't exhibit complications associated with impaired wheelchair transfer mobility, such as depression, altered health maintenance, and falls.
▪ Patient maintains or improves muscle strength and joint ROM.
▪ Patient achieves highest level of mobility possible (independence with regard to wheelchair transfer, ability to transfer to wheelchair with assistance, verbalization of needs regarding wheelchair transfer).
▪ Patient maintains safety during wheelchair transfer.
▪ Patient adapts to alteration in ability to perform wheelchair transfer.
▪ Patient demonstrates understanding of wheelchair transfer techniques.
▪ Patient participates in social and occupational activities to the greatest extent possible.

Documentation

▪ Patient's mobility status
▪ Presence of complications
▪ Evidence of alterations in patient's ability to perform wheelchair transfer
▪ Patient's statements regarding difficulties in wheelchair transfer
▪ Instruction of transfer techniques
▪ Patient's and family members' return demonstration of skills
▪ Patient's response to nursing interventions
▪ Evaluations for expected outcomes

Reference

Gavin-Dreschnack, D., et al. "Wheelchair-related Falls: Current Evidence and Directions for Improved Quality Care," *Journal of Nursing Care Quality* 20(2): 119-27, April-June 2005.

Risk for

TRAUMA

related to external factors (chemical, environmental, physical agents)

Definition

Accentuated risk of accidental tissue injury, such as burns and fractures

Assessment

▪ Health history, including accidents, allergies, exposure to pollutants, falls, hyperthermia, hypothermia, poisoning, sensory or perceptual changes (auditory, gustatory, kinesthetic, olfactory, tactile, and visual), seizures, and trauma

■ Circumstances of current situation that might lead to injury from surgery or from chemical, physical, or human agents

■ Neurologic status, including level of consciousness, mental status, and orientation

■ Laboratory studies, including clotting factors, hemoglobin level, hematocrit, and platelet and white blood cell counts

Risk factors
■ Lack of safety precautions
■ Unsafe home environment
− Pot handles facing toward front of stove
− Obstructed passageways
− Overloaded fuse boxes
− Litter or liquid spills in a passageway
− Defective appliances
− Bathing in very hot water
− Bathtub without hand grip or antislip equipment
− Entering unlighted rooms
− Unsturdy or absent stair rails
− Use of unsteady chairs or ladders
− Slippery floors
− Unanchored rugs
■ Poor vision
■ Balancing difficulties
■ Weakness

Expected outcomes
■ Patient will avoid injury.
■ Patient will state understanding of safety precautions.
■ Patient will use assistive devices correctly (walker or cane, for example).

Suggested NOC outcomes
Balance; Coordinated Movement; Fall Prevention Behavior; Knowledge: Fall Prevention; Risk Control; Safe Home Environment

Interventions and rationales
■ Observe, record, and report falls, seizures, and unsafe practices. *Accurate assessment promotes appropriate interventions; documentation ensures continuity of care.*
■ Monitor and record patient's respiratory status. *Trauma increases respiratory rate; other respiratory effects depend on the nature of the trauma.*
■ Monitor and record patient's neurologic status *to detect changes and to report deteriorated status.*
■ If patient has a seizure, remain with him, loosen restrictive clothing, and protect him from environmental hazards. Don't restrain him or pry his mouth open. Keep an oral airway at the bedside and maintain a patent airway. Turn patient to his side after the seizure stops and suction if secretions occlude the airway. Record seizure characteristics, including onset, duration, and body movements. Reorient patient to his surroundings and allow a rest period. *Remaining with patient pro-*

vides safety and information for accurate documentation of the event. Loosening clothing and proper positioning may prevent further harm.

■ Keep the side rails up at all times *to protect patient and provide a sense of security.*

■ Keep the bed in a low position except when providing direct care *to minimize the effects of a possible fall.*

■ Emphasize the importance of asking for help before getting up. *Illness or injury may have weakened patient.*

■ Help debilitated, weak, or unsteady patient to get out of bed. Ensure that the floor is dry and that furniture and litter don't block patient's way *to help prevent falls.*

■ When using soft restraints, don't secure them too tightly *to avoid skin burns.*

■ Use leather restraints following facility policy; pad them well before applying. Release each extremity on a rotation basis every hour; check for skin burns. *Such restraints should be used only when other kinds are ineffective.*

■ Instruct patient and family members in safety practices such as correct use of a walker, crutches, or cane. *These enable patient and family members to take an active role in health care and maintain a safe environment.*

Suggested NIC interventions

Environmental Management: Safety; Fall Prevention; Health Education; Pressure Ulcer Prevention; Seizure Precautions; Surveillance: Safety; Teaching: Disease Process

Evaluations for expected outcomes

■ Patient remains free from injury.
■ Patient identifies specific safety precautions.
■ Patient demonstrates proper use of assistive devices (specify).

Documentation

■ Patient's statements that indicate potential for injury
■ Physical findings
■ Observations or knowledge of unsafe practices
■ Interventions performed to prevent injury
■ Patient's response to nursing interventions
■ Evaluations for expected outcomes

Reference

Poe, S.S., et al. "An Evidence-based Approach to Fall Risk Assessment, Prevention, and Management: Lessons Learned," *Journal of Nursing Care Quality* 20(2):107-16, April-June 2005.

Risk for
TRAUMA
related to internal factors

Definition
Accentuated risk of accidental tissue injury, such as burns and fractures

Assessment
■ Health history, including accidents, allergies, exposure to pollutants, falls, hyperthermia, hypothermia, poisoning, sensory or perceptual changes (auditory, gustatory, kinesthetic, olfactory, tactile, and visual), seizures, and trauma
■ Circumstances of current situation that might lead to injury
■ Neurologic status, including level of consciousness, mental status, and orientation
■ Laboratory studies, including albumin and globulin levels, clotting factors, hemoglobin level, hematocrit, and platelet and white blood cell counts

Risk factors
■ Lack of safety precautions
■ Unsafe home environment:
– Pot handles facing toward front of stove
– Obstructed passageways
– Overloaded fuse boxes
– Litter or liquid spills in a passageway
– Defective appliances
– Bathing in very hot water
– Bathtub without hand grip or antislip equipment
– Entering unlighted rooms
– Unsturdy or absent stair rails
– Use of unsteady chairs or ladders
– Slippery floors
– Unanchored rugs
■ Poor vision
■ Balancing difficulties
■ Weakness

Expected outcomes
■ Patient will avoid injury.
■ Patient will voice need for understanding safety precautions.
■ Patient will use safety devices correctly (walker or cane, for example).

Suggested NOC outcomes
Falls Occurrence; Personal Safety Behavior; Physical Injury Severity; Risk Control; Safe Home Environment; Tissue Integrity: Skin & Mucous Membranes

Interventions and rationales

■ Observe, record, and report falls, seizures, and unsafe practices. *Accurate assessment promotes appropriate interventions; documentation ensures continuity of care.*
■ Monitor and record patient's respiratory status. *Trauma increases the respiratory rate; other respiratory effects depend on the nature of the trauma.*
■ Monitor and record patient's neurologic status *to assess changes and to report deteriorated status.*
■ For seizures:
– Keep the side rails up *to protect patient and provide a sense of security.*
– Pad the side rails *to protect patient.*
– Protect patient from further injury during seizure *to ensure well-being.*
– Position patient on his side *to prevent aspiration.*
– Record such seizure characteristics as onset, duration, and body movements *to help pinpoint the involved area of the brain and guide treatment.*
– If patient is confused and walking about after the seizure ends, walk with him and guide him back to his bed; don't try to restrain him *to prevent injury.*
■ To prevent falls:
– Keep the bed rails up *to enhance safety.*
– Maintain the bed in a low position except when providing direct care *to reduce the risk of injury.*
– Emphasize the importance of asking for help before getting up. *Illness or injury may have weakened patient.*
– Provide help in ambulating and going to the bathroom *to ensure safety.*
– Anticipate times when falls occur (during the night, after administering a diuretic, while patient is sitting in a chair) and monitor patient closely *to prevent injuries.*
■ Instruct patient and family members in the use of such assistive devices as a cane, walker, crutches, and wheelchair *to ensure their proper use and to provide patient with a feeling of security.*
■ Provide patient and family members with information about necessary safety precautions *to enable patient and family members to take an active role in health care and maintain a safe environment.*

Suggested NIC interventions

Environmental Management: Safety; Fall Prevention; Home Maintenance Assistance; Risk Identification; Seizure Precautions

Evaluations for expected outcomes

■ Patient remains free from injury during specific time frame.
■ Patient identifies need for specific safety precautions.
■ Patient demonstrates proper use of assistive devices (specify).

Documentation

■ Patient's statements about situation that indicate potential for injury
■ Physical findings
■ Record of falls, seizures, and unsafe practices
■ Interventions that reduce risk of injury

- Patient's response to nursing interventions
- Evaluations for expected outcomes

Reference

McCarter-Bayer, A., et al. "Preventing Falls in Acute Care: An Innovative Approach," *Journal of Gerontological Nursing* 31(3):25-33, March 2005.

Impaired
URINARY ELIMINATION
related to anatomical obstruction

Definition

Disturbance in urinary elimination

Assessment

- History of urinary tract disease, trauma, surgery, or previous urethral infection
- Age
- Gender
- Vital signs
- Genitourinary status, including characteristics of urine, excretory urography, pain or discomfort, palpation of bladder, urinalysis, and voiding patterns
- Fluid and electrolyte status, including blood urea nitrogen and creatinine levels, intake and output, mucous membranes (inspection), serum electrolyte levels, skin turgor, and urine specific gravity
- Nutritional status, including appetite, constipation, dietary intake, elimination habits, current weight and change from normal, and rectal examination
- Sexuality status, including capability, concerns, habits, and sexual partners
- Psychosocial status, including coping skills, patient's perception of health problem, self-concept (body image), family members, and stressors (such as finances and job)

Defining characteristics

- Dysuria
- Frequency
- Hesitancy
- Incontinence
- Nocturia
- Retention
- Urgency

Expected outcomes

- Patient will maintain fluid balance; intake will equal output.
- Patient will voice increased comfort.
- Patient will voice understanding of treatment.
- Patient will have few if any complications.

■ Patient will discuss impact of urologic disorder on himself and family members.

■ Patient will demonstrate skill in managing urinary elimination problem.

■ Patient will maintain urinary continence.

Suggested NOC outcomes

Urinary Continence; Urinary Elimination

Interventions and rationales

■ Observe patient's voiding pattern. Document urine color and characteristics, intake and output, and patient's daily weight. Report any changes. *Accurate intake and output measurements are essential for correct fluid replacement therapy. Urine characteristics help verify diagnosis.*

■ Administer appropriate care for the urologic condition and monitor progress (for example, strain urine). Report favorable and adverse responses to the treatment regimen. *Appropriate care helps patient recover from the underlying disorder. Reporting responses to treatment allows modification of the treatment, as needed.*

■ Observe bowel habits.

– Check for constipation.

– Check for fecal impaction; if present, disimpact and institute a bowel regimen. *These measures promote comfort and prevent loss of rectal muscle tone from prolonged distention.*

■ If patient requires surgery, give appropriate preoperative and postoperative instructions and care. *Accurate information allows patient to understand the procedure and builds trust in caregivers.*

■ Explain reasons for therapy and intended effects to patient and family members *to increase patient's understanding and build trust in caregivers.* If patient needs urinary diversion, prepare him for a change in body appearance (instruct patient and family members how to care for the ostomy site postoperatively). *Preparation and appropriate information helps patient and family members cope with changes.*

■ Provide supportive measures, as indicated.

– Administer pain medication and monitor patient *to reduce pain and assess the effects of medication.*

– Encourage fluids, as ordered, *to moisten mucous membranes and dilute chemical materials within the body.*

– Refer patient to a dietitian for instructions on diet. *Dietary changes may decrease urinary infections.*

– Assist with general hygiene and comfort measures, as needed. *Cleanliness prevents bacterial growth and promotes comfort.*

– Maintain the patency of catheters, drainage bags, and other urinary elimination equipment *to avoid reflux and risk of infection and ensure the effectiveness of therapy.*

– Provide meatal care according to facility policy *to promote cleanliness and comfort and reduce the risk of infection.*

■ Encourage patient to ventilate feelings and concerns related to his urologic problem. *Active listening conveys respect for patient; ventilation helps pinpoint patient's fears.*

■ Refer patient and family members to a psychiatric liaison nurse, sex counselor, or support group, when appropriate. *These resources help patient gain knowledge of himself and the situation, reduce anxiety, and promote personal growth. Community resources usually provide support and care not available in other health agencies.*

■ Explain the urologic condition to patient and family members, including instructions on preventive measures, if appropriate. Prepare for discharge according to individual needs. *Accurate health knowledge increases patient's ability to maintain health. Involving family members assures patient that he'll be cared for.*

Suggested NIC interventions

Anxiety Reduction; Fluid Management; Urinary Elimination Management; Urinary Retention Care; Weight Management

Evaluations for expected outcomes

■ Patient's fluid intake equals output.

■ Patient expresses feelings of comfort.

■ Patient voices understanding of treatment, including urinary diversion therapy, if appropriate.

■ Patient doesn't show evidence of skin breakdown, infection, or other complications.

■ Patient discusses disease, signs and symptoms, complications, treatments, and adjustments to lifestyle caused by altered urinary pattern.

■ Patient demonstrates proficiency in steps necessary to manage urinary elimination problems.

■ Patient maintains urinary continence.

Documentation

■ Observations of urologic condition and response to treatment regimen

■ Interventions to provide supportive care and patient's response

■ Instructions given to patient and family members on urologic problem, response to instructions, and demonstrated ability to manage patient's urinary elimination needs

■ Patient's expression of concern about urologic problem and its impact on body image and lifestyle; patient's motivation to participate in self-care

■ Evaluations for expected outcomes

Reference

Wilde, M.H., and Dougherty, M.C. "Awareness of Urine Flow in People with Long-term Urinary Catheters," *Journal of Wound, Ostomy and Continence Nursing* 33(2):164-74, March-April 2006.

Impaired
URINARY ELIMINATION
related to sensory motor impairment

Definition
Disturbance in urine elimination

Assessment
- History of urinary tract disease, trauma, surgery, or infection
- History of sensory or neuromuscular impairment
- Vital signs
- Genitourinary status, including characteristics of urine, cystometry, pain or discomfort, palpation of bladder, postcatheterization, presence and amount of residual urine, use of urinary assistive devices, urinalysis, and voiding pattern
- Fluid and electrolyte status, including blood urea nitrogen, creatinine, and serum electrolyte levels; inspection of mucous membranes; intake and output; skin turgor; and urine specific gravity
- Neuromuscular status, including degree of neuromuscular function, motor ability to start and stop urinary stream, and sensory ability to perceive bladder fullness
- Sexuality status, including capability, concerns, habits, and sexual partners
- Psychosocial status, including coping skills, family members, patient's perception of health problem, self-concept, and stressors (such as finances and job)

Defining characteristics
- Dysuria
- Frequency
- Hesitancy
- Incontinence
- Nocturia
- Retention
- Urgency

Expected outcomes
- Patient will maintain fluid balance; intake will equal output.
- Patient will voice increased comfort.
- Patient will have few if any complications.
- Patient and family members will demonstrate skill in managing urinary elimination problem.
- Patient will express feelings about condition.
- Patient will discuss impact of urologic disorder on himself and family members.
- Patient and family members will identify resources to assist with care following discharge.

Suggested NOC outcomes

Symptom Control; Urinary Continence; Urinary Elimination

Interventions and rationales

■ Monitor patient's neuromuscular status and voiding pattern; document and re-port intake and output. *Accurate intake and output measurements are essential for correct fluid replacement therapy. Data form the basis for a complete evaluation to diagnose the cause.*

■ Provide appropriate care for the urologic condition and monitor progress. Re-port responses to treatment. *Appropriate care helps patient recover from the under-lying disorder. Reporting responses to treatment allows modification of treatment, as needed.*

■ Assist with bladder elimination procedure, as indicated.

– For bladder training, place patient on the commode or toilet every 2 hours while awake and once during the night. Maintain regular fluid intake while pa-tient is awake. Provide privacy. Teach patient how to perform Kegel exercises to strengthen sphincter control. *These measures aid adaptation to routine physiologic function. Women with good muscle tone can improve levator muscle action signifi-cantly if they perform Kegel exercises regularly.*

– For intermittent catheterization, catheterize patient using clean or sterile tech-nique every ___ hours. Record amount voided spontaneously and amount ob-tained with catheterization (for example: 7 a.m., spontaneous void of 200 ml; catheter void of 150 ml). Record bladder balance daily. *These measures promote normal voiding, prevent infection, and help maintain integrity of ureterovesical func-tion. Catheterization schedule is based on flow sheet data and can provide a baseline chart.*

– Bladder balance = Amount of residual urine/Amount of voided urine

– For external catheterization (in a male patient), monitor patency. Apply a con-dom catheter according to the established policy. *Applying a foam strip in a spiral fashion increases the adhesive surface and reduces the risk of impairing circulation.* Avoid constriction. Observe the skin condition of the penis, and clean with soap and water at least twice daily. *These measures prevent infection and ensure thera-peutic effectiveness.*

– For an indwelling urinary catheter, monitor patency. Keep the tubing free from kinks and keep the drainage bag below the level of the bladder *to avoid urine re-flux.* Clean the urinary meatus according to the established policy, and maintain a closed drainage system *to prevent skin irritation and bacteriuria.* Secure the catheter to patient's leg (female) or abdomen (male); avoid tension on the sphinc-ter. *Anchoring the catheter avoids straining the trigone muscle of the bladder and prevents friction leading to inflammation.*

– For a suprapubic catheter, monitor patency. Change the dressing and clean the catheter site according to policy. Keep the tubing free from kinks; keep the drainage bag below bladder level. Maintain a closed drainage system. *Suprapubic drainage allows increased patient mobility and reduces the risk of bladder infection.*

■ Provide supportive measures.

– Administer pain medication and monitor patient *to reduce pain and assess the effects of medication.*

– Encourage fluid intake up to 3,000 ml every 24 hours (unless contraindicated) *to moisten mucous membranes and dilute chemical materials within the body.*

– Provide privacy during the toileting procedure *to avoid inhibiting elimination.*

– Respond to patient's call bell quickly, assign patient to the bed next to the bathroom, and have patient wear easily removed clothing (such as a gown rather than pajamas). *These measures reduce delay and impediments to the voiding routine.*

■ Alert patient and family members to the signs and symptoms of a full bladder: restlessness, abdominal discomfort, sweating, and chills. *Adequate education increases patient's and family members' ability to maintain health level and to prevent patient from harming himself.*

■ Instruct patient and family members on catheterization techniques to be used at home; provide time for return demonstrations until they can perform the procedure well. *Knowledge of procedures and rationales reduces anxiety and promotes comfort. Demonstrations may progress through several sessions until patient can perform independently.*

■ Instruct patient and family members on the signs and symptoms of autonomic dysreflexia (headache, cold sweat, nausea, and elevated blood pressure) and how to manage it (by checking for a kinked indwelling catheter, catheterizing, and elevating the head of the bed). Instruct patient and family members to call the physician or facility immediately if symptoms don't subside with initial treatment. *Autonomic dysreflexia, a medical emergency, is a pathologic reflex condition characterized by exaggerated autonomic responses to stimuli.*

■ Encourage patient to express his feelings and concerns related to his urologic problem. *Active listening conveys respect for patient; ventilation helps pinpoint patient's fears.*

■ Refer patient and family members to a psychiatric liaison nurse, sex counselor, home health care agency, or support group, when appropriate. *These resources help patient gain knowledge of himself and his situation, reduce anxiety, and help promote personal growth. Community resources usually provide care and support not available in other health agencies.*

Suggested NIC interventions

Fluid Management; Urinary Bladder Training; Urinary Catheterization; Urinary Elimination Management

Evaluations for expected outcomes

■ Patient's fluid intake equals output.

■ Patient expresses feeling of comfort.

■ Patient doesn't develop infection, swelling of penis, skin breakdown, or other complications, and urinalysis remains normal.

■ Patient and family members demonstrate skill in managing urinary elimination problem, including catheterization techniques to be used at home.

■ Patient expresses feelings about condition.

■ Patient expresses understanding of urologic disorder and its effect on his family and lifestyle after discharge.

■ Patient and family members identify and contact home health care agency, support group, or other resources, as needed.

Documentation
■ Observations of urologic condition and response to treatment regimen
■ Interventions to provide supportive care and patient's response
■ Instructions given to patient and family members, their understanding of instructions, and demonstrated ability to manage patient's urinary elimination
■ Patient's expression of concern about urologic problem and impact on body image and lifestyle; patient's motivation to participate in self-care
■ Evaluations for expected outcomes

Reference
Nordling, J. "Sensory Bladder Disorders," *International Journal of Clinical Practice* (151):38-42, December 2006.

URINARY RETENTION
related to obstruction, sensory, or neuromuscular impairment

Definition
Incomplete emptying of bladder

Assessment
■ History of sensory or neuromuscular impairment, prostate enlargement, surgery, urethral trauma or tumor, or urinary tract disease
■ Age
■ Gender
■ Vital signs
■ Genitourinary status, including pain or discomfort, palpation of bladder, residual urine volume after voiding, urethral obstruction (prostate hyperplasia or masses, fecal impaction, masses, and swelling), urinalysis, urine characteristics, and voiding patterns
■ Fluid and electrolyte status, including inspection of mucous membranes, intake and output, skin turgor, urine specific gravity, and serum electrolyte, blood urea nitrogen, and creatinine levels
■ Medication history
■ Neuromuscular status, including anal sphincter tone, motor ability to start and stop stream, neuromuscular function, and sensory ability to perceive bladder fullness and voiding
■ Sexuality status, including capability and concerns or partner's concerns
■ Psychosocial status, including coping skills, patient's or family members' perception of problem, self-concept, and stressors (such as finances and job)

Defining characteristics
■ Bladder distention
■ Dysuria
■ High residual urine
■ Overflow incontinence (continuous dribbling)

■ Sensation of bladder fullness

■ Small, frequent voiding or no urine output

Expected outcomes

■ Patient will maintain fluid balance, with intake equal to output.

■ Patient will voice increased comfort.

■ Patient will voice understanding of treatment.

■ Patient will have few if any complications.

■ Patient's urinalysis will remain normal.

■ Patient will avoid bladder distention.

■ Patient and family members will demonstrate skill in managing urine retention.

■ Patient will discuss impact of urologic disorder on himself and family members.

■ Patient and family members will identify resources to assist with care following discharge.

Suggested NOC outcomes

Knowledge: Treatment Regimen; Symptom Control; Symptom Severity; Urinary Continence; Urinary Elimination;

Interventions and rationales

■ Monitor intake and output. Report if intake exceeds output. *Accurate intake and output measurements are essential for correct fluid replacement therapy.*

■ Monitor voiding pattern. *Data on time, place, amount, and patient's awareness of micturition are needed to establish a pattern of incontinence.*

■ Assist with the ordered bladder elimination procedure as follows:

– voiding techniques. Perform Credé's or Valsalva's maneuver every 2 to 3 hours *to increase bladder pressure to pass urine.* Repeat until empty.

– intermittent catheterization. Catheterize using clean or sterile technique every 2 hours. Record amount voided spontaneously and amount obtained with catheterization. *These measures promote normal voiding, prevent infection, and help maintain the integrity of ureterovesical function.*

– use of an indwelling urinary catheter. Monitor patency and avoid kinks in tubing. Keep the drainage bag below bladder level *to avoid urine reflux.* Perform catheter care according to established policy and maintain a closed drainage system *to prevent skin irritation and bacteriuria.* Secure the catheter to patient's leg (female) or abdomen (male), avoiding tension on the sphincter. *Anchoring the catheter prevents straining of the bladder's trigone muscle and prevents friction leading to inflammation.*

– use of a suprapubic catheter. Change dressings according to facility policy. Monitor patency and avoid kinks in the tubing. Keep drainage bag below bladder level. Maintain closed drainage system. *Suprapubic drainage allows for increased mobility and reduces the risk of bladder infection.*

■ Administer pain medication, as ordered, and monitor patient *to reduce pain and assess the medication's effects.*

■ For fecal impaction, disimpact and institute a bowel regimen *to promote comfort and prevent the loss of rectal muscle tone from prolonged distention.*

■ Encourage a high fluid intake 2½ qt (2 L)/day, unless contraindicated, *to moisten mucous membranes and dilute chemical materials within the body.* Limit fluid intake after 7 p.m. *to prevent nocturia.*

■ Monitor therapeutic and adverse effects of prescribed medications *for early recognition and treatment of drug reactions.*

■ If patient requires surgery, give appropriate preoperative and postoperative instructions and care *to increase patient's understanding.* If he'll undergo urinary diversions, prepare him for a change in body image. *Preparation and appropriate information helps patient and family members cope with changes.*

■ Instruct patient and family members on voiding techniques to be used at home. Provide for return demonstrations until they can perform the procedure well. *Knowledge of procedures and rationales reduces anxiety and promotes comfort. Demonstrations may progress through several sessions until patient can perform independently.*

■ Encourage patient and family members to share feelings and concerns related to urologic problems. *Ventilation helps pinpoint patient's fears and establishes an environment of trust in which patient and family members can begin to deal with the situation.*

■ Refer patient and family members to a psychiatric liaison nurse, enterostomal therapist, sex counselor, support group, or home health care agency, when appropriate. *These resources help patient gain knowledge of himself and his situation, reduce anxiety, and help promote personal growth. Community resources usually provide services not available at other health agencies.*

Suggested NIC interventions

Distraction; Perineal Care; Urinary Bladder Training; Urinary Catheterization: Intermittent; Urinary Elimination Management

Evaluations for expected outcomes

■ Patient's fluid intake equals output.

■ Patient expresses feelings of comfort.

■ Patient expresses understanding of treatment, including ordered bladder elimination procedure and surgery, if appropriate.

■ Patient doesn't experience skin breakdown or other complications.

■ Patient's urinalysis remains normal.

■ Patient avoids bladder distention.

■ Patient and family members demonstrate skill in managing urine retention, including voiding techniques to be used at home.

■ Patient expresses at least one fear, one concern, and one positive feeling about urologic problem. If appropriate, patient expresses feelings and fears about surgery.

■ Patient or family contacts home health care agency, support group, or other resources, as needed.

Documentation
- Observations of urologic condition and response to treatment regimen
- Interventions to provide supportive care and patient's response
- Instructions given to patient and family members on urologic problem and their returned response and demonstrated ability to manage patient's urinary elimination
- Patient's concerns about urologic problem and its impact on body image and lifestyle; motivation to participate in self-care
- Evaluations for expected outcomes

Reference
O'Dell, K.K., and Labin, L.C. "Common Problems of Urination in Nonpregnant Women: Causes, Current Management, and Prevention Strategies," *Journal of Midwifery & Women's Health* 51(3):159-73, May-June 2006.

Impaired spontaneous
VENTILATION
related to respiratory muscle fatigue

Definition
Decreased energy reserves result in an individual's inability to maintain breathing adequate to support life

Assessment
- Health history, including previous respiratory problems
- Respiratory status, including rate, rhythm, and depth of respirations; chest excursion and symmetry; presence of cyanosis; and use of accessory muscles
- Effectiveness of cough in clearing secretions
- Suctioning demands, including frequency and tolerance
- Sputum characteristics, including appearance, consistency, color, and odor
- Neuromuscular strength and endurance
- Mental and emotional status, including cognitive state and ability to follow directions
- Laboratory values, including arterial blood gas (ABG) levels (baseline and ongoing), complete blood count, serum electrolyte levels, coagulation studies, serum and sputum cultures, and sensitivity tests
- Vital signs
- Functional status, including ability to perform activities of daily living (ADLs)
- Related or concurrent events that may contribute to respiratory distress, such as bleeding, hypervolemia, hypovolemia, and sepsis

Defining characteristics
- Apprehension
- Decreased arterial oxygen saturation
- Decreased cooperation

- Decreased partial pressure of arterial oxygen (Pao_2)
- Decreased tidal volume
- Dyspnea
- Increased metabolic rate
- Increased partial pressure of arterial carbon dioxide
- Increased restlessness
- Increased use of accessory muscles
- Tachycardia

Expected outcomes
- Patient's respiratory rate will remain within 5 breaths/minute of baseline.
- Patient's ABG levels will be normal.
- Patient will indicate feeling comfortable and won't report pain, dyspnea, or fatigue.
- Patient will carry out ADLs with minimal supplemental oxygen.
- Patient's breathing pattern will return to baseline.
- Patient's Pao_2 will remain within normal limits as his activity level increases.
- Patient will breathe spontaneously after ventilator support is withdrawn.

Suggested NOC outcomes
Anxiety Level; Endurance; Energy Conservation; Respiratory Status: Gas Exchange; Respiratory Status: Ventilation; Vital Signs

Interventions and rationales
- Monitor patient's vital signs every 15 minutes to 1 hour *to detect tachypnea and tachycardia, early indicators of respiratory distress.*
- Monitor patient for nasal flaring, change in depth and pattern of breathing, use of accessory muscles, and cyanosis *to detect signs of severe respiratory distress.*
- Monitor ABG levels and report deviations promptly *to determine the need for changes to the therapeutic regimen.*
- Monitor hemoglobin (Hb) level and hematocrit (HCT). *Low Hb level and HCT indicate decreased oxygen-carrying capacity of the blood.*
- Begin oxygen support using the smallest concentration needed to make patient comfortable. Monitor closely *to avoid oxygen toxicity.*
- Place patient in Fowler's position *to increase comfort and to promote adequate chest expansion and diaphragmatic excursion, thereby decreasing work of breathing.*
- Help patient progress gradually from bed rest to increased activity *to improve patient's sense of well-being.* Monitor vital signs and ABG levels closely. If respiratory status is compromised, return patient to bed rest *to decrease basal metabolic rate and lower oxygen demands.*
- Explain procedures to patient. Describe specific sensations he may experience during each procedure *to decrease anxiety.*
- Anticipate possible complications. Keep in mind that if patient decompensates while on 100% fraction of inspired oxygen nonrebreather mask, he may require endotracheal intubation. *Anticipating complications facilitates prompt intervention.*
- If patient requires intubation, monitor him for spontaneous breathing and gradually wean him from the ventilator. *Progressive weaning helps patient to adjust physiologically and emotionally to increased work of breathing.*

■ Avoid respiratory depressants, such as opioids, sedatives, and paralytics, *to facilitate patient's recovery.*

Suggested NIC interventions

Acid-Base Management; Airway Suctioning; Artificial Airway Management; Aspiration Precautions; Coping Enhancement; Mechanical Ventilation; Oxygen Therapy; Positioning; Respiratory Monitoring; Self-Care Assistance

Evaluations for expected outcomes

■ Patient's respiratory rate is within 5 breaths/minute of baseline.
■ Patient's ABG levels are normal.
■ Patient indicates feeling comfortable and doesn't report pain, dyspnea, or fatigue.
■ Patient carries out ADLs with minimal supplemental oxygen.
■ Patient's breathing pattern returns to baseline.
■ Patient's Pao_2 remains within normal limits when his activity level increases.
■ Patient breathes spontaneously after ventilator support is withdrawn.

Documentation

■ Patient's reports of malaise, dyspnea, restlessness, chest pain, dizziness, or light-headedness
■ Patient's response to nursing interventions
■ Patient's response to initiation of oxygen therapy and progressive changes in therapy
■ Laboratory data, including ABG levels
■ Respiratory status (baseline and ongoing)
■ Subtle personality changes
■ Changes in breath sounds revealed by auscultation
■ Evaluations for expected outcomes

Reference

Houseman, G., and Kelley, M. "Early Respiratory Insufficiency in the ALS Patient: A Case Study," *The Journal of Neuroscience Nursing* 37(4):216-18, August 2005.

Dysfunctional
VENTILATORY WEANING RESPONSE

Definition

Inability to adjust to lowered levels of mechanical ventilator support that interrupts and prolongs the weaning process

Assessment

■ Health history, including previous respiratory problems

■ Nutritional status, including caloric intake and type of and tolerance for feeding

■ Neurologic status, including mental status and level of consciousness (LOC)

■ Emotional status, including signs of anxiety or stress

■ Laboratory values, including arterial blood gas (ABG) levels (baseline and on-going), serum electrolyte and blood glucose levels, complete blood count, blood and sputum culture, and sensitivity tests

■ Weaning parameters and current ventilator settings

■ Respiratory status, including respiratory rate, pattern, character, and depth; chest expansion and symmetry; sputum characteristics (color, amount, odor, and consistency); cough effectiveness; presence of cyanosis in mucous membranes and nail beds; and auscultation of breath sounds

■ Need for suctioning, including frequency and patient's response

■ Musculoskeletal status, including muscle mass, strength, and endurance level

■ Cognitive state, including patient's ability to follow directions and readiness to learn

■ Recent administration of potential respiratory-depressant medications, such as opioids, sedatives, and neuromuscular blockers

■ Vital signs

■ Pulse oximetry readings

Defining characteristics

■ Mild dysfunctional weaning response
- Breathing discomfort
- Expressed increased need for oxygen
- Fatigue
- Increased concentration on breathing
- Queries about possible machine malfunction
- Restlessness
- Slight increase in respiratory response above baseline

■ Moderate dysfunctional weaning response
- Apprehension
- Changes in skin color (paleness and mild cyanosis)
- Decreased air entry on auscultation
- Diaphoresis
- Hypervigilance to activities related to ventilator functioning
- Inability to cooperate
- Inability to respond to coaching
- Increase in blood pressure (no more than 20 mm Hg above baseline)
- Increase in heart rate (no more than 20 beats/minute above baseline)
- Increase in respiratory rate (no more than 5 breaths/minute above baseline)
- Slight respiratory accessory muscle use
- Wide-eyed

■ Severe dysfunctional weaning response
- Adventitious breath sounds
- Agitation
- Audible airway secretions
- Breathing uncoordinated with ventilator

– Cyanosis
– Decreased LOC
– Deteriorating ABG levels
– Full use of respiratory accessory muscles
– Increased blood pressure (more than 20 mm Hg above baseline)
– Increased heart rate (more than 20 beats/minute above baseline)
– Paradoxical abdominal breathing
– Profuse diaphoresis
– Shallow, gasping breaths
– Significant increase in respiratory rate

Expected outcomes

■ Patient will maintain respiratory rate within 5 breaths/minute of baseline during weaning period.
■ Patient's ABG levels will remain within acceptable limits (specify).
■ Patient's mental status and emotional state will remain stable during gradual withdrawal of ventilatory support.
■ Patient will express comfort with progressive ventilator changes.
■ Patient will experience no dyspnea, fatigue, or pain during progressive ventilator changes.
■ Patient will remain within adequate weaning parameters:
– Tidal volume: 4 to 5 cc/kg
– Negative inspiratory force: greater than or equal to –20 cm H_2O
– Vital capacity: 10 to 15 cc/kg
– Minute ventilation: 6 to 10 L
■ Patient's cough will effectively clear secretions.

Suggested NOC outcomes

Anxiety Self-Control; Client Satisfaction: Technical Aspects of Care; Depression Self-Control; Respiratory Status: Gas Exchange; Respiratory Status: Ventilation; Risk Control; Vital Signs

Interventions and rationales

■ Monitor patient's vital signs every hour when changing ventilator settings. *Fever, tachycardia, tachypnea, and elevated blood pressure may indicate hypoxemia.*
■ Auscultate for breath sounds every 2 hours and report deviations. *Adventitious sounds may precede respiratory failure.*
■ Place patient in a comfortable position (preferably Fowler's) *to facilitate adequate chest expansion and drainage.*
■ Describe all weaning procedures to patient. Explain to patient that he may experience changes in his breathing rate and pattern, increased difficulty breathing, and fatigue *to decrease anxiety.*
■ If patient is receiving intermittent mandatory ventilation (IMV), begin to decrease IMV by increments of 2 breaths/minute. This process may take place over days or weeks. *Lowering IMV encourages patient to take his own breaths, thereby exercising respiratory muscles.*

■ Monitor ABG levels with every ventilator change *to assess for adequate oxygenation and acid-base balance.*

■ Include periods of rest between ventilator changes, especially at night, *to reduce tissue oxygen demand.*

■ If patient tolerates IMV of 2 to 4 breaths/minute, try pressure support ventilation (PSV). *PSV prolongs positive airway pressure during inspiration, allowing patient to regulate his own respiratory rate and tidal volume.*

■ When patient is breathing adequately without IMV, place him on continuous positive airway pressure (CPAP) of 5 cm H_2O *to prevent alveolar collapse.*

■ When patient tolerates CPAP, place him on T-piece (T-bar) of 30% to 50% fraction of inspired oxygen. *This allows patient to breathe on his own, continue to receive oxygen, and remain intubated in the event of respiratory compromise.*

■ When patient tolerates longer weaning periods, incorporate activities of daily living into his daily routine *to increase muscular strength and endurance.*

■ When patient has satisfactory respiratory status, weaning parameters, and ABG levels, assist with the removal of the ventilator tubes and keep the oxygen mask on hand *to prevent respiratory compromise.*

■ Assess patient for stridor, respiratory distress, and dysphonia and report these findings to the physician *to monitor the need for renewed ventilatory assistance.*

■ Perform chest physiotherapy and suctioning, as needed, *to maintain a patent airway.*

■ Monitor the respiratory effects of medications closely and evaluate the response to bronchodilators *to detect respiratory status compromise.* Avoid respiratory depressants.

Suggested NIC interventions

Acid-Base Management; Airway Management; Anxiety Reduction; Aspiration Precautions; Mechanical Ventilatory Weaning; Respiratory Monitoring; Support System Enhancement; Teaching: Procedure/Treatment; Vital Signs Monitoring

Evaluations for expected outcomes

■ Patient's respiratory rate is within 5 breaths/minute of baseline during weaning period.

■ Patient's ABG levels are within specified acceptable limits.

■ Patient maintains stable mental and emotional status during withdrawal of ventilatory support.

■ Patient expresses comfort with progressive ventilator changes.

■ Patient doesn't experience dyspnea, fatigue, or pain during progressive ventilator changes.

■ Patient remains within adequate weaning parameters.

■ Patient's cough effectively clears secretions.

Documentation

■ Patient's reports of malaise, anxiety, restlessness, breathlessness, and unusual pain

■ Patient's response to ventilator changes

■ Subtle changes in patient's mental or emotional status
■ Laboratory data, including ABG levels
■ Patient's response to nursing interventions, including positioning, chest physio-therapy, and suctioning
■ Patient's response to medications, including opioids, bronchodilators, and neu-romuscular blockers
■ Respiratory rate, pattern, and depth, including changes from baseline
■ Evaluations for expected outcomes

Reference
Pruitt, B. "Weaning Patients from Mechanical Ventilation," *Nursing* 36(9):36-41, September 2006.

Impaired
WALKING
related to neuromuscular dysfunction

Definition
Limitation of independent movement on foot

Assessment
■ Age
■ Gender
■ Vital signs
■ History of stroke, spinal cord injury, head injury, multiple sclerosis, Guillain-Barré syndrome, or Parkinson's disease
■ Medication history
■ Musculoskeletal status, including coordination, gait, muscle size and strength, muscle tone, range of motion (ROM), and functional mobility as follows:
0 = completely independent
1 = requires use of equipment or device
2 = requires help, supervision, or teaching from another person
3 = requires help from another person and equipment or device
4 = dependent; doesn't participate in activity
■ Neurologic status, including level of consciousness, motor ability, and sensory ability
■ Endurance level — for example, how far the patient can walk before tiring

Defining characteristics
■ Impaired ability to:
– Climb stairs
– Walk on an incline or decline
– Walk on uneven surfaces
– Walk required distances

Expected outcomes

■ Patient won't exhibit complications associated with impaired walking, such as alteration in skin integrity, contractures, venous stasis, or thrombus formation.
■ Patient will maintain or improve muscle strength and joint ROM.
■ Patient will achieve highest level of ambulation possible (independence using wheelchair, ambulation with device, ambulation without device).
■ Patient will maintain safety during ambulation.
■ Patient will demonstrate ability to use equipment or devices safely.
■ Patient will adapt to alteration in walking.
■ Patient will participate in social and occupational activities.
■ Patient will demonstrate understanding of specific interventions related to coping with alteration in walking.
■ Patient will utilize community resources to promote and maintain highest level of mobility.

Suggested NOC outcomes

Ambulation; Balance; Coordinated Movement; Endurance; Fall Prevention Behavior; Mobility; Safe Home Environment; Self-Care: Activities of Daily Living (ADL)

Interventions and rationales

■ Perform ROM exercises for joints of affected limbs, unless contraindicated, at least once per shift. Progress from passive to active ROM, as tolerated, *to prevent joint contractures and muscle atrophy.*
■ Make sure that patient maintains anatomically correct and functional body positioning. Encourage repositioning every 2 hours when patient is in bed. Establish a turning schedule for dependent patients. *Proper positioning relieves pressure, thereby preventing skin breakdown and fluid accumulation in dependent extremities.*
■ Identify patient's level of independence using the functional mobility scale. Communicate the findings to the staff *to provide continuity and preserve documented level of independence.*
■ Implement a preambulation program (for example, turning in bed, sitting on the side of the bed, sitting up in a chair) *to increase independence and patient's self-esteem.*
■ Monitor and record daily evidence of complications related to altered walking, such as contractures, venous stasis, skin breakdown, or thrombus formation. *Patient with a history of neuromuscular dysfunction is at risk for complications.*
■ Perform a medical regimen to manage or prevent complications (for example, administration of prophylactic heparin for venous thrombosis) *to promote patient's health and well-being.*
■ Provide progressive ambulation up to the limits imposed by patient's condition *to maintain muscle tone and prevent complications associated with immobility.*
■ Refer patient to a physical therapist for development of a program to promote walking *to assist with rehabilitation of musculoskeletal deficits.*
■ Encourage attendance at physical therapy sessions and reinforce prescribed activities by using the same equipment, devices, and techniques used in therapy ses-

sions. Request a written copy of patient's ambulation program to use as a reference. *These measures maintain continuity and help ensure patient's safety.*

■ Instruct patient and family members in ambulation techniques and measures *to prevent complications to help prepare patient and family for discharge.*

■ Demonstrate ambulation regimen and note the date. Have patient and family members perform a return demonstration *to ensure continuity of care and use of proper technique.*

■ Assist in identifying resources, such as a community stroke program, sports associations for the disabled, or the National Multiple Sclerosis Society, *to promote patient's reintegration into the community.*

Suggested NIC interventions

Energy Management; Exercise Promotion: Strength Training; Exercise Therapy: Ambulation; Self-Care Assistance

Evaluations for expected outcomes

■ Patient doesn't exhibit complications associated with impaired walking, such as alteration in skin integrity, contractures, venous stasis, or thrombus formation.

■ Patient maintains or improves muscle strength and joint ROM.

■ Patient achieves highest level of ambulation possible (independence using wheelchair, ambulation with device, ambulation without device).

■ Patient maintains safety during ambulation.

■ Patient demonstrates ability to use equipment or devices safely.

■ Patient adapts to alteration in walking.

■ Patient participates in social and occupational activities.

■ Patient demonstrates understanding of specific interventions related to coping with alteration in walking.

■ Patient utilizes community resources to promote and maintain highest level of mobility.

Documentation

■ Patient's ambulation status, presence of complications, and response to ambulation program

■ Patient's statements regarding loss of ambulation ability, current ambulation ability, and goals set for improved ambulation ability

■ Patient teaching

■ Return demonstration of skills for carrying out ambulation program

■ Patient's response to nursing interventions

■ Evaluations for expected outcomes

Reference

Watters, C.L., and Moran, W.P. "Hip Fractures — A Joint Effort," *Orthopedic Nursing* 25(3):157-65, May-June 2006.

II Adolescent health

INTRODUCTION

This section focuses on providing nursing care for adolescent patients. The tremendous physiologic and cognitive changes that occur between ages 10 and 18 are commonly accompanied by overpowering emotional turmoil.

Because the adolescent patient commonly struggles with issues of independence and identity, be particularly sensitive to this when taking his history. Be alert to language; adolescents particularly resent being "talked down to." Let the patient decide the level of parental involvement. Although some adolescents prize their independence, others still need parental support during physical examination and history taking. However, if possible, perform at least part of the nursing assessment in private to allow for open discussion of highly personal issues such as sexuality.

Many adolescents feel invulnerable, and this places them at high risk for such health problems as drug and alcohol abuse, sexually transmitted diseases, and trauma. When talking with the adolescent patient, explore feelings of personal invulnerability and discuss potential consequences.

When planning interventions, think of ways to foster independence and promote self-esteem while helping the adolescent obtain needed support from parents, health care providers, and others. Refer to care plans included in the sections on Adult Health and Child Health as well. Use every opportunity to teach the adolescent patient about health promotion. Increased knowledge allows the adolescent to assume responsibility for himself.

Adolescence can be a trying time for families as well. In addition to asking direct questions about family relationships, be alert to nonverbal and verbal indications of conflict. Also, be aware that parents may be struggling with their adolescent's newly found independence and may need your help as well.

Disturbed
BODY IMAGE
related to an eating disorder

Definition
Confusion in mental picture of one's physical self

Assessment
- Age
- Gender
- Health history, including previous eating disorders; dieting; physical, emotional, or sexual abuse; and episodes of emesis
- Exercise pattern, including type and duration
- Cardiovascular status, including skin color and temperature, heart rate and rhythm, blood pressure, and complete blood count
- Nutritional status, including daily food intake, food likes and dislikes, meal preparation, and knowledge of dietary requirements; height and weight (and weight fluctuations) over past year; and serum albumin, lymphocyte, and electrolyte levels
- Psychological status, including expressions of need for control or perceived loss of self-control, behavioral changes, expressions of helplessness, recent emotional crisis, stress, and body image
- Perception of ideal feminine or masculine form
- Family status, including role performance, perception of role within family, and attitudes and perceptions related to food, body image, success, and control
- Use of diuretics and laxatives

Defining characteristics
- Actual change in structure or function
- Expression of feelings and perceptions that reflect an altered view of one's body in appearance, structure, or function
- Behaviors of avoiding, monitoring, or acknowledging one's body
- Hiding or overexposing body part (intentional or unintentional)
- Missing body part
- Nonverbal response to actual or perceived change in structure or function
- Not looking at or touching body part
- Trauma to nonfunctioning part
- Preoccupation with change or loss
- Personalization of part or loss by name
- Depersonalization of part or loss by impersonal pronouns
- Extension of body boundary to incorporate environmental objects
- Negative feelings about body
- Verbalization of change in lifestyle
- Focus on past strength, function, or appearance
- Fear of rejection by others
- Emphasis on remaining strengths

■ Heightened achievement

Expected outcomes
■ Adolescent will comply with prescribed treatment.
■ Adolescent will express feelings associated with food, exercise, weight loss, and medical condition.
■ Adolescent will describe perception of personal daily caloric needs.
■ Adolescent will express understanding that current eating and exercise patterns are self-destructive.
■ Adolescent will consume appropriate number of calories each day.
■ Adolescent will ask for help in controlling destructive behavior.
■ Adolescent will participate in decisions about care and treatment.
■ Adolescent will participate in support group for people with eating disorders.
■ Adolescent will express insight into reasons behind current eating patterns and other self-destructive behaviors.
■ Adolescent will learn and implement new coping behaviors.
■ Adolescent will express positive feelings about self.
■ Adolescent will express satisfaction with parental involvement in care.

Suggested NOC outcomes
Body Image; Child Development: Adolescence; Grief Resolution; Nutritional Status; Psychosocial Adjustment: Life Change; Self-Esteem; Weight: Body Mass

Interventions and rationales
■ Implement the adolescent's prescribed therapy *to help restore health and body function.*
■ Monitor and record the adolescent's vital signs, weight, and electrolyte levels *to detect abnormal values and prevent complications.*
■ Obtain a referral for dietary consultation *to identify caloric intake, necessary diet modifications, and goals for weight gain and stabilization.*
■ Obtain a referral for psychiatric evaluation *to identify problems related to altered body image, poor self-esteem, and inappropriate coping.*
■ Convey a positive, caring attitude to the adolescent and take steps to ensure continuity of care throughout treatment *to ensure safety and foster a trusting therapeutic relationship.*
■ Encourage the adolescent to participate in self-care and, as appropriate, to make decisions about therapy *to foster a sense of control and involvement in restoring health.*
■ Tell the adolescent that you accept her as a person and provide reassurance that she can overcome her problems *to validate self-perception and enhance confidence.*
■ Maintain communication throughout the adolescent's course of treatment *to assess coping mechanisms and level of self-esteem.*
■ Encourage the adolescent to express feelings about self, eating, exercise, hospitalization, and medical condition *to correct misconceptions, help her clarify her thoughts, and reinforce realistic self-appraisal.*
■ Reinforce appropriate behaviors *to encourage the adolescent to comply with therapy and to participate in care.*

■ Use behavior modification strategies consistently *to enable the adolescent to predict consequences of behavior.*

■ Avoid using coercive techniques to make the adolescent participate in care or adhere to rules. *Use of coercion may encourage the adolescent to view manipulative behavior as acceptable.*

■ Monitor food consumption and record intake *to ensure that the adolescent consumes prescribed calories.*

■ Monitor the adolescent in the bathroom *to detect episodes of purging.*

■ Without conveying an attitude of distrust, watch for signs of noncompliance with the medical regimen. Emphasize that prescribed caloric intake is necessary to maintain health and won't lead to obesity. *This promotes early detection of self-destructive behavior and may improve the adolescent's sense of control.*

■ Inform the adolescent of her progress throughout hospitalization *to increase her awareness of achievements and motivate her to keep trying.*

■ Help the adolescent to identify positive aspects of her appearance *to improve self-esteem by correcting distorted perceptions about body image.*

■ Help direct the adolescent's need for control away from body image and eating behaviors by encouraging her participation in appropriate diversional activities *to channel her energies into new areas in which she can take pride.*

■ Encourage the adolescent's participation in group discussions with peers who also have eating disorders *to foster insight and group support.*

■ Help the adolescent identify appropriate coping strategies. Discuss previously effective strategies *to help her substitute them for maladaptive ones.*

■ Encourage parents to demonstrate emotional support for the adolescent throughout the course of treatment *to strengthen the family support system.*

■ Encourage parents to participate in a support group with other parents of children with eating disorders *to provide a forum for expressing feelings and obtaining support from individuals who can understand their concerns.*

■ Teach parents how to detect signs that their child may be relapsing into self-destructive behaviors *to help them identify the need for early assistance and enhance their confidence in their ability to protect their child from harm.*

Suggested NIC interventions

Active Listening; Body Image Enhancement; Coping Enhancement; Counseling; Developmental Enhancement: Adolescent; Parent Education: Adolescent; Support Group; Therapy Group

Evaluations for expected outcomes

■ Adolescent complies with prescribed treatment regimen.

■ Adolescent expresses feelings associated with food, exercise, weight loss, and medical condition.

■ Adolescent describes her perception of personal daily caloric needs.

■ Adolescent expresses understanding that her current eating and exercise patterns are self-destructive.

■ Adolescent consumes appropriate number of calories each day.

■ Adolescent asks for help in controlling destructive behavior.

■ Adolescent participates in decisions related to care and treatment.

■ Adolescent participates in support group for people with eating disorders.

■ Adolescent expresses insight into reasons behind her eating patterns and other self-destructive behaviors.
■ Adolescent learns and implements new coping behaviors.
■ Adolescent expresses positive feelings about self.
■ Adolescent expresses satisfaction with parental involvement in care.

Documentation
■ Vital signs
■ Weight (recorded daily or weekly according to facility's protocol)
■ Amount of food consumed at each meal
■ Adolescent's description of herself
■ Observations of rituals related to food and exercise
■ Adolescent's participation in and response to support group
■ Observations of self-destructive behaviors, such as forced emesis or use of laxatives or diuretics
■ Observations of manipulative behaviors
■ Coping mechanisms
■ Exercise patterns
■ Behavior modification techniques used by caregivers
■ Adolescent's response to treatment protocol
■ Adolescent's response to nursing interventions
■ Evidence of changes in adolescent's self-perception
■ Evaluations for expected outcomes

Reference
Harris, M., and Cumella, E.J. "Eating Disorders Across the Life Span," *Journal of Psychosocial and Mental Health Services* 44(4):20-26, April 2006.

Risk for
CAREGIVER ROLE STRAIN
related to developmental state

Definition
Adolescent's inability to meet developmental needs because of responsibilities to act as caregiver

Assessment
■ Adolescent caregiver's physical and mental status, including age, sex, and developmental stage; level of cognitive functioning; emotional functioning; and self-care abilities
■ Care recipient's physical and mental status, including age, sex, illness, self-care limitations, mobility limitations, level of cognitive functioning, and relationship to adolescent (parent, sibling, or other)
■ Family status, including role performance and perception of role within family

- Available resources, including finances, emotional support system, community services, and health-related services, such as geriatric day care and home health nursing assistants
- Home environment, including structural barriers, layout of home, need for medical equipment or devices, and availability of transportation
- Cultural, ethnic, and religious background
- Perceived and actual obligations of adolescent
- Effect of caregiver responsibilities on adolescent
- Adolescent's coping skills, problem-solving abilities, and ability to participate in hobbies and preferred activities

Risk factors

- Codependency (between caregiver and recipient)
- Competing role commitments (caregiver)
- Developmental delay or disability (caregiver or recipient)
- Discharge of family member with significant home care needs (care recipient)
- Drug or alcohol addiction (caregiver or recipient)
- Inadequate housing, transportation, community services, or equipment for providing care
- Isolation (caregiver)
- Lack of developmental readiness for caregiver role
- Lack of experience (caregiver)
- Lack of respite or recreation (caregiver)
- Numerous, complex caregiving tasks
- Premature birth or congenital defect (recipient)
- Presence of abuse or violence (recipient)
- Probability of long duration of caregiving

Expected outcomes

- Adolescent will identify current stressors.
- Adolescent will identify and implement adaptive coping strategies.
- Adolescent will identify personal developmental needs and tasks.
- Adolescent will contact sources of support to help provide care.
- Adolescent will allot time each day for respite, recreation, and personal developmental activities.
- Adolescent will report reduced stress related to caregiver duties.

Suggested NOC outcomes

Caregiver Emotional Health; Caregiver Home Care Readiness; Caregiver Lifestyle Disruption; Caregiver-Patient Relationship; Caregiver Physical Health; Caregiver Stressors; Stress Level

Interventions and rationales

- Assess developmental stage and needs of the adolescent caregiver *to provide a basis for developing interventions that reduce caregiver role strain. During adolescence, individuals begin establishing their identity by trying various roles without assuming complete responsibility for them. The imposed role of caregiver impedes this developmental task.*

■ Help the adolescent identify current stressors. Discuss how her responsibility to act as a caregiver places limits on her lifestyle *to evaluate the degree of caregiver role strain.*

■ Encourage the adolescent to discuss coping skills used previously *to reinforce her confidence in her ability to manage the current situation and explore new ways to apply coping strategies.*

■ Help the adolescent identify informal sources of support, such as family members, support groups, or church groups that can help with caregiver tasks, *to provide opportunities for respite from caregiver activities.*

■ Teach the adolescent about formal sources of support, such as home health care agencies, social workers, physicians, clinics, and day-care centers, *to allow the adolescent to fulfill other obligations such as attending school.*

■ Encourage regular participation in enjoyable activities, such as sports, hobbies, reading, or social gatherings. *Incorporating enjoyable activities into the daily schedule helps discipline the adolescent to take needed breaks from caregiver responsibilities.*

■ Provide the adolescent with information about available support groups, and encourage participation. *Support groups provide an outlet for expressing feelings and foster a sense of support and belonging.*

■ Assess the adolescent's view of her actual and perceived responsibilities as a caregiver and correct any misconceptions. *Emotional ties to the care recipient, confusion about roles within the family, or codependence may cloud the adolescent caregiver's perceptions. Your input helps her develop a more objective view of the situation.*

Suggested NIC interventions

Caregiver Support; Coping Enhancement; Decision-Making Support; Family Involvement Promotion; Family Mobilization; Referral; Spiritual Support; Support Group

Evaluations for expected outcomes

■ Adolescent describes her emotional response to stressors in her life.
■ Adolescent identifies and uses adaptive coping strategies.
■ Adolescent identifies personal developmental needs and tasks.
■ Adolescent uses available support systems.
■ Adolescent schedules respite periods for personal developmental needs and recreation.
■ Adolescent reports reduced stress from caregiver responsibilities.

Documentation

■ Care recipient's physical and mental status and adolescent caregiver's responsibility for providing care
■ Current stressors identified by adolescent
■ Risk factors (developmental, situational, psychological, and pathophysiologic) for caregiver role strain
■ Adolescent's statements indicating intention to take actions to minimize stress, such as joining support group, seeking help from support services, and scheduling periods of respite

- Observations of adolescent's response to stress
- Coping strategies identified by adolescent and nurse
- Referrals provided
- Evaluations for expected outcomes

Reference
Siskowski, C. "Young Caregivers: Effect of Family Health Situations on School Performance," *The Journal of School Nursing* 22(3):163-69, June 2006.

DECISIONAL CONFLICT
related to sexual activity

Definition
Uncertainty about whether to engage in sexual activity

Assessment
- Age
- Gender
- Developmental stage, including physical maturity, cognition, beliefs, values, and ethics
- Family system, including nuclear family, extended family, birth order, family roles, and evidence of conflict
- History of sexual experiences, including experimentation, trauma, and other experiences
- Psychological status, including level of function, coping mechanisms, support systems, self-image, self-esteem, and attitude toward physical appearance
- Sociocultural status, including level of education, ethnicity, and religious affiliation
- Sexual orientation

Defining characteristics
- Delayed decision making
- Expressed feelings of distress and questioning of values and beliefs while attempting to decide
- Expressed uncertainty
- Focus on self
- Lack of experience or interference with decision making
- Physical indications of distress (such as increased heart rate, muscle tension, and restlessness)
- Vacillation between choices
- Verbalization of undesired consequences of alternative decisions

Expected outcomes
- Adolescent will express feelings about sexuality and sexual activity.

■ Adolescent will discuss conflicts between personal values and social pressures to be sexually active.

■ Adolescent will identify desirable and undesirable consequences of sexual activity.

■ Adolescent will describe family conflicts and will explore their potential effect on sexual conduct.

■ Adolescent will accept help from parents, other family members, friends, and health professionals.

■ Adolescent will report confidence in choosing sexual behavior consistent with personal values.

Suggested NOC outcomes

Coping; Decision-Making; Information Processing; Participation in Health Care Decisions; Personal Autonomy

Interventions and rationales

■ Visit the adolescent frequently and encourage frequent visits by family members *to promote a trusting therapeutic relationship and ease anxiety and fears.*

■ Encourage expressions of feelings about social and sexual patterns *to improve recognition of feelings and foster open discussion.*

■ Assess the adolescent's knowledge of sex and sexuality. Discuss sexual behavior and its potential consequences. Provide information about safer sex practices, birth control, and abstinence. *Correct information about sexual practices reduces the adolescent's confusion about whether to be sexually active.*

■ Listen attentively and remain nonjudgmental as the adolescent describes personal fears, values, and desires. *Nonjudgmental, active listening demonstrates your unconditional positive regard for the adolescent.*

■ Provide guidance as the adolescent explores options for sexual activity *to promote confidence in decision-making capabilities.*

■ Discuss peer pressure. Ask if the adolescent feels strong social pressure to be sexually active. Ask about other ways peers exert influence, and explore ways of coping with peer pressure. *The adolescent must learn to deal with peer pressure.*

■ Discuss family conflicts. Ask the adolescent if troubled family relationships are pushing her to become sexually active. *The adolescent may seek in sexual relationships love she doesn't receive from family members.*

■ Respect the adolescent's right to make choices based on personal values, desires, religious beliefs, cultural norms, and sexual preference *to foster autonomy and self-confidence.*

■ Help the adolescent identify a support network (friends, family, community services, and church or synagogue groups) and encourage their use in decision making *to help the adolescent make decisions and resolve conflicts in an emotionally supportive environment.*

Suggested NIC interventions

Counseling; Decision-Making Support; Mutual Goal Setting; Self-Responsibility Facilitation; Teaching: Individual

Evaluations for expected outcomes
■ Adolescent expresses feelings related to sexuality and sexual activity.
■ Adolescent describes conflicts between personal values and social pressure to become sexually active.
■ Adolescent expresses increased understanding of options regarding sexual activity and their potential consequences.
■ Adolescent discusses possible influences, including peer pressure and conflicts with family, on decision to be sexually active.
■ Adolescent identifies support network and uses it to aid decision making.
■ Adolescent reports feeling more comfortable with ability to make decisions regarding sexuality and sexual activity.

Documentation
■ Adolescent's statements indicating conflict over decision about whether to be sexually active
■ Adolescent's cognitive, emotional, and behavioral functioning
■ Adolescent's knowledge of birth control and safer sex practices
■ Nursing interventions to help adolescent make choices regarding sexuality and sexual conflict
■ Adolescent's response to interventions
■ Evaluations for expected outcomes

References
Hutchinson, M.K. "The Parent-Teen Sexual Risk Communication Scale (PTSRC-III): Instrument Development and Psychometrics," *Nursing Research* 56(1):1-8, January-February 2007.

Knauth, D.G., et al. "Effect of Differentiation of Self on Adolescent Risk Behavior: Test of the Theoretical Model," *Nursing Research* 55(5):336-45, September-October 2006.

DECISIONAL CONFLICT
related to substance use

Definition
Uncertainty about whether to use illicit drugs

Assessment
■ Age
■ Physical maturity
■ Sociocultural factors, including level of education, financial status, and ethnic group
■ Family history, including family roles, coping patterns, family's ability to meet adolescent's physical and emotional needs, and history of substance abuse in family members
■ Level of functioning (cognitive, emotional, and behavioral)

■ Coping mechanisms
■ Available support systems
■ Evidence of drug use, including drug toxicology screening, urinalysis, personality changes, and social withdrawal

Defining characteristics
■ Delayed decision making
■ Expressed feelings of distress and questioning of values and beliefs while attempting to decide
■ Expressed uncertainty
■ Focus on self
■ Lack of experience or interference with decision making
■ Physical indications of distress (such as increased heart rate, muscle tension, and restlessness)
■ Vacillation between choices
■ Verbalization of undesired consequences of alternative decisions

Expected outcomes
■ Adolescent will discuss conflict over drug use.
■ Adolescent will describe conflict between personal values and options and external value systems (parental, societal, peer, and legal).
■ Adolescent will identify perceived desirable and undesirable consequences of drug use.
■ Adolescent will accept assistance from parents, other family members, friends, and health care providers.
■ Adolescent will report increased comfort with making choices about drug use that are consistent with personal values.

Suggested NOC outcomes

Decision-Making; Family Functioning; Family Social Climate; Information Processing; Participation in Health Care Decisions

Interventions and rationales
■ Visit the adolescent frequently, scheduling a specific amount of time each day, *to promote trust and provide time when the adolescent can discuss feelings confidentially.*
■ Make the adolescent aware that you're willing to discuss all topics, including substance use. Assure him that all information will be kept confidential *to encourage honest discussion of concerns.*
■ Encourage the adolescent to explore feelings related to drug use, school, family, friends, and other vital topics. Remain nonjudgmental and be willing to listen to his values, beliefs, and concerns *to demonstrate that you regard him as a worthwhile person with valid values and beliefs.*
■ Ask the adolescent to describe family and home life *to assess for family conflict that may be creating emotional distress.* Provide referrals for family counseling if needed.
■ Ask the adolescent if peers pressure him to use drugs. Explore ways of coping with peer pressure. *The adolescent must learn to deal with peer pressure.*

■ Discuss the adolescent's self-esteem and explore ways of building self-esteem *to strengthen the adolescent's ability to deal with peer pressure.*

■ Help the adolescent explore alternative recreational activities, such as sports, art, music, community service, or participation in church or synagogue groups, *to help develop alternatives to substance use.*

■ Teach the adolescent about the health and legal consequences of substance abuse. *Accurate information will help him make informed, rational decisions.*

■ Encourage the adolescent to identify and use a support network (family, friends, clinics, school nurse, or other health care providers). *A support network can help the adolescent make decisions and resolve conflicts in an emotionally supportive environment.*

■ Refer the adolescent for long-term counseling if necessary. *Long-standing emotional conflicts may require in-depth intervention.*

Suggested NIC interventions

Counseling; Decision-Making Support; Learning Facilitation; Patient Contracting; Support System Enhancement

Evaluations for expected outcomes

■ Adolescent discusses conflict over whether to use drugs.

■ Adolescent discusses peer pressure, family conflict, or other factors that may be influencing him to use drugs.

■ Adolescent identifies health and legal consequences of drug use.

■ Adolescent identifies available sources of emotional support and requests help, if needed.

■ Adolescent reports increased self-esteem and ability to deal with peer pressure.

Documentation

■ Evidence of drug use

■ Adolescent's stated feelings about drug use

■ Adolescent's level of cognitive, emotional, and behavioral functioning

■ Interventions performed to help adolescent make choices about drug use

■ Adolescent's response to interventions

■ Evaluations for expected outcomes

References

Raphel, S. "Enormity of U.S. Substance Abuse and the Risks Children Face," *Journal of Child and Adolescent Psychiatric Nursing* 18(4):198-200, October-December 2005.

Terry-McElrath, Y.M., et al. "Substance Abuse Counseling Services in Secondary Schools: A National Study of Schools and Students, 1999-2003," *The Journal of School Health* 75(9):334-41, November 2005.

Ineffective
HEALTH MAINTENANCE
related to lack of ability to make deliberate and thoughtful choices

Definition
Inability to identify, manage, or seek out help to maintain health

Assessment
- Age
- Gender
- Developmental stage, including cognitive ability and physical maturity
- Level of knowledge about type 1 diabetes mellitus, routine health practices, preventive needs and safety measures, and treatment and follow-up
- Level of motivation to perform self-care
- Current health status, including height, weight, recent illnesses, and adolescent's perception of personal health status
- Social status, including lifestyle, activity level, sports, interests, and socioeconomic status
- Family health history, including history of diabetes mellitus

Defining characteristics
- Demonstrated lack of adaptive behaviors (internal or external environmental changes)
- Demonstrated lack of knowledge regarding basic health practices
- History of lack of health-seeking behaviors
- Reported or observed impairment of personal support systems
- Reported or observed inability to take responsibility for meeting basic health practices in any or all functional pattern areas
- Reported or observed lack of equipment or financial and other resources

Expected outcomes
- Adolescent will describe feelings about self-management of type 1 diabetes mellitus.
- Adolescent will describe disease process.
- Adolescent will describe influence of peer pressure on his health care practices.
- Adolescent will describe proper techniques for managing signs and symptoms of hypoglycemia, hyperglycemia, and ketosis.
- Adolescent will demonstrate ability to perform self-care activities, such as properly administering insulin and choosing appropriate foods.
- Adolescent won't exhibit signs or symptoms of hypoglycemia, hyperglycemia, or ketosis.

Suggested NOC outcomes
Health Beliefs: Perceived Resources; Health Promoting Behavior; Health Seeking Behavior; Knowledge: Health Behavior; Knowledge: Treatment Regimen; Risk Detection; Symptom Control

Interventions and rationales

■ Evaluate the adolescent's understanding of type 1 diabetes mellitus and attitude about the need to manage it. *This will help you determine which teaching interventions to use.*

■ Correct any misconceptions about type 1 diabetes mellitus and the therapeutic regimen. Use teaching materials appropriate for the adolescent's age *to increase his knowledge of his condition and instill confidence in his ability to manage it.*

■ Discuss peer pressure. Ask the adolescent if he feels that social pressure causes him to ignore his diet or avoid self-administering insulin. Ask if he feels embarrassed about his disorder. Explore ways of coping with peer pressure. *The adolescent must learn to deal with peer pressure.*

■ Observe as the adolescent performs self-care activities *to assess his skills and overall progress.*

■ Teach the adolescent how to interpret glycosylated hemoglobin results and correlate these values with the degree of metabolic control *to increase autonomy and decision-making skills.*

■ Provide written materials that cover each teaching topic. *These materials help reinforce learning and can refresh the adolescent's memory later.*

■ Describe resources available to help the adolescent manage his disorder. Consider arranging a visit with the hospital dietitian or diabetes counselor *to reinforce teaching.*

■ Work with the adolescent to develop an exercise plan *to prevent hypoglycemia.* The plan should identify a support person capable of assisting during a hypoglycemic episode and should include:
– obtaining blood glucose level before and after exercise
– consuming extra food before exercise (if blood glucose falls between 80 and 180 mg/dl) in form of carbohydrates
– abstaining from strenuous exercise if blood glucose is elevated
– wearing medical identification bracelet
– carrying quick-acting sugar in case hypoglycemia occurs.
These measures ensure the adolescent's safety while allowing participation in activities.

■ Discuss how to manage diabetes during illness. For example, explain that infections may lead to hyperglycemia or ketosis and that early detection of infection can reduce the severity of these episodes. Also, explain that fever, nausea, vomiting, and diarrhea require modifications in the prescribed diet such as substituting juice for raw fruits. Teach the adolescent to check over-the-counter medications, such as cold remedies, for sugar content and to avoid products high in sugar. Explain the importance of following the prescribed regimen for increasing insulin dosage in relation to blood glucose test results. *These measures help provide a sense of control, ensure safety, and prevent complications.*

■ Teach the adolescent to recognize signs and symptoms he must report to his health care provider *to improve management skills and ensure safety.*

■ Discuss possible complications, such as atherosclerosis, which most commonly affects eyes, kidneys, and lower extremities; and diabetic neuropathy, which may lead to loss of sensation, function, and paresthesia. *Understanding possible major complications may encourage the adolescent to adhere to the prescribed regimen.*

■ Encourage the adolescent to contact a support group sponsored by the Juvenile Diabetes Association *to provide peer support.*

Suggested NIC interventions

Health Education; Patient Contracting; Self-Modification Assistance; Self-Responsibility Facilitation; Support System Enhancement; Teaching: Disease Process

Evaluations for expected outcomes

■ Adolescent expresses feelings about self-management of type 1 diabetes mellitus.
■ Adolescent accurately describes disease process.
■ Adolescent discusses influence of peer pressure on his health care practices.
■ Adolescent demonstrates techniques for managing signs and symptoms of hypoglycemia, hyperglycemia, and ketosis.
■ Adolescent demonstrates proficiency in self-care activities, including administering insulin and selecting appropriate foods.
■ Adolescent doesn't exhibit signs or symptoms of hypoglycemia, hyperglycemia, or ketosis.

Documentation

■ Adolescent's statements indicating his understanding of type 1 diabetes mellitus, health-promoting activities, management techniques during exercise and illness, and necessary self-care skills
■ Adolescent's statements indicating disregard for consequences of failing to properly manage type 1 diabetes mellitus
■ Adolescent's response to interventions and teaching
■ Literature provided to adolescent about managing his disorder
■ Observations of adolescent's demonstrations of self-care techniques
■ Referrals to community resources or hospital services
■ Evaluations for expected outcomes

References

Cheung, R., et al. "Quality of Life in Adolescents with Type 1 Diabetes Who Participate in Diabetes Camp," *The Journal of School Nursing* 22(1):53-58, February 2006.

Schilling, L.S., et al. "Changing Patterns of Self-management in Youth with Type 1 Diabetes," *Journal of Pediatric Nursing* 21(6):412-24, December 2006.

Risk for
POISONING
related to substance abuse

Definition
Accentuated risk of accidental ingestion of drugs, alcohol, or other potentially hazardous substances in doses sufficient to cause poisoning

Assessment
- Age
- Gender
- Developmental stage, including cognitive ability and physical maturity
- Medication history (prescription and over-the-counter)
- Physical status, including evidence or history of renal or hepatic impairment, eating disorders, or substance abuse
- Family status, including living arrangement, family dynamics, history or current evidence of substance abuse, and financial status
- Social status, including peer group and related social pressures and level of activity
- Knowledge of risks associated with use of drugs, alcohol, or other potentially hazardous substances (such as fumes from glue, nitrous oxide propellants, or lighter fuel gases)
- Psychological status, including evidence of depression or depressive disorder, feelings of isolation, history of attempted suicide, and level of self-esteem
- Results of laboratory tests

Risk factors
- Cognitive or emotional difficulties
- Dangerous products stored within easy reach
- Drugs stored in unlocked cabinets or large supplies of drugs stored in home
- Insufficient finances
- Lack of proper precautions
- Lack of safety or drug education
- Use of illegal drugs contaminated with poisonous additives

Expected outcomes
- Adolescent will express understanding of harmful and potentially lethal effects of substance abuse.
- Adolescent will remain free from toxicity and other injuries during hospital stay.
- Adolescent will identify stressors and feelings that precipitate episodes of substance abuse.
- Adolescent will demonstrate two or more constructive techniques for coping with stressors.
- Adolescent will describe prescribed medication regimen, including dosage and administration schedule, and will demonstrate compliance.

■ Adolescent will describe available community resources and will express intention to contact them.

Suggested NOC outcomes

Family Physical Environment; Personal Safety Behavior; Risk Control; Risk Control: Drug Use; Safe Home Environment

Interventions and rationales

■ Follow a medical regimen to treat toxicity or other injury caused by substance abuse *to ensure the adolescent's safety and promote recovery.*

■ Teach the adolescent about the harmful and potentially lethal effects of abusing drugs, alcohol, or other dangerous substances *to enhance his knowledge, which may help him make better-informed decisions.* Provide appropriate written materials. *Written materials reinforce teaching and allow review after discharge.*

■ Help the adolescent identify stressors, such as depression, peer pressure, or family dysfunction, that may precipitate substance abuse *to provide a basis for developing strategies to prevent future episodes.*

■ Describe available community resources to help prevent or treat substance abuse. *Support services and groups can provide the adolescent with safe settings in which to explore problems and feelings and develop adaptive methods of coping.*

■ If medication is prescribed for the adolescent, explain the reason for the medication. Discuss administration techniques, schedule, dosage, cautions, and possible adverse effects *to promote compliance with the medication regimen.*

Suggested NIC interventions

Environmental Risk Protection; Health Education; Substance Use Prevention; Surveillance: Safety

Evaluations for expected outcomes

■ Adolescent describes harmful and potentially lethal effects of substance abuse.

■ Adolescent remains free from toxicity caused by use of drugs, alcohol, or other hazardous substances.

■ Adolescent describes stressors and feelings that precipitate episodes of substance abuse.

■ Adolescent demonstrates two or more constructive techniques for coping with such stressors as depression, peer pressure, and family dysfunction.

■ Adolescent describes prescribed medication regimen and demonstrates compliance.

■ Adolescent describes available community resources and expresses intention to contact appropriate support services.

Documentation

■ Interventions to treat toxicity or other injury
■ Factors that increase adolescent's risk of drug toxicity
■ Knowledge deficits and learning objectives
■ Teaching topics, materials, and methods
■ Adolescent's response to nursing interventions

- Indications that adolescent is using adaptive techniques to cope with stress, anxiety, peer pressure, or dysfunctional family
- Referrals to community resources or professionals for ongoing counseling
- Evaluations for expected outcomes

Reference

Fok, M.S., and Wong, D.Y. "A Pilot Study on Enhancing Positive Coping Behaviour in Early Adolescents Using a School-based Project," *Journal of Child Health Care* 9(4):301-13, December 2005.

Situational low
SELF-ESTEEM
related to problematic relationship with parents

Definition

Development of a negative perception of self-worth in response to a current situation

Assessment

- Age
- Gender
- Level of education
- Family history, including marital status of parents, financial status, family rules, ability of family to modify rules, consequences when rules are broken, how family members communicate, quality of communication, methods of conflict resolution, family alliances, family stability, ability of family to meet adolescent's physical and emotional needs, and disparities between adolescent's needs and family's ability to meet them
- Goals and values, including extent to which family permits adolescent to pursue individual goals and values
- Family genogram
- Parental status, including level of education, knowledge of normal growth and development, ability to agree on appropriate discipline, stability of parental relationship, and understanding of adolescent's self-esteem disturbance
- Adolescent's psychological status, including changes in appetite, energy level, motivation, personal hygiene, self-image, self-esteem, and sleep patterns; alcohol or drug abuse; reaction to puberty; quality of relationships with authority figures; and scholastic performance

Defining characteristics

- Behavior inconsistent with values
- Developmental changes
- Disturbed body image
- Failures and rejections
- Functional impairment
- Lack of recognition

- Loss
- Social role changes

Expected outcomes

- Adolescent and parents will describe areas of conflict.
- Adolescent will begin to express feelings openly to family members.
- Parents will encourage and support adolescent's attempt at expression of feelings.
- Adolescent will describe positive qualities about self.
- Parents will describe positive qualities of adolescent and family unit.
- Adolescent and parents will state plans for continued outpatient family treatment.

Suggested NOC outcomes

Body Image; Child Development: Adolescence; Depression Level; Motivation; Quality of Life; Self-Esteem

Interventions and rationales

- Provide a secure, structured environment for the adolescent and his parents *to foster open discussion of family conflicts.*
- Educate all family members about the schedule, purpose, and goals of individual and family treatment. *Awareness of expectations and rationale for treatment will enhance cooperation.*
- Encourage the adolescent to participate in group activities, group therapy, and individual counseling *to provide opportunities to develop enhanced self-esteem.*
- Encourage the adolescent to express feelings directly, such as "I'm mad because of my curfew." *Such statements help him get in touch with his feelings and talk about them.*
- Tell parents that their child is learning to express his feelings directly. *Because family communication patterns are deeply ingrained, parents may need time to adjust to their child's assertiveness.*
- Help parents understand the value of talking about feelings *to encourage them to express emotions appropriately and to discourage them from punishing their child for expressing his feelings toward them.*
- Provide the adolescent with a small notebook in which he can write positive events as they occur *to encourage him to focus on his strengths and to enhance self-esteem.*
- Teach parents to reward and praise the adolescent for expressing his feelings *to enhance his self-esteem.*
- Use role-playing to teach the adolescent different ways to respond to specific family conflicts. *This will help him develop problem-solving and negotiating skills.*
- Communicate with the outpatient clinician *to plan continued treatment for family.*
- Emphasize to the adolescent and parents the need for continued support and family therapy after discharge *to enhance compliance.*

Suggested NIC interventions

Developmental Enhancement: Adolescent; Family Support; Hope Instilla-tion; Mood Management; Self-Esteem Enhancement; Values Clarification

Evaluations for expected outcomes
- Adolescent and parents begin to talk about difficulties at home.
- Adolescent begins to express feelings directly to family members.
- Parents demonstrate support for adolescent's expression of feelings.
- Adolescent uses positive statements about self.
- Parents make positive statements about adolescent and family as a whole.
- Parents and adolescent agree to participate in outpatient treatment.

Documentation
- Specific family conflicts as described by adolescent and parents
- Adolescent's and parents' behavior when interacting with each other
- Nursing interventions to facilitate family communication and expression of feelings
- Frequency of family visits and therapy appointments
- Adolescent's description of his own strengths
- Referrals for continued treatment after discharge
- Evaluations for expected outcomes

Reference
Riesch, S.K., et al. "Parent-Child Communication Processes: Preventing Children's Health-risk Behavior," *Journal for Specialists in Pediatric Nursing* 11(1):41-56, January 2006.

SOCIAL ISOLATION

related to behavior that fails to conform to social norms

Definition
Aloneness experienced by the individual and perceived as imposed by others and as a negative or threatening state

Assessment
- Age
- Gender
- Developmental stage
- Level of education
- Reason for hospitalization (physiologic or psychiatric)
- Attitudes of family, friends, teachers, and other important individuals toward adolescent
- Available support systems

■ Factors contributing to social isolation, including delayed physical development, immaturity, altered mental status, changes in behavior or cognition, illness, and history of trauma
■ Self-esteem
■ Coping and problem-solving ability
■ Evidence of substance abuse
■ Current and past stressors
■ Sociocultural factors, including ethnic and religious background

Defining characteristics
■ Culturally unacceptable behavior
■ Description of lifestyle as solitary or circumscribed by membership in subculture
■ Evidence of physical or mental disability or altered state of wellness
■ Expressed feelings of being different from others
■ Expressed feelings of rejection or aloneness
■ Expressed frustration over inability to meet expectations of others
■ Inappropriate or immature interests or activities
■ Insecurity in public
■ Lack of family, friends, and social groups
■ Lack of purpose in life
■ Preoccupation with own thoughts
■ Projection of hostility in voice and behavior
■ Repetitive, meaningless actions
■ Sad, dull affect
■ Uncommunicative and withdrawn behavior (with poor eye contact)

Expected outcomes
■ Adolescent will express feelings of social isolation.
■ Adolescent will identify causes of social isolation.
■ Adolescent will participate in planning social activities.
■ Adolescent will identify personal behaviors that are considered socially unacceptable and will acknowledge the need for change.
■ Adolescent will demonstrate more socially acceptable behaviors.
■ Adolescent will exhibit effective interpersonal communication skills.
■ Adolescent will report feeling less isolated as social interaction improves and will report improved sense of self-esteem.

Suggested NOC outcomes

Aggression Self-Control; Communication; Family Social Climate; Leisure Participation; Loneliness Severity; Social Interaction Skills; Social Involvement; Social Support

Interventions and rationales
■ Assign a primary nurse to the adolescent *to enhance continuity of care, establish a trusting relationship, and provide an opportunity to practice developing a one-on-one relationship.*

■ Arrange uninterrupted time to talk with the adolescent during each visit. Listen to his concerns and feelings. Provide honest feedback (positive and negative) about his behavior *to encourage appropriate behaviors and reinforce awareness of inappropriate ones. Feedback is essential to behavior modification.*

■ Provide guidance as the adolescent explores possible causes for his sense of social isolation. Help him identify inappropriate behaviors, and teach him ways to improve communication and interpersonal skills *to foster socially acceptable behavior. When the adolescent becomes aware of the connection between unacceptable behavior patterns and his feelings of isolation, he may be more willing to learn new skills and behaviors.*

■ Make a contract with the adolescent that requires him to demonstrate one new behavior within a specific period. Reward successful changes in behavior. *Contracts can enhance self-esteem by giving the adolescent responsibility for making constructive changes and allowing enough time to practice new behavior and communication skills without fear of criticism if he falls short. Successful completion of the contract provides positive reinforcement.*

■ Demonstrate appropriate communication skills and behaviors in all interactions with the adolescent *to provide an example of appropriate behavior and reinforce teaching concepts.*

■ Engage the adolescent in role-playing activities that simulate social situations. Provide encouragement and positive reinforcement and avoid criticism *to provide an opportunity to rehearse new skills in a safe environment, which reduces anxiety and boosts self-confidence.*

■ Encourage the adolescent to participate in group activities and one-on-one interactions with staff members. *Gradual increases in social interaction help reduce the adolescent's feelings of social isolation and instill confidence in newly developed communication and interpersonal skills.*

■ Talk to the adolescent about community resources, such as social services or support groups, that can provide ongoing support. Provide names, addresses, and phone numbers whenever possible. *This provides the adolescent with ongoing opportunities for social interaction in a supportive environment.*

Suggested NIC interventions

Behavior Modification: Social Skills; Coping Enhancement; Counseling; Emotional Support; Socialization Enhancement; Support Group; Support System Enhancement; Therapy Group

Evaluations for expected outcomes

■ Adolescent expresses feelings of social isolation and desire for help.

■ Adolescent identifies causes of social isolation.

■ Adolescent takes part in planning social activities.

■ Adolescent identifies socially unacceptable personal behaviors and acknowledges the need for change.

■ Adolescent demonstrates more socially appropriate behaviors.

■ Adolescent exhibits effective communication skills.

■ Adolescent reports increased social interaction, decreased feelings of isolation, and improved self-esteem.

Documentation
- Observations of adolescent's behavior and communication skills
- Adolescent's description of causes for impaired social interaction
- Nursing interventions to promote behavior modification and improved socialization
- Adolescent's response to interventions
- Resources and referrals provided to adolescent or family members
- Evaluations for expected outcomes

Reference
Mahon, N.E., et al. "A Meta-analytic Study of Predictors for Loneliness During Adolescence," *Nursing Research* 55(5):308-15, September-October 2006.

Risk for
TRAUMA
related to feelings of personal invulnerability

Definition
Accentuated risk of accidental tissue injury, such as burns or fractures

Assessment
- Age
- Gender
- Level of education
- Developmental factors, including tendency to test independence and take risks (especially in company of peers), feelings of indestructibility, high level of energy, need for peer approval, and access to potential safety hazards (such as complex machinery or tools, farm equipment, car, motorcycle, jet ski, or snowmobile)
- Health history, including allergies, sports accidents, auditory or visual impairments, and seizure disorders
- Social history, including academic performance, sports, hobbies, social activities, and occupation
- Neurologic status, including level of consciousness and orientation

Risk factors
- Access to alcohol, drugs (prescription, over-the-counter, or illicit), poisons, or other toxic substances
- Access to vehicles
- Developmental stage and level of maturity
- Frequent unsupervised activities with peers
- History of chronic or periodic substance abuse
- Lack of experience operating a car, motorcycle, or other vehicle or poor understanding of safety issues related to operating a vehicle (such as driving at excessive speed or after using alcohol or drugs)
- Participation in contact sports

■ Use of complex power tools or machinery (at work, school, or home)

Expected outcomes

■ Adolescent will recover from injury while in hospital.
■ Adolescent won't experience additional injury while in hospital.
■ Adolescent will identify risks and behaviors he should avoid.
■ Adolescent will state understanding of appropriate safety precautions (for example, obeying speed limits, following fire prevention precautions, never driving while intoxicated, wearing helmet or seat belt, and using protective clothing or equipment).
■ Adolescent will state intention to adopt appropriate safety precautions.

Suggested NOC outcomes

Knowledge: Personal Safety; Personal Safety Behavior; Risk Control; Risk Detection

Interventions and rationales

■ Follow a medical regimen to treat the adolescent's injury *to promote recovery.*
■ Document risk factors and unsafe practices discovered through observation or through discussions with the adolescent *to plan effective interventions.*
■ Select teaching topics that will help the adolescent prevent future injuries and promote personal health — for example, automotive and motorcycle safety, proper use of protective equipment in sports, or alcohol and drug awareness. *Teaching the adolescent increases his knowledge and reinforces the notion that he's responsible for ensuring personal safety.*
■ Demonstrate the use of appropriate safety equipment, such as protective sports gear, and have the adolescent perform a return demonstration *to reinforce learning.*
■ Include the adolescent's parents or guardian in teaching sessions. *If properly informed, family and friends can help the adolescent improve safety practices.*

Suggested NIC interventions

Environmental Management: Safety; Environmental Risk Protection; Health Education; Risk Identification; Surveillance

Evaluations for expected outcomes

■ Adolescent recovers from existing injuries, if present.
■ Adolescent remains free from further injury during hospital stay.
■ Adolescent identifies risks and behaviors he should avoid.
■ Adolescent demonstrates proper use of safety devices and equipment, as appropriate (for example, using protective sports gear, seat belt, and motorcycle helmet).
■ Adolescent states intention to adopt safety precautions.

Documentation

■ Adolescent's statements indicating lack of awareness of or disregard for safety practices

- Physical findings
- Observations of unsafe practices
- Medical treatment for existing injuries
- Nursing interventions to reduce adolescent's risk of future injury
- Adolescent's response to interventions
- Evaluations for expected outcomes

Reference
Garzon, L.S., et al. "The School Nurse's Role in Prevention of Student Use of Performance-enhancing Supplements," *The Journal of School Health* 76(5):159-63, May 2006.

Risk for self-directed
VIOLENCE
related to suicide attempt

Definition
At-risk behaviors in which individual demonstrates that he can be physically, emotionally, or sexually harmful to self

Assessment
- Age
- Gender
- Developmental stage
- Availability of weapons or toxic substances
- Mood and affect, including persistent depression; feelings of worthlessness, hopelessness, helplessness, isolation, inadequacy, and humiliation; deterioration in school work; and flat, distant, remote affect
- Behavioral changes, including loss of interest in personal appearance, overeating or eating too little, verbal or written cues or preoccupation with death, threats of suicide, acting out (such as sexual promiscuity, delinquency, or running away), low energy level, sleep disturbances, frequent naps, irritability, somatic and physical complaints, antisocial or self-destructive behavior, tendency to be accident-prone, and acts of self-mutilation
- Psychological status, including loss of interest in hobbies and preferred activities, refusal to attend school (cutting class and truancy), social withdrawal and isolation, academic problems, and feelings of rejection by peers and social group

Risk factors
- Access to lethal weapon
- Dysfunctional family
- Excessive stress and anxiety
- Expressed or implied statements indicating desire to commit suicide
- Feelings of worthlessness, hopelessness, loneliness, and helplessness
- History of suicide attempts

■ Low self-esteem
■ Poor impulse control
■ Real or perceived threatened loss of important person or possession
■ Recent stressful event, such as parents' divorce or death in family
■ Recent suicide of close friend or relative
■ Severe depression
■ Substance abuse or withdrawal

Expected outcomes
■ Adolescent won't harm self while in hospital.
■ Adolescent will recover from suicidal episode.
■ Adolescent will discuss feelings that precipitated suicide attempt.
■ Adolescent will attend therapy sessions with mental health professional.
■ Adolescent will describe available resources for crisis prevention and management.
■ Adolescent will report improved feelings of self-worth.

Suggested NOC outcomes

Depression Self-Control; Impulse Self-Control; Mood Equilibrium; Quality of Life; Self-Mutilation Restraint; Suicide Self-Restraint; Will to Live

Interventions and rationales
■ Take all suicide threats seriously. *Early intervention reduces the likelihood of a suicide attempt.*
■ Ask the adolescent directly, "Have you thought about killing yourself?" If he says yes, ask, "What do you plan to do?" *Suicide risk increases if the adolescent has definite plan.*
■ Remove any objects that the adolescent could use to injure himself, such as razors, belts, glass objects, and pills, *to ensure his safety.*
■ Arrange supervision (preferably one-on-one) for the adolescent according to facility policy. *This ensures compliance with legal requirements to protect the adolescent while demonstrating staff concern.*
■ Make a contract with the adolescent that he won't harm himself for a specific period. Continue negotiating until there's no evidence of suicidal ideation. *A contract puts the subject of suicide in the open, places some responsibility for safety on the adolescent, and demonstrates your regard for the adolescent as worthwhile.*
■ Supervise administration of all prescribed medications, and be aware of their actions and possible adverse effects. *Medications may be a treatment alternative. By watching as they're administered, you prevent the adolescent from hoarding doses (sometimes called "cheeking"), thus ensuring his safety.*
■ Convey a caring, nonjudgmental attitude when talking with the adolescent. *This demonstrates your unconditional positive regard and helps establish a trusting relationship.*
■ Listen carefully to the adolescent as he talks. Don't challenge his statements or reinforce denial of the current situation. *This communicates caring, support, and understanding without reinforcing denial, which usually masks underlying suicidal feelings.*

■ Encourage the adolescent to set a goal of cooperating with psychiatric intervention. *Ambivalence about psychiatric care or refusal to attend sessions indicates that the adolescent is still in denial.*

■ Provide the adolescent and his family members with telephone numbers for crisis prevention centers, suicide hot lines, counselors, and other community support services. *Having many alternatives for support helps reduce the adolescent's anxiety.*

Suggested NIC interventions

Behavior Management: Self-Harm; Counseling; Crisis Intervention; Family Involvement Promotion; Mutual Goal Setting; Suicide Prevention; Support Group

Evaluations for expected outcomes

■ Adolescent doesn't harm self during hospital stay.
■ Adolescent recovers from suicide attempt.
■ Adolescent discusses feelings and reasons for attempting suicide.
■ Adolescent attends counseling sessions with mental health professional.
■ Adolescent describes crisis prevention resources, such as hot-line telephone number, local crisis center, or name of therapist.
■ Adolescent expresses improved sense of self-worth.

Documentation

■ Adolescent's description of his feelings before and after suicide attempt
■ Observations of adolescent's behavior, mood, and affect
■ Nursing interventions to reduce or prevent self-destructive behavior
■ Adolescent's response to interventions
■ Evaluations for expected outcomes

References

Murray, B.L., and Wright, K. "Integration of a Suicide Risk Assessment and Intervention Approach: The Perspective of Youth," *Journal of Psychiatric and Mental Health Nursing* 13(2):157-64, April 2006.

Puskar, K.R., et al. "Self-cutting Behaviors in Adolescents," *Journal of Emergency Nursing* 32(5):444-46, October 2006.

III Child health

INTRODUCTION

This section focuses on providing care for children — helping them maintain optimal health and achieve their full developmental potential. Your first task is to establish rapport with the child and family under your care. When talking to the child, show understanding and use simple language. If he's frightened, turning portions of your examination into a game may help to calm him. Talk to the child about toys, hobbies, or other subjects of interest, and be generous with compliments.

Your care plan should emphasize working with the entire family. Obtaining accurate assessment information, for example, usually requires the cooperation and trust of family members.

During each stage of growth and development, the child must master specific physical, cognitive, and developmental tasks. Assessment should include an evaluation of the child's growth and developmental level as well as an examination of body systems. Other assessment areas include family roles and relationships, parenting style, stressors, coping patterns, religion, cultural background, living conditions, and financial status. You'll also want to explore how the child and family members perceive the health problem.

After analyzing the assessment data, you'll formulate nursing diagnoses. Your diagnoses should state the child's actual health problems or health problems for which the child is at risk; they may take into account physiologic, psychosocial, or cognitive aspects of the child's well-being. Your nursing care plan will stem from these diagnoses.

When developing interventions, include steps to encourage the child and family members to participate in care. Some families may need encouragement just to ask questions about the child's status; others may want to become involved in treatment-related decisions. To foster participation, be sensitive to the family's values, ideas, and beliefs. Provide referrals to appropriate social service agencies and other community resources. Keep in mind that your ultimate goal is to make the child and family as self-sufficient as possible in managing the health problem.

Periodically evaluate the child's and family's progress as you implement your care plan. If you carefully monitor the effectiveness of interventions, you'll readily see what revisions you need to make to the care plan.

Risk for
ASPIRATION
related to impaired swallowing

Definition
At risk for entry of GI secretions, oropharyngeal secretions, solids, or fluids into the tracheobronchial passages

Assessment
- Respiratory status, including rate, depth, and pattern of respirations; auscultation of breath sounds; frequency and effectiveness of cough; ability to handle secretions; palpation for fremitus; percussion of lung fields; and sputum characteristics (color, consistency, amount, and odor)
- Neurologic status, including mental status and level of consciousness (LOC)
- GI status, including presence or absence of gag and swallowing reflex, gastroesophageal reflux, and continuous or intermittent tube feedings
- Diagnostic studies, including arterial blood gas levels, chest X-rays, and cardiorespiratory monitoring

Risk factors
- Decreased GI motility
- Delayed gastric emptying
- Depressed cough and gag reflexes
- Feeding or GI tubes
- Impaired swallowing
- Incompetent lower esophageal sphincter
- Increased gastric residual
- Increased intragastric pressure
- Medication administration
- Reduced LOC
- Situations hindering elevation of upper body
- Surgery or trauma to face, mouth, or neck
- Tracheostomy or endotracheal tube
- Wired jaws

Expected outcomes
- Auscultation will reveal clear breath sounds.
- Auscultation will reveal presence of bowel sounds.
- Child will maintain patent airway.
- Child will breathe easily, cough effectively, and show no signs of respiratory distress or infection.
- Family members will demonstrate measures to prevent aspiration.
- Child's respiratory rate will remain within normal limits for age.
- Family members will describe plan for home care (for example, removing objects that a child could choke on).

Suggested NOC outcomes

Aspiration Prevention; Knowledge: Treatment Procedure(s); Respiratory Status: Ventilation; Risk Control; Swallowing Status

Interventions and rationales

■ Assess the child for gag and swallowing reflexes. *Impaired reflexes may cause aspiration.*

■ Assess respiratory status at least every 4 hours or according to established standards; begin cardiopulmonary monitoring *to detect signs of possible aspiration (increased respiratory rate, cough, sputum production, and diminished breath sounds).*

■ Auscultate bowel sounds every 4 hours and report changes. *Delayed gastric emptying may cause regurgitation of stomach contents.*

■ Elevate the head of the bed or place the child in Fowler's position *to aid breathing.*

■ Help the child turn, cough, and deep breathe every 2 to 4 hours. Perform postural drainage, percussion, and vibration every 4 hours, or as ordered. Suction, as needed, *to stimulate cough and clear upper and lower airways. These measures promote drainage of secretions and full expansion of lungs.*

■ Perform chest physiotherapy before feeding the child *to decrease the risk of emesis leading to aspiration.*

■ Hold an infant with his head elevated during feeding, and position him in an infant seat after feeding. *Such positioning uses gravity to prevent regurgitation of stomach contents and promotes lung expansion.*

■ Recognize the progression of airway compromise and report your findings *to detect complications early.*

■ Encourage fluids within prescribed restrictions. Provide humidification, as ordered (such as an oxygen tent or nebulizer). *Fluids and humidification liquefy secretions.*

■ Place the child in the lateral or prone position. Change the child's position at least every 2 hours *to reduce the potential for aspiration by allowing secretions and blood to drain.*

■ Instruct the child and family members in the home care plan. *The child and family members must demonstrate the ability to ensure adequate home care before discharge.*

Suggested NIC interventions

Airway Management; Aspiration Precautions; Feeding; Positioning; Respiratory Monitoring; Vital Signs Monitoring; Vomiting Management

Evaluations for expected outcomes

■ Auscultation reveals clear breath sounds.

■ Auscultation reveals presence of bowel sounds.

■ Child maintains airway patency.

■ Child breathes easily, coughs effectively, and shows no signs of respiratory distress or infection.

■ Family members demonstrate measures to prevent aspiration in child (for example, correct positioning of infant during and after feeding).

■ Child's respiratory rate remains within normal limits for age.
■ Family members describe plan for home care.

Documentation
■ Child's ability to handle oral secretions and feedings
■ Observation of respiratory status and response to treatment regimen
■ Child's and family members' abilities to carry out home care plan
■ Evaluations for expected outcomes

Reference
Thoyre, S.M., et al. "The Early Feeding Skills Assessment for Preterm Infants," *Neonatal Network* 24(3):7-16, May-June 2005.

Disturbed
BODY IMAGE
related to surgery

Definition
Confusion in mental picture of one's physical self functioning

Assessment
■ Physiologic changes
■ Behavioral changes
■ Child's and family members' perceptions of health problem
■ Child's developmental stage
■ Child's eating pattern, sleeping pattern, and usual play activities

Defining characteristics
■ Behaviors of avoiding, monitoring, or acknowledging one's body
■ Behavior of hiding or overexposing body part (intentional or unintentional)
■ Change in social involvement
■ Expressed negative feelings about body
■ Expressions of actual or perceived change in appearance, structure, or function
■ Extension of body boundary to incorporate environmental objects
■ Loss of body part
■ Preoccupation with change or loss
■ Refusal to acknowledge change
■ Refusal to look at or touch body part
■ Trauma to nonfunctioning part

Expected outcomes
■ Child will acknowledge change in body appearance or function.
≡ Child will express positive feelings about self.
■ Family members will acknowledge change in child's appearance or body functioning and will verbalize acceptance of child.

Suggested NOC outcomes

Acceptance: Health Status; Body Image; Child Development: Middle Childhood; Coping; Psychosocial Adjustment: Life Change; Self-Esteem

Interventions and rationales

■ Hold, rock, or touch the child frequently *to give the child awareness of body integrity.*

■ Provide an opportunity for the child to interact with peers who have experienced similar health problem *to decrease the child's feelings of isolation and sense of being different from others.*

■ Give the child as much freedom as possible. If restraints are called for, use the minimum restraint necessary to prevent injury. *Providing the least restrictive environment enhances the child's control over his surroundings and provides an opportunity to release feelings through physical activity.*

■ Explain medical procedures in age-appropriate language. For a child younger than age 7, use dolls and actual medical equipment to describe procedures. *A child in the preoperational stage of development understands best by seeing and manipulating objects.* For an older child, use body diagrams to illustrate what changes will and won't appear in the body as a result of medical treatment or disease progression. *Illustration is one technique to reinforce learning.*

■ For a young child, cover injection sites with adhesive bandages. *A child in the preoperational stage of development may hold the misconception that injections create holes that allow blood to drain out. Adhesive bandages may help reinforce the child's sense of body integrity.*

■ Encourage a young child to participate in play activities *to allow the child to act out feelings that he may not have the verbal or cognitive skills to express.*

■ Set aside time with the older school-age child to discuss his feelings *to assess perceptions, clarify misconceptions, and provide an opportunity to ventilate emotions.*

■ Ensure privacy during procedures *to accommodate the heightened sense of modesty that children develop beginning in early school-age years.*

■ Encourage family members to express feelings and concerns about changes in the child's body appearance or function. Provide accurate information and answer questions thoroughly. *Encouraging open discussion enables you to provide emotional support and may help ease family members' anxiety.*

Suggested NIC interventions

Coping Enhancement; Developmental Enhancement: Child; Parent Education: Childrearing Family; Risk Identification; Self-Esteem Enhancement

Evaluations for expected outcomes

■ Child expresses understanding of changes in body.

■ Child expresses positive feelings about self.

■ Family members acknowledge change, verbalize positive feelings about child, and display warmth and affection by holding, comforting, and hugging child as appropriate for child's age.

Documentation
- Child's statements about appearance
- Family members' statements about changes in child's body structure or function
- Account of child's behavior during medical procedures and in play activities
- Observations of family members' behavior toward child and participation in care
- Evaluations for expected outcomes

Reference
Gray, E.H., et al. "Stoma Care in the School Setting," *The Journal of School Nursing* 22(2):74-80, April 2006.

Risk for imbalanced
BODY TEMPERATURE
related to dehydration

Definition
State of being at risk for failure to maintain body temperature within normal range

Assessment
- Age
- Vital signs, including pattern of temperature fluctuation
- Hydration status, including mucous membranes, skin turgor, and fontanels (in infants)
- Respiratory status, including respiratory rate and depth, dyspnea, and use of accessory muscles
- Neurologic status, including incidence of seizures, cerebrospinal fluid infection, abscess, hemorrhage, and history of trauma or cranial surgery
- Nutritional status, including decreased intake and vomiting
- Medication history, including effects of drugs or toxins
- Evidence of disturbance in the temperature-regulating centers of brain

Risk factors
- Altered metabolic rate
- Clothing not appropriate for environmental temperature
- Dehydration
- Exposure to cold or hot environment
- Extremes of age or weight
- Illness or trauma that affects temperature regulation
- Inactivity or vigorous activity
- Use of medication that causes vasoconstriction or vasodilation
- Use of sedation

Expected outcomes
- Child will maintain body temperature of 98.6° to 99.5° F (37° C to 37.5° C).
- Child will maintain weight within 5% of baseline.
- Child will maintain balanced intake and output within normal limits for age.
- Child's urine specific gravity will remain between 1.010 and 1.015.

Suggested NOC outcomes

Hydration; Medication Response; Thermoregulation

Interventions and rationales
- Assess the child's temperature every 4 hours. Use a temperature-taking method appropriate for the child's age and size (rectal or axillary for an infant or toddler, axillary or oral for a preschooler, and oral for a school-age child). *Prolonged elevation of temperature above 104° F (40° C) may produce dehydration and harmful central nervous system effects.*
- Weigh the child daily every morning and record the results. *A decrease in weight may indicate dehydration.*
- Maintain adequate fluid intake by offering small amounts of flavored fluids at frequent intervals; record intake and output every shift. *Fever increases the child's fluid requirements by increasing the metabolic rate. High-calorie liquids, such as colas, fruit juices, and flavored water sweetened with corn syrup, help prevent dehydration.*
- Administer antipyretics, as ordered, and monitor effectiveness. *Antipyretics act on the hypothalamus to regulate body temperature.*
- Check and record urine specific gravity with each voiding. *Urine specific gravity increases with dehydration.* Adequate urine output and urine specific gravity between 1.010 and 1.015 indicates sufficient hydration for children.
- Give a tepid sponge bath for increased temperature *to increase vaporization from skin and decrease body temperature.*
- Teach parents to dress the child in lightweight clothing when the child has elevated body temperature *to allow perspiration to evaporate, thereby releasing body heat.*

Suggested NIC interventions

Fever Treatment; Medication Management; Temperature Regulation; Vital Signs Monitoring

Evaluations for expected outcomes
- Child maintains body temperature of 98.6° to 99.5° F (37° to 37.5° C).
- Child maintains baseline weight.
- Child maintains balanced intake and output within normal limits for age.
- Child maintains urine specific gravity of 1.010 to 1.015.

Documentation
- Observation of physical findings
- Nursing interventions, including administration of medications
- Child's body temperature (recorded every 4 hours)

■ Child's weight, urine output, and urine specific gravity
■ Child's response (behavioral, cognitive, and physiologic) to interventions, including administration of antipyretics
■ Evaluations for expected outcomes

Reference

Braun, C.A. "Accuracy of Pacifier Thermometers in Young Children," *Pediatric Nursing* 32(5):413-18, September-October 2006.

Ineffective
BREATHING PATTERN
related to decreased energy/fatigue

Definition

Inspiration or expiration that doesn't provide adequate ventilation

Assessment

■ Age
■ Allergies
■ History of respiratory disorders
■ Respiratory status, including rate and depth of respiration, symmetry of chest expansion, use of accessory muscles, nasal flaring, presence of cough, anteroposterior chest diameter, palpation for fremitus, percussion of lung fields, auscultation of breath sounds, pulmonary function studies, arterial blood gas (ABG) monitoring, and pulse oximetry readings
■ Cardiovascular status, including history of congenital or acquired heart disease
■ Neurologic status, including mental status and level of consciousness
■ Emotional well-being
■ Knowledge, including understanding of physical condition and physical, mental, and emotional readiness to learn

Defining characteristics

■ Altered chest excursion
■ Altered respiratory rate
– Ages 1 to 4: 20 or greater than 30
– Ages 5 to 14: 14 or 25
■ Decreased vital capacity
■ Depth of breathing
– Adult tidal volume: 500 ml at rest
– Infant tidal volume: 6 to 8 ml/kg
■ Dyspnea
■ Nasal flaring
■ Orthopnea
■ Prolonged expiratory phase
■ Pursed-lip breathing

- Shortness of breath
- Timing ratio
- Use of accessory muscles

Expected outcomes

- .Auscultation won't reveal abnormal breath sounds.
- Child's oxygen saturation (SaO_2) level will remain above 95%.
- Child's respiratory status will remain within normal limits for age.
- Child will demonstrate adequate breathing pattern, with easy, unlabored respirations.
- Child will demonstrate correct technique in pursed-lip breathing, abdominal breathing, and relaxation techniques.
- Child or family member will demonstrate correct technique to use in medication administration, oxygen administration, and airway suctioning.
- Child will participate in age-appropriate play activities without increased respiratory difficulty.
- Family members will develop effective care plan for child's return home.

Suggested NOC outcomes

Anxiety Level; Energy Conservation; Respiratory Status: Airway Patency; Respiratory Status: Ventilation; Vital Signs

Interventions and rationales

- Assess respiratory rate and depth every 2 to 4 hours; monitor for nasal flaring, chest retractions, and cyanosis *to detect early signs of respiratory compromise.*
- Monitor ABG values and pulse oximetry readings *to evaluate oxygenation and respiratory status.*
- Auscultate breath sounds every 2 to 4 hours *to detect decreased or adventitious breath sounds;* report changes.
- Administer oxygen, as ordered, *to help reduce hypoxemia and relieve respiratory distress.*
- Force fluids *to liquefy secretions and prevent dehydration related to increased respiratory rate.*
- Provide nebulizer treatment, vaporizer, or mist tent therapy, as ordered, *to liquefy secretions.*
- Provide postural drainage and chest percussion every 4 hours before meals *to facilitate removal of secretions.*
- Suction airway, as needed, *to remove secretions.*
- Place the child in Fowler's position, raising the head of the bed. Place an overbed table padded with a pillow in front of the child and have him extend his arms over the table *to promote lung expansion.*
- Remain with the child and offer reassurance during periods of respiratory difficulty *to relieve anxiety.*
- Administer bronchodilators and antibiotics, as ordered. *Dilation of bronchi allows greater passageway for air. Antibiotics treat infection.* Monitor effectiveness and check for adverse reactions *to ensure the safety and efficacy of therapy.*

■ Prohibit parents and other visitors from smoking in the child's room and explain why. *Smoking depletes the room of its natural oxygen supply and poses a serious fire hazard in a room with oxygen equipment.*

■ Schedule necessary care activities to provide frequent rest periods *to prevent fatigue and reduce oxygen demand.* Allow adequate playtime. *All children require play for normal growth and development.*

■ Assist with activities of daily living, as necessary, *to help the child conserve energy and avoid fatigue.*

■ Identify the child's developmental level and select appropriate teaching methods. For a preschooler or early school-age child, use stuffed animals, puppets, and drawings. *A preschooler uses sensory experiences to understand information.* For an older school-age child, use demonstration and audiovisual materials such as body outline. *A child in this age-group has the ability to think logically but not abstractly.*

■ Limit the number of new skills taught each day according to the child's age and ability. Teach a preschooler one skill per day and a school-age child, two skills per day. *Limiting daily teaching avoids overloading the child with new information and enhances learning.*

■ Teach the child pursed-lip breathing, abdominal breathing, and relaxation techniques. *These measures allow the child to participate in maintaining his health status and improve ventilation.*

■ Discuss with the child and family members ways to conserve energy while carrying out the daily routine *to prepare the child for discharge from the hospital.*

■ Help the family plan for care at home. Discuss medication administration, use of assistive equipment, and available community resources. Also discuss the signs and symptoms of complications and when to report them. *Increasing the family's knowledge improves the likelihood of compliance with medical treatment, thereby decreasing the risk of recurrence of breathing problems.*

Suggested NIC interventions

Acid-Base Management; Airway Management; Chest Physiotherapy; Energy Management; Oxygen Therapy; Positioning; Respiratory Monitoring; Smoking Cessation Assistance

Evaluations for expected outcomes

■ Auscultation reveals normal breath sounds.

■ Pulse oximetry readings reveal Sao_2 above 95%.

■ Child's respiratory status remains within normal limits for age.

■ Child demonstrates adequate breathing pattern and unlabored respirations.

■ Child demonstrates correct technique in pursed-lip breathing, abdominal breathing, and relaxation techniques.

■ Family members demonstrate correct technique in medication administration, oxygen administration, and suctioning.

■ Child participates in age-appropriate play activities without increased respiratory difficulty.

■ Family members describe care plan they'll implement upon child's return home.

Documentation
- Child's expressions of comfort in breathing
- Child's and family members' understanding of medical diagnosis and readiness to learn
- Child's and family members' responses to teaching
- Physical findings from pulmonary assessment
- Interventions performed
- Child's and family members' responses to nursing interventions
- Evaluations for expected outcomes

Reference
Marcoux, K.K. "Current Management of Status Asthmaticus in the Pediatric ICU," *Critical Care Nursing Clinics of North America* 17(4):463-79, December 2005.

Disabled family
COPING
related to long-term illness of a child

Definition
Behavior of significant person (family member or other primary person) that disables his capabilities and the client's capacities to effectively address tasks essential to either person's adaptation to the health challenge

Assessment
- Child's illness, including severity, duration, and impact on family
- Family process, including number and ages of children, usual patterns of interaction, roles of parents and children, communication patterns, relationship changes (such as separation, divorce, or remarriage), and past response to crisis
- Family members' understanding of child's present health status
- Family resources (financial, social, and spiritual)
- Parental status, including perception of child's behavior, past responses to stress, child care provisions, history of inappropriate parenting, and history of destructive behavior or substance abuse
- Alteration in child's growth and development resulting from illness or dysfunctional parenting
- Transportation limitations, including geographic distances to health resources

Defining characteristics
- Agitation, depression, aggression, and hostility (child)
- Assumption of illness symptoms of child (family member)
- Decisions or actions that harm family's economic or social well-being (parent)
- Desertion of child (parent)
- Development of helplessness and dependence (child)
- Distorted perception of child's health problem, including extreme denial about its existence or severity (parent)

- Impaired individualization (child)
- Impaired restructuring of meaningful life for self (family member)
- Intolerance of child's physical ailments or psychological weaknesses (parent)
- Maintenance of usual routines (parent)
- Neglect of child's basic human needs and illness treatment (parent)
- Neglect of relationships with other family members (parent)
- Prolonged excessive concern for child (parent)
- Rejection of child (parent)

Expected outcomes

- Family members will identify factors that trigger stress and inappropriate behavior.
- Family members will make use of appropriate sources of support.
- Family members will interact appropriately with staff members and each other.
- Parents will meet their children's developmental needs.
- Family members will express feelings and individual needs.
- All children in the family will meet developmental milestones appropriate for their ages.
- Family members will meet child's health care needs.

Suggested NOC outcomes

Caregiver Emotional Health; Caregiver-Patient Relationship; Caregiving Endurance Potential; Family Coping; Family Health Status; Family Social Climate; Family Support During Treatment

Interventions and rationales

- Assess the family history *to identify the family's strengths and limitations.*
- Determine if family members are prepared to accept help. *Changes in behavior won't take place until family members are ready.*
- Communicate only brief amounts of information to family members at any one time. *Family members under stress usually can't grasp large amounts of information.*
- Help the family identify which tasks to tackle now and which to put off until the stress level decreases. *Performing easy, familiar activities decreases discomfort during times of stress.*
- Encourage family members to allow open expression of feelings and to avoid passing judgment on one another. *Family members need to be able to communicate openly without putting each other on the defensive.*
- Identify instances of successful communication among family members *to single out and encourage positive behavior.*
- Use play activity to promote self-esteem in children. *Parents commonly forget the developmental needs of children during crisis. If one child is seriously ill, parents may ignore siblings.*
- Help family members identify situations that trigger inappropriate behavior. *Family members must learn to recognize their tolerance threshold to react appropriately.*
- Help family members identify coping mechanisms used successfully in the past *to enable them to develop appropriate responses without learning new behaviors.*

■ Help family members identify options when confronted with difficult decisions. *Members of dysfunctional families commonly believe they lack choices.*
■ Teach parents about the health care and developmental needs of their child. *Family-centered care is essential for an ill child.*
■ Provide referrals to appropriate social service agencies *to help family members find additional resources.*

Suggested NIC interventions

Anger Control Assistance; Caregiver Support; Family Involvement Promotion; Family Therapy; Mutual Goal Setting; Normalization Promotion; Support Group

Evaluations for expected outcomes

■ Family members state specific factors that lead to inappropriate behavior.
■ Family members state their plans for contacting sources of support.
■ Family members interact (with each other and staff) with appropriate verbal and nonverbal behavior.
■ Parents meet their children's developmental needs.
■ Family members express feelings and try to meet each others' emotional needs.
■ Children show evidence of achieving age-appropriate developmental tasks.
■ Family members meet chronically ill child's health care needs.

Documentation

■ Observation of family members' interactions with each other and with outsiders
■ Observations of family members' reactions to stress
■ Examples of communication between family members
■ Parents' understanding of normal childhood growth and development
■ Interventions performed to help improve family members' coping skills
■ Family members' level of participation in care of ill child
■ Referrals to community resources
■ Evaluations for expected outcomes

Reference

Hummelinck, A., and Pollack, K. "Parents' Information Needs About the Treatment of Their Chronically Ill Child: A Qualitative Study, "*Patient Education and Counseling* 62(2):228-34, August 2006.

Impaired
DENTITION

related to ineffective oral hygiene

Definition

Disruption in tooth development and eruption patterns or structural integrity of individual teeth

Assessment

- Child's age (chronological and developmental) and gender
- Dental health history, including primary and secondary tooth development; frequency of visits to the dentist; frequency of brushing; condition of teeth (such as presence of caries, extractions, plaque, malocclusion, and evulsion), gums, lips, tongue, and mucous membranes; and signs of salivary dysfunction (such as fissuring at corners of mouth, sore mucous membranes, dryness and cracking of lips, crusting of tongue and palate, and paresthesia of tongue or mucous membrane)
- Health history, including medication history, X-ray treatments, infection, allergies, trauma, lead poisoning, rubella, nephrotic illness, and malnutrition
- Nutritional status, including amount of sugar in diet
- Socioeconomic conditions, including access to dental health care
- Environmental conditions, including lack of fluoride in drinking water
- Family status, including willingness and ability of child's primary caregiver to supervise or perform dental health measures and to take child to dental appointments

Defining characteristics

- Caries
- Extractions
- Evidence of periodontal disease
- Evulsion
- Inability or unwillingness of parents or caregiver to provide child with dental care
- Lack of access to dental care
- Lack of knowledge of appropriate dental hygiene practices
- Malocclusion
- Plaque
- Toothache
- Loose teeth
- Premature loss of primary teeth
- Tooth fractures
- Erosion of enamel

Expected outcomes

- Child will brush teeth with minimal supervision.
- Child will demonstrate good brushing technique.
- Child won't show evidence of dental caries, periodontal disease, or malocclusion.
- Child will reduce quantity of cariogenic foods in his diet.
- Child's teeth will show evidence of good daily oral hygiene.

Suggested NOC outcomes

Oral Hygiene; Self-Care: Oral Hygiene

Interventions and rationales

■ Teach the child principles of good dental hygiene using teaching methods appropriate to his age-group *to foster compliance.*

■ Demonstrate good brushing technique. Stress the importance of having teeth feel clean rather than the need to follow a specific procedure. Help the child establish a schedule for brushing. If necessary, provide direct assistance as well as demonstrations *to reinforce good dental hygiene habits.*

■ Teach the child and his parents or caregiver, if necessary, about the relationship between his diet and dental health. For example, show the child pictures of foods that promote good dental health (such as milk) and pictures of foods that promote tooth decay (such as those containing refined sugar, honey, or molasses). If the child can read food labels, teach him to identify and avoid products with excessive sucrose *to increase the child's awareness of cariogenic foods and encourage better eating habits and more frequent brushing.*

■ If assessment reveals evidence of dental caries, periodontal disease, malocclusion, or other conditions requiring dental care, contact the child's parents *to ensure they're aware of impaired dentition and the need for follow-up care.* Provide a referral to a dentist *to ensure professional care.*

■ Assess whether the child's parents are able and willing to assist in meeting the child's needs regarding dental health. Provide referrals to community resources that may help family members obtain dental care. *The high cost of dental care may cause some families to neglect dental care needs.*

■ If the child is prone to dental problems, emphasize the need for more meticulous home dental care *to avoid further deterioration of the child's teeth and gums.*

■ Schedule an appointment to determine whether the child's parents or caregiver have followed up on your referral to a dentist *to ensure continuity of care.*

Suggested NIC interventions

Oral Health Maintenance; Oral Health Promotion; Teaching: Individual

Evaluations for expected outcomes

■ Child assumes responsibility for brushing teeth with minimal supervision.
■ Child demonstrates good brushing technique.
■ Child shows no evidence of dental caries, periodontal disease, or malocclusion.
■ Child reduces quantity of cariogenic foods in his diet.
■ Child's teeth show evidence of good daily oral hygiene.

Documentation

■ Dental health history
■ Evidence of dental problems
■ Teaching sessions with child and parents or caregiver
■ Evidence of improvement in child's dental hygiene
■ Child's response to nursing interventions
■ Evaluations for expected outcomes

Reference
Melvin, C.S. "A Collaborative Community-based Oral Care Program for School-age Children," *Clinical Nurse Specialist* 20(1):18-22, January-February 2006.

DIARRHEA
related to malabsorption

Definition
Passage of loose, unformed stools

Assessment
- History of bowel disorder or surgery
- GI status, including nausea and vomiting, usual bowel patterns, changes in bowel patterns, stool characteristics (color, amount, consistency, and presence of blood or mucus), pain, inspection of abdomen, auscultation of bowel sounds, and palpation for masses and tenderness
- Medication history, including use of antibiotics
- Nutritional status, including dietary intake, appetite, weight, and changes to usual diet
- Fluid and electrolyte status, including intake and output, urine specific gravity, skin turgor, mucous membranes, and serum potassium and sodium levels
- Skin integrity

Defining characteristics
- Abdominal pain and cramping
- At least three loose, liquid stools per day
- Hyperactive bowel sounds
- Urgency

Expected outcomes
- Child will exhibit normal elimination pattern for age.
- Child will maintain balanced intake and output within normal limits for age.
- Auscultation will reveal normal bowel sounds.
- Child will maintain body temperature of 98.6° to 99.5° F (37° C to 37.5° C).
- Child's urine specific gravity will be between 1.010 and 1.015.
- Child's skin will remain intact.
- Caregivers will demonstrate appropriate skin care techniques.

Suggested NOC outcomes
Bowel Continence; Bowel Elimination; Electrolyte & Acid/Base Balance; Fluid Balance; Hydration; Symptom Severity

Interventions and rationales
- Assess the frequency and characteristics of stools, and auscultate bowel sounds every 4 hours *to monitor the treatment's effectiveness.*

■ Monitor and record intake and output, urine specific gravity (with each voiding), skin turgor, condition of mucous membranes, presence of tears, and condition of fontanels (in infants) *to monitor hydration status and the need for fluid replacement.*

■ Record daily weight before the first feeding each morning *to determine if the child is suffering from dehydration. Weight loss of 5% or more in 1 day may indicate dehydration.*

■ As ordered, offer an oral replacement solution such as dextrose and electrolytes (Pedialyte) or clear liquids in small amounts (5 to 15 ml) every 10 to 15 minutes, waiting 20 to 30 minutes after voiding of loose stools, *to decrease intestinal irritation and the likelihood of further diarrhea.*

■ Don't offer fruit juices or carbonated fluids. *The high glucose content and osmolar load associated with these beverages may stimulate further episodes of diarrhea.*

■ Offer the child the BRAT diet (banana, rice, apple, and toast) 4 hours after last loose stool *to help meet the child's nutritional needs without exacerbating diarrhea.*

■ Check the skin in the perianal area after each stool. Change the diaper frequently and clean skin thoroughly *to prevent skin breakdown.*

■ Apply protective ointment to the diaper area *to provide a barrier between the child's skin and stools.*

■ Monitor the child's temperature every 2 to 4 hours *to detect fever, which may be associated with fluid loss and inflammation.* Measure the temperature using axillary or oral routes *because the use of a rectal thermometer may stimulate further diarrhea.*

■ Teach caregivers the importance of frequent diaper changes and meticulous skin care for the child. Instruct them not to use powder in the diaper area *to avoid caking and subsequent skin breakdown.*

Suggested NIC interventions

Diarrhea Management; Electrolyte Management; Fluid Management; Nutrition Management; Skin Care: Topical Treatments; Skin Surveillance

Evaluations for expected outcomes
■ Child regains normal elimination pattern.
■ Child maintains balanced intake and output within normal limits for age.
■ Auscultation reveals normal bowel sounds.
■ Child remains afebrile.
■ Child's urine specific gravity remains between 1.010 and 1.015.
■ Child's skin remains intact, without signs of redness or irritation.
■ Caregivers demonstrate appropriate skin care techniques.

Documentation
■ Frequency and characteristics of stool
■ Appearance of skin
■ Intake and output
■ Weight (recorded daily)
■ Evidence of caregivers' knowledge of dietary management and skin care techniques
■ Evaluations for expected outcomes

Reference

Koslap-Petraco, M.B. "Homecare Issues in Rotavirus Gastroenteritis," *Journal of the American Academy of Nurse Practitioners* 18(9):422-28, September 2006.

Deficient
DIVERSIONAL ACTIVITY
related to prolonged illness and separation from friends and family

Definition
Decreased stimulation from (or interest or engagement in) recreational or leisure activities

Assessment
- Level of comfort, including mobility and activity tolerance
- Cardiovascular status, including heart rate and rhythm, blood pressure, history of murmurs, cardiac disease
- Respiratory status, including respiratory rate at rest and during activity, shortness of breath, cyanosis, wheezing
- Neurologic status, including level of consciousness, orientation, mood, behavior, memory, and coordination
- Psychosocial status, including presence of family members, social interaction, cultural and ethnic background, hobbies, interests, and changes or adaptations needed to carry out activities
- Environment, including isolation and availability of diversional activities
- Developmental level (physical, cognitive, psychosocial, and linguistic) and learning needs

Defining characteristics
- Environmental limitations (such as hospitalization) or physical limitations affecting participation in usual activities
- Statements of boredom or wishing for something to do

Expected outcomes
- Child will select and participate in age-appropriate play.
- Child will express enjoyment in selected play activity.
- Child will achieve age-appropriate developmental tasks.

Suggested NOC outcomes
Leisure Participation; Motivation; Play Participation; Social Involvement

Interventions and rationales
- Provide various toys, supplies, and activities for the child's use. Make sure items are appropriate to the child's age, developmental level, and environment. *Ready access to diversional activities entices the child to make use of time alone. Age-appropriate items are geared to the child's cognitive, motor, and safety needs.*

■ Encourage family members to bring the child's favorite toys, family pictures, or other objects from home. Provide space in the child's room for cards and gifts from family and friends. Encourage the parents to tape-record stories for their child and provide a tape player so the child can listen *to maintain a sense of attachment to the family and provide a sense of security.*

■ Encourage the child to visit the playroom and participate in individual and group activities. *Participating in play activities helps the child meet developmental needs.*

■ Discuss the child's diversional activity deficit with a play therapist *to enable the play therapist to better address the child's special needs.*

■ Schedule time to personally engage the child in therapeutic or developmental play. Schedule play periods for day and evening shifts. *This ensures that the child has ample opportunity for diversional activity and prevents the child from being isolated for prolonged periods. Participation in play will also strengthen your relationship with the child.*

■ For a child confined to bed, provide creative, challenging games. For example, make a fishing pole with large safe hook and challenge the child to pick up items around the room; glue Velcro on soft balls and create a "dart board" on the wall; or make string-and-paper-cup "telephones" to use with other patients in the room. *Creative play encourages age-appropriate behavior, helps make the environment more enjoyable and challenging, and gives the child greater control and independence.*

■ Provide opportunities for therapeutic play. For example, encourage the child to play with safe hospital equipment, play nurse or doctor, play house, pound clay, or perform "procedures" on a doll. *Therapeutic play offers the child an opportunity to express fears, fantasies, sadness, and misconceptions; to learn more about his illness and its treatment; and to release pent-up feelings safely. This helps the child develop a better sense of control and enhances his ability to cope with hospitalization and treatment.*

■ Provide art and craft supplies for the preschool or school-age child *to enhance the child's creativity, provide an emotional outlet, and encourage the development of initiative and industry.*

Suggested NIC interventions

Energy Management; Recreation Therapy; Self-Responsibility Facilitation; Socialization Enhancement; Therapeutic Play; Visitation Facilitation

Evaluations for expected outcomes

■ Child voluntarily participates in age-appropriate activities.
■ Child expresses contentment with activities.
■ Child achieves age-appropriate developmental tasks.

Documentation

■ Child's expressions of boredom and desire for activity
■ Assessment of child's physical, cognitive, and psychosocial developmental abilities
■ Evaluation of child's physical, educational, and psychosocial need for activity
■ Nursing interventions directed at providing diversional activity

- Child's response to play
- Evaluations for expected outcomes

Reference
Wikstrom, B.M. "Communicating via Expressive Arts: The Natural Medium of Self-expression for Hospitalized Children," *Pediatric Nursing* 31(6):480-85, November-December 2005.

FEAR
related to separation from familiar environment and people

Definition
Response to perceived threat that's consciously recognized as a danger

Assessment
- Age
- Psychosocial factors, including child's understanding of his illness and treatment plan, verbal and nonverbal indicators of fear, and availability of family and friends
- Changes in behavior, eating, or sleeping patterns
- Physiologic manifestations of fear, including temperature, pulse rate, blood pressure, respiratory rate, and skin color and temperature

Defining characteristics
- Aggression
- Bed-wetting
- Expressed feelings of alarm, apprehension, dread, horror, panic, or terror
- Identification of and concentration on object of fear
- Immediate response to object of fear
- Impulsive behavior
- Increased alertness
- Increased tension, worrying, and wariness
- Jitteriness
- Wide-eyed

Expected outcomes
- Child will identify sources of fear.
- Child will demonstrate effective use of coping mechanisms.
- Child will seek comfort from parents.
- Child will express understanding of medical procedures.
- Child's vital signs will remain within normal limits for age.
- Child will exhibit fewer physiologic or behavioral manifestations of fear.

Suggested NOC outcomes
Anxiety Self-Control; Comfort Level; Coping; Fear Level; Fear Self-Control

Interventions and rationales

■ Acknowledge the child's fear. *Bringing feelings out allows for discussion and identification of coping strategies.*

■ Don't dismiss fear or blithely reassure the child that "everything will be all right." *Refusing to acknowledge fear or giving false reassurance impairs coping.*

■ Spend as much time as possible talking with the child. For infants and toddlers, use nonverbal communication, such as holding and rocking. *Establishing rapport encourages the child to express his feelings and provides comfort.*

■ Help the child identify sources of *fear to enable him to put his emotions into perspective.*

■ Provide the child with accurate information about his condition and scheduled procedures and treatments. Orient the child to the facility's sights and sounds. *Accurate information dispels misconceptions that can fuel fear.*

■ Encourage the parents and family members to stay with the child as much as possible and participate in his care, as appropriate, *to enhance the child's ability to cope and decrease fear caused by separation.*

Suggested NIC interventions

Coping Enhancement; Counseling; Emotional Support; Presence; Security Enhancement

Evaluations for expected outcomes

■ Child verbalizes known sources of fear.
■ Child demonstrates effective use of coping mechanisms.
■ Child expresses feelings of comfort.
■ Child expresses understanding of medical procedures.
■ Child's vital signs remain within normal limits for age.
■ Child exhibits marked decrease in physiologic and behavioral manifestations of fear.

Documentation

■ Child's verbal and behavioral expressions of fear
■ Physiologic manifestations of fear
■ Interventions performed to reduce fear
■ Child's response to interventions
■ Family's involvement in child's care
■ Child's response to family involvement
■ Evaluations for expected outcomes

Reference

Justus, R., et al. "Preparing Children and Families for Surgery: Mount Sinai's Multidisciplinary Perspective," *Pediatric Nursing* 32(1):35-43, January-February 2006.

Deficient
FLUID VOLUME
related to active fluid volume loss

Definition
Decreased intravascular, interstitial, or intracellular fluid, with no sodium loss

Assessment
- Age
- Height and weight
- History of diarrhea or vomiting
- GI status, including usual bowel patterns, changes in bowel patterns, stool characteristics (color, amount, size, consistency, and frequency), auscultation of bowel sounds, and inspection of abdomen
- Stool culture, ova, and parasites
- Nutritional status, including dietary intake, changes from usual pattern, appetite, current weight, and recent weight changes
- Fluid and electrolyte status, including intake and output, urine specific gravity, skin turgor, mucous membranes, serum sodium and potassium and blood urea nitrogen levels, and hematocrit (HCT)
- Medication history, including use of laxatives, enemas, and antibiotics
- Neurologic status, including level of consciousness
- Presence of sick children or adults at home, school, or day care
- Respiratory status, including increased respiratory rate
- Child's and family members' knowledge of factors that cause vomiting or diarrhea

Defining characteristics
- Changes in mental status
- Decreased pulse volume and pressure
- Decreased urine output
- Dry skin and mucous membranes
- Increased body temperature
- Increased HCT
- Increased pulse rate
- Increased urine concentration
- Low blood pressure
- Poor turgor of skin or tongue
- Sudden weight loss
- Thirst
- Weakness

Expected outcomes
- Child will maintain normal weight.
- Child's intake and output will be balanced and within normal limits for age.
- Child's electrolyte values will remain within normal limits for age.

■ Child will maintain urine specific gravity of 1.010 to 1.015.
■ Child will exhibit moist mucous membranes, good skin turgor, and flat fontanels (in infant).
■ Child will exhibit normal elimination patterns for age.
■ Child will retain feedings and won't experience emesis.

Suggested NOC outcomes

Electrolyte and Acid/Base Balance; Fluid Balance; Hydration; Nutritional Status: Food & Fluid Intake; Vital Signs

Interventions and rationales

■ Record intake and output every shift. Include urine, stools, vomitus, nasogastric or chest tube drainage, and any other output *to obtain fluid status. Increased output and decreased intake indicate fluid deficit.*
■ Weigh the child each morning before the first feeding. *Weight loss of 5% per day indicates fluid deficit.*
■ Assess skin turgor, mucous membranes, and fontanels (in infant) every shift. *Fluid loss occurs first in extracellular spaces, resulting in poor skin turgor, dry mucous membranes, and sunken fontanels.*
■ Monitor vital signs every 4 hours or more frequently, if needed. *Fever and increased respiratory rate contribute to fluid loss. A weak, thready pulse and a drop in blood pressure indicate dehydration.*
■ Check urine specific gravity every voiding. *Increased specific gravity indicates lack of fluids to dilute urine.*
■ Monitor laboratory study results (electrolytes, pH, and HCT). *During fluid loss, electrolytes are excreted, which may lead to electrolyte imbalance.*
■ Assess the child's behavior and activity level every shift. *A child with dehydration may develop anorexia, decreased activity level, and general malaise.*
■ After diarrhea and vomiting have decreased, offer small amounts (5 to 15 ml) of clear fluids frequently *to replace fluid loss without causing further GI irritation.*
■ If the child is permitted nothing by mouth, provide mouth care every 4 hours, and as needed, *to help keep mucous membranes moist. In infants, oral care and a pacifier help meet the developmental need for sucking.*
■ Monitor I.V. fluid infusion every hour. *Because fluid balance is less stable in young children, an infusion rate that's too fast or too slow can lead to fluid imbalance more rapidly than in adults.*
■ Secure the I.V. site by wrapping it in a soft bandage *to protect the site and allow the child free movement of the extremity.*

Suggested NIC interventions

Fluid/Electrolyte Management; Intravenous (IV) Therapy; Urinary Elimination Management; Vital Signs Monitoring

Evaluations for expected outcomes

■ Child maintains normal weight.
■ Child exhibits balance of intake and output within normal limits for age.
■ Child's electrolyte levels, pH, and HCT remain within age-appropriate ranges.

■ Child's urine specific gravity remains between 1.010 and 1.015.
■ Child exhibits moist mucous membranes, good skin turgor, and flat fontanels (in infant).
■ Child experiences normal elimination patterns for age.
■ Child retains feedings without emesis.

Documentation

■ Intake and output
■ Weight (recorded daily)
■ Skin turgor, mucous membranes, vital signs, and other physical findings
■ Urine specific gravity and other laboratory values
■ Interventions and child's response
■ Evaluations for expected outcomes

Reference

Boluyt, N., et al. "Fluid Resuscitation in Neonatal and Pediatric Hypovolemic Shock: A Dutch Pediatric Society Evidence-based Clinical Practice Guideline," *Intensive Care Medicine* 32(7):995-1003, July 2006.

Risk for deficient
FLUID VOLUME
related to presence of risk factors influencing fluid needs

Definition

At risk for experiencing vascular, cellular, or intracellular dehydration

Assessment

■ Age
■ History of problems that can cause excessive fluid loss, such as vomiting, diarrhea, hemorrhage, and ketoacidosis
■ Vital signs
■ Level of consciousness
■ Fluid and electrolyte status, including intake and output, urine specific gravity, skin turgor, mucous membranes, fontanels (in infant), electrolyte levels, and blood urea nitrogen levels
■ GI status, including usual bowel patterns, changes in bowel patterns, stool characteristics (color, amount, consistency, and frequency), auscultation of bowel sounds, and inspection of abdomen
■ Nutritional status, including dietary intake, changes from usual pattern, appetite, current weight, and recent weight changes
■ Psychosocial status, including developmental level, stressors (such as school, disease process, family discord, or separation from family), and coping mechanisms
■ Respiratory status, including increased respiratory rate

■ Child's and family members' knowledge of factors that cause vomiting or diarrhea

Risk factors
■ Conditions that influence fluid needs (such as a hypermetabolic state)
■ Deficient knowledge related to fluid volume
■ Excessive loss of fluid from normal routes (such as from diarrhea)
■ Extremes of age or weight
■ Factors that affect intake of, absorption of, or access to fluids (such as immobility)
■ Loss of fluid through abnormal routes (such as a drainage tube)
■ Medications that cause fluid loss

Expected outcomes
■ Child will maintain weight.
■ Child's urine specific gravity will remain between 1.010 and 1.015.
■ Child's intake and output will be balanced and within normal limits for age.
■ Child will exhibit good skin turgor, moist mucous membranes, and flat fontanels (in infant).
■ Child will exhibit appropriate elimination patterns for age.
■ Child won't show signs of fluid and electrolyte imbalance.
■ Child will retain feedings without experiencing emesis.

Suggested NOC outcomes
Appetite; Electrolyte & Acid/Base Balance; Fluid Balance; Hydration; Nutritional Status: Food & Fluid Intake; Urinary Elimination

Interventions and rationales
■ Record intake and output every shift. Include urine, stools, vomitus, nasogastric or chest tube drainage, and any other output *to obtain fluid status. Increased output and decreased intake result in fluid deficits.*
■ Weigh the child each morning before the first feeding. *Weight loss of 5% per day indicates fluid deficit.*
■ Assess skin turgor, mucous membranes, and fontanels (in infant) every shift. *Fluid loss first occurs in extracellular spaces, resulting in poor skin turgor, dry mucous membranes, and sunken fontanels.*
■ Monitor vital signs at least every 4 hours or more frequently, if needed. *Increased temperature and increased respiratory rate contribute to fluid loss. A weak, thready pulse and drop in blood pressure indicate dehydration.*
■ Check urine specific gravity every voiding. *Increased specific gravity indicates lack of fluids to dilute urine.*
■ Monitor laboratory studies (electrolytes, pH, and hematocrit [HCT]). *During fluid loss, electrolytes are excreted, which may lead to electrolyte imbalance.*
■ Assess the child's behavior and activity level every shift. *A child with dehydration may develop anorexia, decreased activity level, and general malaise.*
■ When diarrhea and vomiting have decreased, offer small amounts (5 to 15 ml) of clear fluids *to replace fluid loss without causing further GI irritation.*

■ If the child is permitted nothing by mouth, provide mouth care every 4 hours, and as needed, *to help keep mucous membranes moist. In infants, oral care and pacifier help meet the developmental need for sucking.*

■ Monitor I.V. fluid infusion every hour. *Because fluid balance is less stable in young children, infusing too rapidly or too slowly can lead to fluid imbalance more quickly than in adults.*

■ Secure the I.V. site by wrapping it in a soft bandage *to protect the site and allow the child to move his hand or arm freely.*

Suggested NIC interventions

Electrolyte Management; Fluid Management; Intravenous (IV) Therapy; Nutrition Management; Vital Signs Monitoring

Evaluations for expected outcomes

■ Child maintains weight.
■ Child's urine specific gravity remains between 1.010 and 1.015.
■ Child exhibits balanced intake and output within normal limits for age.
■ Child exhibits good skin turgor, moist mucous membranes, and flat fontanels (in infant).
■ Child has appropriate elimination patterns for age.
■ Child's electrolyte values, pH, and HCT remain within age-appropriate ranges.
■ Child retains feedings without experiencing emesis.

Documentation

■ Intake and output
■ Weight (recorded daily)
■ Skin turgor, mucous membranes, vital signs, and other physical findings
■ Urine specific gravity and other laboratory values
■ Interventions and child's response
■ Evaluations for expected outcomes

Reference

Mecham, N. "Early Recognition and Treatment of Shock in the Pediatric Patient," *Journal of Trauma Nursing* 13(1):17-21, January-March 2006.

GRIEVING

related to potential loss

Definition

Intellectual and emotional responses and behaviors by which individuals, families, and communities work through the process of modifying self-concept based on the perception of potential loss

Assessment

■ Child's state of grief and mourning

- Child's developmental level
- Perceived value of loss
- Usual patterns of coping with loss
- Behavioral manifestations of grieving
- Somatic problems associated with grieving process, including changes in appetite, sleep pattern, and activity level
- Available support systems

Defining characteristics
- Altered activity level
- Altered communication pattern
- Anger
- Changes in eating habits
- Changes in sleep or dream patterns
- Denial of significance of potential loss
- Difficulty taking on new or different roles
- Expressions of distress at potential loss
- Expressed feelings of guilt or bargaining with a higher power
- Resolution of grief before occurrence of loss
- Sorrow

Expected outcomes
- Child will express feelings in nondestructive manner.
- Child will seek emotional support from family members to help cope with loss.
- Child will take advantage of available resources, such as participation in play therapy, to help cope with loss.
- Parents will express understanding of grieving process.
- Parents will participate in care of child and interact positively with child.

Suggested NOC outcomes
Communication; Coping; Depression Level; Family Coping; Family Integrity; Grief Resolution; Psychosocial Adjustment: Life Change

Interventions and rationales
- Encourage the child to express his feelings through drawing, puppetry, or gross motor play *to provide a safe outlet for pent-up emotions. A child doesn't have the verbal and cognitive skills to express feelings and needs alternative means of expression. Allow the child to express grief in his own way; intervene only to prevent physically destructive behavior.*
- Plan to spend time each shift with the child. If the child doesn't wish to talk, spend the time in silence *to convey concern, understanding, and support.*
- Reassure the child that it's all right to be angry or sad. Assess whether the child feels responsible for the loss, and clear up misconceptions *to help alleviate guilt feelings.*
- Reassure the family that grief is a normal reaction to loss; explain the stages of the grieving process and normal responses. Help parents understand that the child's feelings and behavior are normal under the present circumstances. *Understanding the grieving process will enhance the family's ability to cope.*

■ Encourage parents and siblings to participate in the care of the child. Remind them of child's need for emotional support at this time. *The child may fear he'll no longer be loved or cared for after the loss. It's crucial that the child receive emotional reassurance.*

■ Offer the child simple choices related to care issues *to give the child a sense of control and to meet his developmental needs for initiative and industry.*

■ Encourage the child and family members to develop coping strategies for dealing with loss, such as participating in diversional activities, reminiscing, or seeking out support groups *to facilitate the grieving process.*

■ Provide positive feedback for effective coping behavior *to help the child and family members regain self-confidence.*

Suggested NIC interventions

Active Listening; Anticipatory Guidance; Coping Enhancement; Family Support; Family Therapy; Grief Work Facilitation; Hope Instillation; Spiritual Support

Evaluations for expected outcomes

■ Child expresses feelings in nondestructive manner.

■ Child's verbal expressions and behavior indicate that he knows he'll receive emotional support from family and won't be blamed, punished, or abandoned because of loss.

■ Child uses available resources to help cope with loss.

■ Parents express understanding of grieving process.

■ Parents participate in care of child and interact positively with child.

Documentation

■ Child's verbal expressions and behavior

■ Child's eating, sleeping, and activity patterns

■ Observation of emotional responses

■ Child's attempts to gain control, such as making decisions and using support systems

■ Interaction between parents and child

■ Nursing interventions and child's response to them

■ Evaluations for expected outcomes

Reference

Donnelly, J.P., et al. "The Needs of Children with Life-limiting Conditions: A Healthcare-provider-based Model," *The American Journal of Hospice & Palliative Care* 22(4):259-67, July-August 2005.

Risk for disproportionate
GROWTH

Definition
At risk for growth above the 97th percentile or below the 3rd percentile for age, crossing two percentile channels; disproportionate growth

Assessment
- Age
- Gender
- Physiologic status, including basal metabolic rate, temperature, motor development, sleep patterns (time and quality of sleep), activity level, and vision and hearing screening
- Growth history, including changes in child's size and form, current height and weight, percentile on pediatric growth grid, body proportions, bone development (determined through X-ray examination), tooth development, organ systems development, neuroendocrine function (growth hormone, thyroid hormone, and androgen levels), genetic abnormalities that may affect growth, prenatal influences (fetal exposure to alcohol or illicit drugs, maternal smoking, or malnutrition), birth trauma (possible oxygen deprivation or nerve injuries), and breast-feeding or bottle-feeding
- Environmental factors, including chemical or radiation exposure, lead exposure, passive inhalation of tobacco smoke, and exposure to water, air, or food contaminants
- Nutritional status, including dietary intake, appetite, ability to feed self or availability of feeding assistance, and consumption of adequate calories and appropriate number and size of servings for child's age and sex (based on the U.S. Department of Agriculture's Food Guide Pyramid)
- Social status, including family structure, type and quality of parents' or guardian's interactions with child, peer relationships (if age-appropriate), and socioeconomic status
- Cultural information, including nationality, ethnicity, religious affiliation, and beliefs and practices regarding health and child rearing
- Health history, including psychiatric or medical diagnoses and use of over-the-counter or prescription medications

Risk factors
- Altered nutritional status
- Any disease that persists over time, especially during critical periods of development
- Environmental hazards, such as chemical or radiation exposure, lead exposure, passive inhalation of tobacco smoke, and exposure to water, air, or food contaminants
- Genetic abnormalities
- Inability to digest and absorb nutrients

■ Neuroendocrine factors, such as altered levels of growth or thyroid hormones or androgens
■ Prenatal influences, such as maternal exposure to drugs or alcohol, severe maternal malnutrition, and maternal smoking
■ Financial or socioeconomic hardship

Expected outcomes

■ Child will grow and gain weight as expected based on growth-chart norms for age and gender.
■ Child will consume _____ calories and _____ ml of fluids representing ____ servings (specify for each food group).
■ Child will sleep _____ hours daily.
■ Child will maintain age-appropriate activity level.
■ Child and parents or guardian will identify risk factors that may lead to disproportionate growth.
■ Child and parents or guardian will state understanding of preventive measures to reduce risk of disproportionate growth.

Suggested NOC outcomes

Appetite; Body Image; Child Development: Middle Childhood; Growth; Risk Control; Weight: Body Mass

Interventions and rationales

■ Weigh and measure the child and review the growth-chart curve *to establish current height and weight values and compare the results with growth history.*
■ Collaborate with the dietary department to establish a meal program that meets the child's nutritional needs. Educate the child and parents or guardian on nutritional requirements for the child's age and gender. Discuss the various meals available to the child at home *to promote growth.*
■ Establish a routine sleep schedule for the child. Provide a comfortable environment that promotes rest *to ensure adequate duration and quality of sleep and to initiate a routine sleep pattern that may be continued when the child returns home.* Naps may be recommended, depending on the child's age.
■ Identify age-appropriate activities and exercises for the child *to stimulate bone growth and muscle development and to promote cardiovascular health.*
■ Teach the child and parents or guardian about risk factors associated with disproportionate growth, such as poor nutrition, lack of regular sleep, environmental hazards, or lack of age-appropriate activities. Help them identify preventive measures to be taken in the home *to promote continuity of care.*
■ Encourage healthy, loving interactions between the child and family. Model healthy, positive interactions with the child for parents. *Disproportionate growth may be associated with emotional deprivation.*
■ If a medical or psychiatric illness places the child at risk for disproportionate growth, make sure the child gets adequate follow-up medical care *to ensure appropriate, professional care.* If the parents or guardian can't afford care, assist with obtaining access to community resources *to promote continuity of care.*

■ If financial hardship interferes with the family's ability to provide for the child, offer a referral to a social worker *to improve the family's access to community resources.*

Suggested NIC interventions

Active Listening; Behavior Modification; Coping Enhancement; Counseling; Nutritional Management; Patient Contracting; Weight Management

Evaluations for expected outcomes

■ Child continues to grow and gain weight as expected based on growth-chart norms for age and gender.
■ Child consumes _____ calories and _____ ml of fluids representing _____ servings (specify for each food group).
■ Child sleeps _____ hours daily.
■ Child maintains activity level appropriate for age.
■ Child and parents or guardian identify risk factors that may lead to disproportionate growth.
■ Child and parents or guardian express understanding of preventive measures to reduce risk of disproportionate growth.

Documentation

■ Child's age, gender, height, and weight
■ Growth history
■ Presence of risk factors for disproportionate growth
■ Input and output
■ Daily appetite level
■ Duration of sleep (including any disruptions in sleep cycle)
■ Child's level of participation in activities and the type of activities
■ Teaching provided to child and parents or guardian regarding disproportionate growth
■ Parents' or guardian's response to teaching, including statements indicating understanding of disproportionate growth, ability to identify risk factors for disproportionate growth, and understanding of need to make alterations in child's environment and daily schedule
■ Follow-up care plan and referrals
■ Evaluations for expected outcomes

Reference

Gregory, K. "Update on Nutrition for Preterm and Full-Term Infants," *Journal of Obstetric, Gynocologic, and Neonatal Nursing* 34(1):98-108, January-February 2005.

Delayed
GROWTH AND DEVELOPMENT
related to physical disability or environmental deprivation

Definition
Deviations from age-group norms

Assessment
- Child's age, both chronological and developmental
- Nature of physical disability
- Past experience with hospitalization
- Family history, including parents' educational level and knowledge of child development, family member roles and support systems, and resources and home environment
- Child's abilities, including communication skills, motor skills, socialization skills, and cognitive abilities

Defining characteristics
- Altered physical growth
- Delay or difficulty in performing motor, social, or expressive skills typical of age-group
- Flat affect
- Listlessness and decreased responses
- Inability to perform self-care activities or maintain self-control at age-appropriate level

Expected outcomes
- Child will demonstrate skills appropriate for age.
- Child will participate in developmental stimulation program to increase skill levels.
- Parents will express understanding of norms for growth and development.
- Parents will use community resources to promote child's development.
- Parents will provide play activities to promote child's development.

Suggested NOC outcomes
Child Development: Middle Childhood; Growth; Physical Maturation: Female; Physical Maturation: Male

Interventions and rationales
- Monitor the child's height, weight, nutritional intake, and cardiovascular and pulmonary status *to ensure the child is healthy enough to participate in an activity.*
- Provide appropriate play activities, such as building blocks, dolls, crayons, or games, *to promote development.* Select play activities and related materials according to the child's abilities rather than chronological age *to promote use of existing skills as a basis for mastering higher skill levels.*

■ Teach selected activities to parents and family members, and encourage frequent play with the child. *Parents need to reinforce learning at home.*

■ Monitor developmental progress at regular intervals *to detect changes in the level of functioning and, as appropriate, adapt activity program.*

■ Provide parents with referrals to appropriate community resources, including sources of financial assistance, child care, and suppliers of adaptive equipment, *to ensure the child's right to receive remedial and educational care in accordance with his disability, as guaranteed by federal law.*

Suggested NIC interventions

Developmental Enhancement: Child; Health Screening; Nutrition Management; Risk Identification; Self-Responsibility Facilitation

Evaluations for expected outcomes

■ Child demonstrates skills appropriate for age.

■ Child participates in developmental stimulation program to increase skill levels.

■ Parents express understanding of developmental norms and means to promote child's development.

■ Parents use community resources to obtain adaptive equipment and appropriate educational opportunities for child.

■ Parents provide play activities that offer developmental stimulation for child.

Documentation

■ Assessment of child's developmental level

■ Evidence of parents' knowledge of child's abilities and motivation to promote development

■ Interventions performed to stimulate development

■ Child's response to nursing interventions

■ Evaluations for expected outcomes

Reference

Wagner, J., et al. "Nurses' Utilization of Parent Questionnaires for Developmental Screening," *Pediatric Nursing* 32(5):409-12, September-October 2006.

HYPERTHERMIA

related to illness

Definition

Elevation of body temperature above normal range

Assessment

■ History of present illness

■ History of exposure to communicable disease

■ Age, gestational age at birth

■ Health history, including chronic disease or disability, pathologic conditions known to cause dehydration, recent traumatic event, exposure to sources of infection (intrauterine or extrauterine), exposure to communicable diseases, and other related events

■ Medication history

■ Physiologic manifestations of fever, including vital signs, skin temperature, and skin color

■ Fluid and electrolyte status, including skin turgor, intake and output, mucous membranes, serum electrolyte levels, and urine specific gravity

■ Laboratory studies, including white blood cell count and culture and sensitivity findings

■ Neurologic status, including level of consciousness (LOC) and history of seizures

■ Skin integrity, including presence of open lesions and rashes

Defining characteristics

■ Body temperature above 99.5° F (37.5° C)

■ Flushed, warm skin

■ Increased respiratory and heart rates

■ Mild to severe dehydration

■ Possible seizures

Expected outcomes

■ Child will remain afebrile.

■ Child will maintain adequate hydration, with balanced intake and output within normal limits for age, urine specific gravity between 1.010 and 1.015, and moist mucous membranes, good skin turgor, and flat fontanels (in infant).

■ Child will remain alert and responsive and won't show evidence of seizure activity or decreased LOC.

■ Parents will identify risk factors for infection and state measures to prevent infection.

■ Parents will demonstrate correct technique for assessing temperature.

■ Parents will identify appropriate measures to reduce fever and prevent dehydration.

Suggested NOC outcomes

Hydration; Infection Severity; Thermoregulation; Vital Signs

Interventions and rationales

■ Take an axillary or oral temperature every 1 to 4 hours and 1 hour after administration of antipyretics. Record measurements and identify the route *to obtain an accurate core temperature.*

■ Administer antipyretics, as ordered, and record effectiveness. *Antipyretics act on the hypothalamus to regulate temperature.* Avoid using aspirin. *Aspirin use in children with viral symptoms, especially with flulike symptoms or varicella (chickenpox), has been linked to Reye's syndrome.*

■ Use nonpharmacologic measures to reduce high fever, such as removing sheets, blankets, and most clothing (except diapers and underwear); placing cool cloths on the axillae and groin; and sponging with tepid water. Explain these measures to the child and family members. *Nonpharmacologic measures lower body temperature and promote comfort. Sponging reduces body temperature by increasing evaporation from skin. Tepid water is used because cold water increases shivering, thereby increasing metabolic rate and causing the temperature to rise.*

■ Use a hypothermia blanket if the child's temperature rises above 103° F (39.4° C). Monitor vital signs every 15 minutes for 1 hour and then as indicated. *Too-rapid reduction of fever can cause vascular collapse in young children.* Turn off the blanket if shivering occurs. *Because shivering increases metabolic rate, it's counterproductive to cooling therapy.*

■ Monitor heart rate and rhythm, blood pressure, respiratory rate, LOC and responsiveness, and capillary refill time every 1 to 4 hours *to evaluate the effectiveness of interventions and monitor for complications such as seizures.*

■ Determine the child's preferences for oral fluids and encourage the child to drink as much as possible, unless contraindicated. Monitor and record intake and output, and administer I.V. fluids, if indicated. *Because insensible fluid loss increases by 10% for every 0.5° F (1° C) increase in temperature, the child must increase fluid intake to prevent dehydration.*

■ Discuss precipitating factors with the parents or primary caregiver. Teach the parents:
– how to take a temperature correctly
– ways to prevent fever, such as increased fluid intake
– not to overdress a young child.
Effective teaching will help prevent future episodes of hyperthermia.

■ Describe the complications of fever to the parents and explain which signs and symptoms they need to report to a physician. *Early recognition and treatment of fever reduces the risk of complications, such as dehydration and febrile seizures.*

Suggested NIC interventions

Fever Treatment; Fluid Management; Infection Control; Temperature Regulation; Vital Signs Monitoring

Evaluations for expected outcomes

■ Child remains afebrile.
■ Child maintains adequate hydration.
■ Child remains alert and responsive and doesn't exhibit evidence of seizure activity.
■ Parents identify risk factors for infection and state measures to prevent infection.
■ Parents demonstrate correct technique for assessing temperature.
■ Parents identify appropriate measures to reduce fever and prevent dehydration.

Documentation

■ Observations of physical findings
■ Nursing interventions, including administration of medications
■ Child's response (behavioral, cognitive, and physiologic) to interventions, including administration of antipyretics
■ Evaluations for expected outcomes

Reference

Light, P.A., et al. "Nursing Telephone Triage and its Influence on Parents' Choice of Care for Febrile Children," *Journal of Pediatric Nursing* 20(6):424-29, December 2005.

Total urinary
INCONTINENCE
related to neuropathy, trauma, or disease affecting spinal nerves

Definition

Involuntary, continuous, and unpredictable loss of urine

Assessment

- History of trauma, surgery, congenital anomalies, and disease
- History of sensory or neuromuscular impairment
- Vital signs
- Age
- Gender
- Urination status, including usual urination pattern, frequency, and awareness of need
- Genitourinary status, including palpation of bladder, previous bladder elimination procedures, urinalysis, urine characteristics, use of urinary assistive devices, and voiding pattern
- Fluid and electrolyte status, including fluid intake and output, mucous membranes, skin turgor, serum electrolyte levels, and urine specific gravity
- Neuromuscular status, including degree of neuromuscular function, motor ability to start or stop urine stream, and sensory ability to perceive bladder fullness
- Nutritional status, including usual dietary pattern, appetite, tolerance or intolerance of foods, and current weight
- Activity status, including usual play patterns
- Appearance of skin

Defining characteristics

- Constant flow of urine occurring at unpredictable times without distention or uninhibited bladder contractions or spasms
- Lack of awareness of incontinence, perineal fullness, or bladder filling
- Nocturia
- Unsuccessful incontinence treatments

Expected outcomes

- Child will maintain fluid balance, with intake equal to output.
- Child will urinate when placed on commode or toilet at specified time.
- Child's skin will remain clean and intact.
- Parents will express understanding of bladder care.

■ Parents will express understanding of need to regulate fluid intake to promote continence.
■ Parents and child will demonstrate correct catheterization technique.

Suggested NOC outcomes

Self-Care: Hygiene; Tissue Integrity: Skin & Mucous Membranes; Urinary Continence; Urinary Elimination

Interventions and rationales

■ Monitor and document the child's voiding pattern and intake and output. *Careful monitoring allows you to identify problems and individualize interventions.*
■ Assist with specific bladder elimination procedures, as ordered, such as:
– external catheterization. Apply the catheter according to established procedure. Maintain patency and avoid constriction. Clean the penis or vagina with soap and water at least twice daily. *An external catheter keeps skin dry and protected from contact with urine. Clean skin helps prevent skin breakdown and infection.*
– insertion of indwelling urinary catheter. Insert according to established procedure and monitor patency; keep tubing free from kinks *to avoid drainage pooling and ensure effective drainage.* Keep the drainage bag below bladder level *to prevent urine reflux into the bladder.* Maintain closed drainage *to prevent bacteria from infiltrating into the bladder.* Secure the catheter to the child's leg (in females) or abdomen (in males) *to avoid tension on the bladder and urinary sphincter.*
– insertion of suprapubic catheter. Monitor patency, change the dressing, and perform catheter care according to established protocols *to help prevent skin irritation and breakdown.* Maintain closed drainage *to prevent bacterial infiltration.*
– use of incontinence aids, including diapers, pads and pants, drip collector, linen protector, or absorbent pouch to cover penis. Use as alternatives to indwelling devices. *Incontinence aids prevent soiling of clothes and linen, reduce embarrassment, and draw urine away from skin. Compared to indwelling devices, incontinence aids allow for greater mobility and carry a decreased risk of infection.*
– intermittent self-catheterization. Assess the child's readiness to learn self-catheterization. Instruct the child or family member in the technique and request a return demonstration *to evaluate understanding and ability;* maintain sterile technique in the hospital and clean technique at home *to prevent infection.*
■ Establish a regular pattern for urination; for example, after breakfast each morning, place the child on the toilet or commode. *Regular urinary care encourages adaptation and routine physiologic function.*
■ Teach the parents the urinary care routine *to foster continuity of care.*
■ Teach the parents to regulate the child's fluid intake according to a specific schedule *to encourage voiding at appropriate times.* Limit fluid intake after dinner *to reduce the need to void at night.*
■ Clean and dry the perianal area after each incontinent episode *to prevent skin breakdown and promote comfort.*

Suggested NIC interventions

Fluid Management; Perineal Care; Skin Surveillance; Urinary Catheterization; Urinary Incontinence Care

Evaluations for expected outcomes

■ Child maintains adequate fluid balance, as evidenced by intake and output, urine specific gravity, and skin turgor.

■ Child urinates when placed on commode or toilet.

■ Child's skin remains clean, dry, and intact.

■ Parents express understanding of bladder care.

■ Parents express understanding of need to regulate fluid intake to maintain continence and plan appropriate diet for child.

■ Parents and child demonstrate correct catheterization technique.

Documentation

■ Observations of incontinence and child's response to treatment

■ Nursing interventions performed and child's response to them

■ Instructions given to child and family members and their demonstrated ability to perform bladder program

■ Observations of skin integrity

■ Evaluations for expected outcomes

Reference

Zickler, C.F., and Richardson, V. "Achieving Continence in Children with Neurogenic Bowel and Bladder," *Journal of Pediatric Health Care* 18(6):276-83, November-December 2004.

Risk for
INJURY

related to developmental factors

Definition

At risk of injury as a result of environmental conditions interacting with the individual's adaptive and defensive resources

Assessment

■ Age

■ Environmental factors, including toxic substances within reach of child, stairs not blocked, and unsafe play equipment

■ Developmental status, including cognitive abilities (language and reasoning), sensory perception, response to stimuli (pain, touch, and warmth), level of independence, and motor skills

■ Child's and family members' understanding of safety practices

■ Behavior

■ Laboratory studies, including toxicology screening

Risk factors

■ Abnormal blood profile

■ Altered mobility

- Confusion
- Disorientation
- Exposure to biological or chemical hazards
- Malnutrition
- Mode of transportation
- Nutrients
- Physical (design structure)
- Skin breakdown

Expected outcomes
- Child will remain free from physical injury.
- During hospitalization, staff members will keep toxic substances out of child's reach, have equipment inspected for safety, and remove unsafe equipment.
- Child and family members will express understanding of safety measures.
- Family members will take action to eliminate household safety hazards.

Suggested NOC outcomes
Immune Status; Parenting: Psychosocial Safety; Risk Control; Risk Detection; Safe Home Environment

Interventions and rationales
- Assess and document any motor, mental, or sensory deficits *to identify specific safety needs.*
- Keep frequently used items within the child's easy reach *to help prevent falls.*
- Encourage the use of necessary assistive devices, such as hearing aids, glasses, and leg braces, *to enhance safety and help prevent injury.*
- Orient the child to his immediate environment, as necessary, *to promote mobility and improve safety.*
- Assess the amount of supervision the child needs to ensure safety. *Maintaining supervision is especially important if the child is hyperactive, disoriented, or unconscious.*
- Keep the bed side rails up at all times *to prevent falls.*
- Keep the bed in low position except when providing direct care *to ease getting in and out of bed and to reduce the danger of falling.*
- Use locks on wheelchairs, stretchers, and beds, when appropriate, *to immobilize equipment and enhance safety.*
- Ensure that all equipment, medical supplies, and toys in the child's room are appropriate for his developmental age. Make sure the infant's or toddler's room doesn't contain small objects, sharp instruments, or sharp furniture corners *to reduce the risk of injury.*
- Promote electrical safety. Apply electrical outlet covers to all unused outlets. Inspect all electrical appliances brought from home and have them approved by a safety officer before use. Don't place liquids, jellies, or creams on electrical appliances. Finally, test all electrical equipment before using on a child. *Electrical appliances pose potential hazards for child and staff members.*
- Instruct the child and family members in standard safety practices, including:
- wiping up spills immediately

– providing nonslip surfaces in hallways, on stairs, and in bathtubs and shower stalls
– draining all water from bathtubs immediately after a bath
– placing toxic substances in locked cabinets or out of reach of the child. *Teaching promotes household safety.*

Suggested NIC interventions

Health Education; Parent Education: Childrearing Family; Risk Identification

Evaluations for expected outcomes

■ Child remains free from physical injury.
■ During hospitalization, staff members keep toxic substances out of child's reach, have equipment inspected for safety, and remove unsafe equipment.
■ Child and family members express understanding of safety measures.
■ Family members eliminate safety hazards from home.

Documentation

■ Statements by child or family members that indicate high risk of injury
■ Assessment of home environment
■ Observation of physical findings
■ Child's and family members' knowledge of safety practices
■ Nursing interventions to reduce the risk of injury
■ Child's and family members' responses to interventions
■ Evaluations for expected outcomes

Reference

McCullagh, M.C. "Home Modification," *AJN* 106(10):54-63, October 2006.

Deficient
KNOWLEDGE

related to unfamiliarity with information resources

Definition

Absence or deficiency of cognitive information related to a specific topic

Assessment

■ Age
■ Developmental status, including learning ability (affective, cognitive, and psychomotor domains), decision-making ability, and developmental stage
■ Psychosocial status, including family's resources, health beliefs and attitudes, interest in learning, knowledge and skill regarding current health problem, obstacles to learning, support systems (willingness and ability of others to help child), and usual coping pattern

■ Neurologic status, including level of consciousness, memory, mental status, and orientation
■ Parents' understanding of child's illness, including severity, prescribed treatment, and overall health needs

Defining characteristics
■ Inability to follow through with instruction
■ Inability to perform well on test
■ Inappropriate or exaggerated behaviors (hysteria, hostility, agitation, apathy)
■ Verbalization of problem

Expected outcomes
■ Child and family members will communicate need to gain knowledge and establish realistic learning goals.
■ Child and family members will demonstrate understanding of what they have been taught.
■ Child and family members will demonstrate ability to perform recently learned health-related behaviors.
■ Child and family members will verbalize their intention to make needed changes in lifestyle.

Suggested NOC outcomes
Information Processing; Knowledge: Child Physical Safety; Knowledge: Energy Conservation; Knowledge: Health Behavior; Knowledge: Health Resources

Interventions and rationales
■ Establish an environment of mutual trust and respect *to enhance learning.* Communicate openly and honestly with the child and encourage the parents and others to visit regularly *to enhance the child's feelings of trust in the staff and comfort within the hospital environment.*
■ Identify the child's level of cognitive, physical, linguistic, and perceptual development *to establish appropriate learning goals.*
■ Select teaching methods appropriate to the child's developmental level:
– For a preschooler or early school-age child, use stuffed animals or puppets. *A child in this age-group uses his senses and manipulation of objects to learn.*
– For an older school-age child, use demonstration techniques, role-playing, and illustrations. Relate new terms and concepts to the child's experiences. For example, to explain ventricular septal defect you might say "your heart is like a house with four rooms and a door to one of the rooms isn't working right." *At this age a child thinks concretely and best understands explanations related to past experiences.*
■ Limit the number of new skills taught each day according to the child's age and ability. *Limiting daily teaching helps to avoid overloading the child with new information.* Keep in mind that a young child who successfully learns single concepts may still have difficulty determining when to apply learned rules.
■ Develop a daily schedule for the hospitalized child with plans for rest, meals, play, and performing learned skills. *Establishing routines provides a more con-*

trolled, pleasant environment for the child and thereby fosters learning. Play is a valuable component of any child's life.

■ Encourage family members to participate in planning the child's daily schedule, making it as similar as possible to a typical day at home. *Involving the child's family helps reinforce the skills necessary for home care after discharge.*

■ Regularly discuss progress toward goal achievement with the child and family members. Make changes in the care plan as necessary. *Evaluation helps to reinforce effective learning techniques and identify ineffective techniques. It allows analysis of progress and redirection of activities as necessary.*

■ Have the child and family members demonstrate learned skills. *Return demonstration allows you to evaluate learning and helps the child and family members gain confidence in new skills.*

Suggested NIC interventions

Discharge Planning; Family Support; Health Education; Health System Guidance; Learning Facilitation; Learning Readiness Enhancement; Parent Education: Childrearing Family; Support System Enhancement

Evaluations for expected outcomes

■ Child and family members communicate need to gain knowledge and establish realistic learning goals.
■ Child and family members express understanding of material being taught.
■ Child and family members demonstrate ability to perform new health-related behaviors correctly.
■ Child and family members express intention to institute needed changes in child's lifestyle.

Documentation

■ Child's and family members' knowledge and skills
■ Child's and family members' statements that indicate knowledge deficit
■ Child's and family members' expressions that indicate motivation to learn
■ Learning objectives
■ Teaching methods used
■ Information taught
■ Skills demonstrated
■ Response to teaching
■ Evaluations for expected outcomes

Reference

Nuutila, L., and Salantera, S. "Children with Long-term Illness: Parents' Experiences of Care," *Journal of Pediatric Nursing* 21(2):153-60, April 2006.

Imbalanced
NUTRITION: LESS THAN BODY REQUIREMENTS
related to inability to absorb nutrients or insufficient intake

Definition
Insufficient intake or absorption of nutrients that results in changed body weight and inability to meet metabolic needs

Assessment
- Age
- Developmental level
- GI status, including usual bowel patterns, change in bowel habits, stool characteristics (color, amount, size, and consistency), pain or discomfort, nausea and vomiting, history of GI disorder or surgery, presence of colic, inspection of abdomen, palpation for masses and tenderness, percussion for tympany and dullness, auscultation of bowel sounds, and sucking and swallowing ability (of infants)
- Medication history, including use of antibiotics
- Nutritional status, including dietary history, change in type of food tolerated, height, weight, physical growth percentile (from pediatric growth grid), meal preparation, sociocultural influences, usual dietary pattern, weight fluctuations in past year, and weight maintenance as height increases
- Change in intrapersonal or interpersonal factors, including desire to eat and rate of food consumption
- Psychosocial status, including body image (perception of observer and self-perception), level of attachment with primary caregiver, and family's financial resources
- Laboratory studies, including hemoglobin levels and hematocrit
- Health status, including heart rate, respiratory status, integumentary status, and oral mucosa
- Presence and type of tube feedings
- Activity level and mood

Defining characteristics
- Abdominal pain or cramping, with or without disorder
- Aversion to or lack of interest in eating
- Body weight 20% or more under ideal weight
- Diarrhea and steatorrhea
- Hyperactive bowel sounds
- Inadequate food intake (less than recommended daily allowances)
- Loss of body weight despite adequate food intake
- Pale conjunctivae and mucous membranes
- Perceived inability to ingest food
- Poor muscle tone
- Satiety immediately after eating
- Sore, inflamed buccal cavity

Expected outcomes

▪ Child will exhibit no further weight loss and, if malnourished, will gain 2.2 lb (1 kg) per week.

▪ Child will take in _____ calories per day and will retain feedings without emesis.

▪ Child and family members will express understanding of total parenteral nutrition (TPN), if appropriate, or demonstrate understanding of other feeding techniques essential to daily nutritional requirements.

▪ Family members will express willingness to continue feeding regimen at home.

Suggested NOC outcomes

Appetite; Health Beliefs; Nutritional Status; Nutritional Status: Food & Fluid Intake; Nutritional Status: Nutrient Intake; Self-Care: Eating; Weight Control

Interventions and rationales

▪ Provide a diet that meets child's daily caloric requirements. Daily caloric intake depends on age, metabolic status, and activity level. General guidelines include:

– younger than age 6 months—108 kcal/kg/day

– ages 6 to 12 months—98 kcal/kg/day

– ages 1 to 3—1,300 kcal/day

– ages 4 to 6—1,800 kcal/day

– ages 7 to 10—2,000 kcal/day

– ages 11 to 14—2,500 kcal/day

– ages 15 to 18—3,000 kcal/day.

A diet meeting the child's caloric requirements helps meet the child's maintenance and growth needs.

▪ Provide small, frequent feedings *to reduce fatigue and improve intake.*

▪ For infants older than age 6 months, offer solid foods before formula or breast milk. Place solid foods in the center of the tongue, using a small spoon to press downward slightly *to facilitate swallowing. Older infants and young toddlers may resist solid foods, preferring milk or formula.*

▪ Record and describe food intake. Refer family members to a dietitian or nutritional support team for dietary management. *A dietitian or nutritional support team can individualize the child's diet within prescribed restrictions.*

▪ Promote adequate rest *to reduce fatigue and improve the child's ability and desire to eat.*

▪ Obtain and record the child's weight each morning before the first feeding *to accurately monitor the response to therapy.*

▪ Provide parenteral fluids, as ordered, *to ensure adequate fluid and electrolyte levels.*

▪ Monitor electrolyte values and report abnormalities. *Poor nutritional status may cause electrolyte imbalances.*

▪ Monitor and record the amount, color, consistency, and presence of occult blood in emesis and stools. *Characteristics of vomitus and stools provide clues to nutrient absorption.*

▪ If the child is receiving tube feedings:

– Use a continuous infusion pump, if possible, *to help prevent diarrhea, fatigue, and stimulation of vagal response. A continuous infusion pump also helps prevent reduction in the cough or gag reflex and overstimulation of the stomach.*
– Provide an infant with opportunities to suck on a pacifier *to satisfy oral needs.*
– Check feeding tube placement before each feeding *to verify tube placement in the GI tract rather than in the lung.*
– Begin the regimen with small amounts and diluted concentrations *to decrease diarrhea and improve absorption.* Increase volume and concentration, as tolerated.
– Keep the head of the bed elevated during feedings *to reduce the risk of aspiration.*
– Teach the parents the correct technique for tube feeding *to ensure compliance with the feeding regimen at home.*
■ If the child is receiving TPN:
– Carefully monitor delivery of TPN *to promote effective therapy and prevent circulatory overload.*
– Monitor blood glucose level, urine specific gravity, and urine glucose, protein, and metabolite levels at least every shift *to detect metabolic complications, osmotic diuresis, hypoglycemia, and pulmonary edema.*
– Provide or assist with oral hygiene *to enhance the child's comfort and improve appetite.*
– Teach the parents the correct technique for maintaining TPN infusion at home *to ensure the parents continue the feeding regimen after discharge.*

Suggested NIC interventions

Enteral Tube Feeding; Nutrition Management; Referral; Total Parenteral Nutrition (TPN) Administration; Weight Gain Assistance; Weight Management

Evaluations for expected outcomes
■ Child's weight stabilizes or increases.
■ Child takes in enough calories and essential nutrients and retains feedings.
■ Child and family members demonstrate understanding of nutritional principles and requirements, feeding techniques, and special needs.
■ Family members express willingness to continue feeding regimen at home.

Documentation
■ Child's weight (recorded daily)
■ Child's sucking and swallowing reflexes
■ Intake and output
■ Incidence of emesis or diarrhea
■ Characteristics of emesis or stools
■ Presence of complications
■ Statements by child and family members that indicate understanding of feeding protocol
■ Evaluations for expected outcomes

Reference

Premji, S.S. "Enteral Feeding for High-risk Neonates: A Digest for Nurses into Putative Risk and Benefits to Ensure Safe and Comfortable Care," *The Journal of Perinatal & Neonatal Nursing* 19(1):59-71, January-March 2005.

Acute
PAIN
related to physical, biological, or chemical agents

Definition

An unpleasant sensory and emotional experience arising from actual or potential tissue damage or described in terms of such damage; pain may be of sudden or slow onset, vary in intensity from mild to severe, and be constant or recurring; duration of pain is less than 6 months; and period of pain has an anticipated or predictable end

Assessment

- Age
- Gender
- Descriptive characteristics of pain, including location, quality, intensity rated on a pictorial assessment scale, temporal factors, and sources of relief
- Physiologic variables, including pain tolerance
- Psychological variables, such as body image, personality, previous experience with pain, anxiety, and secondary gain
- Sociocultural variables, including cognitive style, culture, ethnicity, attitude, values, and birth order
- Environmental variables, such as setting and time

Defining characteristics

- Alteration in muscle tone (may range from listless to rigid)
- Autonomic responses (diaphoresis; blood pressure, pulse rate, and respiratory rate changes; and dilated pupils)
- Changes in appetite and eating
- Communication (verbal or coded) of pain
- Distracting behavior (such as pacing, seeking out other people, or performing repetitive activities)
- Expressions of pain (such as moaning and crying)
- Facial mask of pain (grimacing)
- Guarding or protective behavior
- Narrowed focus (including altered time perception, withdrawal from social contacts, and impaired thought processes)
- Self-focusing
- Sleep disturbance

Expected outcomes

■ Child will express feeling of improved comfort or demonstrate pain relief through playful, smiling, responsive behavior.
■ Child will identify measures effective in relieving pain.
■ Parents will express awareness of child's pain and will perform measures to comfort child.

Suggested NOC outcomes

Anxiety Level; Comfort Level; Pain Control; Pain Level; Stress Level; Symptom Control

Interventions and rationales

■ Assess the child's physical symptoms and behavioral cues. If appropriate, encourage the child to describe pain on a pictorial scale depicting a happy face (no pain) and a series of grimacing faces gradually increasing to a sad face with tears (worst pain possible). *A young child lacks verbal skills to describe variations in pain sensation. Pain scales and observation of nonverbal behavior provide alternative means to assess pain in a young child.*
■ Administer analgesics, as ordered, and document the effectiveness and adverse effects. *Analgesics depress the central nervous system, thereby reducing pain.*
■ Using a pain flow chart, record the time of medication administration and results of pain assessment every hour until the next dose *to monitor the therapy's effectiveness.*
■ Demonstrate acceptance when the child reveals pain. *This helps establish a trusting relationship with the child and encourages open expression of feelings. A child may deny pain to appear "good."*
■ Provide comfort measures, such as massage, repositioning, and instruction in deep breathing and relaxation techniques. *Nonpharmacologic techniques decrease the focus on pain and may enhance the effectiveness of analgesics by reducing muscle tension.*
■ Apply heat or cold, as appropriate, to the pain site. *Applying heat relaxes muscles and decreases pain. Applying cold results in vasoconstriction, decreasing the inflammatory response and reducing pain.*
■ Provide diversional activities, such as books, toys, and arts and crafts. *Because of their immature cognitive functioning and short attention span, young children may be distracted from pain by diversional activities. Older children are less easily distracted.*
■ Provide honest information to the child before potentially painful procedures. Tell the child the reasons for the pain and how long it should last. *Honest information builds trust and fosters a sense of control over pain.*
■ Help the child obtain uninterrupted rest periods. *Adequate rest promotes the child's well-being and enhances the effectiveness of pain medication.*
■ Discuss the child's pain with his parents or primary caregiver and enlist their help in pain assessment and management. Ascertain the parents' usual means of providing comfort to the child. *Because parents are most familiar with a child's usual behavior, they can offer valuable information to assist pain assessment and management.*

■ Try to anticipate the onset of pain. Provide prescribed medication before painful procedures such as dressing changes or activities such as deep breathing. *Careful pain management can improve relief and may enable the child to cope better with procedures.*

■ Encourage the child to report which pain-relief measures prove most effective *to give the child a sense of control and promote effective modification of therapy.*

Suggested NIC interventions

Analgesic Administration; Coping Enhancement; Emotional Support; Medication Management; Mood Management; Pain Management; Sleep Enhancement

Evaluations for expected outcomes

■ Child demonstrates reduced pain, as evidenced by verbal reports of pain relief, absence of behavioral signs of pain, and resumption of activities of daily living (age-appropriate diversional activities, social interaction, and adequate nutritional intake and rest).

■ Child identifies most effective pain relief measures.

■ Parents respond to child's expression of pain and provide comfort to child.

Documentation

■ Child's description of pain, feelings about pain, and statements about pain relief

■ Observations of child's physical and psychological responses to pain

■ Comfort measures and medications provided to reduce pain

■ Effectiveness of interventions

■ Information taught to child and family members about pain and pain relief

■ Additional interventions provided to assist child with pain control

■ Evaluations for expected outcomes

Reference

Dlugosz, C.K., et al. "Appropriate Use of Nonprescription Analgesics in Pediatric Patients," *Journal of Pediatric Health Care* 20(5):316-25, September-October 2006.

Risk for impaired
PARENT/INFANT/CHILD ATTACHMENT

Definition

Disrupted interaction between parents and a child that interferes with the development of a protective, nurturing relationship

Assessment

■ Family status, including marital status, composition of family, ages of family members, ability of family to meet physical and emotional needs of its members, evidence of abuse, and health history

■ Parental status, including level of education, knowledge of normal growth and development, stability of relationship, and available support systems

■ Parents' psychological status, including energy level, motivation, recent life changes, psychiatric history, maternal history of drug abuse, and alcohol or antidepressant use by either partner

■ Child's neurologic status, including muscle tone and reflexes; infant lethargy, irritability, seizures, or tremors; and Brazelton Neonatal Behavioral Assessment, Dubowitz Gestational Age Assessment, and Bayley Scales of Infant Development

■ Child's sensory status, including vision or hearing loss, visual and auditory-evoked potentials, and audiometric tests

■ Sleep pattern, including infant's usual hours of sleep

Risk factors

■ Anxiety over parental role

■ Illness in infant that doesn't allow initiation of contact with parents

■ Inability of parents to meet their personal needs

■ Lack of privacy

■ Physical barriers

■ Separation

■ Substance abuse

Expected outcomes

■ Parents will initiate positive interaction with child.

■ Parents will hold child and talk to him.

■ Parents will express confidence in their ability to respond to child's needs.

■ Parents will respond appropriately to child.

■ Parents will express positive feelings about child.

■ Parents will express confidence in their ability to care for child.

■ Parents will recognize when they need assistance.

■ Child will respond positively to parents, show interest in their faces, and become calm when soothed by them.

Suggested NOC outcomes

Parenting Performance; Role Performance

Interventions and rationales

■ Perform an ongoing assessment of parent and child interaction *to evaluate whether parent-child attachment is proceeding normally.*

■ Speak positively about the child in the parents' presence *to encourage the parents to develop positive view of the child.*

■ Maintain eye contact with the child when caring for him, talk to him, and touch him appropriately *to demonstrate healthy interactions with the child.*

■ Help the parents learn to understand behavioral cues from the child. For example, the child may become fussy when he's ready for a nap or may pull his ear if he has an earache. *Developing better understanding of their child's behavior will decrease the parents' frustration and help them to care more effectively for the child.*

■ Provide the parents and the child with privacy *to promote attachment.*

■ Assess the parents' knowledge of child care and development *to develop an appropriate teaching plan.*

■ Teach the parents to provide physical care for the child *to increase their sense of competence and self-confidence.*

■ Encourage the parents to make eye contact with the child, caress and talk to him in soothing tone, call him by name, and make positive remarks about him *to foster a healthy parent-child attachment and to help ensure the child's well-being.*

■ Observe the parents; note whether their responses to the child are appropriate. Compliment them when they exhibit successful parenting skills *to increase their confidence.*

■ Discuss life changes precipitated by birth *to help the parents express their frustrations and feelings about role changes.* Topics may include altered finances, changes in living space, care-taking arrangements, and new roles and responsibilities for parents and siblings.

■ Provide the parents with sources of ongoing support and care *to ensure adequate follow-up.*

■ Assess the home environment. Discuss adaptations the parents need to make. *Adaptations in the home environment may be needed to help the parents properly care for their child.*

Suggested NIC interventions

Abuse Protection Support: Child; Coping Enhancement; Developmental Enhancement: Child; Parenting Promotion

Evaluations for expected outcomes

■ Parents initiate positive interactions with child.

■ Parents make eye contact with child, caress and talk to him, and call him by name.

■ Parents express confidence in their ability to meet child's needs.

■ Parents respond appropriately to child's behavioral cues, provide stimulation when he's alert and ready, don't overstimulate him, and recognize when he needs to nap.

■ Parents express positive feelings about child.

■ Parents express confidence in ability to care for child at home.

■ Parents recognize when they need assistance and make plans to contact appropriate resources.

■ Child responds positively to parents, shows interest in their faces, and becomes calm when soothed by them.

Documentation

■ Description of parent and child interactions

■ Nursing interventions to promote attachment

■ Parents' response to nursing interventions

■ Child's response to modifications in parents' behavior
■ Evaluations for expected outcomes

Reference

Delaney, K.R. "Learning to Observe Relationships and Coping," *Journal of Child and Adolescent Psychiatric Nursing* 19(4):194-202, November 2006.

PARENTAL ROLE CONFLICT

related to child's hospitalization

Definition

State in which one or both parents experience role confusion and conflict in response to crisis

Assessment

■ Parental status, including age and maturity; apprehension, fear, and guilt; coping mechanisms employed; developmental state of family and other children; knowledge of normal growth and development of children; past response to crises; understanding of child's present condition; previous parent-child relationship; spiritual practices of parents and family; stability of parental relationship; and support systems available to parent
■ Parent-child interaction, including eye contact, response to appearance (such as bandages, deformities, and hospital equipment), smiling, touching, and verbalization
■ Child's health status, including severity of illness and health care needs
■ Child's level of development

Defining characteristics

■ Disruption in care-taking routines
■ Expressed concern about changes in parental role and family functioning, communication, and health
■ Expressed feeling of inadequacy to provide for child's needs
■ Expressed loss of control over decisions relating to child
■ Expressed or demonstrated feelings of guilt, anger, fear, anxiety, and frustration about effect of child's illness on family
■ Reluctance to participate in usual caregiving activities, even with support

Expected outcomes

■ Parents will communicate feelings about present situation.
■ Parents will participate in their child's daily care.
■ Parents will express feelings of greater control and ability to contribute more to child's well-being.
■ Parents will express knowledge of child's developmental needs.
■ Parents will hold, touch, and convey warmth and affection to child.
■ Parents will use available support systems or agencies to assist in coping.

Suggested NOC outcomes

Caregiver Adaptation to Patient Institutionalization; Caregiver Home Care Readiness; Coping; Family Coping; Family Normalization

Interventions and rationales

■ Orient the parents or primary caregivers to the hospital environment, visiting procedures, medical equipment, and staff. *Familiarity decreases anxiety.*

■ Provide family-centered care by obtaining the parents' input for the child's care. *Parents can meet many of the child's needs better than staff.* Involve the parents in the child's care conferences and in the physical care of the child. *Participation may decrease the parents' feelings of helplessness.*

■ Teach the parents normal childhood physical and psychological development *to prepare the parents to deal with changes.*

■ Encourage parental involvement in appropriate support groups or agencies when necessary or ordered. *Such groups can provide emotional support and help reduce feelings of being overwhelmed.*

■ Ask the parents if they have questions about the child's status and provide information, as requested, *to reduce feelings of helplessness.*

■ Provide for the needs of the parents, as appropriate. Offer facilities for showering, sleeping, and eating. Be available to care for the child if the parents need an opportunity to rest. *Helping the parents meet their needs will empower them to meet child care demands.*

Suggested NIC interventions

Caregiver Support; Coping Enhancement; Family Involvement Promotion; Family Presence Facilitation; Family Process Maintenance; Role Enhancement

Evaluations for expected outcomes

■ Parents communicate feelings about present situation.
■ Parents participate in their child's daily care.
■ Parents express feelings of control in present situation.
■ Parents communicate knowledge of child's developmental needs.
■ Parents hold, touch, and express warmth and affection to child.
■ Parents contact support systems or community agencies to assist in coping.

Documentation

■ Observations of parents' ability to cope and their level of involvement in child's hospital care and daily needs
■ Interventions performed to help parents lower stress and cope with situation
■ Referrals to outside agencies or support groups
■ Child's medical and emotional state
■ Evaluations for expected outcomes

References

Corlett, J. and Twycross, A. "Negotiation of Parental Roles Within Family-centered Care: A Review of the Research," *Journal of Clinical Nursing* 15(10):1308-16, October 2006.

Miceli, P.J. and Clark, P.A. "Your Patient — My Child: Seven Priorities for Improving Pediatric Care from the Parent's Perspective," *Journal of Nursing Care Quality* 20(10):43-53, January-March 2005.

PARENTAL ROLE CONFLICT

related to home care of a child with special needs

Definition
State in which one or both parents experience role confusion and crisis in response to the special needs of a child at home

Assessment
- Extent of child's special needs
- Parental status, including age and maturity, developmental state of family, authority within family, employment status, financial needs, marital status, stability of parental relationship, knowledge of normal growth and development, understanding of child's condition and prognosis, expectations regarding child, participation in community, past response to crises, and coping mechanisms
- Available support systems, including other family members, friends, visiting nurses, and community resources
- Parent-child interaction
- Parent-child relationship before development of special needs and any changes that have occurred
- Religious practices of parents and family
- Presence of conflict between family's lifestyle and child's needs
- Home environment

Defining characteristics
- Disruption in care-taking routines
- Expressed concern about changes in parental role and family functioning, communication, and health
- Expressed feeling of inadequacy to provide for child's needs
- Expressed loss of control over decisions relating to child
- Expressed or demonstrated feelings of guilt, anger, fear, anxiety, and frustration about effect of child's illness on family
- Reluctance to participate in usual caregiving activities, even with support

Expected outcomes
- Parents will seek out and accept external support, education, and assistance in caring for child at home.
- Parents will demonstrate knowledge of child's developmental needs.

■ Parents will begin to provide physical, emotional, and developmental care to child at home.

■ Parents will seek assistance in meeting their own emotional and developmental needs.

■ Parents will express feelings of greater control and capability in meeting their child's needs.

■ Siblings will voice their emotional needs.

Suggested NOC outcomes

Caregiver Home Care Readiness; Coping; Family Coping; Family Functioning; Family Resiliency; Parenting Performance

Interventions and rationales

■ Provide family-centered care by involving parents in their child's care. Explain their rights as primary caregivers. Provide information to help them make informed decisions. Give them an opportunity to support the child during painful procedures. *Parents can better meet the needs of their child than staff members can. Parents need to receive proper information and have their own needs met before they can meet the child's needs.*

■ Promote the emotional well-being of parents by providing respite care, encouraging parents to spend time away from the child to enhance their marital relationship, and providing information about additional sources of support. *Encouraging parents to pay attention to their own emotional needs will enhance their ability to care for their child.*

■ Listen to the parents, child, and siblings openly and without passing judgment *to gain their trust.*

■ Help parents develop realistic expectations of their child and formulate achievable short-term goals based on the child's needs and abilities *to reduce frustration and feelings of helplessness.*

■ Ensure attention to all of the child's normal health needs, including dental care, immunizations, safety, and educational and nutritional needs. *A chronically ill child needs total health care, not just illness-related interventions.*

■ Pay attention to the needs of siblings at home. Devote time to discussing their feelings about having a brother or sister with special needs. How do their friends react? Contact their school nurse for assistance. Encourage them to help care for their brother or sister, but make sure activities are age-appropriate. *Becoming involved will help siblings achieve greater self-esteem and enhance their sense of control.*

■ Advocate normal growth and development for the child with special needs. Encourage visits by friends and discourage overprotective behavior *to help the child obtain social acceptance. Increased social interaction will encourage parents, siblings, and others to view the child as a unique individual instead of a burden. This, in turn, will help promote the child's self-esteem.*

■ Act as a liaison between the family and the multidisciplinary health care team, equipment vendors, community agencies, and third-party payers. *An organized approach with one central coordinator decreases stress for the family and enhances continuity of care.*

Suggested NIC interventions

Crisis Intervention; Decision-Making Support; Family Process Maintenance; Limit Setting; Mutual Goal Setting; Parenting Promotion; Role Enhancement

Evaluations for expected outcomes

■ Parents seek out and use community resources to assist in meeting child's physical, psychological, and educational needs.

■ Parents express increased knowledge of their child's needs and demonstrate comfort in caring for child at home.

■ Parents provide appropriate physical, emotional, and developmental care to child at home.

■ Parents seek help to meet their own emotional and developmental needs.

■ Parents express feelings of greater control and capability in meeting child's needs.

■ Siblings come to terms with having brother or sister with special needs.

Documentation

■ Family members' expressions of feelings about their role in caring for child at home

■ Observations of parent-child interaction

■ Physical and psychological status of child with special needs

■ Nursing interventions to resolve parental role conflict in home

■ Parents', child's, and siblings' responses to interventions

■ Evaluations for expected outcomes

Reference

Loretta Secco, M., et al. "Factors Affecting Parenting Stress Among Biologically Vulnerable Toddlers," *Issues in Comprehensive Pediatric Nursing* 29(3):131-56, July-September 2006.

Impaired
PARENTING

related to lack of knowledge about parenting skills

Definition

Inability of a nurturing figure to promote optimum growth and development in an infant or child

Assessment

■ Parental status, including age, degree of apprehension, developmental state, family roles, and relationship with spouse or significant other

■ Gender and health status of other children

■ Parents' knowledge of child care and normal growth and development

■ Previous bonding history

■ Interaction of parent and infant or child, including care practices, eye contact, smiling, touching, verbalization, visual and voice responses, and response to appearance, disabilities, and gender of child

■ Psychosocial status, including financial stressors and previous experience, work demands, and support of family, friends, and significant other

Defining characteristics

■ Child: behavioral disorders, failure to thrive, frequent accidents and illness, history of trauma or abuse, lack of attachment, no separation anxiety, poor academic performance, poor cognitive development, poor social competence, tendency to run away

■ Parents: evidence of inflexibility in meeting child's needs; evidence of neglectful behavior toward or abandonment of child; expressed frustration over inability to fulfill role; expressed inability to control child; expressed inability to meet child's needs; expressed negative feeling about child; inadequate child health maintenance; inappropriate child care arrangements; inappropriate visual, tactile, or auditory stimulation for child; inconsistent caregiving; inconsistent management of child's behavior; poor or inappropriate caregiving skills; poor parent-child interaction, with little cuddling; punitive or abusive behavior toward child; rejection of or hostility toward child; unsafe home environment; weak or no attachment to child

Expected outcomes

■ Parents will establish eye, physical, and verbal contact with infant or child.
■ Parents will voice satisfaction with infant or child.
■ Parents will demonstrate correct feeding, bathing, and dressing techniques.
■ Parents will express willingness to work to maintain relationship with each other.
■ Parents will state plans for well-child care.
■ Parents will express knowledge of developmental norms.
■ Parents will provide play activities for child.
■ Parents will identify ways to express anger and frustration that don't harm child.

Suggested NOC outcomes

Caregiver Performance: Direct Care; Child Development: Middle Childhood; Family Coping; Family Functioning; Parenting: Early/Middle Childhood Physical Safety; Parenting Performance

Interventions and rationales

■ Involve parents in the care of the infant or child immediately *to promote attachment to the child.*

■ Provide opportunities for care-taking by allowing parents to share a room with their infant or child or by extending visitation periods. *Participation in care increases a parent's feeling of self-esteem and self-worth.*

■ Educate parents about:

– normal growth and development

- breast-feeding or bottle-feeding techniques
- infant care, such as bathing and dressing
- routine well-child care
- signs and symptoms of illness
- the child's need for tactile and sensory stimulation.

Knowledge of normal growth and development may decrease unrealistic expectations and increase chances of successful parenting.

■ When caring for the child in the parents' presence, act as a role model for effective parenting skills. *Lack of knowledge of routine child care practices and growth and developmental norms significantly contributes to child abuse. Demonstration is a more effective means of teaching parenting skills than lecturing.*

■ Encourage questions about care-taking and provide appropriate information *to allay anxiety and monitor knowledge retention.*

■ Praise parents when they display appropriate parenting skills *to provide positive reinforcement.*

■ Refer parents to a family support group and other community resources such as Parents Anonymous. *Battering parents typically lack a support system and have a sense of being alone. A support group may help ease isolation.*

■ Encourage verbalization of the infant's or child's impact on family life. *Ventilation of feelings helps parents deal more effectively with the stress of child care.*

■ Be alert for signs and symptoms of child abuse, including neglect, uncleanliness, and frequent accidents or withdrawn, fearful behavior on the part of the child. Report actual or suspected child abuse to appropriate authorities. *Reporting child abuse is your professional duty. The United States legally requires nurses to report abuse.*

Suggested NIC interventions

Coping Enhancement; Family Process Maintenance; Family Support; Mutual Goal Setting; Parent Education: Childrearing Family; Role Enhancement

Evaluations for expected outcomes

■ Parents make appropriate physical, verbal, and eye contact when interacting with infant or child.
■ Parents make statements indicating satisfaction with infant or child.
■ Parents demonstrate correct feeding, bathing, and dressing techniques.
■ Parents express willingness to maintain their relationship with each other.
■ Parents bring infant for routine well-child care.
■ Parents verbalize knowledge of developmental norms.
■ Parents provide play activities for child.
■ Parents identify ways to express anger and frustration that don't harm child.

Documentation

■ Parents' expressions of feelings about child
■ Parents' expressions of concern about their performance as parents
■ Observation of parental visits, bonding, care-taking, and knowledge level
■ Instructions given to parents and parents' understanding of their responsibilities

- Infant's weight
- Evaluations for expected outcomes

Reference
Tucker, S., et al. "Lessons Learned in Translating Research Evidence on Early Intervention Programs into Clinical Care," *The American Journal of Maternal Child Nursing* 31(5):325-31, September-October 2006.

Risk for impaired
PARENTING
related to lack of or poor parental role model

Definition
Presence of risk factors that may interfere with primary caregiver's ability to promote optimum growth and development in an infant or child

Assessment
- Ages of caregiver and child
- Caregiver's psychosocial status, including developmental state, educational level, family roles, presence or absence of spouse or significant other, financial stressors, previous parenting experience, work demands, and support of family, friends, or significant other
- Interaction between caregiver and infant or child, including care practices, eye contact, response to appearance and gender of infant, smiling, touching, verbalization, and visual and voice responses

Risk factors
- Change in family unit
- Father of child not involved
- Financial difficulties
- History of being abused
- Inability to put child's needs before own
- Inadequate child care arrangements
- Lack of access to resources
- Lack of family cohesiveness
- Lack of or poor parental role model
- Lack of social support network
- Lack of transportation
- Lack of value of parenthood
- Legal difficulties
- Low self-esteem
- Low socioeconomic class
- Maladaptive coping strategies
- Marital conflict, declining satisfaction
- Poor home environment

- Poor problem-solving skills
- Poverty
- Relocation
- Role strain or overload
- Single parent
- Social isolation
- Stress
- Unemployment or job problems
- Unplanned or unwanted pregnancy

Adult

- Inability to recognize and act on infant cues
- Lack of cognitive readiness for parenthood
- Lack of knowledge about child development
- Lack of knowledge about child health maintenance
- Lack of knowledge about parenting skills
- Low cognitive functioning
- Low educational level or attainment
- Poor communication skills
- Preference for physical punishment
- Unrealistic expectations of child

Physiological

- Physical illness

Infant or child

- Altered perceptual abilities
- Attention deficit hyperactivity disorder
- Difficult temperament
- Handicapping condition or developmental delay
- Illness
- Lack of goodness of fit (temperament) with parental expectations
- Multiple births
- Not gender desired
- Premature birth
- Prolonged separation from parent
- Separation from parent at birth
- Unplanned or unwanted child

Psychological

- Depression
- Difficult labor or delivery
- Disability
- High number or closely spaced children
- History of mental illness
- History of substance abuse or dependence
- Lack of, or late, prenatal care
- Separation from infant or child

■ Sleep deprivation or disruption
■ Young age, especially adolescent

Expected outcomes

■ Caregiver will establish eye, physical, and verbal contact with infant or child.
■ Caregiver will demonstrate correct feeding, bathing, and dressing techniques.
■ Caregiver will state plans to bring infant or child to clinic for routine physical and psychological examinations.
■ Caregiver will express understanding of developmental norms.
■ Caregiver will provide age-appropriate play activities.

Suggested NOC outcomes

Caregiver Performance: Direct Care; Family Coping; Family Functioning; Parenting Performance

Interventions and rationales

■ Assess the amount of developmental stimulation provided by the caregiver. For example, use the Home Observation for Measurement of the Environment (HOME) Inventory on a home visit *to assess whether the home environment is developmentally stimulating.*
■ Instruct the caregiver in the basics of infant and child care. *Research shows that the primary source of information about parenting is the caregiver's own parents. If a caregiver lacks an effective role model, you may need to supply basic information about parenting.*
■ When caring for the child in the caregiver's presence, act as a role model for effective parenting skills. Demonstrate comfort measures, such as rocking the infant, and show the caregiver how to hold the infant in an *en face* position *to familiarize the caregiver with routine child-care practices.*
■ Teach the caregiver about normal growth and development, and identify ages at which the child should master developmental tasks such as rolling over, crawling, and walking. *This will help the caregiver monitor the child's growth and development and practice appropriate safety precautions, such as blocking stairways, securing crib side rails, and preventing other accidents.* Also discuss problem behaviors associated with specific ages, such as colic, temper tantrums, and sleeping difficulties, *to further enhance the caregiver's understanding of developmental norms.*
■ Discuss the child's need for tactile and sensory stimulation. Demonstrate play activities that promote developmental skills, such as shaking a rattle in front of an infant to build eye-and-hand coordination or placing a mobile above an infant to encourage visual tracking and trunk and head control. *Sensory experiences promote cognitive development.*
■ Familiarize the caregiver with techniques for detecting symptoms of illness in an infant or child, including:
– taking temperatures and reading thermometers
– assessing the child's respiratory status
– observing for behavioral cues of illness, such as increased crying, rubbing ears, or drawing legs to abdomen.
Knowledge of how to monitor the child's health status will assist in the diagnosis and early treatment of problems.

■ Encourage the caregiver to ask questions about infant and child care. Identify the questions parents commonly ask about infant care, such as cord care, feeding techniques, and bathing. Reassure the caregiver that other parents also need to ask basic questions. *A caregiver who lacks effective parenting role models may not know what questions to ask or may hesitate to ask questions because of embarrassment.*

■ Praise the caregiver for display of appropriate parenting skills *to provide positive reinforcement.*

■ Emphasize the importance of making regular visits to a health care professional, even when the child appears healthy. *Routine visits allow early detection of developmental delays and provision of preventive care, such as immunizations.*

■ As necessary, refer the caregiver and family to a physician, nurse practitioner, or social services for follow-up *to ensure continuity of care.*

Suggested NIC interventions

Counseling; Family Integrity Promotion: Childbearing Family; Family Process Maintenance; Family Support; Parenting Promotion

Evaluations for expected outcomes

■ Caregiver makes appropriate eye, physical, and verbal contact with infant or child.

■ Caregiver demonstrates correct feeding, bathing, and dressing techniques.

■ Caregiver brings infant or child to clinic for routine examinations.

■ Caregiver expresses understanding of developmental norms and accurately assesses child's developmental status and needs.

■ Caregiver provides age-appropriate play activities.

Documentation

■ Evidence of neglect of infant or child
■ Observations of caregiver's skills and knowledge level
■ Presence or absence of caregiver-child bonding behaviors
■ Questions asked by caregiver about care of infant or child
■ Instructions given to caregiver and caregiver's response
■ Evaluations for expected outcomes

Reference

Tucker, S., et al. "Lessons Learned in Translating Research Evidence on Early Intervention Programs into Clinical Care," *The American Journal of Maternal Child Nursing* 31(5):325-31, September-October 2006.

Bathing or hygiene
SELF-CARE DEFICIT
related to developmental delay

Definition

Inability to carry out aspects of self-care, such as bathing and personal hygiene

Assessment

- Age
- History of neurologic, sensory, or developmental impairment
- Self-care abilities, including knowledge and use of adaptive equipment, preparation of equipment and supplies, and technical or mechanical skills
- Musculoskeletal status, including range of motion, muscle tone, gait, muscle size and strength, functional capabilities, and mechanical restrictions (such as splints, casts, or traction)
- Neurologic status, including cognition, communication ability, insight or judgment, level of consciousness, memory, motor ability, orientation, and sensory ability
- Psychosocial status, including child's affective reaction to imbalances between motor abilities and cognitive reasoning abilities, usual lifestyle, and parents' perception of developmental delay

Defining characteristics

- Impaired ability to get into and out of bathroom
- Impaired ability to obtain bath supplies
- Impaired ability to obtain or get to water source
- Impaired ability to regulate water temperature or flow
- Impaired ability to wash or dry body

Expected outcomes

- Child's skin will remain clean, dry, and intact.
- Child and family members will voice feelings about self-care deficit.
- Child or family member will demonstrate ability to perform bathing and hygiene.
- Child or family member will perform self-care program daily.

Suggested NOC outcomes

Coordinated Movement; Psychomotor Energy; Self-Care: Bathing; Self-Care: Hygiene

Interventions and rationales

- Assess the child's functional, cognitive, and perceptual level at established intervals. Document and report any changes. *Ongoing assessment allows you to identify changing needs and adjust interventions accordingly.*
- Provide the prescribed treatment for the child's underlying condition. Monitor and report progress *to provide a basis for the care plan.*
- Monitor completion of bathing and hygiene *to evaluate self-care abilities and identify areas of need.* Provide help only when the child has difficulty.
- Teach the child and family members bathing and hygiene techniques. Have them perform return demonstrations *to identify problem areas and build self-confidence.*
- Allow ample time to perform self-care. Encourage the child to complete each task. Provide constructive feedback. *Rushing creates unnecessary stress and pro-*

motes failure. *Completing a task without assistance promotes self-confidence. Positive feedback encourages progress.*

■ Provide privacy for self-care activities. *Modesty becomes important to children around age 6.*

■ Provide safety equipment *to promote safety.*

■ Refer the child and family to support groups or community services *to provide continued assistance for efforts to promote self-care independence.*

Suggested NIC interventions

Bathing; Decision-Making Support; Energy Management; Self-Care Assistance: Bathing/Hygiene; Teaching: Individual

Evaluations for expected outcomes

■ Child's skin remains clean, dry, and intact.

■ Child and family members voice feelings about self-care deficit.

■ Child or family member displays competence in performing bathing and hygiene through return demonstration.

■ Child or family member performs self-care program daily.

Documentation

■ Child's expressions of frustration or feelings of inadequacy

■ Family members' expressions of concern regarding child's inability to carry out bathing and hygiene

■ Child's response to treatment of underlying condition

■ Child's motor and sensory status

■ Observations of child's impaired self-care ability

■ Interventions to promote self-care skills and provide supportive care

■ Instructions to child and family members, their understanding of instructions, and their demonstrated ability to carry out bathing and hygiene

■ Child's and family members' responses to nursing interventions

■ Evaluations for expected outcomes

Reference

Moss, J. "Development of a Functional Ability Scale for Children and Young People with Myalgic Encephalopathy (ME)/Chronic Fatigue Syndrome (CFS)," *Journal of Child Health Care* 9(1):20-30, March 2005.

Dressing or grooming
SELF-CARE DEFICIT
related to developmental delay

Definition

Inability to carry out activities associated with dressing and grooming

Assessment
- Age
- History of neurologic, sensory, or developmental impairment
- Self-care abilities, including knowledge and use of adaptive equipment, preparation of equipment and supplies, and technical or mechanical skills
- Musculoskeletal status, including range of motion, muscle tone, gait, muscle size and strength, functional capabilities, and mechanical restrictions (such as splints, casts, or traction)
- Neurologic status, including cognition, communication ability, insight or judgment, level of consciousness, memory, motor ability, orientation, and sensory ability
- Psychosocial status, including child's affective reaction to imbalances between motor abilities and cognitive reasoning abilities, usual lifestyle, and parents' perception of developmental delay

Defining characteristics
- Impaired ability to clothe part or all of body
- Impaired ability to fasten clothing (such as inability to use zippers)
- Impaired ability to obtain or replace items of clothing
- Impaired ability to put on or take off specific articles of clothing (such as socks or shoes)
- Inability to choose clothing
- Inability to maintain appearance at satisfactory level
- Inability to pick up clothing
- Inability to use assistive devices

Expected outcomes
- Child will be dressed and well groomed each day.
- Child and family members will express feelings and concerns regarding child's self-care deficit.
- Child or family member will display competence in performing dressing and grooming skills through return demonstration.
- Child or family member will perform self-care program daily.

Suggested NOC outcomes
Body Image; Energy Conservation; Self-Care: Dressing; Self-Care: Hygiene

Interventions and rationales
- Assess the child's functional, cognitive, and perceptual level at periodic intervals. Document and report any changes. *Ongoing assessment allows you to identify changing needs and adjust interventions accordingly.*
- Provide the prescribed treatment for the child's underlying condition. Monitor and report progress *to provide a basis for the care plan.*
- Monitor completion of dressing and grooming *to evaluate self-care abilities and identify areas of need.* Provide help only when the child has difficulty. *Appropriate assistance provides an opportunity to teach self-care and promote good habits.*

■ Suggest clothing that the child can manage easily, such as clothing slightly larger than regular size or pants and shoes with Velcro fasteners *to foster independence and improve self-esteem.*

■ Instruct the child and family members in dressing and grooming techniques. Have them perform return demonstrations *to identify problem areas and build self-confidence.*

■ Allow ample time to perform self-care. Encourage the child to complete each task. Provide constructive feedback. *Rushing creates unnecessary stress and promotes failure. Completing a task without help promotes self-confidence. Positive feedback encourages progress.*

■ Provide privacy for dressing and grooming. *Modesty becomes important to children around age 6.*

■ Refer the child and family to support groups or community services *to provide ongoing assistance.*

Suggested NIC interventions

Body Image Enhancement; Dressing; Energy Management; Hair Care; Nail Care; Self-Care Assistance: IADL

Evaluations for expected outcomes

■ Child is dressed and well groomed each day.

■ Child and family members voice feelings regarding deficit in grooming and dressing skills.

■ Child or family member displays competence in performing dressing and grooming skills through return demonstration.

■ Child or family member performs self-care program daily.

Documentation

■ Child's expressions of frustration or feelings of inadequacy

■ Family members' expressions of feelings and concerns regarding child's inability to carry out dressing and grooming

■ Child's response to treatment of underlying condition

■ Child's motor and sensory status

■ Interventions to promote self-care skills and provide supportive care

■ Instructions provided to child and family members, their understanding of instructions, and their demonstrated ability to carry out dressing and grooming

■ Child's and family members' responses to nursing interventions

■ Evaluations for expected outcomes

Reference

Lindblad, B.M., et al. "Being Invigorated in Parenthood: Parents' Experience of Being Supported by Professionals When Having a Disabled Child," *Journal of Pediatric Nursing* 20(4):288-97, August 2005.

Feeding
SELF-CARE DEFICIT
related to developmental delay

Definition

Inability to carry out feeding routine

Assessment

- Age
- History of injury or disease associated with musculoskeletal impairment
- Self-care abilities, including knowledge and use of adaptive equipment, preparation of equipment and supplies, and technical and mechanical skills
- Musculoskeletal status, including coordination, functional ability, muscle tone and strength, range of motion, and mechanical restrictions (such as cast, splint, or traction)
- Neurologic status, including cognition, communication ability, level of consciousness, motor ability, and sensory status
- Nutritional status, including weight and food preferences
- Psychosocial status, including child's affective reaction to imbalances between motor abilities and cognitive reasoning abilities, usual lifestyle, and parents' perception of developmental delay

Defining characteristics

- Inability to bring food from receptacle to mouth
- Inability to chew food
- Inability to complete meals
- Inability to get food onto utensil
- Inability to handle cup or glass
- Inability to handle utensils
- Inability to ingest food safely and in socially acceptable manner
- Inability to ingest sufficient food
- Inability to open containers
- Inability to prepare food
- Inability to swallow food
- Inability to use assistive devices

Expected outcomes

- Child will consume adequate calories and maintain desired weight.
- Auscultation will reveal clear breath sounds.
- Child and family members will express feelings and concerns.
- Child or family member will demonstrate correct feeding technique.

Suggested NOC outcomes

Appetite; Cognition; Nutritional Status; Nutritional Status: Food & Fluid Intake; Self-Care Status; Self-Care: Eating; Swallowing Status

Interventions and rationales

■ Assess the child's functional, cognitive, and perceptual level at periodic intervals. Document and report any changes. *Ongoing assessment allows you to identify changing needs and adjust interventions accordingly.*

■ Provide the prescribed treatment for the child's underlying condition. Monitor and report progress *to provide a basis for the care plan.*

■ Weigh the child daily and record results *to assess nutritional status.*

■ Determine the type of food the child handles most and tolerates best (finger foods, soft or liquid diet) *to enhance self-feeding ability.*

■ Monitor and record breath sounds every 4 hours. Report any evidence of crackles, wheezing, or rhonchi *to detect aspiration.*

■ Monitor the feeding routine *to evaluate self-care abilities and identify areas of need.* Assist only if necessary; for example, cut food into bite-size portions. *Appropriate assistance provides an opportunity to teach self-care and promote good habits.*

■ Instruct the child and family members in the feeding routine. Have them perform return demonstrations *to build self-confidence.*

■ Allow ample time to perform self-care activities. Encourage the child to complete each task. Provide constructive feedback. *Rushing creates unnecessary stress and promotes failure. Completing a task without assistance promotes self-confidence. Positive feedback encourages progress.*

■ Position the child in the upright sitting position. Use supportive devices, as needed, to maintain the child's posture. Sit at eye level with the child. *These measures help decrease the risk of aspiration. Sitting at eye level helps prevent the child from hyperextending his neck, which may increase the risk of aspiration.*

■ Teach specific tasks (such as grasping a spoon, opening the mouth, closing the lips around a utensil, or swallowing) rather than the total feeding skill. Use behavior modification techniques of praise and reward to mark accomplishments. *Children may not have cognitive or motor abilities to complete the total skill. Breaking down behavior into smaller units increases the likelihood of success.*

Suggested NIC interventions

Energy Management; Nutrition Management; Nutritional Counseling; Self-Care Assistance: Feeding

Evaluations for expected outcomes

■ Child maintains weight above 5th percentile on pediatric growth charts.

■ Aspiration doesn't occur as evidenced by clear breath sounds heard during auscultation.

■ Child and family members voice feelings regarding feeding routine.

■ Child or family member demonstrates correct feeding technique.

Documentation

■ Child's expressions of frustration or feelings of inadequacy

■ Family members' expressions of concern

■ Child's response to treatment of underlying condition

■ Child's motor and sensory status

■ Interventions performed to promote self-care skills and provide supportive care

■ Instructions provided to child and family members, their understanding of instructions, and their demonstrated ability to carry out feeding routine
■ Child's and family members' responses to nursing interventions
■ Evaluations for expected outcomes

Reference
Redstone, F., and West, J.F. "The Importance of Postural Control for Feeding," *Pediatric Nursing* 30(2):97-100, March-April 2004.

Toileting
SELF-CARE DEFICIT
related to developmental delay

Definition
Inability to carry out aspects of self-care associated with bowel and urine elimination

Assessment
■ Developmental factors, including age, maturity, and smooth-muscle control
■ History of neurologic, sensory, or developmental impairment
■ Self-care abilities, including knowledge and use of adaptive equipment, preparation of equipment and supplies, and technical or mechanical skills
■ Musculoskeletal status, including range of motion, muscle tone, gait, muscle size and strength, functional capabilities, and mechanical restrictions (such as splints, casts, or traction)
■ Neurologic status, including cognition, communication ability, insight or judgment, level of consciousness, memory, motor ability, orientation, and sensory ability
■ Psychosocial status, including child's affective reaction to imbalances between motor abilities and cognitive reasoning abilities, usual lifestyle, and parents' perception of developmental delay

Defining characteristics
■ Inability to carry out proper toilet hygiene
■ Inability to flush toilet or empty commode
■ Inability to get to toilet or commode
■ Inability to manipulate clothing for toileting
■ Inability to sit on or rise from toilet or commode

Expected outcomes
■ Child will maintain normal urine and bowel elimination patterns for age.
■ Child and family members will voice feelings about impaired toileting ability.
■ Child and family members will demonstrate correct toileting activities.
■ Child's skin will remain clean, dry, and intact.

Suggested NOC outcomes

Balance; Coordinated Movement; Self-Care: Hygiene; Self-Care: Toileting; Self-Direction of Care

Interventions and rationales

■ Observe the child's functional, cognitive, and perceptual level. Document and report any changes. *Ongoing assessment allows you to identify changing needs and adjust interventions accordingly.*

■ Provide the prescribed treatment for the child's underlying condition. Monitor and report progress *to provide a basis for the care plan.*

■ Monitor intake and output *to detect fluid and electrolyte imbalances.*

■ Assess skin condition, especially in the perianal area, *to detect evidence of skin breakdown.*

■ Assist with toileting when necessary. As much as possible, allow the child to perform the toilet routine independently *to enhance toileting ability and promote feelings of control.*

■ Teach the child and family members the toileting routine. Have the child and family members demonstrate the toileting routine under supervision. *Return demonstration allows you to evaluate learning and increases the child's and family members' confidence.*

■ Provide privacy for toileting activities. *Modesty becomes important to children around age 6.*

■ Assist with specific bladder elimination procedures, such as intermittent self-catheterization, as prescribed. Assess the child's readiness to learn self-catheterization. Instruct the child or family members in the technique and request a return demonstration *to evaluate understanding and ability.* Maintain sterile technique in the hospital and clean technique at home *to prevent infection.*

■ Assist with the use of incontinence aids, such as diapers, pads, and pants, which may be prescribed as an alternative to indwelling devices. *Incontinence aids prevent the soiling of clothes and linen, reduce embarrassment, and draw urine away from skin.*

■ Establish a regular pattern for bowel care. For example, after breakfast, place the child on the toilet or commode for 1 hour after inserting a glycerin suppository; allow the child to remain upright for 30 minutes, and then clean the anal area. *Regular bowel care encourages routine physiologic function.*

■ Teach the parents the bowel care routine *to foster compliance.*

■ Maintain a diet log *to identify irritant foods,* and then eliminate such foods from the child's diet *to promote regular bowel function.* Teach parents the need to regulate the child's intake of foods and fluids that cause diarrhea or constipation *to encourage healthful nutritional patterns.*

■ Teach parents to regulate the child's fluid intake according to a specific schedule and to limit fluid intake after dinner *to encourage voiding at appropriate times.*

Suggested NIC interventions

Bowel Training; Self-Care Assistance: Bathing/Hygiene; Urinary Elimination Management

Evaluations for expected outcomes

■ Child maintains normal elimination patterns for age.
■ Child and family members express feelings associated with child's toileting routine.
■ Child and family members demonstrate correct toileting activities.
■ Child's skin remains intact with no evidence of breakdown.

Documentation

■ Child's expressions of feelings of inadequacy or depression
■ Family members' concerns about child's inability to carry out toileting activities
■ Child's response to treatment of underlying condition
■ Child's motor and sensory status
■ Interventions to promote self-care skills and to provide supportive care
■ Child's and family members' responses to nursing interventions
■ Instructions to child and family members, their understanding of instructions, and demonstrated ability to carry out toileting routine
■ Evaluations for expected outcomes

Reference

Merenda, L.A., and Hickey, K. "Key Elements of Bladder and Bowel Management for Children with Spinal Cord Injuries," *SCI Nursing* 22(1):8-14, Spring 2005.

Ineffective
THERMOREGULATION

related to child's illness or trauma

Definition

Temperature fluctuations between hyperthermia and hypothermia

Assessment

■ Age
■ History of illness or injury, including related events, such as exposure to infection (intrauterine or extrauterine)
■ Perinatal history, including asphyxia
■ Health history, including chronic disease or disability
■ Medication history, including antibiotics, steroids, nonsteroidal anti-inflammatory drugs
■ Vital signs, including temperature, pulse, blood pressure, and respirations
■ Skin color and temperature
■ Fluid and electrolyte status, including skin turgor, intake and output, mucous membranes, serum electrolyte levels, and urine specific gravity
■ Neurologic status, including level of consciousness
≡ Nutritional status, including willingness and ability to eat, current weight, and weight gain pattern (on growth chart)

Defining characteristics

- Cyanotic nail beds
- Fluctuations in body temperature above or below normal range
- Flushed skin
- Hypertension
- Increased capillary refill time
- Increased respiratory or heart rate
- Mild shivering
- Moderate pallor
- Piloerection
- Seizures
- Warm or cool skin

Expected outcomes

- Child will maintain body temperature at normal levels (96.8° to 99° F [36° to 37.2° C]).
- Child's fluid intake and output will remain balanced and within normal limits for age.
- Child will maintain adequate glucose intake and will consume ___ calories per day.
- Child and family members will identify risk factors and describe measures to prevent dehydration.
- Family members will demonstrate procedure for assessing axillary or oral temperature accurately.
- Family members will demonstrate measures to care for child with fever.

Suggested NOC outcomes

Hydration; Thermoregulation; Vital Signs

Interventions and rationales

- Take an axillary or oral temperature every 1 to 4 hours. Avoid taking rectal temperatures. Record the temperature and route. *Physically and psychologically safer than rectal thermometers, axillary and oral thermometers provide an accurate core temperature.*
- If the child has a fever, remove sheets, blankets, and most clothing (except diapers and underwear). Place cool cloths on the axilla and groin. Perform a tepid sponging procedure. Use a hypothermia blanket for a temperature above 103° F (39.4° C). Set the blanket temperature at 41° F (5° C). Discontinue if shivering occurs *because shivering increases the metabolic rate and supports fever.* Monitor vital signs every 15 minutes for 1 hour, and as indicated, *because decreasing body temperature too rapidly can cause vascular collapse. These steps reduce excessive fever.*
- Monitor heart rate, rhythm, and respiratory rate. *Careful monitoring determines the need for more aggressive intervention.*
- Calculate the child's fluid, glucose, and electrolyte requirements. Administer I.V. fluids as indicated. Monitor and record intake and output *to compensate for an increase in metabolic rate and to prevent dehydration. Insensible fluid losses increase by 10% for every 0.5° F (1° C) rise in temperature.*

■ If the child's body temperature is below 96.8° F (36° C), use a warming blanket. Set the blanket temperature at 100.4° F (38° C). Keep the child wrapped in blankets and cover the child's head. *The body surface area, particularly the head, is proportionally larger in a young child; adequate covering will prevent heat loss. These steps combat hypothermia.*

■ Teach parents how to take an accurate temperature and have parents provide a return demonstration *to ensure accurate monitoring after discharge.*

■ Determine the child's preferences for oral fluids. Push fluids in a manner appropriate to the child's age and level of development. *A well-hydrated child's temperature returns to normal range more quickly.*

■ Discuss factors that precipitate neurogenic temperature drift with family members *to prevent future episodes.*

Suggested NIC interventions

Environmental Management; Fever Treatment; Fluid Management; Temperature Regulation; Vital Signs Monitoring

Evaluations for expected outcomes

■ Child's temperature remains within normal limits.

■ Child maintains balanced fluid intake and output within normal limits for age.

■ Child maintains adequate glucose and caloric intake.

■ Child and family members identify risk factors and describe measures to prevent dehydration.

■ Family members demonstrate ability to measure axillary or oral temperature accurately.

■ Family members demonstrate measures to care for child with fever.

Documentation

■ Observations of physical findings

■ Nursing interventions performed

■ Medications administered

■ Child's response to nursing interventions

■ Evaluations for expected outcomes

Reference

Chang, A., et al. "Minimizing Complications Related to Fever in the Postoperative Pediatric Oncology Patient," *Journal of Pediatric Oncology Nursing* 23(2):75-81, March-April 2006.

Impaired

VERBAL COMMUNICATION

related to developmental factors

Definition

Decreased, delayed, or absent ability to receive, transmit, and use a system of symbols

Assessment

■ Age

■ Health history, including past respiratory, neurologic, or musculoskeletal disorders or surgery

■ Respiratory status, including dyspnea, use of accessory muscles, and respiratory pattern

■ Neurologic status, including mental status and speech (pattern, signing, and such communication aids as artificial larynx, computer-assisted speech device, pen and pencil, picture board, and alphabet board)

■ Musculoskeletal status, including range of motion and manual dexterity

■ Parental status, including understanding of normal speech development, level of frustration with child's speech impairment, and coping skills

Defining characteristics

■ Difficulty comprehending and maintaining usual communication pattern

■ Difficulty expressing thoughts verbally (aphasia, dysphasia, apraxia, dyslexia)

■ Difficulty forming words or sentences (aphonia, dyslalia, dysarthria)

■ Difficulty using or inability to use facial expressions or body language

■ Disorientation

■ Dyspnea

■ Impaired articulation

■ Inability or lack of desire to speak

■ Inability to speak dominant language

■ Inappropriate verbalizations

■ Lack of eye contact or poor selective attention

■ Visual deficit (partial or total)

Expected outcomes

■ Family members will express desire to better understand child's communication impairment.

■ Family members will demonstrate understanding of verbal development in children and alternative communication techniques.

■ Child will communicate needs.

Suggested NOC outcomes

Cognition; Information Processing

Interventions and rationales

■ Teach parents to:

– talk to, read to, and play music for the child

– repeat the sounds the child makes

– point to objects and name them

– use generative speech ("What would you like to wear today?") rather than directive speech ("Do you want to wear the red shirt?").

These measures stimulate language development. Generative speech requires the child to generate words rather than simply responding with yes or no.

■ Describe to family members the alternative methods of assessing the needs of a speech-delayed child. A toddler or preschooler may communicate his needs through role playing with dolls and stuffed animals. A preschooler or school-age child may communicate through drawing. Parents may use pictorial (faces) pain scale to assess an ill child's level of discomfort. *These techniques will enable the family to better understand their speech-impaired child.*

■ Assess the family members' level of understanding of the speech development process. Tell them that a toddler has limited receptive language skills and should be given one direction at a time. A preschooler has limited vocabulary and may communicate through gestures and symbols. Further explain that each child develops speech at a different rate. *These measures increase family members' understanding of the child's speech impairment.*

Suggested NIC interventions

Anxiety Reduction; Communication Enhancement: Speech Deficit; Presence; Touch

Evaluations for expected outcomes

■ Family members describe stages of speech development.
■ Family members demonstrate alternative methods of assessing needs of speech-delayed child.
■ Child communicates needs.

Documentation

■ Family members' understanding of speech development process
■ Family members' demonstration of alternative methods of assessing needs of speech-delayed child
■ Family members' understanding of alternative methods of communicating with child
■ Nursing interventions and family's and child's response to them
■ Evaluations for expected outcomes

Reference

Olswang, L.B., et al. "Communication in Young Children with Motor Impairments: Teaching Caregivers to Teach," *Seminars in Speech and Language* 27(3):199-214, August 2006.

IV Maternal-neonatal health

INTRODUCTION

This section covers maternal, fetal, and neonatal care, with an emphasis on meeting the changing needs of the mother, child, and family. Because of the dynamic nature of pregnancy and childbirth, you'll need to be flexible in your care planning. Expect to form new nursing diagnoses continually during the time that you're providing care.

During pregnancy, you'll assess maternal factors, such as age, past experience with pregnancy and delivery, health history, reaction to fetal movement, and nutritional status. Keep in mind that the mother's health status directly affects the fetus's well-being.

After birth, you'll assess neonatal factors, such as Apgar scores, gestational age, weight in relation to gestational age, vital signs, feeding patterns, muscle tone, condition of fontanels, and characteristics of the neonate's cry.

Throughout your assessment, maintain a family-centered, holistic approach. Assess family status. Be aware of how pregnancy and the neonate's arrival affect parents, siblings, and the rest of the family. Evaluate how well the mother, father, siblings, and other family members bond with the neonate.

Use information gathered during assessment to develop appropriate nursing diagnoses. In this section, you'll find nursing diagnoses and related etiologies for the prenatal period, labor and delivery, and the postpartum period. Neonatal health is covered as well. These nursing diagnoses state actual or potential health problems of the developing family, focusing on the physiologic and psychosocial needs of its members.

When implementing your care plan, reinforce your interventions with thorough patient teaching. Encourage family members to become involved in the planning and implementation of care. Stay attuned to their changing educational needs, and remain sensitive to the new mother and supportive of her emotional concerns.

Inform other members of the health care team of your nursing goals, and enlist their support, as needed. Keep colleagues informed about the family's progress in attaining goals.

Evaluate the care plan frequently. This will allow you to determine the need for revisions promptly, thereby ensuring that the care plan accurately reflects the developing family's current needs.

ANXIETY

related to hospitalization and birth process

Definition

Vague, uneasy feeling of discomfort or dread accompanied by an autonomic response(the source often nonspecific or unknown to the individual); a feeling of apprehension caused by anticipation of danger; an alerting signal that warns of impending danger and enables the individual to take measures to deal with threat

Assessment

- History of stress-related signs or symptoms
- Cultural influences
- Current worries, fears, and concerns
- Expectations of labor experience, including knowledge and past experience
- Behavior, including reaction to fetal movement and uterine activity, motor activity, excessive or extraneous movements, and interactions with nurse and significant others
- Cognitive status, including ability to concentrate, learn, and remember
- Physiologic status
- Usual coping methods
- Mood
- Personality
- Progress of labor

Defining characteristics

- Excessive attention to fetal movement or uterine activity
- Excessive or uncontrolled reaction to labor contractions
- Expressed concern about pregnancy or birth
- Expressed fear of unspecified negative outcome
- Expressed feelings of helplessness or incapacity
- Fear, apprehension, and wariness
- Inability to concentrate, understand, or remember
- Increased muscle tension in body or face
- Perspiration
- Rapid pulse rate
- Restlessness, shakiness, trembling, jittery behavior, and extraneous movements

Expected outcomes

- Patient will express feelings of anxiety.
- Patient will identify causes of anxiety.
- Patient will make use of available emotional support.
- Patient will show fewer signs of anxiety.
- Patient will identify positive aspects of her efforts to cope during childbirth.
- Patient will acquire increased knowledge about childbirth and will be better prepared to cope with future births.

Suggested NOC outcomes

Anxiety Self-Control; Concentration; Coping; Social Interaction Skills; Symptom Control

Interventions and rationales

■ Assess the patient's knowledge, experience, and expectations of labor *to learn the precise source of anxiety and increase the effectiveness of interventions.*

■ Discuss normal labor progression with the patient, and explain what to expect during labor *to increase the patient's knowledge about normal progression of labor and understanding of her own experience.*

■ Involve the patient in making decisions about care *to reduce the sense of powerlessness that some women experience during labor.*

■ Share information on labor progression, vital signs, and the neonate's condition with the patient *to provide reassurance of normality and increase her sense of participation.*

■ Interpret environmental sights and sounds (electronic fetal monitor strip, fetal monitor sounds, and activities on unit) for the patient *to make the environment seem less threatening.*

■ Attend to the patient's comfort needs *to increase trust and reduce anxiety.*

■ Encourage the patient to employ coping skills used successfully in the past *to enhance her sense of control.*

■ Teach new coping skills (relaxation, breathing techniques, and positioning) *to diminish anxiety by increasing the patient's sense of power and control.* Review these skills with the patient periodically *because anxiety impairs recall.*

■ Organize your work to spend as much time as possible with the patient *to provide comfort and assistance, thereby promoting the patient's sense of security.*

■ Allow family members to participate in care *to provide comfort and help the patient cope with labor.*

Suggested NIC interventions

Anxiety Reduction; Calming Technique; Simple Relaxation Therapy; Spiritual Support

Evaluations for expected outcomes

■ Patient expresses feelings of anxiety about pregnancy or birth.

■ Patient identifies causes of anxiety.

■ Patient communicates with nurse or family members to gain reassurance, information, or emotional support.

■ Patient's physiologic or behavioral signs return to normal.

■ Patient, verbally or nonverbally, indicates that giving birth was a positive experience and expresses satisfaction with her behavior while giving birth.

■ Patient verbalizes increased knowledge about childbirth and displays confidence in her ability to cope with future births.

Documentation

■ Patient's expressions of anxiety

■ Patient's statements of reasons for anxiety

■ Observation of physical or behavioral signs of anxiety
■ Interventions to assist patient with coping
■ Patient's response to interventions
■ Evaluations for expected outcomes

Reference

Baldwin, K.A. "Comparison of Selected Outcomes of Centering Pregnancy versus Traditional Prenatal Care," *Journal of Midwifery & Women' Health* 51(4):266-72, July-August 2006.

Risk for
ASPIRATION
related to neonate's immature cough or gag reflex

Definition

At risk for entry of GI secretions, oropharyngeal secretions, or exogenous fluids into neonate's tracheobronchial passages

Assessment

■ Gestational age
■ Neonate's weight in relation to gestational age
■ Maternal sedation before delivery and effects of maternal sedation on labor
■ Neonate's health status, including preexisting conditions, anomalies, intrauterine environment, urologic status, cardiovascular status, respiratory status, and GI status
■ Laboratory studies of neonate, including fluid, electrolyte, and arterial blood gas levels
■ Neonate's vital signs
■ Neonate's nutritional status, including continuous or intermittent gavage feeding

Risk factors

■ Decreased GI motility
■ Delayed gastric emptying
■ Depressed cough and gag reflexes
■ Feeding or GI tubes
■ Impaired swallowing
■ Incompetent lower esophageal sphincter
■ Increased gastric residual contents
■ Increased intragastric pressure
■ Medication administration
■ Reduced level of consciousness
■ Situations hindering elevation of upper body
■ Surgery or trauma to face, mouth, or neck
■ Tracheostomy or endotracheal tube

Expected outcomes

■ Neonate will receive suctioning, as needed, and will maintain clear airway.
■ Neonate won't exhibit gastric distention.
■ Neonate will demonstrate minimal to moderate quantity of nasopharyngeal and oropharyngeal secretions.
■ Neonate will tolerate initial feeding.
■ Neonate won't demonstrate any color changes during feeding.
■ Neonate will demonstrate appropriate suck and swallow reflex.
■ Neonate will have no adventitious breath sounds.
■ Neonate won't exhibit signs and symptoms of aspiration.

Suggested NOC outcomes

Aspiration Prevention; Respiratory Status: Airway Patency; Respiratory Status: Ventilation; Risk Detection; Swallowing Status

Interventions and rationales

■ Regularly assess the neonate's respiratory status until stable *to evaluate respiratory system transition to extrauterine life.*
■ Monitor vital signs, according to facility protocol, and report changes *to determine multisystem adjustment to extrauterine existence.*
■ Suction as needed *to keep the upper and lower airways clear.* If the neonate aspirates meconium, assist the physician with laryngoscopy to suction below the vocal cords. If you're in the delivery room, suction the oropharynx and nasopharynx with a bulb syringe, DeLee catheter, or suction catheter attached to wall suction. *These measures may prevent additional respiratory compromise.*
■ Perform a head-to-toe physical assessment *to detect abnormalities in other body systems that may affect respiratory effort.*
■ Withhold oral feedings if signs of respiratory distress occur. Provide I.V. fluids, as ordered. *Sucking may place additional stress on the neonate in respiratory distress and may lead to aspiration.*
■ When offering the initial feeding, observe for suck and swallow reflex, gag and cough reflex, and color changes. Have suction equipment available and ready to use. *Early detection of difficulty may prevent neonatal morbidity and mortality.*
■ If the neonate is receiving gavage feeding:
– Keep the head of the bed elevated during and after feedings, unless contraindicated.
– Ensure proper positioning of the neonate before feeding or administering medication.
– Monitor residual gastric contents and follow parameters for withholding feedings.
– Once per shift, measure abdominal girth to check for distention; stop gavage feeding immediately if you suspect aspiration. Keep suction apparatus at the bedside and suction, as needed. Turn the neonate on his right side.
Preventive measures reduce the risk of aspiration.
■ Review laboratory results and report abnormalities. *Early identification of abnormal laboratory values reduces the risk of aspiration.*
■ Explain to the parents the reasons for these interventions *to gain parental understanding and cooperation, which contributes to a positive outcome.*

■ Instruct the parents in feeding techniques that will help prevent a distended abdomen leading to aspiration. Tell them to avoid overfeeding and to burp the neonate at frequent intervals (after intake of ½ to 1 oz [14.5 to 29.5 ml]). Instruct the parents to position the neonate on his right side with the head of the bed elevated for 30 to 60 minutes after feeding. *Providing instructions encourages parental understanding and cooperation.*

Suggested NIC interventions

Aspiration Precautions; Positioning; Respiratory Monitoring; Vital Signs Monitoring; Vomiting Management

Evaluations for expected outcomes

■ Neonate receives suctioning as needed and maintains patent airway.
■ Neonate doesn't exhibit gastric distention.
■ Neonate has minimal to moderate nasopharyngeal and oropharyngeal secretions.
■ Neonate tolerates initial feeding.
■ Neonate doesn't demonstrate color changes during feeding.
■ Neonate has appropriate suck and swallow reflex.
■ Neonate has no adventitious breath sounds.
■ Neonate shows no signs or symptoms of aspiration.

Documentation

■ Neonate's tolerance of initial feeding and of gavage feedings
■ Residual gastric contents after gavage feeding
■ Incidents of vomiting, aspiration, or both
■ Breath sounds
■ Observations of physical findings
■ Interventions performed to prevent aspiration
■ Evaluations for expected outcomes

Reference

White-Traut, R.C., et al. "Feeding Readiness in Preterm Infants: The Relationship between Preterm Behavioral State and Feeding Readiness Behaviors and Efficiency during Transition from Gavage to Oral Feeding," *The American Journal of Maternal Child Nursing* 30(1):52-59, January-February 2005.

Effective
BREAST-FEEDING

related to basic breast-feeding knowledge

Definition

State in which mother, neonate, and family exhibit proficiency and satisfaction with breast-feeding process

Assessment

■ Maternal status, including age and maturity, parity, level of prenatal breast-feeding preparation, past breast-feeding experience, previous postpartum history, physical condition (actual or perceived inadequate milk supply and comfort level), and psychosocial factors (apprehension level, body image, stress from family and career, sociocultural views of breast-feeding, and emotional support from significant others)

■ Neonatal status, including satisfaction and contentment, growth rate, age-weight relationship, urine output, quantity and characteristics of stools, and ability to latch onto breasts

Defining characteristics

■ Ability to position infant at breast to promote successful latching on (mother)
■ Adequate elimination pattern for age (infant)
■ Appropriate weight pattern for age (infant)
■ Eagerness to nurse (infant)
■ Effective communication pattern (mother and infant)
■ Evidence of contentment after feeding (infant)
■ Expressed satisfaction with breast-feeding process (mother)
■ Regular and sustained sucking and swallowing at breast (infant)
■ Signs and symptoms of oxytocin release (mother)

Expected outcomes

■ Mother will breast-feed neonate successfully and will experience satisfaction with breast-feeding process.
■ Neonate will feed successfully on both breasts and appear satisfied.
■ Neonate will grow and develop in pace with accepted standards.
■ Mother will continue breast-feeding neonate after early postpartum period.

Suggested NOC outcomes

Breast-feeding Establishment: Infant; Breast-feeding Establishment: Maternal; Breast-feeding Maintenance; Breast-feeding Weaning; Hydration; Knowledge: Breast-feeding

Interventions and rationales

■ Assess the mother's knowledge and experience of breast-feeding *to focus teaching on specific learning needs.*
■ Educate the mother and selected support person about breast-feeding techniques:
– Clean hands and breasts before nursing.
– Position the neonate for feeding (the neonate should be able to grasp most of the areola).
– Change positions to decrease nipple tenderness and use both breasts at each feeding.
– Remove the neonate from the breast by breaking suction; avoiding setting time limits in the early stage.
Greater understanding of techniques improves chances for success.

■ Teach the mother how to use warm showers and compresses, relaxation and guided imagery, infant suckling, holding the infant close to breasts, and listening to the infant cry *to stimulate letdown.*

■ Educate the mother about nutritional needs. She requires a well-balanced diet plus an additional 500 calories and two extra glasses of fluid each day *to maintain an adequate milk supply.* She should limit caffeine and avoid foods that make her uncomfortable.

■ Teach the mother what to expect from a breast-feeding neonate *to prepare the mother for care of the neonate at home.* The neonate should pass one to six stools and wet six to eight diapers per day. Stools should be soft to liquid and nonodorous. The neonate should feed every 2 to 3 hours, or as needed, and appear content and satisfied after feeding. Explain that the neonate also requires nonnutritive sucking.

■ Assist the mother and family in planning for home care. The mother needs to rest when the neonate sleeps, practice self-care, learn techniques for expressing and storing breast milk, and recognize signs of engorgement and infection. Family members should understand importance of helping and supporting the mother in her desire to breast-feed. *A mother who stops breast-feeding after she returns home and resumes work usually does so because of fatigue.*

■ Provide quiet and privacy *to enhance development of breast-feeding skills.*

■ Encourage mother to express concerns about breast-feeding *to reduce anxiety.*

■ Offer mother information about breast-feeding support groups *to help meet emotional and learning needs.*

Suggested NIC interventions

Breast-feeding Assistance; Family Support; Lactation Counseling; Nutrition Management; Parent Education: Infant

Evaluations for expected outcomes

■ Mother breast-feeds neonate successfully and expresses satisfaction with breast-feeding.

■ Neonate feeds on both breasts and appears satisfied.

■ Neonate's weight and length remain consistent and within 10th and 90th percentiles on pediatric growth grid.

■ Mother continues to breast-feed infant after discharge from hospital.

Documentation

■ Mother's expressions about breast-feeding experience

■ Observations of breast-feeding techniques and mother-infant interaction during breast-feeding

■ Teaching and instructions given

■ Neonate's growth and weight

■ Referrals to support groups

■ Mother's plans for breast-feeding after discharge

■ Evaluations for expected outcomes

Reference

Noel-Weiss, J., et al. "Developing a Prenatal Breastfeeding Workshop to Support Maternal Breastfeeding Self-efficacy," *Journal of Obstetric, Gynecologic, and Neonatal Nursing* 35(3):349-57, May-June 2006.

Ineffective
BREAST-FEEDING
related to dissatisfaction with breast-feeding process

Definition
State in which mother, neonate, or family experience dissatisfaction or difficulty with breast-feeding process

Assessment
- Maternal status, including age and maturity, relationships with significant others, previous bonding history, parity, level of prenatal breast-feeding preparation, knowledge or previous breast-feeding experience, physical condition (actual or perceived inadequate milk supply, nipple shape, and comfort level), and psychosocial factors (apprehension level, body image and perceptions, stress from family and career, sociocultural views of breast-feeding, and emotional support from significant others)
- Neonatal status, including satisfaction and contentment, growth rate, and age-weight relationship

Defining characteristics
- Actual or perceived inadequate milk supply (mother)
- Arching and crying when at breast (infant)
- Evidence of inadequate intake (infant)
- Fussiness and crying within first hour after feeding (infant)
- Inability to latch on to nipple correctly (infant)
- Inadequate opportunity for suckling (infant)
- Insufficient emptying of each breast (mother)
- Lack of observable signs of oxytocin release (mother)
- Lack of response to other comfort measures (infant)
- Lack of sustained suckling at breast (infant)
- Persistently sore nipples after first week of breast-feeding (mother)
- Resistance to latching on (infant)
- Unsatisfactory breast-feeding process (mother and infant)

Expected outcomes
- Mother will express physical and psychological comfort with breast-feeding techniques and practice.
- Mother will show decreased anxiety and apprehension.
- Neonate will feed successfully on both breasts and appear satisfied for at least 2 hours after feeding.

- Neonate will grow and thrive.
- Mother will state at least one resource for breast-feeding support.

Suggested NOC outcomes

Breast-feeding Establishment: Infant; Breast-feeding Establishment: Maternal; Breast-feeding Maintenance; Fluid Balance; Hydration; Knowledge: Breast-feeding

Interventions and rationales

- Educate the mother in breast care and breast-feeding techniques. *This reduces anxiety and enhances proper nutrition of the neonate.*
- Be available, yet discreet, during breast-feeding. *Assessment of the mother's technique can reveal problem areas.* Encourage the mother to ask questions *to increase understanding and reduce anxiety.*
- Teach techniques for encouraging the let-down reflex, including:
- warm shower
- breast massage
- physically caring for the neonate
- holding the neonate close to the breasts.
These measures reduce anxiety and promote the let-down reflex.
- Provide the mother and infant with a quiet, private, comfortable environment with decreased external stressors *to promote successful breast-feeding.*
- Encourage the expression of fears and anxieties between the mother and significant other *to reduce anxiety and increase the mother's sense of control.*
- Offer information about the importance of adequate nutrition and fluid intake while breast-feeding *in order to meet the infant's demand for breast milk.*
- Offer written information, a reading list, or information about breast-feeding support groups *to help meet the mother's emotional and learning needs.*

Suggested NIC interventions

Breast-feeding Assistance; Emotional Support; Lactation Counseling; Nutrition Management; Parent Education: Infant; Support Group

Evaluations for expected outcomes

- Mother expresses physical and psychological comfort with breast-feeding techniques and practice.
- Mother displays decreased anxiety and apprehension.
- Neonate feeds successfully on both breasts and appears satisfied for at least 2 hours after feeding.
- Neonate grows and thrives.
- Mother states at least one available resource for breast-feeding support.

Documentation

- Mother's expressions of comfort with breast-feeding ability
- Observations of bonding and breast-feeding process
- Teaching and instructions given

- Referrals to support groups
- Neonate growth and weight
- Evaluations for expected outcomes

Reference

Lewallen, L.P., et al. "Toward a Clinically Useful Method of Predicting Early Breast-feeding Attrition," *Applied Nursing Research* 19(3):144-48, August 2006.

Ineffective
BREAST-FEEDING
related to limited maternal experience

Definition

State in which mother, neonate, or family experiences dissatisfaction or difficulty with breast-feeding process

Assessment

- Maternal status, including age and maturity, relationship with significant other, previous bonding history, parity, level of prenatal breast-feeding preparation, knowledge or previous breast-feeding experience, and physical condition (actual or perceived inadequate milk supply, nipple shape, and comfort level)
- Psychosocial status, including apprehension level, body image and perceptions, stressors such as family and career, sociocultural views of breast-feeding, and emotional support from significant other
- Neonatal status, including satisfaction and contentment, growth rate, age-weight relationship, neurologic status, respiratory status, suck reflex, presence of factors that interfere with proper sucking (cleft lip or palate), and previous feedings with artificial nipples

Defining characteristics

- Actual or perceived inadequate milk supply (mother)
- Arching and crying when at breast (infant)
- Evidence of inadequate intake (infant)
- Fussiness and crying within first hour after feeding (infant)
- Inability to latch on to nipple correctly (infant)
- Inadequate opportunity for suckling (infant)
- Insufficient emptying of each breast (mother)
- Lack of observable signs of oxytocin release (mother)
- Lack of response to other comfort measures (infant)
- Lack of sustained suckling at breast (infant)
- Persistently sore nipples after first week of breast-feeding (mother)
- Resistance to latching on (infant)
- Unsatisfactory breast-feeding process (mother and infant)

Expected outcomes

- Mother will express understanding of breast-feeding techniques and practice.
- Mother will display decreased anxiety and apprehension.
- Mother and neonate will experience successful breast-feeding.
- Neonate's initial weight loss will be within accepted norms.
- Neonate's nutritional needs will be met.

Suggested NOC outcomes

Anxiety Self-Control; Breast-feeding Establishment: Maternal; Breast-feeding Maintenance; Knowledge: Breast-feeding; Knowledge: Infant Care; Swallowing Status

Interventions and rationales

- Assess the mother's knowledge *to help direct your interventions.*
- Educate the mother in breast care and breast-feeding techniques *to reduce anxiety and help ensure proper nutrition of the neonate.*
- Provide appropriate pamphlets and audiovisual aids *to help meet the mother's learning needs. The mother can review written material at her own pace; audiovisual materials illustrate proper technique.*
- Determine the mother's level of anxiety or ambivalence related to breast-feeding. *Anxiety and ambivalence can interfere with the mother's ability to learn and with the let-down reflex.*
- Teach techniques for encouraging the let-down reflex, including:
- warm shower
- breast massage
- relaxation and guided imagery
- infant suckling
- holding the neonate close to the breasts.
These measures reduce anxiety and facilitate the let-down reflex.
- Remain with the mother and neonate during several feedings *to pinpoint problem areas.* Encourage the mother to ask questions *to increase understanding and reduce anxiety.*
- Evaluate the position of the neonate's tongue during breast-feeding. *To produce proper sucking motion, the neonate's tongue must be down during breast-feeding, with the nipple directly on top.*
- Instruct the mother to offer the breast as soon as possible after the neonate awakens and not to wait until the neonate is crying vigorously. *Getting an extremely upset neonate to breast-feed effectively is difficult.*
- Evaluate need for a nipple shield and instruct the mother in its use. *Nipple shields help draw out partially inverted nipples.*
- Make sure the neonate is awake and alert when feeding; unwrap, as needed. *A tightly wrapped, sleepy neonate won't be alert enough to suckle sufficiently.*
- Sprinkle glucose water on the nipples before feeding, if needed. *When making preliminary attempts at breast-feeding, the neonate may open his mouth on tasting glucose water. The mother can then direct and attach the neonate's open mouth to the nipple.*

■ Evaluate the neonate for anomalies that may interfere with breast-feeding ability *to plan comprehensive treatment and teaching.*

■ Instruct the mother in proper breast care techniques, such as wearing a supportive bra, using cream, washing, and air-drying. *Proper breast care helps prevent nipple drying, cracking, soreness, and bleeding, which can interfere with effective breast-feeding.*

■ Instruct the mother on ways to alleviate breast engorgement. *Breast engorgement can prevent the neonate from effectively latching on to the nipple.*

■ Review the principles of milk production and identify factors that can alter production or quality of breast milk, such as emotional upset and intake of alcohol, drugs, and certain foods. *Any substance the mother ingests passes through to the breast milk. The mother must be aware of possible dangerous adverse effects.*

■ Provide positive reinforcement for the mother's efforts *to decrease anxiety and enhance feelings of self-esteem and success.*

■ Provide the mother with information about breast-feeding support groups. *Participation in a support group after discharge can help meet the mother's emotional and learning needs.*

Suggested NIC interventions

Breast-feeding Assistance; Coping Enhancement; Emotional Support; Lactation Counseling; Learning Facilitation; Parent Education: Infant

Evaluations for expected outcomes

■ Mother properly positions neonate during breast-feeding, uses appropriate techniques to encourage attachment to nipple, and (if applicable) correctly uses supplemental devices.

■ Mother expresses decreased anxiety and increased enthusiasm for breast-feeding.

■ Neonate feeds successfully on both breasts and appears satisfied for at least 2 hours after feeding.

■ Neonate's initial weight loss remains within accepted norms.

■ Neonate's nutritional needs are met.

Documentation

■ Mother's level of knowledge related to breast-feeding

■ Mother's expressions of dissatisfaction with breast-feeding ability

■ Mother's emotional response to breast-feeding

■ Mother's breast care practices

■ Maternal conditions that may interfere with breast-feeding, such as inverted nipples or mammaplasty

■ Mother's and neonate's behavior during and after breast-feeding, including positioning of neonate, neonate's response to being put to breast, and neonate's level of satisfaction

■ Mother's use of such devices as nipple shield

■ Frequency and duration of feedings

■ Neonate's growth, weight, output, and any supplemental feedings administered

■ Teaching and instructions given and mother's response to instructions

■ Goals established by mother

- Referrals to support groups
- Mother's and neonate's responses to nursing interventions
- Evaluations for expected outcomes

Reference
Lewallen, L.P., et al. "Breastfeeding Support and Early Cessation," *Journal of Obstetric, Gynecologic, and Neonatal Nursing* 35(2):166-72, March-April 2006.

Interrupted
BREAST-FEEDING
related to a contraindicating condition

Definition
Break in the continuity of breast-feeding resulting from an inability or inadvisability to put the baby to the breast for feeding

Assessment
- Maternal status, including age and maturity, employment hours, relationship with significant other, parity, level of prenatal breast-feeding knowledge or experience, and physical condition (comfort level, nipple shape, presence of infection, and use of medication)
- Neonatal status, including age-weight relationship, growth rate, neurologic status, respiratory status, suck reflex, and factors that interfere with proper sucking (such as cleft lip or palate)

Defining characteristics
- Continued desire to maintain lactation and provide breast milk for infant's nutritional needs (mother)
- Failure to receive nourishment at breast for some or all feedings (infant)
- Lack of knowledge about expressing and storing breast milk (mother)
- Separation of mother and infant

Expected outcomes
- Mother will express her understanding of factors that necessitate interruption in breast-feeding.
- Mother will express comfort with her decision about whether to resume breast-feeding.
- Mother will express and store breast milk appropriately.
- Mother will resume breast-feeding when interfering factors cease.
- Mother will have adequate milk supply when breast-feeding resumes.
- Mother will obtain relief from discomfort associated with engorgement.
- Infant's nutritional needs will be met.

Suggested NOC outcomes

Breast-feeding Maintenance; Knowledge: Breast-feeding; Motivation; Parent-Infant Attachment; Parenting Performance; Role Performance

Interventions and rationales

■ Assess the mother's understanding of reasons for interrupting breast-feeding *to evaluate the need for additional instruction.*

■ Reassure the mother that the neonate's nutritional needs will be met through other methods *to allay her anxiety.*

■ Assess the mother's desire to resume breast-feeding *to help plan interventions.*

■ Provide appropriate educational materials, including audiovisual aids and written materials. *Audiovisual aids demonstrate proper expressing and storing techniques; written material allows the mother to review information at her own pace.*

■ Instruct the mother in techniques for expressing and storing breast milk *to ensure adequate milk supply.*

■ Recommend the use of a breast pump according to the following guidelines *to provide maximum stimulation and prolactin production:*

– Initiate pumping 24 to 48 hours after delivery.

– Pump a minimum of five times per day.

– Pump a minimum of 100 minutes per day.

– Pump long enough to soften the breasts each time, regardless of duration.

■ Encourage the mother to save her breast milk in a sterile container and store it in the refrigerator or freezer for future feedings. *Preserving breast milk ensures that the neonate receives maternal antibodies and helps to encourage maternal involvement in neonatal care.*

■ If the mother must pump for a prolonged period, encourage her to use a piston-style electric pump. *Using an electric pump rather than a hand pump produces milk with a higher fat content.*

■ If the mother intends to resume breast-feeding, instruct her in ways to relieve breast engorgement *to prevent discomfort that may keep the neonate from sucking effectively.*

■ If appropriate, instruct the mother in the use of devices such as a nipple shield, *which is designed to alter flat or inverted nipples, a condition that may interfere with successful breast-feeding.*

■ Review the mother's daily routine *to advise her how to incorporate breast-feeding into her schedule.*

■ Provide the mother with information about breast-feeding support groups. *A support group can help the mother obtain needed emotional support and continue learning.*

■ If the mother doesn't intend to resume breast-feeding, advise her to wear a supportive bra, apply ice, and take a mild analgesic, such as acetaminophen, *to alleviate discomfort associated with engorgement.*

Suggested NIC interventions

Attachment Promotion; Bottle Feeding; Emotional Support; Lactation Counseling; Parent Education: Infant; Teaching: Individual

Evaluations for expected outcomes

■ Mother describes factors that necessitate interruption in breast-feeding.
■ Mother expresses comfort with her decision about whether to resume breast-feeding.
■ Mother demonstrates proper milk expression and storage techniques.
■ Mother resumes breast-feeding when interrupting factors are eliminated.
■ Mother has adequate milk supply when breast-feeding resumes.
■ Mother obtains relief from discomfort associated with engorgement.
■ Infant's nutritional needs are met, as evidenced by appropriate weight gain (for example, 1 oz [28.3 g] per day for first 6 months of life).

Documentation

■ Factors that necessitated interruption in breast-feeding (reassessed periodically to determine status)
■ Mother's expression of feelings about need to interrupt breast-feeding
■ Mother's decision whether to continue breast-feeding when possible
■ Mother's efforts to ensure adequate milk supply
■ Mother's responses to nursing interventions
■ Neonate's growth, weight, and output
■ Referrals to support groups
■ Evaluations for expected outcomes

Reference

Spatz, D.L. "State of the Science: Use of Human Milk and Breast-feeding for Vulnerable Infants," *The Journal of Perinatal & Neonatal Nursing* 20(1):51-55, January-March 2006.

Ineffective
BREATHING PATTERN
related to adjustment to extrauterine existence

Definition

Inspiration and/or expiration that doesn't provide adequate ventilation

Assessment

■ Gestational age
■ Weight in relation to gestational age
■ Maternal sedation before delivery
■ Preexisting conditions, including anomalies, adverse intrauterine environment, and prematurity
■ Health assessment, including laboratory studies and neurologic, cardiovascular, respiratory, integumentary, GI, and fluid and electrolyte status

Defining characteristics

■ Accessory muscle use

- Altered chest excursion
- Altered respiratory rate or depth or both
- Decreased inspiratory-expiratory pressure
- Decreased minute ventilation
- Decreased vital capacity
- Dyspnea
- Nasal flaring
- Retractions
- Shortness of breath

Expected outcomes

- Neonate will establish normal respiratory rate (40 to 60 breaths/minute) within 1 hour of birth.
- Neonate will have no signs of respiratory distress 1 hour after birth.
- Neonate won't require assisted ventilation or supplemental oxygen.
- Neonate will have Apgar score of 8 to 10 at 5 minutes after birth.
- Neonate will make successful transition to extrauterine life with adequate respiratory function.

Suggested NOC outcomes

Respiratory Status: Airway Patency; Respiratory Status: Ventilation; Vital Signs

Interventions and rationales

- Immediately after delivery:
- Vigorously dry the neonate and place him under a radiant warmer.
- Suction the oropharynx and nasopharynx, as needed, with a bulb syringe, DeLee catheter, or suction catheter connected to wall suction.
- Obtain 1-minute and 5-minute Apgar scores.
- Provide whiffs of oxygen, if indicated.
- Remove wet blankets and replace them with dry ones.
- Observe for signs of respiratory distress (nasal flaring, tachypnea, retractions, grunting, and use of accessory muscles for breathing).
- Provide or assist with resuscitative measures, as indicated, including bag and mask; naloxone (Narcan) administration, as ordered, if respiratory distress is secondary to maternal sedation; intubation; and suctioning below the vocal cords under direct visualization. *Respiratory difficulties are responsible for most morbidity and mortality during the neonatal period. Accurate assessment and prompt intervention at delivery are critical to sustaining life.*
- Transfer the neonate to the nursery when he's stable or if he needs more extensive resuscitation measures *to help improve transition to extrauterine life.*
- On admission to the nursery:
- Obtain the neonate's vital signs. Observe central and peripheral color. Note signs of respiratory distress.
- Perform a physical assessment, noting anomalies or other abnormal findings.
- Maintain a neutral thermal environment.

– Obtain a brief obstetric history, including the course of labor and delivery and condition of the neonate before his arrival in the nursery. Note the presence of risk factors.
– Obtain laboratory studies, as ordered.
– Provide resuscitative measures, if needed.
– Continue monitoring vital signs until stable, then routinely or as ordered. *Obtaining baseline data and identifying risk factors will help direct interventions.*
■ Perform chest physiotherapy, as indicated, *to clear the lungs of fluid.*
■ Continually assess the need to repeat suctioning to maintain a patent airway. *Repeated pharyngeal suctioning can prevent aspiration caused by the neonate's immature glottal reflex.*

Suggested NIC interventions

Airway Management; Aspiration Precautions; Respiratory Monitoring; Ventilation Assistance

Evaluations for expected outcomes

■ Neonate establishes respiratory rate of 40 to 60 breaths/minute within 1 hour of birth.
■ Neonate has no signs of respiratory distress 1 hour after birth.
■ Neonate doesn't require assisted ventilation or supplemental oxygen.
■ Neonate has Apgar score of 8 to 10 at 5 minutes after birth.
■ Neonate makes successful transition to extrauterine life with adequate respiratory function.

Documentation

■ Vital signs
■ Physical findings
■ Interventions performed to enhance neonate's ability to breathe effectively
■ Neonate's responses to nursing interventions
■ Evaluations for expected outcomes

Reference

Aylott, M. "The Neonatal Energy Triangle. Part 2: Thermoregulatory and Respiratory Adaption," *Paediatric Nursing* 18(7):38-42, September 2006.

Compromised family
COPING

related to neonatal health problems that exhausts supportive capacity of the parents

Definition

Usually supportive primary person (family member or close friend) provides insufficient, ineffective, or compromised support, comfort, assistance, or encouragement that

may be needed by the patient to manage or master adaptive tasks related to his/her health challenge

Assessment

■ Family process, including normal pattern of interaction among family members; family's understanding and knowledge of neonate's condition; support systems available (financial, social, and spiritual); family's response to past crises, including coping behaviors and problem-solving techniques; recreational activities; and communication patterns used to express anger, affection, and confrontation
■ Neonate's health status
■ Family's perception of present situation
■ Degree of difficulty imposed by care of neonate
■ Possible impact of neonate's health status on family's future structure and lifestyle

Defining characteristics

■ Attempts to care for neonate that meet with unsatisfactory results
■ Display of excessive or inadequate protective behavior
■ Inadequate understanding or knowledge base that interferes with ability to care for neonate
■ Preoccupation with personal reaction to neonate's health problem
■ Withdrawal from neonate at time of need

Expected outcomes

■ Family members will communicate feelings about neonate's condition.
■ Family members will engage in healthy coping behaviors.
■ Family members will become involved in planning for and providing neonate's care.
■ Family members will identify and use available support systems.
■ Family members will set realistic goals for neonate.
■ Family members will express feeling of having greater control over their situation.

Suggested NOC outcomes

Caregiver Emotional Health; Caregiver-Patient Relationship; Caregiver Stressors; Caregiving Endurance Potential; Family Coping; Parent-Infant Attachment; Parenting Performance

Interventions and rationales

■ Encourage family members to voice their feelings about the neonate's condition *to decrease tension by clearing up misunderstandings and misconceptions.*
■ Identify and reduce unnecessary environmental stimuli *to enhance family members' ability to focus on caring for the neonate.*
■ Assess family members' understanding of the neonate's condition. Help them view the situation realistically and understand its future implications. *Setting realistic goals helps the family plan for the future and avoid unnecessary disappointment.*

■ Actively involve family members in learning to care for the neonate *to decrease feelings of helplessness and isolation from the neonate.*

■ Explain the rationale for all treatments and procedures to family members *to help reduce anxiety and enhance cooperation.*

■ Involve the family members in decision making when possible *to increase their feelings of involvement and control.*

■ Provide positive feedback when family members care for the neonate *to increase self-esteem and reinforce their ability to care for the neonate successfully.*

■ Encourage family members to identify and contact support systems and resources, such as extended family, friends, clergy, and community groups, *to decrease the sense of being overwhelmed.*

■ Help family members identify and use appropriate coping behaviors *to reduce anxiety and tension.*

■ Coordinate referrals to other health care professionals, such as a social worker or physical therapist, *to ensure clear communication among health care providers, which enables the neonate to receive appropriate comprehensive care.*

■ Provide family members with up-to-date reports on the neonate's condition *to ease anxiety and help the family plan for future needs.*

Suggested NIC interventions

Caregiver Support; Coping Enhancement; Emotional Support; Family Involvement Promotion; Family Mobilization; Family Support; Spiritual Support

Evaluations for expected outcomes

■ Family members voice their feelings about neonate's condition.
■ Family members identify and use at least two healthy coping behaviors.
■ Family members demonstrate ability to plan for and provide neonate's care.
■ Family members identify and use available support systems.
■ Family members set realistic goals for neonate.
■ Family members express feeling of increased control over their situation.

Documentation

■ Family members' perceptions of neonate's health and long-term implications
■ Observations of family members' behaviors, including interactions with neonate
■ Family members' statements indicating their feelings toward neonate
■ Teaching and referrals given to family members
■ Family members' abilities to meet neonate's physical and emotional needs
■ Consultations with other health care team members
■ Interventions to help family members cope
■ Family members' responses to nursing interventions
■ Evaluations for expected outcomes

Reference

Dyer, K.A. "Identifying, Understanding, and Working with Grieving Parents in the NICU, Part II: Strategies," *Neonatal Network* 24(4):27-40, July-August 2005.

Ineffective
COPING
related to uncertainty about labor and delivery

Definition
Inability to form a valid appraisal of the stressors, inadequate choices of practiced responses, and/or inability to use available resources

Assessment
- Psychosocial status, including age, developmental stage, health beliefs and attitudes, feelings about pregnancy, decision-making ability, usual coping patterns, support systems, income, ability to learn (cognitive, affective, and psychomotor domains), motivation to learn, and obstacles to learning
- Neurologic status, including level of consciousness, orientation, memory, and mental status
- Pain threshold, perception of pain, and response to analgesia or anesthesia
- Labor, including stage and length of labor, complications, patient's ability to concentrate, patient's ability to use breathing techniques, and presence and effectiveness of support person
- Circumstances surrounding delivery, including method of delivery (vaginal [complicated or uncomplicated], cesarean [elective or nonelective], or vaginal birth after previous cesarean delivery), analgesia or anesthesia, presence and effectiveness of support person, and outcome (actual and perceived)
- Previous experience with pregnancy, labor, and delivery and knowledge of birth process
- Medical history, including preexisting and pregnancy-induced conditions

Defining characteristics
- Change in communication pattern
- Decreased use of social support
- Destructive behavior toward self or others
- Expressed inability to cope or inability to ask for help
- Fatigue
- Inability to meet basic needs and role expectations
- Lack of goal-directed behavior, such as inability to attend, difficulty organizing information, poor concentration, and poor problem-solving abilities

Expected outcomes
- Patient will express need to develop better coping behaviors.
- Patient will set realistic learning goals.
- Patient will demonstrate ability to use newly learned coping skills.
- Patient will communicate feelings about pregnancy, labor, and delivery.
- Patient will maintain appropriate sense of control throughout course of labor and delivery.
- Patient will enlist help from support person and nurses to obtain physical and psychological comfort.

■ Patient will demonstrate ability to cope with unexpected change.

Suggested NOC outcomes
Anxiety Self-Control; Coping; Decision-Making; Information Processing; Role Performance; Social Interaction Skills;
Social Support

Interventions and rationales
■ Establish an environment of mutual trust and respect *to enhance the patient's learning.*
■ Negotiate with the patient to develop learning goals *to promote cooperation and foster a sense of control.*
■ Select teaching strategies (discussion, demonstration, role playing, and visual materials) appropriate for the patient's learning style *to encourage compliance.*
■ Teach skills that the patient can use during labor and delivery. Have her give a return demonstration of each new skill. *The patient must thoroughly understand these skills before labor begins because painful contractions will reduce her attention span.*
■ During the first (latent) phase of labor (dilation 1 to 4 cm), take these steps:
– Encourage the patient to ventilate her feelings and to participate in her own care. Offer diversions such as reading materials. Review breathing techniques she can use during labor. *These measures help allay the patient's fears and help her achieve a sense of control.*
– Involve the support person in care and comfort measures *to allay the patient's fears.*
– Provide continuous monitoring *to identify deviations from normal.*
■ During the active phase of labor (dilation 4 to 8 cm), take these steps:
– Encourage the patient to assume a comfortable position *to promote relaxation between contractions.*
– Assist the patient with breathing techniques *to reduce anxiety and prevent hyperventilation.*
– Encourage the support person to participate in patient care and comfort. Allow involvement to the extent that is comfortable to both the woman and the support person (e.g., give back rub, provide ice chips, assist with walking) *to provide continuity of care and encourage a therapeutic relationship.*
– Provide encouragement and instruction between contractions *to foster a sense of control.*
– Administer analgesia, as ordered, *to reduce pain.*
– Provide opportunities for rest between contractions, when appropriate. Reassure the patient about fetal status. *These measures reinforce the patient's ability to cope.*
■ During the transitional phase of labor (dilation 8 to 10 cm), take these steps:
– Assist the patient with breathing during contractions. Advise her not to push until complete dilation occurs.
– Encourage rest between contractions.
– Identify and reduce unnecessary stimuli in the environment.
– Explain all treatments and procedures and answer the patient's questions.

These measures help allay fear and reduce sensory overload.
■ During delivery, provide these measures:
– Instruct the patient in effective pushing techniques *to promote the effectiveness of her bearing-down efforts.*
– Continue to reassure the patient and provide encouragement. Explain the physiologic changes and procedures being performed *to prepare the patient psychologically for delivery.*
– Escort the support person to the delivery room. Explain each step of the process. Instruct the support person in how to effectively coach the patient *to provide further support for the patient and strengthen her ability to cope.*
■ During delivery of the placenta, take these steps:
– Enlist the patient's cooperation in maintaining her position *to facilitate delivery of the placenta.*
– Show the neonate to the patient and explain the care being provided. Reassure the patient about the neonate's condition *to provide emotional support.*
– If permitted, allow the patient and support person to hold the neonate. If the patient desires, allow her to breast-feed the neonate *to promote bonding.*
■ In a cesarean delivery, allow the patient to express her feelings. Explain the procedure and care being provided. Allow the support person to be present before and during delivery, if permitted. *Failure to provide the patient with a source of support and opportunity to express negative feelings may interfere with her ability to cope with the impending tasks of motherhood.*

Suggested NIC interventions

Anticipatory Guidance; Anxiety Reduction; Calming Technique; Coping Enhancement; Decision-Making Support; Emotional Support; Patient Contracting

Evaluations for expected outcomes
■ Patient states need for better coping behaviors.
■ Patient participates in establishing learning goals.
■ Patient successfully uses breathing and relaxation techniques during labor and delivery.
■ Patient becomes more comfortable with expressing feelings about pregnancy, labor, and delivery.
■ Patient maintains appropriate sense of control during labor and delivery.
■ Support person and nurses provide effective comfort to patient during labor and delivery.
■ Patient demonstrates ability to cope with unexpected change.

Documentation
■ Patient's previous knowledge of labor and delivery
■ Patient's expressions indicating her motivation to learn
■ Patient's learning objectives
■ Methods used to teach patient
■ Information taught and skills demonstrated to patient
■ Patient's response to nursing interventions

- Patient's and support person's level of satisfaction with delivery
- Patient's expressions of comfort, discomfort, or both
- Evaluations for expected outcomes

Reference

Campbell, D.A., et al. "A Randomized Control Trial of Continuous Support in Labor by a Lay Doula," *Journal of Obstetric, Gynecologic, and Neonatal Nursing* 35(4):456-64, July-August 2006.

Risk for sudden infant
DEATH SYNDROME

Definition

Presence of risk factors for sudden death of an infant younger than age 1 year

Assessment

- Age, sex, weight, ethnic background
- Perinatal history (gestational age, Apgar score, birth weight, birth order)
- Maternal history (age, socioeconomic status, level of education, parenting experience; smoking, alcohol, and drug history)
- Cardiovascular status (pulse, blood pressure, heart sounds)
- Respiratory status (respiratory rate, quality, depth, breath sounds)
- Neurologic status (alertness, reflexes — especially gag, suck, swallow, response to touch)
- Sleep routines (position, mattress, sleepwear, room temperature, co-bedding)
- Feeding routines (breast- or bottle-fed, ease of feeding, spitting up)

Risk factors

Modifiable

- Delayed or nonattendance of prenatal care
- Infant co-bedding with parents or siblings
- Infant overheating or overwrapping
- Infant placed to sleep in the prone position
- Prenatal or postnatal infant smoke exposure
- Prenatal or postnatal substance abuse (heroin, methadone, cocaine)
- Soft mattress or loose articles in the sleep environment

Potentially modifiable

- Low birth weight
- Low socioeconomic status
- Prematurity
- Young maternal age

Nonmodifiable
■ Ethnicity (for example, African American, Hispanic, or Native American race of mother)
■ Increasing birth order (subsequent siblings as opposed to firstborn)
■ Infants with one or more severe life-threatening events requiring cardiopulmonary resuscitation (CPR)
■ Male sex
■ Multiple births
■ Seasonability of sudden infant death syndrome (SIDS) deaths (higher in winter and fall months)
■ Sibling of two or more SIDS victims

Expected outcomes
■ Parents will be receptive to teaching and guidance.
■ Parents will verbalize understanding of risk factors and provide all precautions possible to prevent disorder.
■ Infant will be placed in proper position on back with head of crib slightly elevated.
■ Infant will be able to move extremities and head freely without restriction or without becoming tangled in loose bedding or articles.
■ Infant will sleep alone in appropriate crib on firm sleep surface.
■ Infant's body temperature will remain within normal limits.
■ Infant will be monitored with apnea monitor during sleep.
■ Parents state that they feel prepared and have the ability to handle emergencies utilizing CPR techniques and 911 services.
■ Parents will handle the stress of knowing they have a high-risk infant with appropriate coping skills.

Suggested NOC outcomes
Risk Control; Risk Detection

Interventions and rationales
■ Educate the family about the risk factors of SIDS *so that they'll be aware of the current practices to reduce risk and prevent its occurrence.*
■ Position the infant on his back when placed in the crib. *Incidence of SIDS is higher among infants placed prone.*
■ Make sure the infant's head is slightly elevated *to decrease abdominal pressure on the diaphragm and allow better expansion of the lungs.*
■ Teach the parents to avoid having loose blankets, toys, or other articles in the crib *to decrease the risk of accidental suffocation.*
■ Make sure the infant lies on a firm surface so he doesn't sink into the mattress, mattress cover, or blanket *to decrease the risk of suffocation.*
■ Avoid overheating the room and wrapping the infant's body in heavy blankets. *Overheating the infant increases the body's demand for oxygen.*
■ Encourage the mother to breast-feed the infant *because this is associated with a lower incidence of SIDS.*
■ When an apnea monitor is ordered for the high-risk infant, teach the parents how to correctly apply the apparatus and leads and ensure that alarms are set cor-

rectly. The machine will sound an alarm if the respiratory rate or heart rate falls below a predetermined level (typically specified by the physician). *The benefit of the monitor can only be achieved if it's utilized appropriately.*

▣ Instruct the parents in the correct application of CPR *to reduce anxiety and promote confidence in technique.*

▣ Assess the level of anxiety in the parents and family members routinely and provide suggestions for coping mechanisms *to assist the family in dealing with the period of vulnerability for the infant.*

▣ Make appropriate referrals for community health nursing and home visits *to allow an opportunity to assess the home situation, care provided, and coping level of the family.*

Suggested NIC interventions

Anticipatory Guidance; Anxiety Reduction; Caregiver Support; Coping Enhancement; Emotional Support; Environmental Management: Safety; Family Integrity Promotion: Childbearing Family; Infant Care; Learning Facilitation; Parent Education: Childrearing Family; Positioning; Risk Identification: Childbearing Family; Teaching: Infant Safety

Evaluations for expected outcomes

▣ Parents listen and cooperate with patient teaching.
▣ Parents readily participate in education regarding SIDS risk factors and management.
▣ Parents utilize appropriate positioning of infant in crib.
▣ Infant moves freely without entanglement or suffocation in crib during sleep.
▣ Parents allow infant to sleep alone on firm surface.
▣ Infant's temperature remains within normal limits.
▣ Apnea monitor is utilized correctly.
▣ Parents utilize CPR and activate emergency services appropriately.
▣ Family members recognize need for heightened coping skills to deal with stress of high-risk infant.

Documentation

▣ Information given to parents regarding SIDS, positioning the infant, and sleeping arrangements
▣ Infant's temperature
▣ Demonstration of apnea monitor
▣ Attendance at CPR class
▣ Evaluations for expected outcomes

Reference

Maindonald, E. "Patient-Education Guide: Sudden Infant Death Syndrome (SIDS)," *Nursing* 35(7):53, July 2005.

Interrupted
FAMILY PROCESSES

related to impending birth

Definition
Change in family relationships and/or functioning

Assessment
- Age of patient and partner
- Availability of family members or friends to help
- Planned or unplanned pregnancy
- Family status, including number and ages of other children, usual patterns of interaction among family members, family members' assumed or expected roles, communication patterns, support systems, financial resources, past responses to change, spiritual resources, and living conditions
- Perceived impact of pregnancy on family unit
- Presence of obstetric or fetal complications or other medical conditions

Defining characteristics
Changes in:
- Assigned tasks and effectiveness in completing those tasks
- Availability for affective responsiveness and intimacy
- Availability for emotional support
- Communication patterns
- Expressions of conflict with or isolation from community resources
- Expressions of conflict within family
- Mutual support
- Participation in problem solving and decision making
- Patterns and rituals
- Power alliances
- Satisfaction with family
- Somatic complaints
- Stress-reduction behaviors

Expected outcomes
- Family members will take on portion of duties carried out by patient, such as housecleaning, heavy lifting, and meal preparation.
- Patient and family members will voice realistic expectations about pregnancy's impact on their future.
- Patient and family members will share their feelings about pregnancy with each other.
- Family members will identify and contact appropriate support systems.
- Family will welcome new member of the family.

Suggested NOC outcomes

Family Coping; Family Functioning; Family Normalization; Family Resiliency; Parenting Performance

Interventions and rationales

■ Encourage family members to express their feelings about the pregnancy. Tell them that a wide range of emotions, ranging from fear to excitement, may accompany a diagnosis of pregnancy. *Pent-up feelings can lead to misunderstanding and resentment.*

■ Provide emotional support to the patient and family members *to help them come to terms with altered roles and responsibilities.*

■ Encourage the pregnant woman to voice her concerns about the pregnancy's potential impact on family structure and finances *to identify unrealistic fears and decrease anxiety.*

■ Arrange and participate in family conferences, as needed. *Some families may require help to improve interpersonal communication.*

■ Refer family members to classes in prepared childbirth or parenting, psychological counseling, or social service and health care agencies, as appropriate, *to provide additional information and support.*

■ Periodically assess the woman's acceptance of pregnancy *to determine the need for further interventions. The mother usually grows to accept the pregnancy as the uterus develops and she feels the fetus kick. She may also fantasize about what the neonate will look like and begin preparing for birth.*

Suggested NIC interventions

Coping Enhancement; Family Integrity Promotion; Family Process Maintenance; Family Support; Normalization Promotion; Parent Education: Childrearing Family

Evaluations for expected outcomes

■ Family members take on portion of patient's duties.
■ Patient and family members voice realistic expectations about emotional and financial impact of pregnancy on family structure.
■ Patient and family members honestly communicate feelings about pregnancy.
■ Patient and family members identify and contact potential support groups or organizations.
■ Neonate is successfully integrated into family.

Documentation

■ Reactions of patient and partner to diagnosis of pregnancy
■ Referrals to outside agencies
■ Patient's adherence to prescribed medical practices
■ Observations of patient's acceptance of and interest in pregnancy as it progresses
■ Interventions to assist patient and family
■ Patient's and family's response to nursing interventions
■ Evaluations for expected outcomes

Reference

Sittner, B.J., et al. "Effects of High-risk Pregnancies on Families," *The American Journal of Maternal Child Nursing* 30(2):121-26, March-April 2005.

Interrupted
FAMILY PROCESSES

related to shift of roles to include new member

Definition

Change in family relationships and/or functioning

Assessment

■ Family status, including assumed or expected roles, communication patterns, developmental stage of family members, number and ages of children, financial resources, past responses to change, available support systems, significant others, and spiritual practices
■ Family members' perceptions of impact of birth on their assumed roles

Defining characteristics

Changes in:
■ Assigned tasks and effectiveness in completing those tasks
■ Availability for affective responsiveness and intimacy
■ Availability for emotional support
■ Communication patterns
■ Expressions of conflict with or isolation from community resources
■ Expressions of conflict within family
■ Mutual support
■ Participation in problem solving and decision making
■ Patterns and rituals
■ Power alliances
■ Satisfaction with family
■ Somatic complaints
■ Stress-reduction behaviors

Expected outcomes

■ Family members will voice feelings about neonate.
■ Family members will express need to assume new or altered roles and adapt to changes within family structure.
■ Family members will contact support groups for help, if needed.
■ Neonate will be successfully welcomed into family structure.

Suggested NOC outcomes

Family Coping; Family Functioning; Family Normalization; Parenting Performance; Social Support

Interventions and rationales

■ Encourage family members to express their feelings about the arrival of the neonate and altered roles and responsibilities *to help clear up misunderstandings and misconceptions.*

■ Explore with family members the ways the neonate will affect family structure and functioning. Topics may include changes in finances and living space, care-taking arrangements, and new roles or responsibilities for parents and siblings. *Discussing legitimate concerns may improve family members' attitudes toward the neonate.*

■ Discuss with family members the degree of sibling preparation and the possi-bility of sibling rivalry. *Siblings must be reassured that they're still vital members of the family.* Encourage siblings to visit the neonate at the hospital *to decrease sepa-ration anxiety, foster a sense of family, and facilitate bonding.*

■ Assess measures taken to prepare the home for the arrival of the neonate. *Lack of preparation may indicate limited financial resources or difficulty accepting the neonate.*

■ Assess the need for help from social services or community agencies and coor-dinate referrals *to ensure ongoing comprehensive care.*

Suggested NIC interventions

Coping Enhancement; Emotional Support; Family Integrity Promotion; Family Process Maintenance; Family Support; Normalization Promotion; Support System Enhancement

Evaluations for expected outcomes

■ Family members share feelings about neonate with each other.

■ Family members assume new or additional responsibilities, as needed, such as preparing meals, assisting with transportation, shopping, cleaning, and providing child care.

■ Family members contact community agencies or support groups for assistance, if needed.

■ Family members come to terms with arrival of neonate.

Documentation

■ Observations of family members' reactions to neonate
■ Family members' statements indicating attitude toward neonate
■ Interventions performed to help family cope with new arrival
■ Family members' response to nursing interventions
■ Referrals to outside agencies
■ Evaluations for expected outcomes

References

St. John, W., et al. "Meeting the Challenge of New Fatherhood during the Early Weeks," *Journal of Obstetric, Gynecologic, and Neonatal Nursing* 34(2):180-89, March-April 2005.

Waterston, T., and Welsh, B. "Helping Fathers Understand their New Infant: A Pilot Study of a Parenting Newsletter," *Community Practitioner* 79(9):293-95, September 2006.

Readiness for enhanced
FAMILY PROCESSES

Definition
A pattern of family functioning that's sufficient to support the well-being of family members and can be strengthened

Assessment
■ Family structure, including perception of self and family, family composition, social roles of family members, family developmental stages, socioeconomics, education, occupation, ethnicity, and cultural and religious beliefs
■ Family health pattern, including perception of health, health management, family developmental tasks, coping mechanisms, health beliefs and values, health status, stressors, and safety
■ Family function, including family interactions, use of resources, decision making, growth and development, responses to affection and concerns

Defining characteristics
■ Activities that support safety and growth of family members
■ Adequate communication
■ Balance between autonomy and cohesiveness
■ Energy level that supports activities of daily living
■ Family adaptation to change
■ Family functioning that meets physical, social, and psychological needs of family members
■ Family resilience
■ Flexible family roles, appropriate for developmental stages
■ Generally positive relationships; interdependent with community; family tasks accomplished
■ Maintenance of family members' boundaries
■ Respect for family members
■ Willingness to enhance family dynamics

Expected outcomes
■ Family members will identify family goals and structured directions.
■ Family members will express enjoyment and satisfaction in their roles in the family.
■ Family members will regularly participate in traditional family activities.
■ Family members will maintain open and positive communications.
■ Family members will maintain a safe home environment.

- Family members will contact community resources for help, if needed.
- Family members will seek regular health screenings and immunizations.
- Family members will identify and acknowledge risk factors.
- Family members will make plans for dealing with life changes and unexpected events.
- Family members will maintain healthy lifestyles by exercising regularly, eating a well-balanced diet, avoiding substance abuse, and using proven holistic health strategies.

Suggested NOC outcomes

Community Competence; Community Health Status; Compliance Behavior; Decision-Making; Family Coping; Family Functioning; Family Health Status; Family Integrity; Family Normalization; Family Participation in Professional Care; Health Beliefs: Perceived Ability to Perform; Health Beliefs: Perceived Control; Health Orientation; Health Promoting Behavior; Hope; Identity; Risk Detection

Interventions and rationales

- Encourage family members to identify individual and family goals and structured directions. *Individual and family goals set the boundaries that are respected by the family members. Family functioning with structured direction should enhance family members' ability to meet their physical, social, and psychological needs.*
- Encourage family members to express enjoyment and satisfaction in their roles in the family *to enhance family dynamics and strengthen family bonds.*
- Assist the family members in coping with changes related to growth and development. *Each transition stage of growth and development is a stressful life event.*
- Explore with the family members traditional activities that all family members will enjoy doing together. *Sharing traditional family activities increases loyalty, security, and a sense of belonging for family members.*
- Assess measures taken to maintain open and positive communications. *Healthy communications bridge the gap between members of the family.*
- Assist family to clarify family values and beliefs regarding health and health practices by helping the family identify their values, restate the values, and identify conflicts between values and action. *Values guide actions and have power to motivate behaviors. Value conflicts could lead to noncompliant health practices and interrupt the well-being of family members.*
- Assess measures taken to maintain safety in the home environment. *Environments that are free from environmental hazards, both chemical and physical, assure a sense of security.*
- Assess the stress-coping ability of the family members, individually and as a whole, to determine the strength and weakness status of the individual's and family's stress-coping pattern. Help the family make realistic plans for dealing with life changes and unexpected events. *Preparation for stress enhances the use of coping mechanisms and minimizes the threat.*
- Provide the family with information on social support and community resources. *Social support and community resources enhance the family process, reinforce family strength, and assist when families are experiencing stresses.*

■ Provide the family with information on recommended health screenings and immunizations, and encourage them to schedule regular checkups accordingly to their growth and developmental stages. *Screening is a valuable tool to enhance preventive interventions.*

■ Help the family develop a Genogram to identify genetic risk factors. *Information from a Genogram highlights a family's health patterns, provides knowledge leading to early identification of genetically related diseases, and may delay disease onset.*

■ Educate and encourage family members to exercise regularly, eat a well-balanced diet, avoid substance abuse, and use proven holistic health strategies. *Health-promotion behaviors could maintain optimum health.*

Suggested NIC interventions

Active Listening; Anticipatory Guidance; Attachment Promotion; Behavior Modification: Social Skills; Coping Enhancement; Emotional Support; Environmental Management: Attachment Process; Environmental Management: Comfort; Environmental Management: Safety; Environmental Management: Violence Prevention; Exercise Promotion; Family Involvement Promotion; Family Mobilization; Family Process Maintenance; Family Support; Health Education; Health Screening; Health System Guidance; Hope Instillation; Humor; Meditation Facilitation; Risk Identification; Role Enhancement; Security Enhancement; Self-Esteem Enhancement; Self-Responsibility Facilitation; Socialization Enhancement; Spiritual Support; Support System Enhancement; Truth Telling; Values Clarification

Evaluations for expected outcomes

■ Family functions in a structured and goal-oriented direction.

■ Family members state enjoyment and satisfaction in their roles in the family.

■ Family members regularly participate in traditional family activities.

■ Family members maintain open and positive communications.

■ Family members maintain a safe home environment.

■ Family utilizes various available social support venues as well as community resources to meet the needs of the family and individual family members.

■ Family members participate in regular health screenings and immunizations.

■ Family members identify and acknowledge risk factors.

■ Family members have plans for dealing with life changes and unexpected events.

■ Family members maintain healthy lifestyle by exercising regularly, eating a well-balanced diet, avoiding substance abuse, and using proven holistic health strategies.

Documentation

■ Identification of goals and activities carried out

■ Satisfaction level of family members

■ Use of support services

■ Health visits, patterns of exercise and diet, use of other health-promoting strategies

■ Evaluations for expected outcomes

Reference
Kouri, P., et al. "Pregnant Families' Discussions on the Net—From Virtual Connections Toward Real-life Community," *Journal of Midwifery & Women's Health* 51(4):279-83, July-August 2006.

Deficient
FLUID VOLUME
related to altered intake during labor

Definition
Decreased intravascular, interstitial, and/or intracellular fluid—refers to dehydration, water loss alone without change in sodium

Assessment
■ Vital signs, including temperature, pulse rate, blood pressure, and respirations
■ Fluid and electrolyte status, including weight, intake and output, urine specific gravity, skin turgor, mucous membranes, and electrolyte and blood urea nitrogen levels

Defining characteristics
■ Changes in mental status
■ Decreased pulse volume and pressure
■ Decreased urine output
■ Decreased venous filling
■ Dry skin and mucous membranes
■ Increased body temperature
■ Increased hematocrit
■ Increased pulse rate
■ Increased urine concentration
■ Low blood pressure
■ Poor turgor of skin or tongue
■ Sudden weight loss (except in third-space fluid shifting)
■ Thirst
■ Weakness

Expected outcomes
■ Patient will maintain fluid balance.
■ Patient will demonstrate optimal hydration.
■ Patient will show no signs of dehydration.

Suggested NOC outcomes

Electrolyte & Acid/Base Balance; Fluid Balance; Hydration; Nausea & Vomiting Severity; Urinary Elimination

Interventions and rationales

■ Monitor vital signs as often as policy dictates. *Decreased blood pressure and increased pulse rate may be late signs of fluid volume loss. With gestational hypertension, increased blood pressure may occur.*

■ Assess skin turgor and examine oral mucous membranes for dryness. *Dehydration can cause dry mucous membranes, skin tenting, and dry, cracked lips.*

■ Continuously monitor intake and output. Administer and monitor parenteral fluids. Maintain intake according to order or protocol (usually 125 to 175 ml/hour). Output should approximate intake. *These measures help ensure adequate hydration.*

■ Monitor electrolyte values and report abnormalities. *Hypernatremia may indicate dehydration, requiring I.V. volume replacement. Hypernatremia may also be related to excessive insensible water loss.*

■ Provide the patient with ice chips or a cool, damp, 4″ × 4″ gauze compress *to increase patient comfort and decrease mouth dryness, especially if the patient breathes through her mouth.*

■ Measure the amount and character of vomitus to assess the need for an antiemetic. *When labor begins, blood is rerouted to serve the energy needs of the contracting uterus and blood flow to the GI tract decreases. GI motility and absorption also decrease so that food may remain in the stomach for up to 12 hours. These factors predispose the patient to nausea and vomiting, especially during the transition phase of labor.*

■ As ordered, administer an antiemetic, and evaluate its effectiveness *to help control emesis and prevent excessive fluid loss.*

■ Keep the patient cool and comfortable. Change her gown, as indicated, and apply cool compresses to her face and body *to reduce discomfort caused by diaphoresis.*

■ Position the patient on her left side *to aid kidney perfusion and increase cardiac and urine output.*

■ If urine output is reduced, carefully assess the patient for peripheral edema, hyperreflexia, increased blood pressure, and presence of urine protein. *Decreased urine output, increased blood pressure, hyperreflexia, and peripheral edema may indicate intrapartal gestational hypertension. Proteinuria may result from dehydration, exhaustion, or preeclampsia.*

Suggested NIC interventions

Electrolyte Management: Hypernatremia; Fluid/Electrolyte Management; Fluid Monitoring; Hemodynamic Regulation; Hypovolemia Management; Medication Management

Evaluations for expected outcomes

■ Patient maintains fluid balance, with intake approximately equaling output.

■ Patient maintains optimal hydration.

■ Patient has no signs of dehydration; her mucous membranes remain pink and moist; skin turgor remains optimal; vital signs stay within normal limits; and urine output is at least 30 ml/hour or 100 ml in 4 hours.

Documentation
■ Patient's vital signs
■ Observation of patient's fluid volume status
■ Intake and output
■ Nursing interventions performed to maintain adequate fluid intake
■ Patient's response to nursing interventions
■ Evaluations for expected outcomes

Reference
Tranmer, J.E., et al. "The Effect of Unrestricted Oral Carbohydrate Intake on Labor Progress," *Journal of Obstetric, Gynecologic, and Neonatal Nursing* 34(3):319-28, May-June 2005.

Deficient
FLUID VOLUME
related to postpartum hemorrhage

Definition
Decreased intravascular, interstitial, and/or intracellular fluid — refers to dehydration, water loss alone without change in sodium

Assessment
■ History of problems that can cause fluid loss, such as hemorrhage, vomiting, diarrhea, and indwelling catheters
■ Vital signs
■ Fluid and electrolyte status, including weight, intake and output, urine specific gravity, skin turgor, mucous membranes, and serum electrolyte and blood urea nitrogen levels
■ Laboratory studies, including hemoglobin (Hb) level and hematocrit (HCT)
■ Factors that place patient at high risk for postpartum hemorrhage, including grand multipara, overdistended uterus, prolonged labor, previous history of postpartum hemorrhage, traumatic delivery, uterine fibroids, overstimulation with oxytocin, and bleeding disorders

Defining characteristics
■ Changes in mental status
■ Decreased pulse volume and pressure
■ Decreased urine output
■ Decreased venous filling
■ Dry skin and mucous membranes
■ Increased body temperature

- Increased HCT
- Increased pulse rate
- Increased urine concentration
- Low blood pressure
- Poor turgor of skin or tongue
- Sudden weight loss (except in third-space fluid shifting)
- Thirst
- Weakness

Expected outcomes
- Patient's vital signs will remain stable.
- Patient's hematology studies will be within normal range.
- Patient's uterus will remain firm.
- Medical personnel will quickly identify signs of possible shock and initiate treatment.
- Patient's bladder won't become distended.
- Patient's blood volume will return to normal.

Suggested NOC outcomes

Blood Loss Severity; Electrolyte & Acid/Base Balance; Fluid Balance; Hydration; Risk Detection; Urinary Elimination

Interventions and rationales
- Immediately after delivery, monitor the color, amount, and consistency of the lochia every 15 minutes for 1 hour, then every 4 hours for 24 hours, then every shift until discharge. Weigh or count sanitary pads if the lochia is excessive. *Hemorrhage is the most common cause of mortality during childbirth.*
- Monitor and record vital signs every 15 minutes for 1 hour, then every 4 hours for 24 hours, then every shift until discharge *to detect signs of hemorrhage and shock, such as increased pulse and respiratory rates and decreased blood pressure.*
- Immediately after delivery, palpate the fundus every 15 minutes for 1 hour, then every 4 hours for 24 hours, then every shift until discharge. Note its location and tone. *Palpation of the fundus will enable you to detect uterine atony (lack of normal uterine muscle tone or strength), the most common cause of postpartum hemorrhage.*
- Gently massage a boggy fundus; avoid overstimulation. *Gentle stimulation can help the fundus to become firm; overstimulation can cause relaxation.*
- Explain to the patient the process of involution and the need to palpate the fundus. Teach the patient to assess and gently massage the fundus and to notify you if bogginess persists. *Explaining normal postpartum physiologic adjustments can decrease the patient's anxiety and increase cooperation.*
- Evaluate postpartum hematology studies and report abnormal results. Consider whether the patient needs typing and crossmatching for transfusion. *Comparison of postdelivery Hb and HCT with previous results provides information about the amount of blood loss and allows time to plan interventions, such as requesting blood from a blood bank.*

■ Administer fluids, blood or blood products, or plasma expanders, as ordered, *to replace lost blood volume.* Monitor for adverse reactions.

■ Monitor the patient's intake and output every shift. Note bladder distention and catheterize, as ordered. *A distended bladder interferes with the involution of the uterus.*

■ Administer oxytocic agents, such as oxytocin (Pitocin), methylergonovine (Methergine), and ergonovine (Ergotrate), as ordered, and evaluate their effectiveness. *Oxytocic agents stimulate uterine musculature, controlling postpartum hemorrhage and atony.*

■ Regularly assess the patient for signs and symptoms of shock, including rapid, thready pulse; increased respiratory rate; decreased blood pressure and urine output; and cold, clammy, pale skin. *Prompt recognition and treatment of shock limits the amount of fluid lost and the impact on other body systems.*

Suggested NIC interventions

Acid-Base Management; Bleeding Reduction: Antepartum Uterus; Blood Products Administration; Electrolyte Management; Fluid Monitoring; Hemodynamic Regulation; Intravenous (IV) Therapy; Medication Management; Shock Management; Vital Signs Monitoring

Evaluations for expected outcomes

■ Patient's vital signs remain stable.

■ Results of patient's hematology studies are within normal range.

■ Patient's uterus remains firm.

■ If patient develops shock, medical personnel identify it quickly and promptly start treatment.

■ Patient doesn't develop distended bladder.

■ Patient's blood loss after delivery is less than 500 ml and fluid volume is replenished.

Documentation

■ Estimation of blood loss
■ Signs of possible shock
■ Location and tone of fundus
■ Laboratory results
■ Replacement of lost fluid
■ Nursing interventions to control active blood loss
■ Patient's response to nursing interventions
■ Evaluations for expected outcomes

Reference

MacMullen, N.J., et al. "Red Alert: Perinatal Hemorrhage," *The American Journal of Maternal Child Nursing* 30(1):46-51, January-February 2005.

Delayed
GROWTH AND DEVELOPMENT
related to perinatal insult or injury

Definition
Deviations from age-group norms

Assessment
- Maternal history, including age, use of controlled substances, trauma, and anesthesia or analgesia during labor
- Labor and delivery record
- Neonate status, including gestational age, Apgar scores, vital signs, feeding patterns, muscle tone, condition of fontanels, and characteristics of cry
- Neonate's neurologic status, including reflexes, responsiveness, activity level, and presence of seizures
- Diagnostic tests, including laboratory studies and ultrasound examinations

Defining characteristics
- Altered physical growth
- Diminished or absent reflexes
- Flat affect
- Listlessness and decreased responses
- Inability to perform self-care or self-control activities appropriate for age

Expected outcomes
- Neonate's alteration in growth and development will be evaluated, and supportive measures will be initiated.
- Family members will express realistic expectations for neonate's growth.
- Neonate will receive appropriate physical therapy on regular basis.
- Family members will demonstrate understanding of neonate's special needs.
- Family members will accept referrals to available community resources.

Suggested NOC outcomes
Child Development: 2 Months; Knowledge: Parenting; Parenting Performance; Physical Maturation: Female; Physical Maturation: Male

Interventions and rationales
- Reposition the hypotonic neonate every 2 hours *to prevent skin breakdown and pulmonary complications of immobility.*
- Measure the neonate's head circumference every shift. *An increasing head circumference indicates increased intracranial pressure (ICP).*
- Evaluate and record the activity level every shift. *An altered activity level may indicate such conditions as sepsis, hyperbilirubinemia, increased ICP, or intraventricular hemorrhage.*
- Monitor and report changes in the neonate's neurologic status *to detect exacerbation or lessening of danger signs.*

■ Refer the neonate to an appropriate health care specialist, such as a physical therapist, social worker, developmental specialist, or neurologist. Provide the parents or other family members with information on community resources *to ensure comprehensive care for the neonate.*

■ Provide emotional support to family members who have difficulty accepting the neonate's condition. Assess their goals for the neonate's development. *By offering support and identifying unrealistic goals, you can help family members come to terms with the neonate's condition.*

■ Involve family members in the neonate's daily care, and keep them abreast of the neonate's condition. *Personal involvement promotes bonding, decreases anxiety, and helps prepare for discharge.*

■ Assess the neonate's ability to suck on an ongoing basis. *A weak suck reflex may indicate neurologic defect or a need for nutritional supplementation.*

■ Monitor the neonate's temperature every 4 hours, or as ordered. Maintain a neutral thermal environment *to minimize oxygen consumption, prevent cold stress, and promote growth by decreasing unnecessary caloric use.*

Suggested NIC interventions

Family Process Maintenance; Family Support; Family Therapy; Infant Care; Parenting Promotion

Evaluations for expected outcomes

■ Neonate's alteration in growth and development is evaluated and his nutritional, physical, and safety needs are met.

■ Family members express realistic understanding of neonate's present condition and potential for improvement.

■ Neonate receives appropriate physical therapy on regular basis.

■ Family members demonstrate understanding of and ability to meet neonate's physical and emotional needs.

■ Family members agree to seek help and support from appropriate community resources.

Documentation

■ Observed characteristics of neonate, including seizure activity, characteristics of cry, hypoactive or hyperactive muscle activity, condition of fontanels, presence or absence of reflexes, feeding ability, and vital signs

■ Use of respiratory support

■ Family members' response to neonate's condition

■ Consultations with other health care team members

■ Referrals to outside agencies

■ Nursing interventions and neonate's response

■ Evaluations for expected outcomes

Reference

McGrath, J.M. "Family-Centered Developmental Care Begins Before Birth: Little Things Can Make a Big Difference," *The Journal of Perinatal and Neonatal Nursing* 20(3):195-96, July-September 2006.

HYPOTHERMIA
related to cold, stress, or sepsis

Definition
State in which neonate's body temperature is below normal range

Assessment
- History of present illness
- Gestational age
- Prenatal and intrapartal history
- Presence of maternal risk factors, such as fever, diabetes mellitus, drug use, dystocia, and history of perinatal asphyxia
- Neurologic status, including level of consciousness (LOC) and sensory status
- Cardiovascular status, including core temperature, heart rate and rhythm, blood pressure, and capillary refill time
- Respiratory status, including rate, rhythm, and depth; breath sounds; and arterial blood gas values
- Integumentary status, including temperature, color (central versus peripheral), and turgor
- Nutritional status, including dietary pattern, birth weight, current weight, and recent weight changes
- Fluid and electrolyte status, including intake and output, serum glucose and electrolyte levels, and urine specific gravity
- Psychosocial status, including behavior, parental stressors, parental coping skills, and financial resources

Defining characteristics
- Body temperature below normal range
- Cool, pale skin
- Cyanotic nail beds
- Increased blood pressure and heart rate
- Piloerection
- Shivering
- Slow capillary refill

Expected outcomes
- Neonate will exhibit normal body temperature.
- Neonate will have warm, dry skin and normal capillary refill time.
- Neonate's cardiovascular status will be normal.
- Neonate won't develop complications of hypothermia.
- Neonate won't shiver.
- Neonate won't develop signs of hyperthermia related to radiant heat source.
- Neonate will be weaned from self-contained incubation unit or radiant warmer bed, as tolerated.
- Family members will verbalize knowledge of how hypothermia develops and will state measures to prevent recurrent hypothermia.

■ Family members will demonstrate ability to measure neonate's temperature accurately.

■ Family members will demonstrate willingness to provide adequate home care for neonate.

Suggested NOC outcomes

Thermoregulation: Newborn; Vital Signs

Interventions and rationales

■ Monitor body temperature every 1 to 3 hours by axillary or inguinal route (avoid rectal measurement). Record temperature and route. *Monitoring body temperature helps to detect developing complications.* If using an electronic heat source, such as a radiant warmer, monitor the device's temperature reading hourly and compare it with the neonate's body temperature *to evaluate the effectiveness of interventions.*

■ Monitor and record neurologic status every 1 to 4 hours. *Falling body temperature and slowed metabolic rate may cause decreased LOC.*

■ Monitor and record vital signs every 1 to 4 hours. As ordered, initiate and maintain continuous electronic cardiorespiratory monitoring. *These measures help avert metabolic acidosis and respiratory arrest.*

■ Provide supportive measures:

– Maintain a neutral thermal environment—a narrow range of environmental temperature that maintains a stable core temperature with minimal caloric and oxygen expenditure. Determination of a neutral thermal environment depends on the neonate's age and weight.

– If indicated, place the neonate in an open crib. For mild hypothermia, dress the neonate with an undershirt, diaper, and knitted or stockinette cap and cover him with double blankets.

– Avoid overheating the neonate.

– Keep the diaper area dry.

– Cover all metal or plastic surfaces that could come in contact with the neonate.

– Maintain the room temperature between 75° and 78° F (23.9° and 25.6° C).

– Perform all procedures under a radiant warmer, if possible. Postpone bathing the neonate.

These measures protect the neonate from heat loss.

■ For severe hypothermia, place the neonate in an Isolette or overhead radiant warmer bed, providing these supportive measures:

– Keep the neonate undressed.

– Set the mechanism to the desired skin temperature (96.8° to 97.8° F [36° to 36.6° C]).

– If the neonate is under a radiant warmer, use plastic wrap placed like a blanket to prevent heat and fluid loss. Use a sheet large enough to cover only the neonate. Border it with tape.

– Attach a skin probe to the right upper quadrant of the neonate's abdomen. Don't place it over bone or the rib cage.

– Use a heat shield for a very unstable neonate inside an Isolette.

– Monitor carefully for evaporative loss and insensible fluid loss. Keep in mind that radiant warmer and Isolette therapy increase fluid maintenance needs.

These measures help ensure safe use of a radiant warmer or Isolette.

■ Follow the prescribed treatment regimen for hypothermia, which may include administering an antibiotic in cases of sepsis, administering I.V. fluids, and feeding the neonate small, frequent portions, if appropriate. *Prescribed treatment helps eliminate infection and meet the neonate's fluid and nutrient needs.*

■ Discuss precipitating factors with family members *to help prevent recurrence.*

■ Instruct family members in preventive measures, such as dressing the neonate appropriately and providing adequate nutrition for the neonate's growth needs. If the family requires financial help, refer them to the appropriate social service agency. *These precautions may help protect the neonate from future cold stress episodes.*

Suggested NIC interventions

Circulatory Precautions; Environmental Management; Fluid/Electrolyte Management; Hypothermia Treatment; Newborn Care; Skin Surveillance; Temperature Regulation

Evaluations for expected outcomes

■ Neonate's temperature returns to normal range.

■ Neonate exhibits warm, dry skin and normal capillary refill time.

■ Neonate has normal cardiovascular assessment findings.

■ Neonate doesn't develop complications of hypothermia.

■ Neonate doesn't begin shivering.

■ Neonate doesn't develop signs of hyperthermia related to radiant heat source.

■ Neonate is successfully weaned from Isolette or radiant warmer bed.

■ Family members verbalize understanding of causes of hypothermia and preventive measures.

■ Family members demonstrate proper axillary or inguinal temperature measurement technique.

■ Family members demonstrate willingness to provide adequate home care for neonate.

Documentation

■ Neonate's physical findings, including cardiovascular status, temperature, and shivering

■ Nursing interventions and neonate's response to them

■ Family members' willingness and abilities to provide adequate home care

■ Evaluations for expected outcomes

References

Galligan, M. "Proposed Guidelines for Skin-to-skin Treatment of Neonatal Hypothermia," *The American Journal of Maternal Child Nursing* 31(5):298-304, September-October 2006.

Sherman, T.I., et al. "Optimizing the Neonatal Thermal Environment," *Neonatal Network* 25(4):251-60, July-August 2006.

Disorganized
INFANT BEHAVIOR

related to pain, prematurity, oral problems, motor problems, feeding intolerance, environmental overstimulation, or lack of stimulation

Definition

Disintegrated physiological and neurobehavioral response to the environment

Assessment

■ Cardiovascular status, including pulse and respirations
■ GI status, including feeding pattern, food tolerance, defecation pattern, ability to maintain adequate weight, and abdominal bloating and distention
■ Neurologic status, including muscle tone, neonatal reflexes, excessive crying, lethargy, irritability, seizures, tremors, and assessments such as Brazelton Neonatal Behavioral Assessment and Dubowitz Gestational Age Assessment
■ Sensory status, including responsiveness to visual, tactile, and auditory stimuli and experience with pain
■ Parental status, including knowledge of normal growth and development
■ Sleep status, including sleep patterns and usual hours of sleep
■ Parents' psychological status, including energy level, motivation, self-image, competence, recent life changes, experience with children, and eye contact and interaction with infant

Defining characteristics

■ Bradycardia, tachycardia, or arrhythmias
■ Evidence of problems in behavioral and neurologic development, such as apnea; deficient response to visual and auditory stimuli; excessive crying; excessive yawning; hyperextension of arms and legs; irregular sleep pattern or difficulty obtaining adequate sleep; tremors, startles, and twitches
■ Feeding intolerance (aspiration or emesis)
■ Oximeter reading that reflects desaturation
■ Pale, cyanotic, mottled, or flushed color
■ Time-out signals (such as gaze, grasp, cough, sneeze, hiccup, sigh, slack jaw, open mouth, tongue thrust)

Expected outcomes

■ Parents will learn to identify and understand infant's behavioral cues.
■ Parents will identify their own emotional responses to infant's behavior.
■ Parents will identify means to help infant overcome his behavioral disturbance.
■ Parents will identify ways to improve their ability to cope with infant's responses.
■ Infant will begin to show appropriate signs of maturation.
■ Parents will express positive feelings about their ability to care for infant.
■ Parents will identify resources for help with infant.

Suggested NOC outcomes

Knowledge: Infant Care; Neurological Status; Preterm Infant Organization; Sleep

Interventions and rationales

■ Explain to the parents that infant maturation is a developmental process and that their participation is crucial *to help them understand the importance of nurturing the infant.*

■ Explain to the parents that their actions can help modify some of their infant's behavior. However, make it clear that infant maturation isn't completely within their control. *This explanation may help decrease the parents' feelings of incompetence.*

■ Explain to the parents that infants give behavioral cues that indicate their needs. Discuss appropriate ways to respond to these behavioral cues—for example, providing stimulation that doesn't overwhelm the infant, stopping stimulation when the infant gives behavioral cues (such as yawning, looking away, or becoming agitated), and finding methods to calm the infant if he becomes agitated (such as swaddling, gentle rocking, and quiet vocalizations). Help the parents identify and cope with their responses to the infant's behavioral disturbance *to help them recognize and adjust their response patterns. When the infant doesn't respond positively to them, the parents may feel inadequate or become frustrated. They need to understand that these reactions are normal.*

■ Explore with the parents ways to cope with stress imposed by the infant's behavior *to help them develop better coping skills.*

■ Praise the parents when they demonstrate appropriate methods of interacting with the infant *to provide positive reinforcement.*

■ Provide the parents with information on sources of support and special infant services *to help them cope with their infant's long-term needs.*

Suggested NIC interventions

Environmental Management; Neurologic Monitoring; Newborn Care; Parent Education: Infant; Positioning; Sleep Enhancement

Evaluations for expected outcomes

■ Parents state their understanding of infant's behavioral cues.

■ Parents discuss appropriate ways of responding to infant's behavior and exhibit decreased frustration with infant's behavior.

■ Parents identify ways to help infant overcome his behavioral disturbance by recognizing infant's needs and responding appropriately.

■ Parents report improved ability to cope with stress of caring for infant.

■ Infant begins to show appropriate signs of maturation, such as longer periods of sleep, shorter periods of crying, longer periods of being awake and alert, smoother transitions between behavioral states, and positive responses to parents' interventions.

■ Parents express positive feelings about their ability to care for infant.

■ Parents identify resources for help with infant.

Documentation
- Assessment of factors that may enhance or retard infant behavioral development
- Parents' expressed feelings about caring for infant
- Nursing interventions and infant's response to them
- Evaluations for expected outcomes

Reference
Beal, J.A. "Evidence for Best Practices in the Neonatal Period," *The American Journal of Maternal Child Nursing* 30(6):397-403, November-December 2005.

Readiness for enhanced organized
INFANT BEHAVIOR

Definition
A pattern of modulation of the physiologic and behavioral systems of functioning (such as autonomic, motor, state-organizational, self-regulatory; and attentional-interactional systems) in an infant that's satisfactory but that can be improved resulting in higher levels of integration in response to environmental stimuli

Assessment
- Cardiovascular status, including pulse and respirations
- GI status, including feeding and defecation patterns, food tolerance, ability to maintain adequate weight, and abdominal distention and bloating
- Neurologic status, including excessive crying, poor sleep patterns, lethargy, irritability, seizures, tremors, muscle tone, neonate reflexes, and such assessments as Brazelton Neonatal Behavioral Assessment and Dubowitz Gestational Age Assessment
- Sensory status, including responsiveness to visual, tactile, and auditory stimuli and experience with pain
- Sleep status, including usual hours of sleep
- Parental status, including knowledge of normal growth and development
- Parents' psychological status, including energy level, motivation, experience with children, eye contact and interaction with infant, and Home Observation Measurement of the Environment results

Defining characteristics
- Ability to use some self-regulatory behaviors
- Definite sleep-wake states
- Responsiveness to visual and auditory stimuli
- Stable physiologic measures

Expected outcomes

■ Parents will express understanding of their role in infant's behavioral development.
■ Parents will express confidence in their ability to interpret infant's behavioral cues.
■ Parents will identify means to promote infant's behavioral development.
■ Parents will express positive feelings about their ability to care for infant.
■ Parents will identify resources for help with infant.

Suggested NOC outcomes

Child Development: 2 Months; Knowledge: Infant Care; Neurological Status; Sleep

Interventions and rationales

■ Explain to the parents that infant maturation is a developmental process. Further explain that infants exhibit three behavioral states: sleeping, crying, and being awake and alert. Also explain that infants provide behavioral cues that indicate their needs. *Education will help parents understand the importance of nurturing the infant and prepare them to respond to the infant's behavioral cues.*
■ Explain to the parents that their actions can help promote infant development. Make it clear, however, that infant maturation isn't completely within their control. *This explanation may decrease feelings of anxiety and incompetence and help to prevent unrealistic expectations.*
■ Demonstrate appropriate ways of interacting with the infant, such as moderate stimulation, gentle rocking, and quiet vocalizations, *to help the parents identify the most effective methods of interacting with their child.*
■ Help the parents interpret behavioral cues from their infant *to foster healthy parent-child interaction.* For example, help them recognize when the infant is awake and alert, and point out to them that this is a good time to provide stimulation.
■ Help the parents identify ways they can promote the infant's development, such as providing stimulation by shaking a rattle in front of the infant, talking to the infant in a gentle voice, and looking at the infant when feeding him, *to encourage practices that promote the infant's development. Sensory experiences promote cognitive development.*
■ Explore with the parents ways to cope with stress caused by the infant's behavior *to increase their coping skills.*
■ Praise the parents for their attempts to enhance their interaction with the infant *to provide positive reinforcement.*
■ Provide the parents with information on sources of support and special infant services *to encourage them to continue to foster their infant's development.*

Suggested NIC interventions

Attachment Promotion; Developmental Care; Family Integrity Promotion: Childbearing Family; Infant Care; Sleep Enhancement

Evaluations for expected outcomes

- Parents express understanding of their role in infant's behavioral development.
- Parents express confidence in their ability to recognize infant's behavioral cues.
- Parents identify activities that foster positive responses from infant and provide appropriate sensory and tactile stimulation.
- Parents express positive feelings about their ability to care for infant.
- Parents identify resources for help with infant.

Documentation

- Assessment of factors that may enhance infant's behavioral development
- Parents' expressed feelings about caring for their infant
- Nursing interventions and infant's response to them
- Evaluations for expected outcomes

Reference

Byers, J.F., et al. "A Quasi-experimental Trial on Individualized, Developmentally Supportive Family-centered Care," *Journal of Obstetric, Gynecologic, and Neonatal Nursing* 35(1):105-115, January-February 2006.

Risk for disorganized
INFANT BEHAVIOR

related to pain, prematurity, oral problems, motor problems, feeding intolerance, environmental overstimulation, or lack of stimulation

---

Definition

Risk for alteration in integration and modulation of the physiological and behavioral systems of functioning (such as autonomic, motor, state-organizational, self-regulatory, and attentional-interactional systems)

Assessment

- Cardiovascular status, including pulse and respirations
- GI status, including feeding and defecation patterns, food tolerance, ability to maintain adequate weight, and abdominal bloating and distention
- Neurologic status, including muscle tone, neonate reflexes, excessive crying, lethargy, irritability, seizures, tremors, and such assessments as Brazelton Neonatal Behavioral Assessment and Dubowitz Gestational Age Assessment
- Sensory status, including infant's responsiveness to visual, tactile, and auditory stimuli and experience with pain
- Sleep status, including sleep pattern and usual hours of sleep
- Parental status, including knowledge of normal growth and development
- Parents' psychological status, including energy level, motivation, experience with children, and eye contact and interaction with infant

Risk factors

- Environmental overstimulation

- Invasive or painful procedures
- Lack of containment or boundaries
- Oral or motor problems
- Pain
- Prematurity

Expected outcomes

- Parents will identify factors that place infant at risk for behavioral disturbance.
- Parents will identify potential signs of behavioral disturbance in infant.
- Parents will identify appropriate ways to interact with infant.
- Parents will identify their reactions to infant (including ways of coping with occasional frustration and anger).
- Parents will express positive feelings about their ability to care for infant.
- Parents will identify resources for help with infant.

Suggested NOC outcomes

Child Development: 2 Months; Knowledge: Infant Care; Knowledge: Parenting; Preterm Infant Organization

Interventions and rationales

- Explain to the parents that infant maturation is a developmental process and that their participation is crucial *to help them understand the importance of nurturing the infant.*
- Explain to the parents that their actions can help modify some of their infant's behavior. However, make it clear that infant maturation isn't completely within their control. *This explanation may decrease the parents' feelings of incompetence.*
- Explain to the parents that certain risk factors may interfere with the infant's ability to achieve optimal development. These risk factors include overstimulation, lack of stimulation, lack of physical contact, and painful medical procedures. *Educating the parents will help them understand their role in interpreting the infant's behavioral cues and providing appropriate stimulation.*
- Describe for the parents the potential signs of a behavioral disturbance in the infant: inappropriate responses to stimuli, such as the failure to respond to human contact or tendency to become agitated with human contact; physiologic regulatory problems, such as a breathing disturbance in a premature infant; and apparent inability to interact with the environment. *Education will help the parents recognize if the infant has a problem in behavioral development.*
- Demonstrate appropriate ways of interacting with the infant *to help the parents identify and interpret the infant's behavioral cues and respond appropriately.* For example, help them recognize when the infant is awake and alert, and help them understand when the infant needs more stimulation, such as being spoken to or held.
- Explore with the parents ways to cope with the stress imposed by the infant's behavior *to increase their coping skills.* Help them identify their emotional responses to the infant's behavior *to help them recognize and adjust their response patterns.* Explain that it's normal for parents to experience feelings of inadequacy, frustration, or anger if the infant doesn't respond positively to them.

■ Praise the parents when they demonstrate appropriate methods of interacting with the infant *to provide positive reinforcement.*

■ Provide the parents with information on sources of support and special infant services *to help them cope with the infant's long-term needs.*

Suggested NIC interventions

Infant Care; Newborn Monitoring; Parent Education: Infant; Positioning; Surveillance

Evaluations for expected outcomes

■ Parents identify risk factors for behavioral disturbance.

■ Parents identify potential signs of behavioral disturbance in infant.

■ Parents identify actions that promote their infant's development.

■ Parents report improvement in their ability to cope with the stress of raising an infant.

■ Parents express positive feelings about their ability to care for infant.

■ Parents identify resources for help with infant.

Documentation

■ Assessment of factors that could disturb infant's behavioral development

■ Parents' expression of feelings about caring for infant

■ Nursing interventions and infant's response to them

■ Evaluations for expected outcomes

Reference

Swartz, M.K. "Parenting Preterm Infants: A Meta-Synthesis," *The American Journal of Maternal Child Nursing* 30(2):115-20, March-April 2005.

Ineffective
INFANT FEEDING PATTERN
related to neurologic impairment or developmental delay

Definition

Impaired ability of an infant to suck or coordinate the suck and swallow response

Assessment

■ Perinatal history, including gestational age and Apgar score

■ Suck and swallow reflex, including condition of lip and palate

■ Nutritional status, including intake (type, amount, and frequency of feedings), output (frequency, amount, and characteristics of urine), current weight, weight change since birth, skin turgor, and signs of dehydration

■ Laboratory studies, including glucose and bilirubin levels

■ Parental assessment, including age, maturity level, and previous experience with infant feeding

Defining characteristics

- Inability to coordinate sucking, swallowing, and breathing
- Inability to initiate or sustain effective suck

Expected outcomes

- Neonate won't lose more than 10% of birth weight within first week of life.
- Neonate will gain 4 to 7 oz (113.5 to 198.5 g)/week after first week of life.
- Parents or caregivers will identify factors that interfere with neonate establishing effective feeding pattern.
- Parents will express increased confidence in their ability to perform appropriate feeding techniques.
- Neonate won't become dehydrated.
- Neonate will receive adequate supplemental nutrition until able to suckle sufficiently.
- Neonate will establish effective suck and swallow reflexes that allow for adequate intake of nutrients.

Suggested NOC outcomes

Breast-feeding Establishment: Infant; Breast-feeding Maintenance; Nutritional Status: Food & Fluid Intake

Interventions and rationales

- Weigh the neonate at the same time each day on the same scale *to detect excessive weight loss early.*
- Continuously assess the neonate's sucking pattern *to monitor for ineffective patterns.*
- Assess the parents' knowledge of feeding techniques *to help identify and clear up misconceptions.*
- Assess the parents' level of anxiety about the neonate's feeding difficulty. *Anxiety may interfere with the parents' ability to learn new techniques.*
- Remain with the parents and neonate during the feeding *to identify problem areas and direct interventions.*
- Teach the parents to place the neonate in the upright position during feeding *to prevent aspiration.*
- Teach the parents to unwrap and position a sleepy neonate before feeding *to ensure that the neonate is awake and alert enough to suckle sufficiently.*
- Provide positive reinforcement for the parents' efforts to improve their feeding technique *to decrease anxiety and enhance feelings of success.*
- For bottle-feeding, record the amount ingested at each feeding; for breast-feeding, record the number of minutes the neonate nurses at each breast and the amount of any supplement ingested *to monitor for inadequate caloric and fluid intake.*
- Provide an alternative nipple, such as a preemie nipple. *A preemie nipple has a larger hole and softer texture, which makes it easier for the neonate to obtain formula.*
- For breast-feeding, ensure the neonate's tongue is properly positioned under the mother's nipple *to promote adequate sucking.*

■ Monitor the neonate for poor skin turgor, dry mucous membranes, decreased or concentrated urine, and sunken fontanels and eyeballs *to detect possible dehydration and allow for immediate intervention.*

■ Record the number of stools and amount of urine voided each shift. *An altered bowel elimination pattern may indicate decreased food intake; decreased amounts of concentrated urine may indicate dehydration.*

■ Assess the need for gavage feeding. *The neonate may temporarily require alternative means of obtaining adequate fluids and calories.*

■ Alternate oral and gavage feeding *to conserve the neonate's energy.*

■ If the neonate requires I.V. nourishment, assess the insertion site, amount infused, and infusion rate every hour *to monitor fluid intake and identify possible complications, such as infiltration and phlebitis.*

■ Assess the neonate for neurologic deficits or other pathophysiologic causes of ineffective sucking *to identify the need for more extensive evaluation.*

Suggested NIC interventions

Attachment Promotion; Breast-feeding Assistance; Lactation Counseling; Nonnutritive Sucking

Evaluations for expected outcomes

■ Neonate doesn't lose more than 10% of birth weight within first week of life.

■ Neonate gains 4 to 7 oz per week after first week of life.

■ Parents identify factors that interfere with effective feeding.

■ Parents express increased confidence in their ability to perform appropriate feeding techniques.

■ Neonate maintains urine output of 1 ml/kg/day, urine specific gravity of 1.003 to 1.013, good skin turgor, moist mucous membranes, and soft, flat fontanels.

■ Neonate receives adequate nutrition.

■ Neonate establishes effective sucking reflex and coordinated suck and swallow response.

Documentation

■ Frequency, amount, and type of fluid ingested by neonate

■ Effectiveness of suck reflex

■ Neonate's daily weight

■ Parents' knowledge of feeding techniques, involvement with caregiving, and bonding with neonate

■ Frequency of neonate's bowel elimination and urination

■ Signs of dehydration

■ Nursing interventions

■ Use of special feeding techniques and equipment

■ Parents' and neonate's responses to nursing interventions

■ Evidence of neurologic or other physical impairment in neonate

■ Evaluations for expected outcomes

Reference

Kelly, M.M. "Primary Care Issues for the Healthy Premature Infant," *Journal of Pediatric Health Care* 20(5):293-99, September-October 2006.

Risk for
INFECTION
related to altered primary defenses during the postpartum period

Definition
At increased risk for being invaded by pathologic organisms

Assessment
■ Laboratory studies, including white blood cell (WBC) and platelet count, clotting factors, hemoglobin level, hematocrit, serum albumin level, and cultures of blood, body fluid, sputum, urine, and wound drainage
■ Labor and delivery record, including episiotomy; presence of invasive devices, such as I.V. and urinary catheters; and premature rupture of membranes
■ Presence of medical conditions such as diabetes mellitus that may increase incidence of infection
■ Signs and symptoms of infection, including pallor, fatigue, malaise, anorexia, chills, foul-smelling lochia, calf tenderness, elevated temperature, dysuria, marked abdominal tenderness, and tender, reddened breasts that are warm to the touch

Risk factors
■ Altered immune function
■ Chronic illness
■ Environmental exposure to pathogens
■ Inadequate primary defenses (such as broken skin) or secondary defenses (such as suppressed inflammatory response)
■ Invasive procedures
■ Lack of knowledge about causes of infection
■ Malnutrition
■ Medication use
■ Premature membrane rupture
■ Tissue destruction
■ Trauma

Expected outcomes
■ Patient's vital signs will remain within normal range.
■ Results of laboratory studies won't indicate infection.
■ Patient's respiratory secretions and urine won't show evidence of infection.
■ Patient's episiotomy or abdominal incision site will remain free from infection.
■ Patient's I.V. sites won't become inflamed.
■ Patient will maintain good personal hygiene.
■ Patient will state risk factors that can lead to infection.
■ Patient will remain free from signs and symptoms of infection.

Suggested NOC outcomes
Immune Status; Infection Severity; Knowledge: Infection Control; Risk Detection; Wound Healing: Primary Intention

Interventions and rationales

■ Minimize the patient's risk of infection by:

– washing your hands before and after providing care. *Hand washing is the single best way to avoid spreading pathogens.*

– wearing gloves to maintain asepsis when providing direct care and when in contact with blood or body secretions. *Gloves reduce the possibility of transmitting disease.*

■ After delivery, monitor vital signs every 15 minutes for 1 hour, then every 4 hours for 24 hours, then every shift until discharge. Report abnormal readings. *Elevated temperature, pulse or respiratory rates, or blood pressure may indicate infection. A temperature greater than 100.4° F (38° C) on two consecutive readings after the first 24 hours postdelivery may indicate puerperal sepsis, urinary tract infection, endometritis, mastitis, or other infection.*

■ Monitor the WBC count, as ordered, and promptly report abnormal values. *A total WBC count above 11,000/µl indicates increased production of leukocytes by bone marrow, usually in response to bacterial pathogens.*

■ As ordered, culture urine, respiratory secretions, wound drainage, or blood *to identify pathogens and guide antibiotic therapy.*

■ Instruct the patient in proper personal hygiene, such as use of a sitz bath and perineal irrigation bottle, hand washing, and breast care, *to reduce the risk of infection.* Explain to the patient that the most common site of localized postpartum infection is the episiotomy site. Tell the patient how to apply sanitary pads (front to back) and how to remove them (back to front). Tell her to wipe the perineum after elimination and to clean the perineum from front to back. *These measures decrease bacterial concentration and help prevent genitourinary infections.*

■ Follow the facility's infection-control policy *to minimize the risk of nosocomial infection.*

■ Use strict sterile technique when performing invasive procedures, such as urinary catheterization or I.V. line insertion, *to minimize the risk of introducing pathogens into the body.*

■ Assess the I.V. site every 4 hours, noting the presence of redness or warmth. Change I.V. tubing and site every 72 hours, or as dictated by facility policy. *These measures keep pathogens from entering the body.*

■ Instruct the postoperative patient to deep-breathe and cough *to help remove secretions and prevent respiratory complications.*

■ Ensure adequate nutritional intake. *A diet high in protein, iron, and vitamin C helps promote healing.*

■ Assess the patient for generalized signs and symptoms of infection (pallor, fatigue, malaise, anorexia, and chills) every shift, and instruct her to report danger signs immediately. These include foul-smelling lochia, calf tenderness, elevated temperature, dysuria, marked abdominal tenderness, and tender, reddened breasts that feel warm to the touch. *Prompt detection of infection helps minimize complications.*

Suggested NIC interventions

Allergy Management; Cesarean Section Care; Infection Control; Perineal Care; Postpartal Care

Evaluations for expected outcomes
■ Patient's vital signs remain within normal limits.
■ Patient's WBC count and differential remain within normal range, and cultures don't indicate any pathogens.
■ Patient's respiratory secretions are clear and odorless, and urine is clear yellow, odorless, and sediment-free.
■ Patient's episiotomy or abdominal incision site remains free from infection.
■ Patient's I.V. sites don't become inflamed.
■ Patient performs proper personal hygiene on regular basis.
■ Patient states risk factors that can lead to infection.
■ Patient remains free from infection.

Documentation
■ Vital signs
■ Appearance of episiotomy or abdominal incision site
■ Date, time, and sites of cultures
■ Date, time, and sites of catheter insertions
■ Appearance of invasive catheter and I.V. sites
■ Patient teaching about infection control
■ Interventions performed to reduce risk of infection
■ Patient's response to nursing interventions
■ Evaluations for expected outcomes

Reference
Christenson, M., et al. "Improving Patient Safety: Resource Availability and Application for Reducing the Incidence of Healthcare-associated Infection," *Infection Control and Hospital Epidemiology* 27(3):245-51 March 2006.

Risk for
INFECTION
related to labor and delivery

Definition
At increased risk for being invaded by pathologic organisms

Assessment
■ Vital signs, including fetal heart rate
■ Health history, including previous infections
■ Rupture of membranes, including time of rupture and characteristics of amniotic fluid (amount, color [blood tinged or meconium stained], and odor)
■ Laboratory studies, including white blood cell (WBC) and platelet count, clotting factors, hemoglobin level, hematocrit, serum albumin level, and cultures of blood or body fluid, sputum, urine, and wound drainage

■ Signs and symptoms of chorioamnionitis, including maternal pulse rate over 160 beats/minute, malodorous amniotic fluid, increasing uterine tenderness, and fetal tachycardia

Risk factors
■ Altered immune function
■ Amniotic membrane rupture
■ Chronic illness
■ Environmental exposure to pathogens
■ Inadequate primary defenses (such as broken skin) or secondary defenses (such as suppressed inflammatory response)
■ Invasive procedures
■ Lack of knowledge about causes of infection
■ Malnutrition
■ Medication use
■ Tissue destruction
■ Trauma

Expected outcomes
■ Patient will maintain good hygiene.
■ Patient will remain free from infection.
■ Patient's temperature will remain within normal range.

Suggested NOC outcomes
Immune Status; Infection Severity; Risk Detection; Self-Care: Hygiene; Wound Healing: Primary Intention

Interventions and rationales
■ Monitor and record the patient's temperature every 4 hours before the membranes rupture and every 2 hours after they rupture. *Temperature elevations are an early sign of infection.*
■ Use continuous fetal monitoring to assess the fetal heart rate and variability. Report rates over 160 beats/minute and variability under 3 to 5 beats/minute. *Fetal heart rates over 160 beats/minute and minimal variability may indicate maternal fever.*
■ Wash your hands thoroughly, using proper technique, before and after providing care *to prevent the spread of infection.*
■ Maintain standard precautions. Wear gloves if you might come into contact with the patient's blood and body secretions. *Standard precautions protect you and the patient from the transfer of microorganisms.*
■ Use strict sterile technique when suctioning the lower airway, applying scalp electrodes, or inserting urinary catheters, pressure catheters, or I.V. lines *to reduce the likelihood of nosocomial infections.*
■ After spontaneous or artificial rupture of the membranes, assess the color, amount, and odor of the amniotic fluid and the presence of blood or meconium. *Alterations in the color, amount, and odor of the amniotic fluid may indicate infection. Meconium may indicate a predisposition to intrauterine infection and fetal distress.*

■ After rupture of the membranes, minimize vaginal examinations and always use sterile gloves *to decrease the risk of chorioamnionitis or other uterine infection.*

■ Maintain good patient hygiene. Clean the perineal area from front to back and keep the area dry *to reduce the risk of infection.*

■ Carefully monitor intake and output *to assess for dehydration. Signs and symptoms of infection (tachycardia, dry mucous membranes, and poor skin turgor) may resemble those of dehydration.*

Suggested NIC interventions

High-Risk Pregnancy Care; Infection Control; Infection Protection; Intrapartal Care: High-Risk Delivery; Postpartal Care

Evaluations for expected outcomes

■ Patient maintains good hygiene.

■ Patient remains free from infection, as evidenced by clear, odorless, sediment-free urine; WBC count within acceptable limits for labor and delivery (up to 20,000/µl); and cultures free from pathogens.

■ Patient's temperature ranges from 97° to 99° F (36.1° to 37.2° C).

Documentation

■ Maternal vital signs

■ Fetal heart rate and variability

■ Date, time, and sites of cultures

■ Date, time, and sites of catheter insertions

■ Appearance of all invasive catheter and tube sites and wounds

■ Nursing interventions performed to reduce risk of infection

■ Patient's response to nursing interventions

■ Evaluations for expected outcomes

Reference

Christenson, M., et al. "Improving Patient Safety: Resource Availability and Application for Reducing the Incidence of Healthcare-associated Infection," *Infection Control and Hospital Epidemiology* 27(3):245-51, March 2006.

Risk for
INFECTION

related to neonate's immature immune system

Definition

At increased risk for being invaded by pathologic organisms

Assessment

■ Gestational age

■ Neonate's temperature and vital signs

■ Labor and delivery record, including premature rupture of membranes, characteristics of amniotic fluid (odorous or foul-smelling), and maternal temperature

■ Maternal infections (recent or current), maternal disease or infection during pregnancy, and maternal pathogens passed on during birth process

■ Condition of umbilical cord and skin at base of cord, including redness, odor, and discharge

■ Signs and symptoms of neonatal infection, including lethargy, poor weight gain, restlessness, jaundice, visible lesions, thrush, temperature elevations or unstable low temperature, hypoglycemia, altered feeding patterns, diarrhea, vomiting, and subtle color changes such as cyanosis, mottling, or grayish skin tones

■ Signs of respiratory distress, including grunting, retractions, nasal flaring, and cyanosis

■ Evidence of chronic intrauterine infections, including growth retardation, microcephaly, and hepatosplenomegaly

Risk factors

■ Altered immune function
■ Amniotic membrane rupture
■ Environmental exposure to pathogens
■ Inadequate primary defenses (such as broken skin) or secondary defenses (such as suppressed inflammatory response)
■ Invasive procedures
■ Malnutrition
■ Medication use
■ Tissue destruction
■ Trauma

Expected outcomes

■ Neonate's vital signs will remain within normal range.
■ Neonate will be alert and active.
■ Neonate will remain free from signs and symptoms of infection.
■ Neonate's umbilical cord will heal properly and remain free from infection.
■ Family members will demonstrate good hand-washing technique before handling neonate.

Suggested NOC outcomes

Immune Status; Infection Severity; Infection Severity: Newborn

Interventions and rationales

■ Review the maternal chart and delivery record *to detect risk factors that predispose the neonate to infection.*

■ Assess the neonate's gestational age. *Passive immunity of the neonate via the placenta increases significantly in the last trimester, making the premature neonate much more susceptible to infection.*

■ Follow sterile technique. Remove all rings, bracelets, and wristwatches before handling the neonate. Scrub your hands and arms with an antimicrobial preparation before entering the nursery and after contact with contaminated material.

Wash your hands again after handling the neonate. Instruct the parents and siblings in hand-washing techniques and procedures. *These measures help prevent the spread of pathogens.*

■ Monitor all hospital personnel, parents, and visitors for potential infection *to prevent spreading infection to the neonate.*

■ Organize the nursery. Make sure the aisles are 3′ (1 m) wide and cribs are 18″ (45.7 cm) apart. Keep individual supplies separate for each neonate. *These measures help prevent cross-contamination.*

■ Provide cover gowns for nonnursing personnel who enter the nursery *to prevent the spread of pathogens.*

■ Provide eye prophylaxis as facility policy dictates *to prevent ophthalmia neonatorum or gonococcal or chlamydia infections.*

■ Perform umbilical cord care with each diaper change, as facility policy dictates, *to promote healing, remove urine and stools, and facilitate desiccation process.*

■ Assess respirations, pulse, and blood pressure every 15 minutes for 1 hour, then every hour for 4 hours, then once per shift or more frequently, as indicated. Assess temperature every 4 hours for 24 hours, then every 8 hours, or as indicated. *Unstable vital signs, persistent elevations in temperature, or hypothermia may indicate neonatal infection.*

■ Observe the neonate for signs and symptoms of infection. Notify the physician immediately if signs and symptoms of infection appear *to ensure rapid identification and early treatment.*

■ Observe standard precautions. Wear gloves before the neonate's first bath and when in contact with blood and body secretions. *Following standard precautions prevents cross-contamination and transmission of pathogens, including human immunodeficiency virus.*

■ Encourage the mother to begin breast-feeding early. *Colostrum and breast milk contain high amounts of immunoglobulin (Ig) A, which provides passive immunity to the neonate and helps reduce infection.*

■ As ordered, monitor laboratory studies, including white blood cell (WBC) count, serum levels of IgM, and blood cultures. Culture any lesions, pustules, or drainage. *A decreased WBC count commonly indicates infection in a neonate; elevated IgM levels indicate that an infectious process has occurred in utero. Cultures identify pathogens and help guide antibiotic therapy.*

■ Administer topical, oral, and parenteral antibiotics, as ordered, *to eradicate pathogenic organisms.*

■ Observe the circumcision site for color, healing, and presence of drainage. *A fresh, healing circumcision site is a port of entry for bacteria.*

Suggested NIC interventions

Environmental Management; Infection Control; Infection Protection; Newborn Care; Surveillance; Vital Signs Monitoring

Evaluations for expected outcomes

■ Neonate's vital signs remain within normal range.
■ Neonate is alert and active.
■ Neonate is free from signs and symptoms of infection.

■ Neonate's umbilical cord is clean, dry, and healing.
■ Family members demonstrate proper hand-washing technique before handling neonate.

Documentation

■ Vital signs
■ Appearance of umbilical cord
■ Date, time, and sites of cultures
■ Feeding patterns and weight gain
■ Bowel elimination patterns
■ Condition of oral mucosa
■ Skin color and rashes
■ Activity pattern
■ Interventions performed to reduce risk of infection
■ Neonate's response to nursing interventions
■ Evaluations for expected outcomes

Reference

Couto, R.C., et al. "Risk Factors for Nosocomial Infection in a Neonatal Intensive Care Unit," *Infection Control and Hospital Epidemiology* 27(6):571-75, June 2006.

Risk for
INJURY

related to internal and external neonatal risk factors

Definition

Accentuated risk of injury as a result of environmental conditions interacting with the individual's adaptive and defensive reserves

Assessment

■ Ability of parents to care for neonate
■ Apgar scores
■ Developmental stage (neonate and parents or caregivers)
■ Environment, including air temperature, water temperature, and stability of equipment
■ Labor and delivery record
■ Laboratory studies, including blood glucose and bilirubin levels, white blood cell count, clotting factors, platelet count, hemoglobin level, hematocrit, and maternal and neonatal blood types
■ Neonatal health history, including traumatic delivery, blood dyscrasia, hypothermia, and hyperthermia
■ Neurologic status (neonate and parents or caregivers)
■ Prenatal history

Risk factors

- Extremes in environmental temperature
- Hyperbilirubinemia
- Improper padding of cold surfaces
- Improperly functioning radiant warmer and temperature probe
- Litter or liquid spills on floor
- Malfunctioning equipment
- Parents' or caregiver's cognitive, emotional, or motor difficulties
- Parents' or caregiver's lack of familiarity with information resources
- Placement of neonate near drafts
- Requests for information by parents or family members
- Unsafe handling of neonate
- Water temperature at improper setting for washing neonate

Expected outcomes

- Neonate will have physical and safety needs met.
- Family members will provide safe environment for neonate after discharge.
- Family members will recognize and report dangerous or potentially dangerous situations.
- Neonate won't experience injury.

Suggested NOC outcomes

Parenting: Infant/Toddler Physical Safety; Parenting: Psychosocial Safety; Risk Control; Safe Home Environment

Interventions and rationales

- Assess family members' baseline knowledge of neonatal safety. Instruct them, as needed. *Education in safety techniques minimizes the risk of injury.* Consider which teaching methods (pamphlets, videotapes, or demonstrations) best suit each family member's individual learning style *to facilitate learning.*
- Immediately report malfunctioning equipment to appropriate personnel for replacement or repair *to help prevent accidents.*
- Keep one hand 1″ to 2″ (2.5 to 5 cm) above the neonate when measuring weight *to prevent the neonate from accidentally slipping off the scale.*
- When transporting neonates from the nursery, take one bassinet at a time, if possible, *to improve safety.*
- Discourage family members from walking in the hall while holding the neonate *to avoid falls caused by wet or slippery floors.*
- Discourage the mother from sleeping in bed with the neonate. *While sleeping, she may accidentally turn over onto, or lose her grip on, the neonate.*
- Monitor the neonate's skin color for signs of jaundice every shift. *Hyperbilirubinemia occurs in approximately 50% of neonates. Elevated bilirubin levels can lead to neurologic and developmental difficulties.*
- Test the water temperature before washing the neonate. The temperature shouldn't exceed 100° F (37.8° C). *A neonate's fragile skin can't tolerate high temperatures.*

■ Don't allow ill staff members or visitors to approach the neonate *to prevent transfer of pathogens.*

■ Assess the neonate's potential for injury based on prenatal and labor and delivery records. *Early detection and treatment can minimize injury from intrauterine or perinatal insults.*

■ Never leave neonates unattended in an unprotected area. *Neonates are totally dependent on others for their physical, emotional, and safety needs.*

■ Monitor respiratory and neurologic status as well as laboratory test results. Promptly report abnormal findings *to ensure immediate intervention and prevent complications.*

■ Avoid heat loss to the neonate from evaporation. *Cold stress leads to increased metabolic rate, which can result in oxygen consumption and hypoglycemia.*

■ Review with family members the state regulations regarding car seats before discharge *to decrease the risk of automobile injury or fatality.*

Suggested NIC interventions

Environmental Management; Parent Education: Infant; Risk Identification; Surveillance: Safety

Evaluations for expected outcomes

■ Parents meet neonate's physical and safety needs.

■ Family members express understanding of techniques to ensure neonate's safety, after discharge, and practice safety techniques during neonate's stay in hospital.

■ Family members express understanding of potentially dangerous situations.

■ Neonate doesn't experience injury.

Documentation

■ Neonate's skin color

■ Temperature of radiant warmer and presence of functioning temperature probe

■ Laboratory results

■ Observations of physical findings

■ Observations or knowledge of unsafe practices

■ Instructions given to family members and their responses

■ Interventions performed to prevent injury

■ Neonate's response to nursing interventions

■ Evaluations for expected outcomes

Reference

Thompson, D.G. "Safe Sleep Practices for Hospitalized Infants," *Pediatric Nursing* 31(5):400-403, September-October 2005.

Risk for
INJURY
related to labor

Definition
Accentuated risk of injury as a result of environmental conditions interacting with the individual's adaptive and defensive reserves

Assessment
- Previous pregnancies
- Prenatal history, including prenatal laboratory studies, pelvic measurements, allergies, weight gain, last menses, and estimated date of confinement
- Physical examination, including maternal vital signs, Leopold's maneuvers (to determine fetal position), palpation of uterus (to assess frequency, intensity, and duration of contractions), sterile vaginal examination (to assess ripeness of cervix [Bishop score]), presentation, estimation of maternal pelvis, and fetal heart rate
- Diagnostic studies, including ultrasound to determine gestational age and fetal size, and nonstress test or contraction stress test to assess fetal-placental function
- Laboratory studies, including complete blood count, blood type and Rh factor, platelets, Nitrazine test (to confirm rupture of membranes), and urine protein and glucose levels
- Contraindications to oxytocin stimulation, such as absolute cephalopelvic disproportion, fetal distress, grand multipara, overdistention of uterus from multiple gestation or polyhydramnios, vaginal bleeding, and unfavorable fetal presentation or position

Risk factors
- Dysfunctional labor
- Home far from hospital
- Hypotonic contractions
- Postmaturity
- Previous precipitous delivery
- Prolonged rupture of membranes

Expected outcomes
- Patient will have uterine contractions every 2 to 3 minutes, with intensity of 40 to 60 mm Hg (by internal monitoring).
- Continuous fetal monitoring will show fetal heart rate maintains variability of 6 to 10 beats/minute, with reassuring pattern.
- Patient will achieve good labor pattern, and neonate will be delivered without complications.
- Medical personnel will monitor patient closely for adverse reactions to oxytocin stimulation and will initiate appropriate interventions.
- Patient will maintain fluid balance.
- Patient and fetus will maintain optimal well-being.

Suggested NOC outcomes

Fetal Status: Intrapartum; Maternal Status: Intrapartum; Risk Detection

Interventions and rationales

■ Explain oxytocin protocol to the patient and her support person. Describe how oxytocin-induced contractions may peak more quickly and last longer than spontaneous contractions *to allay apprehension and encourage patient participation.*

■ Before applying a fetal monitor or administering oxytocin, encourage the patient to void. Palpate the bladder every 2 hours for distention. *A full bladder causes discomfort, especially when equipment is placed on the patient's abdomen.*

■ Monitor intake and output, and measure urine specific gravity. *Decreased output with increased specific gravity may indicate urine retention, which may impede fetal descent.*

■ Place the patient in as comfortable a position as possible. Left lateral tilt relieves the pressure of a gravid uterus on the inferior vena cava and promotes blood flow to the placenta. *Correct positioning enhances patient comfort and may help you obtain a clearer fetal monitoring strip.*

■ Apply the fetal monitor and obtain a 15- to 20-minute baseline strip *to ensure adequate assessment of fetal heart rate and contraction pattern.*

■ Use an 18G or 20G catheter when starting a primary I.V. line *to prepare for possible emergency interventions, such as cesarean delivery or blood administration.*

■ Prepare oxytocin, as ordered. Add the drug to a dextrose 5% injection or normal saline solution (initially, 10 units to 1,000 ml of solution). Label the bottle with the patient's name, amount of oxytocin, date and time prepared, and your name. Note that a physician must be present in the facility during oxytocin infusion. *Strict procedure ensures uniform administration and accurate assessment of uterine response.*

■ Piggyback oxytocin solution to the primary I.V. line at the site most proximal to the patient. Use an I.V. infusion pump to control the flow rate. *Insertion at the most proximal site to the patient prevents bolus infusion if oxytocin is stopped and the flow rate of the primary I.V. solution is increased. The infusion pump guarantees exact dose administration.*

■ Begin infusion at the rate of 0.5 to 1 mU/minute. Remain with the patient during the first 20 minutes. *Initiating oxytocin at this rate enables you to evaluate the patient's individual response to stimulation.*

■ Increase the oxytocin infusion by increments of 1 to 2 mU/minute, as ordered, every 30 to 60 minutes until the desired contraction pattern is achieved and the cervix is dilated 5 to 6 cm. Monitor blood pressure before and after each increase in dosage. *Increasing oxytocin slowly avoids hyperstimulation, which can cause fetal distress and uterine hypoxia.*

■ If you increase to an infusion rate of 20 mU/minute without the patient achieving the desired contraction pattern, notify the physician. *Increments above 20 mU/minute increase the risk of hyperstimulation and water intoxication.*

■ Monitor maternal vital signs every 15 to 30 minutes, as indicated by facility policy, *to assess for oxytocin-induced hypertension.*

■ Monitor the contractile pattern and fetal heart rate every 15 minutes. Assess contractions by palpation or intrauterine pressure catheter. At least every 30 minutes, document the heart rate, variability, and fetal monitor strip changes. *Assess-*

ment of the fetal heart rate and variability allows you to detect nonreassuring fetal heart patterns. Palpation of contractions or intrauterine catheter monitoring allows you to monitor uterine activity.

■ If the patient responds poorly to oxytocin infusion, take these steps:

– Check the I.V. mixture.

– Check the lines for patency.

– Increase the oxytocin flow rate, according to facility policy.

– Palpate the uterine fundus for quality, duration, and relaxation of contractions. *Errors in oxytocin mixture and I.V. administration can cause poor uterine response. An unripe cervix or uterus will also diminish the desired response. If the patient's response doesn't improve, the infusion may have to be discontinued after 8 to 12 hours and restarted the next day.*

■ Observe for hypertonicity—contractions lasting longer than 90 seconds and occurring less than 2 minutes apart. When using an intrauterine pressure catheter, a reading greater than 75 mm Hg indicates hypertonicity. *Because hypertonicity is unpredictable, the patient must be monitored carefully.*

■ If you detect hypertonicity, discontinue infusion immediately. Check maternal vital signs and notify the physician. Increase the flow rate of the primary I.V. solution, and position the patient on her left side. *These measures will help arrest hypertonicity.*

■ Monitor continuously for loss of variability, late decelerations, or persistent bradycardia *to detect fetal distress. Fetal distress may result from impaired uteroplacental perfusion caused by increased tonicity of contractions.*

■ If you detect signs of fetal distress, take these steps:

– Discontinue oxytocin infusion *to minimize the risk to the fetus.*

– Administer 8 to 12 L of oxygen via a tight rebreathing mask *to increase the oxygen supply to the fetus.*

– Increase the flow rate of the primary I.V. line *to increase fluids.*

– Reposition the patient on her left or opposite side *to increase placental blood flow.*

– Notify the physician *to expedite medical evaluation of maternal and fetal status.*

– Assess maternal vital signs *to monitor for early signs of distress.*

– Perform or assist with a sterile vaginal examination *to rule out possibility of umbilical cord prolapse.*

– Make sure the patient isn't left unattended *to promote safety.*

■ Assess the patient's intake and output, and monitor the amount of oxytocin administered over the course of stimulation. Total fluid intake shouldn't exceed 125 ml/hour. *Over time, the antidiuretic effects of oxytocin combined with the administration of large volumes of electrolyte-free solutions can lead to water intoxication.*

Suggested NIC interventions

Bleeding Precautions; Electronic Fetal Monitoring: Intrapartum; Environmental Management; Intrapartal Care: High-Risk Delivery; Labor Induction; Medication Administration

Evaluations for expected outcomes

■ Patient has contractions every 2 to 3 minutes that last 30 to 60 seconds and are of moderate intensity with adequate resting tonus.

■ Continuous fetal monitoring shows fetal heart rate maintains variability of 6 to 10 beats/minute, with reassuring pattern.

■ Patient achieves good labor pattern and delivers neonate without complications.

■ Medical personnel monitor patient closely for adverse reactions to oxytocin stimulation and initiate appropriate interventions.

■ Patient maintains fluid balance.

■ Patient and fetus maintain optimal well-being during labor and delivery.

Documentation

■ Patient's vital signs on admission and every 15 to 30 minutes, according to facility policy

■ Baseline assessment of uterine activity (frequency, intensity, interval, duration, and tonus) before oxytocin stimulation and every 30 minutes thereafter via continuous electronic fetal monitoring

■ Assessment of fetal heart rate, including baseline rate, long-term variability, short-term variability (with internal monitoring), accelerations, and periodic changes

■ Patient's physical and emotional response to induction or augmentation of labor or both

■ Nursing interventions to reduce risk of injury to patient or fetus from oxytocin stimulation

■ Patient's response to nursing interventions

■ Evaluations for expected outcomes

Reference

Simpson, K.R. "The Context & Clinical Evidence for Common Nursing Practices During Labor," *The American Journal of Maternal Child Nursing* 30(6):356-63, November-December 2005.

Deficient
KNOWLEDGE

related to lack of information about birth process

Definition

Absence or deficiency of cognitive information related to a specific topic

Assessment

■ Age

■ Psychosocial status, including developmental stage, previous experience with childbearing, expectations of the birth process, interest in learning, and current level of knowledge about pregnancy, birth, and recovery

■ Ability to learn, including cognitive domain, intellectual and conceptual skills, and attention span

■ Support systems, including presence of support person and support person's interest in helping patient and ability to participate in doing so

Defining characteristics
■ Inability to follow through with instruction
■ Inappropriate or exaggerated behaviors (hysteria, hostility, agitation, apathy)
■ Poor performance on test of knowledge
■ Verbalization of problem

Expected outcomes
■ Patient will recognize that increased knowledge and skill will help her cope better with birth process.
■ Patient will demonstrate understanding of what she's taught.
■ Patient will demonstrate ability to perform skills needed for coping with labor.
■ Patient will express realistic expectations about birth process.
■ Patient's level of anxiety about giving birth will be realistic.
■ Patient will express satisfaction with her increased knowledge.

Suggested NOC outcomes
Concentration; Knowledge: Labor & Delivery; Knowledge: Pregnancy; Motivation

Interventions and rationales
■ Find a quiet, private environment for teaching the patient and support person. *Freed from distractions, the patient and support person will learn more effectively.*
■ Establish a trusting relationship with the patient. Develop mutual goals for learning. *These measures will enhance learning.*
■ Select teaching strategies appropriate to the material and patient's learning style (lecture, discussion, demonstration, practice, or audiovisual materials). *Careful selection of teaching strategies will enable you to better meet the patient's needs.*
■ Teach information and skills needed for understanding and coping during birth *to decrease the patient's anxiety and increase her sense of competence.* Evaluate the patient's level of understanding and ability to use knowledge during the birth process.

Suggested NIC interventions
Anticipatory Guidance; Childbirth Preparation; Learning Readiness Enhancement; Teaching: Individual

Evaluations for expected outcomes
■ Patient expresses intention to put knowledge to use during labor.
■ Patient describes birth process in her own words.
■ Patient correctly performs labor skills.
■ Patient expresses realistic expectations of labor.

■ Patient responds to labor without undue anxiety, using breathing, relaxation, and position changes to cope.

■ Patient voices satisfaction with newly acquired knowledge and skills.

Documentation

■ Patient's current understanding about birth process
■ Patient's expression of need for better understanding or skills
■ Learning goals established in cooperation with patient
■ Information and skills taught to patient
■ Teaching method used
■ Patient's response to teaching
■ Patient's mastery of information, including demonstration of new skills
■ Evaluations for expected outcomes

Reference

Elcioglu, O., et al. "How do Accounts of the Patients on Pregnancy and Birth Process Enlighten Medical Team in Terms of Narrative Ethics?" *Patient Education and Counseling* 61(2):253-261, May 2006.

Deficient
KNOWLEDGE
related to neonatal care

Definition

Absence or deficiency of cognitive information related to a specific topic

Assessment

■ Psychosocial status, including age, learning ability (affective, cognitive, and psychomotor domains), decision-making ability, developmental stage, financial resources, health beliefs and attitudes, interest in learning, knowledge and skills regarding neonatal care, obstacles to learning, support systems (willingness and capability of others to help), and usual coping pattern

■ Neurologic status, including level of consciousness, memory, mental status, and orientation

Defining characteristics

■ Inability to follow through with instruction
■ Inappropriate or exaggerated behaviors (hysteria, hostility, agitation, apathy)
■ Poor performance on test of knowledge
■ Verbalization of problem

Expected outcomes

■ Patient will express need to improve her understanding of neonatal care.
■ Patient will set realistic learning goals for developing competence in caring for neonate.

■ Patient will express understanding of neonatal care.

■ Patient will demonstrate ability to care for neonate independently or with minimal assistance.

■ Patient will identify specific learning goals and target dates for mastering new skills.

■ Patient will express intention to adjust lifestyle to accommodate arrival of neonate.

■ Patient or family member will contact community resources when necessary.

■ Family members will take active role in caring for neonate.

Suggested NOC outcomes

Concentration; Information Processing; Knowledge: Infant Care; Knowledge: Postpartum Maternal Health

Interventions and rationales

■ Establish an environment of mutual trust and respect *to enhance learning. Achieving rapport is especially important in light of the maternity patient's short length of stay.*

■ Assess the patient's level of knowledge. Does she have other children? Has she had recent experience caring for a neonate? *Answering these questions will determine whether the patient requires basic information or reinforcement of previous learning.*

■ Negotiate with the patient to develop goals for learning. *Allowing the patient to participate in decision making enhances learning.*

■ Select teaching strategies appropriate for the patient's individual learning style, such as one-on-one discussion and demonstration, attending unit-based neonatal care class, or viewing audiovisual materials. *Choosing an approach that best serves the patient increases the chance for successful learning.*

■ Teach skills that the patient must incorporate into daily life *to ensure the relevance of the learning experience.* Have the patient give a return demonstration of each new skill, such as feeding, diapering, and bathing the neonate, *to increase the patient's comfort level and identify areas of misunderstanding.*

■ Have the patient incorporate learned skills into her daily routine during the hospital stay. Encourage the patient to care for the neonate in the hospital and allow for rooming-in, if possible. *Practicing skills leads to proficiency.* Acknowledge positive efforts *to increase the patient's self-esteem.*

■ Provide the patient with names and telephone numbers of resources (such as a local breast-feeding association or child welfare service) to contact with questions. *The patient may benefit from additional sources of support during her hospital stay as well as after discharge.*

■ Encourage family members to become involved in the care of the neonate *to promote family unity and bonding with the neonate.*

Suggested NIC interventions

Childbirth Preparation; Counseling; Health Education; Learning Facilitation; Referral; Teaching: Infant Safety

Evaluations for expected outcomes

■ Patient expresses need to improve her understanding of neonatal care.

■ Patient sets realistic learning goals.

■ Patient expresses understanding of neonatal care.

■ Patient demonstrates ability to care for neonate, including comfortably holding and playing with neonate, bottle-feeding or breast-feeding and burping neonate at appropriate intervals, caring for circumcision (when applicable) and umbilical cord site, providing scalp care, and bathing and diapering neonate.

■ Patient sets specific learning goals and target dates for mastering new skills.

■ Patient adjusts lifestyle to accommodate arrival of neonate.

■ Patient or family members express willingness to follow up on referrals to community resources.

■ Family members demonstrate willingness to take active role in neonatal care.

Documentation

■ Patient's current level of knowledge and skills

■ Patient's expressions indicating her motivation to learn

■ Patient's learning objectives

■ Methods used to teach patient

■ Teaching provided

■ Skills demonstrated

■ Patient's response to teaching

■ Evaluations for expected outcomes

Reference

Swartz, M.K. "Parenting Preterm Infants: A Meta-synthesis," *The American Journal of Maternal Child Nursing* 30(2):115-20, March-April 2005.

Deficient
KNOWLEDGE
related to postpartum self-care

Definition

Absence or deficiency of cognitive information related to a specific topic

Assessment

■ Psychosocial status, including age, learning ability (affective, cognitive, and psychomotor domains), decision-making ability, developmental stage, financial resources, health beliefs and attitudes, interest in learning, knowledge and skill regarding postpartum self-care, obstacles to learning, support systems (willingness and capability of others to help patient), and usual coping pattern

■ Neurologic status, including level of consciousness, memory, mental status, and orientation

■ Physical ability to perform self-care activities

Defining characteristics
- Inability to follow through with instruction
- Inappropriate or exaggerated behaviors (hysteria, hostility, agitation, apathy)
- Poor performance on test of knowledge
- Verbalization of problem

Expected outcomes
- Patient will communicate desire to learn how to care for herself after delivery.
- Patient will establish realistic learning goals.
- Patient will verbalize or demonstrate understanding of what she has learned about self-care.
- Patient will incorporate newly learned skills into daily routine.
- Patient will make changes in postpartum routine, including seeking help from health care professional, if necessary.

Suggested NOC outcomes
Knowledge: Health Resources; Knowledge: Postpartum Maternal Health

Interventions and rationales
- Establish an environment of mutual trust and respect *to enhance the patient's learning. Establishing rapport is especially important in light of the maternity patient's short length of stay.*
- Assess the patient's level of understanding of postpartum self-care activities *to establish a baseline for learning and provide direction for goal development.*
- Negotiate with the patient target dates for mastering postpartum self-care skills. *Having the patient participate in decision making will promote learning.*
- Select teaching strategies (discussion, demonstration, role playing, or audiovisual materials) best suited for the patient's individual learning style *to enhance learning.*
- Teach skills that the patient must incorporate into her daily postpartum routine, including perineal care, use of a sitz bath, use of witch hazel compresses, application and removal of perineal pads, and breast care. *Relevant topics enhance the patient's motivation to learn.*
- Have the patient give a return demonstration of each new skill *to reinforce learning.*
- Teach the patient about the process of involution *to help her understand postpartum occurrences.*
- Teach the patient the importance of adequate nutrition and hydration *to ensure proper urinary and bowel elimination.*
- Discuss the importance of adequate rest *to promote emotional and physical stability.*
- Have the patient incorporate learned skills into her daily routine during hospitalization. Acknowledge her efforts. *Practicing learned skills will help the patient gain proficiency.*
- Provide the patient with names and telephone numbers of appropriate resource people and community service agencies *to provide further resources to help with problem solving, both during the patient's stay and after discharge.*

Suggested NIC interventions

Health Education; Learning Facilitation; Nutritional Counseling; Postpartal Care; Teaching: Prescribed Activity/Exercise

Evaluations for expected outcomes

- Patient expresses motivation to learn.
- Patient establishes realistic learning goals.
- Patient verbalizes or demonstrates understanding of what she has learned, including process of involution and deviations from normal that she should report, ability to use sitz bath, and knowledge of hemorrhoidal care.
- Patient incorporates skills into her daily routine, including performing breast and perineal care, resuming normal bowel and bladder elimination, and obtaining adequate rest and sleep.
- Patient states intention of making changes in daily routine and seeking help from health care professional, if necessary.

Documentation

- Patient's understanding of and skill in postpartum self-care (including insight into her own abilities)
- Patient's expressions that indicate her motivation to learn
- Learning objectives
- Methods used to teach patient
- Information imparted to patient
- Skills demonstrated to patient
- Patient's response to teaching
- Evaluations for expected outcomes

Reference

Bowman, K.G. "Postpartum Learning Needs," *Journal of Obstetric, Gynecologic, and Neonatal Nursing* 34(4):438-43, July-August 2005.

Deficient
KNOWLEDGE

related to premature labor

Definition

Absence or deficiency of cognitive information related to a specific topic

Assessment

- Age
- Psychosocial status, including decision-making ability, developmental stage, financial resources, health beliefs and attitudes, interest in learning, knowledge and skill regarding pregnancy and birth process, learning ability (affective, cognitive, and psychomotor domains), obstacles to learning, previous experience with pre-

mature labor, support systems (willingness and ability of others to help patient), and usual coping pattern
- Neurologic status, including level of consciousness, memory, mental status, and orientation

Defining characteristics
- Inability to follow through with instruction
- Inappropriate or exaggerated behaviors (hysteria, hostility, agitation, apathy)
- Poor performance on test of knowledge
- Verbalization of problem

Expected outcomes
- Patient will communicate desire to learn about premature labor and will set realistic learning goals.
- Patient will express understanding of causes, signs and symptoms, and management of premature labor.
- Patient will identify and immediately report danger signals during and after hospitalization.
- Patient will voice emotional response to premature labor.
- Patient will use available support systems.
- Patient will cope successfully with premature labor.
- Pregnancy will result in positive outcome.

Suggested NOC outcomes
Communication: Receptive; Knowledge: Labor & Delivery; Knowledge: Pregnancy; Motivation

Interventions and rationales
- Introduce yourself to the patient and support person, and orient them to their surroundings. Explain all procedures beforehand. *These measures reduce the patient's anxiety.*
- Establish an environment of mutual trust and respect *to calm the patient, decreasing uterine stimulation from stress, and to provide an atmosphere conducive to learning.*
- Work with the patient to develop realistic learning goals. *Unrealistic goals will frustrate you and the patient. Failure to achieve goals may reduce the patient's interest in learning.*
- Select the teaching strategy most appropriate for the patient and support person *to enhance learning.*
- Assess the patient's understanding of pregnancy and premature labor *to establish a basis for a nursing care plan and help guide future interventions.*
- Explain the causes, signs and symptoms, and treatment of premature labor to the patient and support person *to prepare them to actively participate in care.* Avoid information overload. *Anxiety may limit the patient's ability to assimilate information.*
- Project a warm, caring attitude and convey a willingness to listen *to encourage the patient to ask questions and voice feelings.*

■ Don't place unrealistic demands on the patient *to avoid exacerbating feelings of inadequacy and anxiety.*

■ Remain with the patient for uninterrupted periods. Assure the patient and support person that they can rely on staff for emotional support *to ease anxiety and establish a therapeutic relationship.*

■ Include the patient in the decision-making process when possible *to give her a sense of participation and control.*

■ Provide positive feedback to the patient *to strengthen her self-esteem.*

■ Provide the patient with information related to her health status and the condition of the fetus. Inform the support person as well. *Continued knowledge of maternal and fetal health status helps relieve anxiety.*

■ Teach the patient the danger signs to report immediately, such as contractions occurring every 10 minutes or less for 1 hour, fluid leaking from the vagina, or lack of or altered fetal movement. *Promptly identifying and reporting danger signs helps avoid premature labor.*

■ If the patient is discharged to home before delivery, review discharge instructions. Emphasize taking prescribed medications; limiting activities, as instructed; and reporting danger signs. *If the patient understands her needs and limitations, she may be able to avoid a recurrence of premature labor.*

Suggested NIC interventions

Childbirth Preparation; High-Risk Pregnancy Care; Teaching: Individual

Evaluations for expected outcomes

■ Patient expresses desire to learn about premature labor and sets realistic learning goals.

■ Patient identifies possible causes and signs and symptoms of premature labor and expresses understanding of methods of managing it.

■ Patient promptly reports danger signs and receives appropriate interventions.

■ Patient expresses emotional response to premature labor.

■ Patient uses available support systems.

■ Patient successfully copes with premature labor as demonstrated by verbal and nonverbal behaviors.

■ Pregnancy results in positive outcome.

Documentation

■ Patient's statements indicating her understanding of premature labor

■ Patient's expressions indicating her motivation to learn

■ Learning objectives

■ Methods used to teach patient and support person

■ Information discussed with patient and support person

■ Patient's and support person's responses to teaching

■ Maternal and fetal physical status

■ Evaluations for expected outcomes

Reference
Palmer, L., and Carty, E. "Deciding When it's Labor: The Experience of Women who Have Received Antepartum Care at Home for Preterm Labor," *Journal of Obstetric, Gynecologic, and Neonatal Nursing* 35(4):509-15, July-August 2006.

Deficient
KNOWLEDGE
related to self-care activities during pregnancy

Definition
Absence or deficiency of cognitive information related to a specific topic

Assessment
- Age
- Psychosocial status, including decision-making ability, developmental stage, financial resources, health beliefs and attitudes, interest in learning, knowledge and skill regarding pregnancy, learning ability (affective, cognitive, and psychomotor domains), obstacles to learning, previous obstetric history, support systems (willingness and ability of others to help patient), and usual coping pattern
- Neurologic status, including level of consciousness, memory, mental status, and orientation

Defining characteristics
- Inability to follow through with instruction
- Inappropriate or exaggerated behaviors (hysteria, hostility, agitation, apathy)
- Poor performance on test of knowledge
- Verbalization of problem

Expected outcomes
- Patient will communicate need for more information about self-care and will set realistic learning goals.
- Patient will demonstrate understanding of material taught.
- Patient will demonstrate ability to perform new health-related behaviors she has learned.
- Patient will continue to practice appropriate health-related behaviors after pregnancy.

Suggested NOC outcomes
Knowledge: Health Resources; Knowledge: Pregnancy

Interventions and rationales
- Establish an environment of mutual trust and respect *to help the patient relax and be receptive to learning.*

■ Negotiate realistic learning goals with the patient. *Unrealistic goals will frustrate you and the patient. Failure to achieve goals may reduce the patient's interest in learning.*

■ Using open-ended questions, assess the patient's knowledge of pregnancy-related health practices *to establish a basis for a nursing care plan and help guide future interventions.*

■ Adapt teaching strategies (discussion, demonstration, role playing, or use of audiovisual materials) to the patient's individual learning style. *Tailoring teaching and content to the patient's learning style helps enhance learning.*

■ Refer the patient to appropriate resource people, agencies, and organizations *to ensure comprehensive care.*

■ Discuss appropriate dental care and instruct the patient to visit a dentist early in pregnancy. *Poor oral hygiene and caries may result from nausea, vomiting, heartburn, and gum hyperemia associated with pregnancy.*

■ Review the possible effects of caffeine, alcohol, addicting drugs, and tobacco on the developing fetus *to help ensure fetal well-being.* Tell the patient that any substance she ingests during pregnancy can affect the fetus. Explain that alcohol may cause developmental anomalies, marijuana and tobacco may cause intrauterine growth retardation and prematurity, and cocaine may cause abruptio placentae in the mother and prematurity, poor feeding patterns, irritability, neural tube defects, and increased respiratory and heart rates in the neonate.

■ Urge the patient to consult her physician or nurse-midwife before taking any medications *to avoid possible teratogenic effects on the fetus.*

■ Review exercise routines designed for pregnant women and, if appropriate, refer the patient to an organized exercise group. *A regular exercise program during pregnancy enhances well-being and helps improve muscle tone in preparation for childbirth.*

■ Review dietary intake for 1 week and instruct the patient in proper nutrition during pregnancy. Explain to the patient that she needs an extra 300 calories each day, for a total of 2,100 to 2,400 calories per day. Refer the patient to a dietitian, if appropriate. *The patient needs more calories to maintain optimal use of protein, allow for fetal and maternal tissue synthesis, and meet increased basal metabolic needs.*

■ Discourage the patient from wearing constrictive clothing and shoes or high-heeled shoes. *High-heeled shoes increase the likelihood of developing low back strain, backache, and poor balance. Constrictive clothing and shoes can alter venous circulation.*

■ Discuss exposure to possible sources of toxic chemicals or gases *to avoid possible teratogenic effects on the developing fetus.*

■ Review the patient's daily routine at home and at work. *The patient may need to alter her routine during pregnancy. For example, if she holds a sedentary job, she should walk about periodically to increase circulation to her legs. If she stands for long periods, she may need to adopt a less physically demanding posture.*

■ Instruct the patient to contact a physician or nurse-midwife immediately if she experiences danger signs or symptoms, including severe vomiting, frequent and severe headaches, epigastric pain, vision disturbances, swelling of fingers or face, altered or absent fetal movements after quickening, signs of vaginal or urinary tract infection, unusual or severe abdominal pain, or fluid discharge from the vagina. *Prompt identification of danger signs reduces the risk of an abnormal pregnancy.*

Suggested NIC interventions

Energy Management; Health Education; Parenting Promotion; Teaching: Prescribed Activity/Exercise; Teaching: Prescribed Diet

Evaluations for expected outcomes
■ Patient communicates need for more information about self-care and establishes realistic learning goals.
■ Patient demonstrates understanding of material taught, including importance of:
– maintaining appropriate diet
– following appropriate exercise regimen
– limiting or stopping smoking (if applicable)
– not consuming illicit drugs or alcohol
– checking with physician or nurse-midwife before taking any medication
– limiting caffeine intake
– obtaining sufficient rest
– avoiding areas that may contain toxic chemicals or gases
– not wearing constrictive clothing and shoes or high-heeled shoes
– reporting danger signals to physician or nurse-midwife
– visiting dentist early in pregnancy
– taking prenatal vitamins as prescribed.
■ Patient demonstrates ability to perform health-related behaviors she has learned during pregnancy.
■ Patient continues to practice appropriate health-related behaviors after pregnancy.

Documentation
■ Patient's knowledge of self-care activities during pregnancy
■ Expressions indicating patient's motivation to learn
■ Learning objectives
■ Teaching methods
■ Subject matter discussed in teaching session
■ Record of dietary intake for 1 week
■ Demonstration and return demonstration of skills
■ Written and audiovisual materials given to patient
■ Patient's response to teaching
■ Evaluations for expected outcomes

References
Herzig, K., et al. "Seizing the 9-month Moment: Addressing Behavioral Risks in Prenatal Patients," *Patient Education and Counseling* 61(2):228-35, May 2006.

Krulewitch, C.J. "Alcohol Consumption during Pregnancy," *Annual Review of Nursing Research* 23:101-34, 2005.

Imbalanced
NUTRITION: LESS THAN BODY REQUIREMENTS
related to ineffective suck reflex

Definition
Intake of nutrients insufficient to meet metabolic needs

Assessment
- Gestational age
- Perinatal history
- Apgar score
- Suck and swallow reflex, including intactness of lips and palate
- GI assessment, including vomiting and regurgitation, stool characteristics (color, amount, consistency, and frequency), inspection of abdomen, auscultation of bowel sounds, palpation for masses, and percussion for tympany or dullness
- Nutritional status, including intake and output, current weight, weight change since delivery, skin turgor, urine characteristics (frequency and amount), signs of dehydration, and feedings (type, amount, and frequency)
- Laboratory studies, including urine glucose levels, urine bilirubin levels, and urine specific gravity
- Maternal assessment, including anesthetic used during labor and delivery, parity, knowledge level, and breast-feeding (condition of nipples and positioning of neonate)

Defining characteristics
- Aversion to or lack of interest in feeding
- Body weight 20% or more under ideal weight
- Diarrhea and steatorrhea
- Evidence of lack of food intake
- Fragile capillaries
- Hyperactive bowel sounds
- Inadequate intake
- Pale conjunctivae and mucous membranes
- Poor muscle tone
- Satiety immediately after feeding
- Signs of abdominal pain or cramping, with or without disorder
- Weakness of muscles required for sucking

Expected outcomes
- Mother will demonstrate effective feeding techniques.
- Neonate won't lose more than 10% of birth weight.
- Neonate will retain entire feeding without vomiting or regurgitating.
- Neonate will ingest 130 to 200 oz/kg and 95 to 145 calories/kg per day.
- Neonate will establish effective suck and swallow reflexes, allowing for adequate nutritional intake.

■ Neonate will maintain good (elastic) skin turgor, moist mucous membranes, urine specific gravity between 1.005 and 1.015, and flat, soft fontanels.
■ Infant will gain at least 1 oz (28.4 g) each day for first 6 months after birth.

Suggested NOC outcomes

Nutritional Status; Nutritional Status: Food & Fluid Intake; Nutritional Status: Nutrient Intake; Weight: Body Mass

Interventions and rationales

■ Obtain the neonate's weight at the same time each day, using the same scale, *to ensure early recognition of excessive weight loss.*
■ If bottle-feeding, record the amount ingested at each feeding. If breast-feeding, record the number of minutes the neonate nurses at each feeding as well as ingestion of any supplement *to aid in early recognition of inadequate caloric and fluid intake.*
■ Assess the parents' knowledge of feeding techniques. As needed, teach the parents how much and how often to feed the neonate, how to prepare formula, how to position the neonate during and after feeding, and how to burp the neonate. *Early detection of knowledge deficits and appropriate instruction help eliminate misconceptions.*
■ Regularly assess the neonate's sucking pattern. Try to correct ineffective sucking patterns *to help eliminate ongoing difficulties.*
■ Provide a preemie nipple or breast shell, as appropriate. *The preemie nipple's larger hole and softer texture make it easier for the neonate to obtain formula. A breast shell helps draw out an inverted nipple.*
■ Make sure the neonate's tongue is properly positioned under the nipple *to enable the neonate to suck adequately.*
■ Make sure the neonate is awake before feeding. Unwrap the blanket and tap the soles of the feet. *A tightly wrapped, drowsy neonate is less likely to be interested in feeding. The neonate must be fully awake and stimulated to suck effectively.*
■ Record the number of stools and amount of urine voided each shift. *Decreased amounts of concentrated urine may indicate dehydration; an altered bowel elimination pattern may indicate decreased food intake.*
■ Monitor the neonate for signs of dehydration, such as poor (inelastic) skin turgor, dry mucous membranes, decreased or concentrated urine, and sunken fontanels and eyeballs, *to establish the need for immediate medical intervention.*
■ Assess the neonate for neurologic or other physical causes of ineffective sucking *to identify the need for more extensive evaluation.*
■ Assess the need for gavage feeding. *The neonate may temporarily require an alternative means of obtaining adequate fluids and calories.*

Suggested NIC interventions

Bottle Feeding; Bowel Management; Fluid Monitoring; Nutrition Management; Teaching: Prescribed Diet; Weight Management

Evaluations for expected outcomes

■ Mother demonstrates effective feeding techniques.

■ Neonate returns to birth weight by 10 days after delivery.

■ Neonate retains entire feeding.

■ Neonate ingests 130 to 200 oz/kg and 95 to 145 calories/kg each day.

■ Neonate establishes effective suck and swallow reflexes.

■ Neonate maintains good skin turgor, moist mucous membranes, urine specific gravity between 1.005 and 1.015, and flat, soft fontanels.

■ Infant gains at least 1 oz each day for first 6 months after birth.

Documentation

■ Frequency, amount, and type of fluid ingested

■ Incidence of vomiting and regurgitation

■ Effectiveness of suck reflex

■ Neonate's daily weight

■ Parent's knowledge, level of caregiving, and bonding with neonate

■ Frequency of bowel elimination and urination

■ Signs of dehydration

■ Nursing interventions and neonate's response

■ Use of special nipple (such as preemie nipple)

■ Results of laboratory studies

■ Presence of physical or neurologic impairment

■ Evaluations for expected outcomes

Reference

Kelly, M.M. "Primary Care Issues for the Healthy Premature Infant," *Journal of Pediatric Health Care* 20(5):293-99, September-October 2006.

Acute
PAIN

related to physiologic changes of pregnancy

Definition

An unpleasant sensory and emotional experience arising from actual or potential tissue damage or described in terms of such damage; pain may be of sudden or slow onset, vary in intensity from mild to severe, and be constant or recurring; pain lasts less than 6 months; and period of pain has an anticipated or predictable end

Assessment

■ Characteristics of pain, including location, quality, intensity on a scale of 1 to 10, temporal factors, and sources of relief

■ Physiologic variables, such as age and pain tolerance

■ Psychological variables, such as body image, personality, previous experience with pain, anxiety, and secondary gain from symptoms

■ Sociocultural variables, such as cognitive style, culture or ethnicity, and attitude and values

■ Environmental variables, such as setting and time

■ Understanding of pregnancy and birth process

Defining characteristics
■ Alteration in muscle tone (may range from listless to rigid)
■ Autonomic responses (diaphoresis; blood pressure, pulse rate, and respiratory rate changes; and dilated pupils)
■ Changes in appetite and eating
■ Communication (verbal or coded) of pain
■ Distracting behavior (such as pacing, seeking out other people, and performing repetitive activities)
■ Expressions of pain (such as moaning and crying)
■ Facial mask of pain (grimacing)
■ Guarding or protective behavior
■ Narrowed focus (including altered time perception, withdrawal from social contact, and impaired thought processes)
■ Self-focusing
■ Sleep disturbance

Expected outcomes
■ Patient will identify characteristics of pain.
■ Patient will articulate factors that intensify pain and will modify behavior accordingly.
■ Patient will carry out appropriate interventions for pain relief.

Suggested NOC outcomes
Client Satisfaction: Symptom Control; Comfort Level; Nausea & Vomiting Severity; Pain Control; Pain Level

Interventions and rationales
■ Provide care for the patient experiencing nausea and vomiting:
– Assess and document the extent of nausea and vomiting *to create a database for nursing interventions and patient teaching.*
– Reassure the patient that nausea will usually subside by the 4th month of pregnancy *to reduce the patient's anxiety level and enhance compliance with nursing interventions.*
– Instruct the patient to eat dry, unsalted crackers before rising in the morning *to prevent nausea resulting from an empty stomach.*
– Tell the patient to avoid greasy or spicy foods. Spicy foods irritate the stomach. *Fats with meals depress gastric motility and digestive enzyme secretion and slow intestinal peristalsis. These effects may lead to gastroesophageal reflux.*
– Tell the patient to avoid cooking odors that predispose her to nausea and to use an electric fan while cooking *to help avoid nausea. Air circulation dilutes odors.*
– Advise the patient to eat six small meals per day instead of three large ones *to avoid overloading the stomach.*
– Advise the patient to eat foods high in carbohydrates. *Such foods are easier to digest.*
– Tell the patient to take iron pills and vitamins after meals *to avoid irritating the stomach.*

– Advise the patient to take frequent walks outdoors. *Walking in fresh air reduces nausea and helps reinforce a positive outlook.*

– Tell the patient to separate food and fluid intake by ½ hour. *Drinking excessive fluids with meals distends stomach, predisposing patient to nausea. Taking fluids between meals also prevents dehydration.*

– Advise the patient to avoid very cold fluids and foods at mealtimes. *Cold fluids and foods may cause nausea and abdominal cramping.*

– Caution the patient to consult a physician before taking over-the-counter medications to treat nausea and vomiting *to avoid harmful effects on fetus.*

■ Provide care for the patient experiencing urinary frequency:

– Assess the patient for frequency and dysuria *to rule out a possible urinary tract infection (UTI).*

– Reassure the patient that urinary frequency is normal in the early and late stages of pregnancy because the enlarging uterus places pressure on the bladder. *Reassurance may reduce the patient's confusion and anxiety.*

– Tell the patient to avoid drinking large amounts of liquids within 2 to 3 hours of bedtime *to prevent frequent nocturnal urination and sleep loss.*

– Instruct the patient to ingest the required amount of liquids early in the day *to reduce the need for evening liquids.*

– Instruct the patient to void when the urge occurs *to prevent bladder distention and urinary stasis, which may predispose patient to UTI.*

– Teach the patient signs and symptoms of UTI. Urge her to report signs and symptoms promptly. *Early detection of UTI allows early treatment and helps prevent complications, such as pyelonephritis and premature labor.*

■ Provide care for the patient experiencing breast fullness and tingling:

– Assess the patient's breast discomfort *to obtain a database for further interventions.*

– Assure the patient that breast changes and discomfort are natural. Tell her that fullness will last the entire pregnancy but that tenderness will resolve after the first trimester. *Reassurance decreases the patient's anxiety level and promotes compliance.*

– Advise the patient to wear a supportive bra with wide, adjustable straps and smooth lining *to decrease irritation and provide support for enlarging breasts.*

– Instruct the patient to avoid tight bras and clothing that may confine breasts. *Pressure increases tenderness, tingling sensations, and discomfort.*

– Teach the patient the anatomy and physiology of breast changes during pregnancy. If indicated, begin preparation for breast-feeding at the end of the third trimester *to enhance breast-feeding experience.*

■ Provide care for the pregnant patient who develops a headache:

– Assess the type and location of the headache and associated signs and symptoms. *Assessment provides information for selection of interventions and clues to the patient's discomfort. The presence of associated factors, such as proteinuria, weight gain, edema, elevated blood pressure, and hyperreflexia, may indicate the occurrence of gestational hypertension.*

– Advise the patient to sleep 8 hours each night and to nap or rest for 2 hours in the afternoon *to alleviate fatigue.*

– Advise the patient to drink 6 to 8 glasses (1,500 to 2,000 ml) of fluid per day to prevent or alleviate a headache resulting from dehydration. *Increasing fluids may eliminate the headache by increasing vascular space and dilating cerebral veins.*

– Instruct the patient to apply cool, wet compresses to the forehead and back of the neck and to massage the neck, shoulders, face, and scalp. *Cool compresses may eliminate headaches resulting from emotional tension and spasms of sternocleido-mastoid muscles of the neck and back.*

– Instruct the patient to take two acetaminophen tablets every 4 to 6 hours, as ordered. Tell her to avoid aspirin because of its anticoagulant action. Remind her to consult a physician before taking over-the-counter medications. *Acetaminophen effectively relieves minor headaches of pregnancy.*

■ Provide care to the patient experiencing heartburn:

– Assess the patient's nutritional habits *to obtain clues to the patient's discomfort and information for selection of interventions.*

– Reassure the patient that normal pregnancy changes can cause heartburn *to decrease anxiety and increase compliance with nursing interventions.*

– Advise the patient to eliminate greasy and spicy foods from her diet and to avoid fats. *Such foods decrease stomach motility and increase the secretion of stomach acids and gastric acidity.*

– Instruct the patient to reduce fluid intake with meals. *Liquids tend to inhibit gastric juices.*

– Instruct the patient to avoid very cold foods. *Very cold foods promote gastric reflux.*

– Instruct the patient to drink cultured milk, such as buttermilk, rather than regular whole milk. *Cultured milk has less fat than regular milk.*

– Instruct the patient in good posture. *Good posture gives the patient's stomach more room to function.*

– Instruct the patient to take small, frequent meals *to avoid overloading the stomach* and to remain upright for 3 to 4 hours after each meal *to decrease the possibility of reflux.*

– Advise the patient to use antacids that are low in sodium *to reduce the risk of tissue edema.* Tell her to take antacids that contain both aluminum and magnesium (such as Maalox and Riopan). *Aluminum-based antacids (such as Amphojel) may cause constipation. Magnesium-based antacids (such as Milk of Magnesia) have laxative effects. Aluminum-magnesium combinations tend to balance these effects.* Tell the patient to avoid antacids that contain sodium bicarbonate *to prevent hypokalemia, metabolic alkalosis, and hypernatremia.*

■ Provide care for the patient with round ligament pain:

– Assess the onset and site of round ligament discomfort and associated uterine activity *to rule out the possibility of premature labor activity.*

– Reassure the patient that round ligament pain is normal during pregnancy and results from the stretching of ligaments that support the expanding uterus. *Reassurance will decrease anxiety and promote cooperation.*

– Instruct the patient to avoid sudden jerky movement, to rise slowly from recumbent positions, and to avoid excessive exercise, standing, or walking. *Sudden, jerky movements or twisting of the torso pulls on round ligaments, causing unilateral or bilateral pain. Excessive exercise, standing, or walking can also strain abdominal muscles.*

■ Provide care to the patient who experiences backache:

– Assess the patient's posture, lifting techniques, and footwear *to pinpoint causes of pain.*

– Instruct the patient to wear low-heeled shoes, maintain good posture, and hold her shoulders back *to increase spinal curvature, which may reduce backache.*

– Instruct the patient in proper body mechanics *to help her avoid stress to her lower back.*

– Tell the patient to rest in a recumbent position or with her legs bent and elevated on a bed or chair *to relieve strain on the lower back.*

– Instruct the patient to perform moderate daily exercise *to tone and maintain muscle strength in the lower back.*

– Discuss the benefits of massaging and applying warm, moist heat to the lower back. *These measures will help relax and soothe tight muscles.*

■ Provide care for the patient with hemorrhoids:

– Assess the patient's diet for fiber, fluids, and iron intake *to plan an appropriate diet that will enhance bowel function.*

– Assess prepregnancy bowel habits and history of hemorrhoids *to provide a database for planning interventions.*

– Instruct the patient to avoid constipation by increasing intake of dietary fiber, bran cereals, and fluids. She should also drink warm water when she arises in the morning. *Avoiding constipation helps prevent straining at stool and lessens the risk of hemorrhoids. Dietary fiber, bran cereals, and fluids increase intestinal peristalsis and facilitate bowel function.*

– Encourage the patient to take sitz baths and to use witch hazel and Epsom salt compresses. *Warm sitz baths cause tissue dilation, increased blood flow, and healing. Witch hazel pads (such as Tucks) and Epsom salt compresses reduce tissue swelling.*

– According to the physician's recommendation, encourage the use of analgesic ointments and topical preparations *to reduce pain.*

– Administer stool softeners, as ordered, *to allow normal evacuation without straining.*

■ Provide care for the pregnant patient with varicosities:

– Assess for the degree of pain, family history, level of exercise, extent of varicosities, and history of varicosities before pregnancy. *Assessing pain helps rule out thrombophlebitis. Assessing the extent of varicosities and the patient's level of exercise helps plan for nursing interventions.*

– Reassure the patient about the cause and usual duration of her discomfort *to decrease anxiety and promote compliance.*

– Tell the patient to rest in a recumbent position, with her legs elevated above body level, twice per day *to promote venous return and avoid stagnation and pooling of venous blood.*

– Instruct the patient to put on supportive stockings before arising in the morning and to raise her legs when putting them on. *Supportive stockings promote venous return and increase comfort.*

– Tell the patient to avoid garters and tight knee-high stockings and not to cross her legs *to reduce the risk of venous pooling and thrombus formation.*

– Advise the patient to perform regular exercise, take frequent walks, and avoid sitting for long periods *to increase blood flow and retard stasis and pooling.*

■ Provide care for the patient suffering from leg cramps:

– Assess the patient's diet for excessive soft drink intake or inadequate dairy protein. *Inadequate dairy protein or excessive intake of soft drinks, which contain large amounts of phosphorus, can disrupt the body's calcium-phosphorus ratio, thereby leading to leg cramps.*

– Reassure the patient that leg cramps are normal during pregnancy *to reduce anxiety and promote compliance.*

– Tell the patient to consult with a physician about supplementing milk intake with aluminum hydroxide (Amphojel). *Taken with milk, aluminum hydroxide helps remove dietary phosphorus from the intestinal tract.*

– Instruct the patient to elevate her legs periodically and to avoid lying prone with toes pointed. *Lying prone with toes pointed predisposes the patient to blood vessel occlusion and subsequent cramping.*

– Tell the patient to exercise and use good body mechanics to prevent leg cramping *by increasing general circulation.*

– Advise the patient to take warm baths at bedtime *to relax muscle fibers and increase blood flow circulation to the muscles.*

– If cramping occurs, tell the patient to straighten the affected leg and dorsiflex the foot. *These measures pull contracted muscle taut, thus relieving a cramp caused by contraction.*

– Caution the patient not to rub the affected calf *to avoid risk of dislodging undetected thrombus.*

■ Provide care for the patient who experiences Braxton Hicks contractions:

– Assess the patient for frequency, strength, and regularity of contractions *to rule out preterm or true labor.*

– Reassure the patient that Braxton Hicks contractions are normal in pregnancy *to reduce anxiety.*

– Instruct the patient to walk. *Walking may cause Braxton Hicks contractions to cease and can help distinguish them from true labor.*

– Advise the patient to assume a left lateral position when at rest *to increase blood flow to the uterus, which may decrease the intensity and frequency of contractions.*

Suggested NIC interventions

Anxiety Reduction; Coping Enhancement; Environmental Management; Pain Management; Teaching: Individual

Evaluations for expected outcomes

■ Patient identifies characteristics of pain.
■ Patient lists factors that intensify pain and modifies behavior accordingly.
■ Patient carries out appropriate interventions for pain relief.

Documentation

■ Patient's description of pain and expression of feelings about pain
■ Observations about patient's physical, psychological, and sociocultural responses to pain
■ Comfort measures and medications provided to reduce pain
■ Effectiveness of pain relief interventions
■ Patient teaching about pain and pain relief
■ Additional nursing interventions performed to assist patient with pain control
■ Evaluations for expected outcomes

References

Granath, A.B., et al. "Water Aerobics Reduces Sick Leave Due to Low Back Pain during Pregnancy," *Journal of Obstetric, Gynecologic, and Neonatal Nursing* 35(4):465-71, July-August 2006.

"Nausea and Vomiting during Pregnancy," *Journal of Midwifery & Women's Health* 51(4):303-304, July-August 2006.

Acute
PAIN

related to physiologic response to labor

Definition

An unpleasant sensory and emotional experience arising from actual or potential tissue damage or described in terms of such damage; pain may be of sudden or slow onset, vary in intensity from mild to severe, and be constant or recurring; pain lasts less than 6 months; and period of pain has an anticipated or predictable end

Assessment

■ Descriptive characteristics of pain, including location, quality, intensity on scale of 1 to 10, temporal factors, and sources of relief
■ Physiologic variables, including age and pain tolerance
■ Psychological variables, including body image, personality, previous experience with pain, anxiety, and secondary gain from symptoms
■ Sociocultural variables, including cognitive style, culture or ethnicity, and attitude and values
■ Environmental variables, including setting and time
■ Understanding and expectations of labor and delivery

Defining characteristics

■ Alteration in muscle tone (may range from listless to rigid)
■ Autonomic responses (diaphoresis; blood pressure, pulse rate, and respiratory rate changes; and dilated pupils)
■ Changes in appetite and eating
■ Communication (verbal or coded) of pain
■ Distracting behavior (such as pacing, seeking out other people, and performing repetitive activities)
■ Expressions of pain (such as moaning and crying)
■ Facial mask of pain (grimacing)
■ Guarding or protective behavior
■ Narrowed focus (including altered time perception, withdrawal from social contact, and impaired thought processes)
■ Self-focusing
■ Sleep disturbance

Expected outcomes

■ Patient will identify characteristics of pain and will describe factors that intensify it.

■ Patient will modify behavior to decrease pain.

■ Patient will express decrease in intensity of discomfort.

■ Patient will experience satisfaction with her performance during labor and delivery.

Suggested NOC outcomes

Client Satisfaction: Symptom Control; Comfort Level; Pain Control; Pain Level

Interventions and rationales

■ Orient the patient on admission to the labor and delivery suite. Show the patient her room and explain the operations of her bed and call bell. Explain admission protocol and the labor process. *These measures will allay the patient's initial anxiety.*

■ Assess the patient's knowledge of the labor process and her current anxiety level *to plan supportive strategies.*

■ Explain available analgesics and anesthesia to the patient and support person. *Awareness that medications are available reduces anxiety.*

■ Encourage the support person to remain with the patient in labor. *A woman in labor will respond more readily to supportive measures offered by a familiar, caring person.*

■ Instruct the patient and support person in techniques to decrease the discomfort of labor:

– Discuss techniques of conscious relaxation. *During labor, relaxation enables the patient to use coping techniques.*

– Tell the patient to concentrate on an internal or external focal point. *A focal point allows controlled thoughts while breathing.*

– Instruct the patient in basic deep chest breathing, which is similar to normal breathing but slower and deeper. *Deep chest breathing creates a sense of relaxation during contractions.*

– Instruct the patient in shallow chest breathing. Tell her to take slow, panting-like breaths. *Slow breathing avoids hyperventilation. Shallow chest breathing lifts the diaphragm from the uterus during contractions, decreasing the intensity of contractions.*

– Instruct the patient in effleurage. *This technique stimulates large diameter sensory nerve fibers and interferes with the transmission of pain impulses to the brain.*

■ In early labor, provide the patient with diversional activities, such as watching television, *to decrease anxiety.*

■ As labor progresses, modify the environment to reduce distractions (close door, turn off television, and close curtains). *These measures help the patient to concentrate during the active phase of labor.*

■ Apply sacral pressure to the patient, if needed, *to decrease back pain.*

■ Help the patient change positions and use pillows *to make herself more comfortable.* Make sure all body parts are supported, with joints slightly flexed. *Frequent position changes reduce stiffness, prevent pressure sores, and promote comfort.*

■ Assess the bladder for distention and encourage the patient to void every 2 hours. *A distended bladder increases the patient's discomfort during contractions and interferes with fetal descent.*

■ Provide frequent mouth care. According to facility protocol, provide ice chips, water-based jelly, or a wet 4″ × 4″ gauze swab for dry lips *to relieve dry mouth and lips caused by breathing techniques and nothing-by-mouth status.*

■ Apply a cool, damp cloth to the patient's forehead *to relieve diaphoresis.*

■ Change the patient's gown and bed linens, as needed. *Diaphoresis and vaginal discharge can dampen the gown and bed and cause discomfort.*

■ Encourage the patient to rest and relax between contractions *to decrease fatigue. Fatigue worsens pain perception and decreases the patient's ability to cope with contractions.*

■ Discuss with the patient and support person which pain medications are available if alternative pain control methods prove inadequate. *The patient may need prescribed analgesics to cope with the labor process.*

Suggested NIC interventions

Calming Technique; Medication Management; Pain Management; Simple Massage; Support System Enhancement

Evaluations for expected outcomes

■ Patient identifies characteristics of pain and describes factors that intensify it.

■ Patient modifies behavior to decrease pain, including using breathing techniques, asking for analgesia, when needed, and assuming more comfortable position.

■ Patient reports decrease in intensity of discomfort.

■ Patient expresses satisfaction with her performance during childbirth.

Documentation

■ Patient's childbirth preparation and plans for giving birth

■ Patient's description of pain

■ Observation of patient's response to labor

■ Nursing interventions to decrease discomfort

■ Patient's response to nursing interventions

■ Evaluations for expected outcomes

Reference

Chang, M.Y., et al. "A Comparison of Massage Effects on Labor Pain using the McGill Pain Questionnaire," *The Journal of Nursing Research* 14(3):190-97, September 2006.

Acute
PAIN

related to postpartum physiologic changes

Definition
An unpleasant sensory and emotional experience arising from actual or potential tissue damage or described in terms of such damage; pain may be of sudden or slow onset, vary in intensity from mild to severe, and be constant or recurring; pain lasts less than 6 months; and period of pain has an anticipated or predictable end

Assessment
- Descriptive characteristics of pain, including location, quality, intensity on scale of 1 to 10, temporal factors, and sources of relief
- Physiologic variables, such as age and pain tolerance
- Psychological variables, such as body image, personality, previous experience with pain, anxiety, and secondary gain from symptoms
- Sociocultural variables, including cognitive style, culture or ethnicity, attitude and values, and birth order
- Environmental variables, such as setting and time
- Physical factors, including perineal pain, sulcus tears, hemorrhoids, hematomas, uterine discomfort, breast fullness and engorgement, nipple soreness or cracking, and episiotomy (type, extension, redness, edema, ecchymosis, discharge, and approximation)

Defining characteristics
- Alteration in muscle tone (may range from listless to rigid)
- Autonomic responses (diaphoresis; blood pressure, pulse rate, and respiratory rate changes; and dilated pupils)
- Changes in appetite and eating
- Communication (verbal or coded) of pain
- Distracting behavior (such as pacing, seeking out other people, and performing repetitive activities)
- Expressions of pain (such as moaning and crying)
- Facial mask of pain (grimacing)
- Guarding or protective behavior
- Narrowed focus (including altered time perception, withdrawal from social contact, and impaired thought processes)
- Self-focusing
- Sleep disturbance

Expected outcomes
- Patient will identify characteristics of pain and will describe factors that intensify it.
- Patient will understand and carry out appropriate interventions for pain relief.
- Patient will expresses comfort and relief from pain.

Suggested NOC outcomes

Client Satisfaction: Symptom Control; Comfort Level; Pain Control; Pain Level

Interventions and rationales

■ Assess the patient's pain symptoms *to obtain information and plan appropriate nursing interventions.*

■ As ordered, administer pain medications *to provide pain relief.*

■ Discuss with the patient the reasons for her discomfort and its expected duration *to decrease anxiety and increase compliance.*

■ Examine the episiotomy site for redness, edema, ecchymosis, drainage, and approximation *to detect trauma to perineal tissues or developing complications.*

■ Inspect the rectum for hemorrhoids. Provide instruction on hemorrhoidal care, as appropriate. Tell the patient to apply ice for 20 minutes every 4 hours, apply a witch hazel compress, and use sitz baths. *Hemorrhoidal care will help decrease patient discomfort. Ice aids in the regression of hemorrhoids and vulval irritation by promoting localized vasoconstriction.*

■ Apply ice packs to the episiotomy site for the first 24 hours *to increase vasoconstriction and reduce edema and discomfort.*

■ Encourage the use of sitz baths. Baths should be cool to cold for the first day and warm (100° to 105° F [37.8° to 40.6° C]) thereafter. The patient should take sitz baths three or four times per day, with each lasting about 20 minutes. *Sitz baths with cold water decrease edema and promote comfort. After 24 hours, moist heat increases circulation to the perineum, reduces edema, promotes healing, and enhances oxygenation and nutrition of tissues.*

■ As ordered, teach the patient how to use sprays, creams, and ointments for the perineal area. *These products penetrate sensory nerve endings, providing a depressant effect on peripheral nerves, thereby reducing the response to sensory stimulation. Astringents, such as witch hazel, shrink tissues and reduce swelling.*

■ Assess for uterine tenderness and the presence and frequency of after-birth pains every hour for first 24 hours, then every shift, as indicated. *In the first 12 hours after birth, uterine contractions are strong and regular. Factors that may intensify contractions include multiparity, breast-feeding, and oxytocin administration.*

■ Encourage the patient to tighten the buttocks before sitting and to sit on a flat, padded surface. She should avoid foam donuts or soft pillows. *Tightening gluteal muscles before sitting reduces stress and direct pressure on the perineum. Because foam donuts separate the buttocks, they may decrease venous blood flow to the affected area, thereby increasing discomfort.*

■ Inspect breast and nipple tissue for engorgement or cracked nipples *to ensure selection of appropriate nursing interventions.*

■ Encourage the breast-feeding mother to wear a supportive bra *to increase comfort* and to position the neonate properly during feedings. She shouldn't use the same position every time. *This will help prevent sore nipples.*

■ If the breast-feeding patient is engorged, instruct her to use warm compresses or take a warm shower before breast-feeding and to breast-feed more often *to relieve discomfort. Warm compresses and showers help stimulate the flow of milk and may help relieve stasis and engorgement.*

■ If the breast-feeding mother's nipples become sore, instruct her to air-dry the nipples for 20 to 30 minutes after feedings *to help toughen the nipples* and to apply breast creams, as ordered, *to soften the nipples and relieve irritation.* If only one nipple is sore or cracked, instruct her to offer the nontender nipple first for several feedings *to reduce potential trauma on the sore nipple.*

■ Tell the non-breast-feeding patient to wear a tight supportive bra or breast binder and apply ice packs, as needed, *to prevent or reduce lactation.*

■ Assess for bladder distention. Implement measures to facilitate voiding, and provide appropriate patient teaching. *Bladder fullness can cause discomfort.*

■ After epidural or spinal anesthesia, assess the patient for spinal headache. Pain is primarily located behind the eyes but may radiate to the temples and occipital area. The supine position decreases pain; sitting or standing increases pain. Don't give pain medications before a medical evaluation of the source of the headache. Increase oral fluids, and notify the physician or anesthesiologist, as indicated. *Epidural or spinal anesthesia may lead to leakage of cerebrospinal fluid (CSF) and subsequent headache. Increasing oral fluids helps to compensate for the loss of CSF.*

■ After a cesarean delivery, provide an abdominal pillow and teach the patient to splint the incision site when moving or coughing *to provide support for the abdominal muscles.*

Suggested NIC interventions

Distraction; Heat/Cold Application; Pain Management; Presence; Simple Relaxation Therapy; Sleep Enhancement

Evaluations for expected outcomes

■ Patient identifies characteristics of pain and describes factors that intensify it.

■ Patient understands and carries out appropriate interventions for pain relief, including taking sitz baths and prescribed medications.

■ Patient expresses comfort and relief from pain.

Documentation

■ Patient's description of physical pain, pain relief, and feelings about pain

■ Nurse's observations about patient's physical, psychological, and sociocultural responses to pain

■ Comfort measures and medications provided to reduce pain

■ Effectiveness of pain relief interventions

■ Information provided to patient about pain and pain relief

■ Additional nursing interventions performed to help patient control pain

■ Evaluations for expected outcomes

Reference

Borders, N. "After the Afterbirth: A Critical Review of Postpartum Health Relative to Method of Delivery," *Journal of Midwifery & Women's Health* 51(4):242-48, July-August 2006.

Impaired
PARENTING
related to inadequate attachment to high-risk neonate

Definition
Inability of the primary caretaker to create, maintain, or regain an environment that promotes the optimum growth and development of a high-risk neonate

Assessment
■ Parental status, including age and maturity, apprehension, parental role models during childhood, knowledge of child care and normal growth and development, previous bonding history, available support systems, coping mechanisms, and feelings about pregnancy and neonate
■ Family status, including age, sex, status, and developmental stage of other children and parents' relationship with each other and with other children
■ Mother's medical condition
■ Neonatal status, including medical condition, separation from parents, and presence of medical equipment
■ Psychosocial status, including financial stressors and work demands

Defining characteristics
■ Neonate:
– Failure to thrive
– Frequent illness
– History of trauma or abuse
– No evidence of attachment
– No separation anxiety
■ Parents:
– Evidence of inflexibility in meeting neonate's needs
– Evidence of neglectful behavior toward or abandonment of neonate
– Expressed frustration of inability to fulfill role
– Expressed inability to meet neonate's needs
– Expressed negative feelings about neonate
– Inadequate child health maintenance
– Inappropriate child care arrangements
– Inappropriate visual, tactile, or auditory stimulation for neonate
– Inconsistent caregiving
– Poor interaction with neonate, with little cuddling
– Poor or inappropriate caregiving skills
– Punitive or abusive behavior toward neonate
– Rejection of or hostility toward neonate
– Unsafe home environment
– Weak or no attachment to neonate

Expected outcomes
■ Parents will establish contact with neonate.

- Parents will communicate feelings and anxieties about neonate's condition and their parenting skills.
- Parents will express willingness to care for neonate and will demonstrate competent parenting skills.
- Parents will demonstrate knowledge of neonate's developmental needs.
- Parents will become involved in planning and providing neonate's care.
- Parents will use available support systems to assist with care of neonate.

Suggested NOC outcomes

Family Coping; Knowledge: Infant Care; Parent-Infant Attachment; Parenting Performance

Interventions and rationales

- Before the parents' first visit to the neonatal intensive care unit (NICU), explain the appearance of the neonate and the presence of supportive devices *to prepare the parents for sights and sounds that may otherwise upset them.*
- Encourage the mother to visit the NICU. Assess whether the mother can physically go, and offer assistance, if necessary. *The mother may hesitate to ask for help or may be unsure of her physical surroundings.*
- Provide the parents with a picture of the neonate *to help them accept the reality of the birth.*
- If the neonate must be transferred to another facility, arrange for the parents to meet the transfer team and visit with the neonate beforehand. *Seeing the neonate and meeting the transfer team will increase the parents' feelings of involvement and help them come to terms with the neonate's condition.*
- Encourage the father or other family member to visit the neonate soon after admittance to the NICU or transfer to another facility, especially if the mother can't visit. *Firsthand reports from a family member about the neonate's condition and physical surroundings will help allay fears of the rest of the family.*
- Assess the parents' level of understanding of the neonate's condition and their expectations *to clear up misunderstandings, allow for prompt intervention, and promote realistic planning.*
- Encourage the parents to express their anxieties related to the neonate's condition and their parenting skills *to identify and clarify misconceptions.*
- Make sure the parents are informed of the neonate's ongoing condition *to help decrease their anxiety and help them plan for the future.*
- Encourage the parents to touch and talk to the neonate and call the neonate by name. Reassure them that touching the infant won't cause any harm. *This will stimulate bonding between the parents and the infant.*
- Allow time for the parents to care for the neonate within the secure environment of the hospital. Provide positive feedback for the parents' efforts to care for the neonate *to increase the parents' self-confidence.*
- Provide the parents with the NICU telephone number and encourage phone calls at any time *to make information about the neonate readily available.*
- Refer the parents to social services, as needed, *to help ensure comprehensive care.*
- Encourage the parents to bring in personal items for the neonate, such as small stuffed animals or pictures of family members, *to encourage emotional bonding with the neonate.*

Suggested NIC interventions

Attachment Promotion; Environmental Management: Attachment Process; Family Integrity Promotion; Infant Care; Parent Education: Infant

Evaluations for expected outcomes

- Parents initiate regular contact with neonate.
- Parents voice their anxieties about neonate's condition and their ability to provide care.
- Parents express willingness to meet neonate's basic needs and, if appropriate, special care needs, and display appropriate caregiving and attachment behaviors, including providing appropriate verbal, tactile, and auditory stimulation for neonate.
- Parents demonstrate knowledge of neonate's developmental needs.
- Parents take part in planning and providing neonate's care.
- Parents express awareness of and willingness to contact available sources of support.

Documentation

- Observations of parents' behavior
- Parents' statements concerning neonate
- Information provided to parents and their level of understanding
- Parents' interactions with neonate
- Parents' willingness to meet neonate's physical and emotional needs
- Consultations with health care team members
- Parents' and neonate's responses to nursing interventions
- Evaluations for expected outcomes

References

Beal, J.A. "Evidence for Best Practices in the Neonatal Period," *The American Journal of Maternal Child Nursing* 30(6):397-403, November-December 2005.

Franklin, C. "The Neonatal Nurse's Role in Parental Attachment in the NICU," *Critical Care Nursing Quarterly* 29(1):81-85, January-March 2006.

Readiness for enhanced
PARENTING

Definition

A pattern of providing an environment for children or other dependent persons that's sufficient to nurture growth and development and can be strengthened

Assessment

- Parental status that includes parents' age and maturity, parental role models during childhood, role satisfaction, adjustment to parental role, ability to relate appropriately to various age levels of children, willingness to adjust to various age needs, social support available, education needs of parent, present parenting skills, coping mechanisms, knowledge of child care and growth and development, discipline methods utilized, bonding and attachment issues

■ Family status, including relationship of parents to each other, relationship of parents to children and to other dependent person(s), sibling relationships, spirituality, community involvement, age-appropriate safety issues, nutritional status, health care practices

■ Psychosocial status including financial, single parent or dual parent family, educational level, employment, environment, stressors, affection and concern, consistency and reliability of parenting techniques

Defining characteristics

■ Willingness to enhance parenting

■ Satisfaction with home environment (children or other dependent persons)

■ Emotional and tacit support of children or other dependent persons; bonding or attachment

■ Fulfillment of physical and emotional needs (children or other dependent persons)

■ Realistic expectations of children or other dependent persons

Expected outcomes

■ Parents will express satisfaction in role of parent.

■ Parents will express confidence in ability to parent.

■ Home will exhibit signs of safe and functional environment.

■ Childcare or dependent persons care routines will be adequate.

■ Children and dependent persons will appear nutritionally healthy.

■ Family will appear to be physically healthy.

■ Family will express belief in a higher spiritual power.

■ Family will express enjoying spending time together.

■ Parents will demonstrate consistency and effectiveness related to discipline.

■ Family will express confidence in social and community resources available related to family needs.

Suggested NOC outcomes

Parent-Infant Attachment; Parenting: Psychosocial Safety

Interventions and rationales

■ Discuss with the parents their perceptions and philosophy related to the role of parents in a family. *Verbalizing perceptions and beliefs provides an opportunity to clarify the parents' thinking.*

■ Offer the parents an opportunity to express their doubts or convictions about the adequacy of their parenting skills. *An open and receptive attitude provides an atmosphere for increased trust and enhanced learning.*

■ Support family efforts as they adapt to the ever-changing issues of family needs. *Recognition of and appreciation for one's efforts enhances motivation to continue to improve skills.*

■ Observe the home environment and discuss the issues of safety and cleanliness, if needed. *Family members need to have privacy and a sense of personal space as well as an environment that's free from environmental hazards, both chemical and physical.*

■ Request that the parents describe a typical day with normal routines related to family dynamics and functioning. *This provides a concrete example for reflection of family functioning.*

■ Discuss the food likes and dislikes of the family. *Parents need to be aware of nutritional preferences in order to increase family compliance for change.*

■ Review the elements of a well-balanced diet for the various age-groups represented in the family. *Different ages and developmental levels have different nutritional needs.*

■ Discuss health care beliefs and practices with regard to the health maintenance of all family members. *Knowledge of sound health care practices enhances the well-being of family members.*

■ Explore the family's value system as well as their spiritual beliefs and practices. *Spirituality and values provide a basis for ethical and moral reasoning and an enhanced meaning to life.*

■ Encourage the family to "play" together. *Laughter and joy increase enjoyment and bonding as well as growth in the family unit.*

■ Praise the family for traditions and activities that they do together. *Sharing meaningful activities increases loyalty, security, and a sense of belonging for family members.*

■ Engage the parents in a discussion of discipline practices and offer suggestions to enhance their present skills. *Discipline needs to be consistent, loving, and have reasonable guidelines. Children want and need limits so as to feel secure and safe.*

■ Explore the parents' perception of social support and community resources available to the family. *Social support and community resources provide guidance and positive reinforcement for parenting techniques and are a source of assistance and strength when families are experiencing stress.*

Suggested NIC interventions

Developmental Enhancement: Child; Family Integrity Promotion: Childbearing Family; Family Involvement Promotion

Evaluations for expected outcomes

■ Parents state enjoyment and satisfaction in the role of parent.

■ Parents relate a positive sense of self and confidence in their ability to parent.

■ Home environment is clean and free from chemical and physical hazards.

■ Family functions in a structured and goal-oriented direction.

■ Family members express participating in regular health and dental checkups.

■ Family members express belief in a higher power and participation in their spiritual community.

■ Family members look forward to family traditions, especially those related to holidays and vacations, and to spending time together as a family at school and community activities.

■ Children are provided with consistent structure and guidelines; they express awareness of family rules and belief that those rules are fair.

■ Family utilizes various social support venues as well as community resources to meet the needs of the family and individual family members.

Documentation

- Parents' feelings and concerns about parenting
- Discipline methods described by parents
- Interventions to assist family with identifying nutritional needs of various age-groups
- Health care teaching for family with different age-groups
- Parents' perception of social and community support and resources
- Evaluations for expected outcomes

Reference

Gage, J.D., et al. "Integrative Review of Parenting in Nursing Research," *Journal of Nursing Scholarship* 38(1):56-62, 2006.

Situational low
SELF-ESTEEM

related to behavior during labor and delivery

Definition

Negative perception of self-worth in response to a current situation

Assessment

- Availability of support
- Patient's and support person's perception of labor and delivery
- Patient history, including past labor and delivery experience, ethnic and cultural background, and usual pattern of coping with stress
- Physiologic and behavioral changes during labor and delivery

Defining characteristics

- Expressed shame or guilt
- Expressions of self-negating thoughts
- Hypersensitivity to slights or criticism
- Perception of self as unable to deal with events
- Projection of blame or responsibility for problems onto others
- Rationalization of personal failures
- Rejection of positive feedback and exaggeration of negative feedback about self

Expected outcomes

- Patient will express feelings about labor and delivery.
- Patient will set realistic goals for her behavior during labor and delivery.
- Patient will receive adequate emotional and physical support during labor and delivery.
- Patient will project positive self-concept through behavioral and verbal expression.

Suggested NOC outcomes

Coping; Psychosocial Adjustment: Life Change; Self-Esteem

Interventions and rationales

■ Encourage the patient and support person to articulate their expectations of the labor and delivery experience *to identify and correct misconceptions early in the couple's experience.*

■ Provide ongoing, positive feedback about the patient's behavior *to clear up misconceptions and increase feelings of self-esteem.*

■ Emphasize realistic goals for behavior during labor and delivery. *Placing unrealistic demands on the patient can lead to feelings of inadequacy and poor self-esteem.*

■ Encourage the support person to express feelings about labor and delivery. *The patient may misunderstand how the support person viewed her behavior during labor.*

■ Encourage the patient to take active role in self-care activities after delivery *to reinforce the patient's ability to care for herself and increase self-esteem.*

Suggested NIC interventions

Active Listening; Coping Enhancement; Emotional Support; Self-Esteem Enhancement

Evaluations for expected outcomes

■ Patient expresses feelings about labor and delivery.

■ Patient expresses realistic understanding of what to expect from her own behavior during labor and delivery.

■ Patient expresses satisfaction with emotional and physical support received during labor and delivery.

■ Patient's behavior and remarks reflect positive self-image.

Documentation

■ Patient's behaviors and expressions that indicate low self-esteem

■ Nurse's perceptions of patient's readiness for decision making

■ Nursing interventions to improve patient's self-concept

■ Patient's response to nursing interventions

■ Patient's willingness to perform self-care activities

■ Patient's expressions of well-being

■ Evaluations for expected outcomes

Reference

Lothian, J. "Birth Plans: The Good, the Bad, and the Future," *Journal of Obstetric, Gynecologic, and Neonatal Nursing* 35(2):295-303, March-April 2006.

Impaired
SKIN INTEGRITY
related to episiotomy or abdominal incision

Definition
Altered epidermis dermis

Assessment
- Age
- Vital signs
- Integumentary status, including color, elasticity, hygiene, lesions, moisture, quantity and distribution of hair, sensation, temperature, texture, and turgor
- Musculoskeletal status, including area affected by anesthetic procedure, joint mobility, muscle strength and mass, paralysis, and range of motion
- Health history, including past skin problems, trauma, surgery, chronic debilitating disease, and immobility
- Nutritional status, including appetite, dietary intake, hydration, present weight, and change from normal
- Laboratory studies, including hemoglobin levels, hematocrit, and serum albumin levels
- Psychosocial status, including coping patterns, family or significant other, mental status, occupation, self-concept, and body image
- Knowledge, including patient's current understanding of her physical condition and physical, mental, and emotional readiness to learn
- Presence of medical condition that may interfere with healing
- Extent of interruption in skin integrity because of delivery

Defining characteristics
- Destruction of skin layers surrounding episiotomy or abdominal incision
- Disruption of skin surfaces
- Invasion by pathogens

Expected outcomes
- Patient will demonstrate understanding of self-care activities.
- Patient will perform skin care routine.
- Patient will identify possible danger signs and report them immediately to physician.
- Patient will regain skin integrity.
- Patient's episiotomy or abdominal incision will heal without infection.
- Patient and partner will express feelings about possible change in body image.

Suggested NOC outcomes

Tissue Integrity: Skin & Mucous Membranes; Wound Healing: Primary Intention

Interventions and rationales

■ Inspect the incision every shift using the REEDA (redness, edema, ecchymosis, discharge, and approximation) method. Document findings. *Frequent assessment can detect signs and symptoms of possible infection.*

■ Perform the prescribed treatment regimen. Monitor progress and report favorable and adverse responses. *Periodic cleaning decreases bacterial concentrations, thus aiding the healing process. Monitoring response to treatment can help identify a possible need for alternative interventions.*

■ Instruct and assist the patient with general hygiene, including hand-washing and toileting practices. *Proper hand washing is the most effective method of disease prevention. Bacteria from hands can easily contaminate other areas.*

■ Instruct and assist the patient in the use of sitz baths (three to four times daily) and perineal irrigation bottle (after each elimination). *Sitz baths aid the healing process by increasing circulation to the perineum and decreasing edema. Perineal irrigation bottles maintain cleanliness, thus decreasing bacterial concentration.*

■ Teach the patient how to apply and remove a maternity perineal pad. Tell her to apply a clean pad from front to back and to remove a soiled pad from back to front *to decrease the risk of contaminating the vaginal area with stools.*

■ Maintain infection control standards *to help minimize the risk of nosocomial infections.*

■ Provide a splinting pillow for the patient with an abdominal incision. *Splinting provides support to the area, minimizing discomfort and encouraging the patient to move and cough.*

■ Help the patient assume a comfortable position *to minimize the incidence of pain-induced immobility.*

■ Inform the patient of the purpose of self-care practices *to increase compliance.*

■ Encourage the patient and partner to discuss the impact of impaired skin integrity. The patient's self-esteem may be lowered because of a scar from the abdominal incision. The patient or partner may be concerned about the effect the episiotomy will have on sexual relations. *Open communication increases understanding between partners.*

■ Instruct the patient and partner in the possible danger signs and symptoms that should be reported to the physician immediately. These include:
– temperature above 100.4° F (38° C) on two consecutive readings
– incisional drainage
– increased discomfort at the episiotomy or incision site
– reddened or warm skin surrounding the episiotomy or incision site.
Prompt reporting of danger signs and symptoms may help prevent major complications.

Suggested NIC interventions

Cesarean Section Care; Incision Site Care; Perineal Care; Skin Surveillance

Evaluations for expected outcomes

■ Patient demonstrates correct self-care practices.
■ Patient performs skin care routine.

- Patient identifies possible danger signs and reports them immediately to physician.
- Patient regains skin integrity.
- Patient's episiotomy or abdominal incision site shows no redness, edema, ecchymosis, or discharge, and edges are approximated.
- Patient and partner communicate feelings about possibly altered body image or sexuality.

Documentation
- Patient's concerns about change in skin integrity
- Patient's willingness and ability to perform self-care practices
- Observations of episiotomy or abdominal incision site and response to treatment regimen
- Presence and type of skin closure method
- Instructions regarding treatment regimen and patient's understanding of instructions
- Prescribed treatment
- Interventions to provide supportive care
- Patient's response to nursing interventions
- Self-care practices performed by patient
- Evaluations for expected outcomes

Reference
Borders, N. "After the Afterbirth: A Critical Review of Postpartum Health Relative to Method of Delivery," *Journal of Midwifery & Women's Health* 51(4):242-48, July-August 2006.

Ineffective
THERMOREGULATION
related to immaturity

Definition
Temperature fluctuation between hypothermia and hyperthermia

Assessment
- Gestational age
- Weight in relation to gestational age
- Neurologic status, including level of consciousness and motor and sensory status
- Cardiovascular status, including blood pressure, capillary refill time, electrocardiogram results, heart rate and rhythm, pulses (apical and peripheral), and temperature
- Respiratory status, including arterial blood gas measurements, breath sounds, and rate, depth, and character of respirations
- Integumentary status, including color, temperature, and turgor

■ Fluid and electrolyte status, including blood urea nitrogen levels, intake and output, serum electrolyte levels, and urine specific gravity
■ Laboratory studies, including clotting factors, hemoglobin levels, hematocrit, and platelet and white blood cell counts
■ Environmental factors that contribute to heat loss, including radiation (loss of heat to objects not in direct contact with neonate), conduction (loss of heat through direct contact with cooler objects), convection (loss of heat from body surface to cooler surrounding air), and evaporation (changing of liquid to vapor)
■ Coexisting conditions and diagnoses
■ Maternal sedation before delivery

Defining characteristics
■ Cyanotic nail beds
■ Fluctuations in body temperature above or below normal range
■ Flushed or mottled skin
■ Hypertension
■ Increased capillary refill time
■ Increased respiratory or heart rate
■ Mild shivering
■ Moderate pallor
■ Piloerection
■ Seizures
■ Warm or cool skin

Expected outcomes
■ Neonate will maintain body temperature at normal levels.
■ Neonate will have warm, dry skin.
■ Neonate will maintain heart rate, respiratory rate, and blood pressure within normal range.
■ Neonate won't exhibit signs of compromised neurologic status.
■ Staff members will take steps to maintain neonate's body temperature at normal level.
■ Parents will recognize and avoid possible sources of heat loss.
■ Parents will express understanding of neonate's thermoregulatory disturbance and thermoregulation.

Suggested NOC outcomes
Hydration; Newborn Adaptation; Thermoregulation: Newborn

Interventions and rationales
■ Monitor the neonate's body temperature after delivery *to obtain a baseline.* According to facility protocol, continue routine monitoring of the neonate's body temperature until discharge *to determine the need for intervention and the effectiveness of therapy. Timely intervention prevents complications related to prolonged cold stress.*

■ Monitor and record the heart rate, respiratory rate, and blood pressure after delivery and routinely thereafter until discharge *to help ensure prompt diagnosis and treatment of conditions that may affect thermoregulation.*

■ Monitor the results of laboratory studies for indications of sepsis or of metabolic or respiratory disorders. *Difficulty maintaining normal body temperature may indicate an underlying disorder. Conditions resulting from cold stress may further interfere with effective thermoregulation. For example, hypoxia, central nervous system trauma, and hypoglycemia may impair the neonate's ability to maintain normal body temperature.*

■ Place the neonate under a radiant warmer device, with a temperature probe. When his temperature is stable, transfer a healthy neonate to a regular open crib. Transfer a sick neonate to a servo-controlled open warmer bed or incubator. *These measures will help minimize oxygen consumption and metabolic rate, cause sweat gland activity to cease, and maintain deep body temperature at appropriate level.*

■ Closely monitor the neonate's temperature and compare it with the temperature of the warming device. Be aware of potential hazards:

– Make sure the temperature probe doesn't become detached from the neonate's skin *to prevent hyperthermia. Overheating increases the metabolic rate and, subsequently, oxygen consumption and may lead to apneic spells, particularly in a premature neonate.*

– Don't place the temperature probe between the neonate and the mattress. *This can result in a falsely high reading, causing the warming device to decrease heat output, thus leading to hypothermia.*

– Maintain an accurate record of environmental and core temperatures. Observe for variations in heater output. *Consistent variations in heater output may be symptomatic of sepsis.*

– Monitor the neonate for signs of dehydration, including inelastic skin turgor, increased urine specific gravity, and dry mucous membranes. *Warming devices may contribute to insensible water loss.*

■ Provide fluids based on the neonate's age, size, and condition. Monitor intake and output, and administer parenteral fluids, as ordered. *The neonate may need an increase in fluids to compensate for water loss caused by an increase in metabolic rate.*

■ Maintain the environmental temperature at a comfortable setting. Take these steps:

– Dry the neonate thoroughly after delivery.

– Provide a bath only when the neonate's temperature is stable. After the bath, return the neonate to an incubator or warmer device until his temperature returns to the normal range.

– Monitor the nursery temperature and humidity.

– Provide heated, nebulized oxygen, when ordered.

– Use an overhead warmer during procedures and extensive examinations.

– Keep the incubator or radiant warmer away from windows and cold walls.

– Ensure that linen and clothing are clean and dry.

– Warm your hands before performing examinations and procedures.

– Warm the examination table and instruments, such as scales and stethoscope, when possible, before exposure to the neonate. *Maintaining the temperature of the external environment reduces the effects of heat loss from the body surface to the environment.*
■ Teach family members about:
– signs and symptoms of altered body temperature, such as cool extremities
– factors in the home that contribute to neonatal heat loss and ways to minimize heat loss
– signs of prolonged heat loss, including poor weight gain
– importance of contacting a health care provider when problems related to temperature regulation arise.
Careful teaching allows family members to take an active role in maintaining the neonate's health.

Suggested NIC interventions

Environmental Management; Fluid Monitoring; Newborn Care; Newborn Monitoring; Temperature Regulation

Evaluations for expected outcomes

■ Neonate's temperature is stable at 96.8° to 98.6° F (36° to 37° C) within 4 hours of birth.
■ Neonate has warm, dry skin.
■ Neonate maintains heart rate, respiratory rate, and blood pressure within normal limits.
■ Neonate exhibits no signs of compromised neurologic status.
■ Staff members keep neonate in neutral thermal environment throughout hospitalization.
■ Parents minimize or eliminate potential for heat loss in home environment and incorporate precautions against ineffective thermoregulation into routine care of neonate.
■ Parents express understanding of neonate's thermoregulatory disturbance and thermoregulation.

Documentation

■ Physical findings
■ Intake and output
■ Laboratory results
■ Vital signs, including blood pressure
■ Environmental temperature
■ Teaching provided to parents regarding thermoregulation
■ Parents' expressions indicating understanding of problems related to thermoregulation
■ Nursing interventions
■ Neonate's response to interventions
■ Evaluations for expected outcomes

Reference
Sherman, T.I., et al. "Optimizing the Neonatal Thermal Environment," *Neonatal Network* 25(4):251-60, July-August 2006.

Impaired
URINARY ELIMINATION
related to sensory impairment during labor

Definition
Disturbance in urine elimination

Assessment
- Vital signs
- History of sensory or neuromuscular impairment, urinary tract trauma, surgery, or infection
- Genitourinary status, including palpation of bladder, voiding pattern, urine characteristics, and presence of pain or discomfort
- Labor and delivery, including anesthesia (regional or local) and oxytocin induction or augmentation
- Fluid and electrolyte status, including skin turgor, intake and output, urine specific gravity, and inspection of mucous membranes
- Neuromuscular status, including ability to perceive bladder fullness

Defining characteristics
- Frequency
- Hesitancy
- Incontinence
- Retention
- Urgency

Expected outcomes
- Patient's vital signs will remain within normal limits.
- Patient will empty bladder regularly, as confirmed by abdominal palpation.
- Patient's intake and output will remain approximately equivalent.
- Patient's urinary function will remain normal and free from complications.

Suggested NOC outcomes
Urinary Continence; Urinary Elimination

Interventions and rationales
- Review the patient's intake and output before and during labor. Note the color, amount, concentration, and urine specific gravity. *Decreased output may indicate dehydration, hemorrhage, gestational hypertension, and excessive oxytocin stimula-*

tion. Urine specific gravity reflects the kidneys' ability to concentrate urine and the patient's hydration status.

■ Assess for dehydration (poor skin turgor; flushed, dry skin; confusion; dry mucous membranes; fever; and rapid, thready pulse). *Dehydration leads to decreased circulatory blood volume and decreased urine output.*

■ Palpate the abdomen above the symphysis pubis every 2 hours *to detect bladder distention and the degree of fullness.*

■ Encourage the patient to void every 2 hours *to promote optimum bladder tone, prevent distention, and assist in promoting fetal descent.*

■ To facilitate voiding, help the patient relax by:

– having her sit in an upright position. Assist her to the bathroom, if appropriate. *An upright or squatting position promotes contraction of the pelvis and intra-abdominal muscles, thereby assisting in sphincter control and bladder contraction.*

– providing privacy *to promote relaxation.*

– pouring warm water over the perineum *to stimulate the urge to void.*

– providing an audible sound of slow-running water. *This technique helps many patients void through power of suggestion.*

■ As ordered, catheterize the patient if she can't void independently. *An overdistended bladder can cause atony and impede fetal descent or can become traumatized by the presenting part of the fetus during delivery.*

Suggested NIC interventions

Prompted Voiding; Urinary Catheterization; Urinary Elimination Management

Evaluations for expected outcomes

■ Patient's vital signs remain within normal range.

■ Patient empties her bladder adequately at least every 2 hours.

■ Patient's intake approximately equals output.

■ Patient's urinary function remains normal and free from complications.

Documentation

■ Intake and output

■ Vital signs

■ Results of bladder assessment

■ Nursing interventions performed to promote voiding

■ Patient's response to nursing interventions

■ Evaluations for expected outcomes

References

Patraca, K. "Measure Bladder Volume without Catheterization," *Nursing* 35(4):46-47, April 2005.

White, G. "Intrapartum and Postpartum Bladder Care," *RCM Midwives* 8(9):393, September 2005.

V Geriatric health

INTRODUCTION

This section focuses on nursing diagnoses and care plans for patients age 65 and older — an age-group that makes up approximately 12.8% of the North American population and is growing twice as fast as younger age-groups.

Traditionally, our culture has valued youth over old age. In keeping with this cultural prejudice, our health care system emphasizes cure over care, acute intervention over long-term rehabilitation, and highly specialized technology over nurturing and support. Not surprisingly, such a system frequently fails to adequately meet the needs of elderly patients. With the older population growing so rapidly, nurses and other health care providers face the challenge of finding newer and better approaches to geriatric care. Nursing diagnoses and associated care plans offer an important alternative framework for meeting the needs of elderly patients.

Holistic geriatric care involves not only helping the patient cope with the effects of aging and chronic illness but also supporting his efforts to maintain self-reliance and autonomy. Your assessment should therefore take into account the patient's psychosocial functioning as well as his physiologic status. Don't neglect to consider such factors as the amount and quality of contact with family and friends, the opportunity to perform meaningful life roles, access to transportation, and available financial resources. Such factors have a tremendous influence on an older patient's well-being.

Because older people now lead longer and more productive lives, geriatric care is increasingly focused on health promotion. Your interventions may include encouraging the patient to make lifestyle changes, such as seeking and maintaining social support, moving to a more healthful environment, and exercising and eating properly. If the patient becomes ill, your task may be to help restore optimal functioning. If recovery is unlikely, your task may be to help the patient adjust to and accept his condition and to make sure he receives necessary assistance.

Always keep in mind that interventions must be tailored to the individual patient's needs. Although aging is common to all, each person ages differently. Factors that influence aging include genetics, culture, nutrition, environment, stress, and lifestyle, among others. Modifying your care plan to meet the patient's individual needs not only leads to better nursing practice but also demonstrates respect for the patient's rich life experiences.

ACTIVITY INTOLERANCE
related to generalized weakness

Definition
Insufficient physical or psychological energy to endure or complete required or desired daily activities

Assessment
■ Usual activity level, including self-care (dressing, feeding self, toileting), transfer, walking, stair climbing, and aids for ambulation
■ Pain
■ Cardiovascular status, including blood pressure, heart rate and rhythm (at rest and with activity), skin temperature and color, edema, and chest pain or discomfort
■ Respiratory status, including arterial blood gas results, auscultation of breath sounds, and rate, rhythm, depth, and pattern of respiration at rest and with activity
■ Musculoskeletal status, including range of motion and muscle size, strength, tone, and functional mobility grades as follows:
0 = completely independent
1 = requires use of equipment or device
2 = requires help, supervision, or teaching from another person
3 = requires help from another person and equipment or device
4 = dependent; doesn't participate in activity
■ Laboratory studies, including complete blood count
■ Environmental factors, including safety hazards
■ History of chronic illnesses (cardiopulmonary, cardiovascular, musculoskeletal, and neuromuscular)
■ Sensory deficits, including hearing, vision, and tactile
■ Psychosocial status, including cognitive and mental status, mood, affect, behavior, family support, and coping style
■ Economic status
■ Medication history, including use of prescription and over-the-counter medications

Defining characteristics
■ Abnormal heart rate or blood pressure in response to activity, arrhythmia or ischemic changes on electrocardiogram, and exertional discomfort or dyspnea
■ Verbal report of fatigue or weakness

Expected outcomes
■ Patient's pulse, respirations, and blood pressure will remain within established parameters.
■ Patient will use assistive devices to carry out activities.
■ Patient will modify activities to adjust to decreased activity tolerance.
■ Patient will seek help in performing activities of daily living (ADLs), as needed.

■ Patient will demonstrate willingness to perform activities needed to follow prescribed care plan.

■ Patient will verbalize acceptance of decreased activity level.

■ Patient will experience less discomfort when ambulating, transferring, or performing other activities.

■ Patient will state plan to use support services.

Suggested NOC outcomes

Activity Tolerance; Endurance; Energy Conservation; Self-Care: Activities of Daily Living (ADL); Self-Care: Instrumental Activities of Daily Living (IADL)

Interventions and rationales

■ Establish realistic goals for improving the patient's activity level, taking into account the patient's physical limitations and energy level *to help improve the patient's quality of life. Keep in mind that in some older patients with chronic conditions, even minimal improvements in activity level are noteworthy.*

■ Demonstrate the use of assistive devices, such as a cane or walker, shopping cart on wheels, or trapeze, *to teach methods of conserving energy and maintaining independence.*

■ Establish progressive goals to increase ambulation, for example:
– ambulate 20' (6.1 m) three times per day for 1 week
– ambulate 40' (12.2 m) three times per day for 1 week
– ambulate 60' (18.3 m) three times per day for 1 week.
Older patients may tire easily; therefore, the activity level should be increased gradually. Monitor vital signs before and after ambulation *to detect cardiovascular insufficiency.*

■ Provide encouragement if the patient achieves even small improvements in his activity level *to help restore self-confidence.*

■ Coordinate the activities of the interdisciplinary team when developing an activity regimen for the patient. For example, the physician can prescribe treatment for the medical condition, a physical therapist can design an exercise program, a dietitian can devise a nutrition plan, and a social worker can locate community resources, such as Meals On Wheels or home health care services. *All of these measures address the patient's physical and psychosocial needs.*

■ Refer a depressed patient to a mental health practitioner *to address the psychosocial problems that may be causing impairment in activity.*

■ Encourage the patient to express his feelings about the decreased energy levels that may accompany advanced age *to enhance acceptance.*

■ Teach the patient about good nutrition and the importance of getting adequate rest *to improve poor health practices.*

■ Monitor the patient's medication regimen regularly *to identify drugs that may cause gait, posture, or ambulatory problems.*

■ Help the patient identify activities that are personally meaningful and develop a realistic plan to incorporate meaningful activities into the daily routine *to heighten satisfaction with energy expenditure.*

■ Encourage the patient to take part in exercise and social activities, as tolerated, *to increase stamina and decrease social isolation.*

■ Modify the environment *to maximize independent activity.* For example, place the bed on the first floor of the home with easy access to the bathroom and instruct the patient to obtain and use energy-saving devices, such as an elevated toilet seat, trapeze bar on the bed, and a chair with arms and a seat that raises the patient to standing position, *to promote independence.*

■ Perform periodic health assessments and monitor for complaints of weakness or fatigue *to assess whether acute illness or exacerbation of chronic condition is causing activity intolerance.*

■ Refer the patient to a home health care agency for follow-up care. Encourage the patient to interview and select home health care personnel *to foster the patient's sense of independence.*

Suggested NIC interventions
Energy Management; Exercise Promotion; Home Maintenance Assistance; Nutrition Management; Self-Care Assistance

Evaluations for expected outcomes
■ Patient's pulse, respirations, and blood pressure are within established parameters.

■ Patient uses assistive devices to carry out activities.

■ Patient demonstrates necessary skills for modifying activity level to adjust to activity intolerance.

■ Patient requests help to complete ADLs, as needed.

■ Patient demonstrates willingness to perform activities needed to follow care plan, including maintaining balanced diet, getting adequate rest, and participating in modified exercise program.

■ Patient's verbal statements indicate that he's learning to accept decreased energy level and to come to terms with the fact that he may not regain his former level of activity.

■ Patient reports experiencing less discomfort and pain when ambulating, transferring, and performing ADLs.

■ Patient states that acceptance of support services won't damage self-esteem or alter independent living efforts.

Documentation
■ Observations of patient's activity level, both deficits and improvements

■ Patient's compliance with treatment regimen and response to multidisciplinary approach

■ Teaching provided to patient and family members and their response

■ Modification of home or facility environment to ease patient's activity level

■ Evaluations for expected outcomes

Reference
Gunn, E., et al. "Exercise and the Heart Failure Patient: Aerobic vs. Strength Training—Is There a Need for Both?" *Progressive Cardiovascular Nursing* 21(3):146-50, Summer 2006.

Disturbed
BODY IMAGE
related to psychosocial factors

Definition
Confusion in mental picture of one's physical self

Assessment
- Sensory acuity, including vision and hearing
- Skin changes, including discoloration (for example, age spots), thinning, sagging, dryness associated with diminished sebaceous gland production, and wrinkling associated with diminished underlying connective structures
- Hair, including thinning and loss of color
- Musculature, including diminished muscle mass, alterations in body shape, and sagging skin
- Mental status, including denial, depression, discouragement, fear, and grief
- Activity level, including activities of daily living and physical exercise

Defining characteristics
- Excessive or inappropriate use of cosmetics to cover signs of aging
- Excessive or inappropriate use of hair-coloring products
- Frequent disparaging remarks about aging and its physical manifestations
- Hypersensitivity to remarks about advancing age
- Inappropriate dress for safety and comfort needs
- Indulgence in dangerous physical activities with intent of demonstrating youthful capabilities
- Personal rigidity or unwillingness to change
- Reluctance or refusal to wear corrective lenses or hearing aids
- Unwillingness or inability to view aging in positive light
- Unwillingness to acknowledge physical changes associated with aging
- Use of cosmetic surgery to reverse signs of aging

Expected outcomes
- Patient will alter skin care routine to reflect age-related changes and will use cosmetics appropriately.
- Patient will identify physical changes caused by aging without disparaging comments.
- Patient will identify at least one positive aspect of aging.
- Patient will use vision and hearing aids appropriately.
- Patient will dress appropriately with regard to safety, comfort, and personal taste.
- Patient will clean and style hair appropriately, without excessive coloring.
- Patient will demonstrate increased flexibility and willingness to consider lifestyle changes.
- Patient will participate in at least one social activity or group regularly.

■ Patient will exercise and engage in other physical activity at level consistent with desire, ability, and safety.

Suggested NOC outcomes

Body Image; Grief Resolution; Self-Esteem

Interventions and rationales

■ Encourage the patient to express his feelings about the physical changes associated with aging. *Active listening conveys a caring and accepting attitude.*

■ Provide information on appropriate self-care activities, such as:

– maintaining a proper diet

– bathing less frequently

– using skin lotions to combat dryness

– exercising appropriately to maintain muscle mass, bone strength, and cardiorespiratory health

– avoiding fractures related to osteoporosis.

Providing accurate self-care information helps the patient establish realistic goals.

■ Encourage the patient to consider new grooming styles or to seek advice from a barber or cosmetologist on "updating" hair and makeup styles. *Attractive, tasteful grooming may help the older patient achieve a sense of control over the aging process.*

■ Provide the patient with referrals for corrective eyewear and hearing aids *to address sensory deficits.*

■ Provide the patient with positive role models. For example, offer to share literature that emphasizes the accomplishments, capabilities, and contributions of older adults *to promote a positive self-image and a more positive view of the elderly population.*

■ During conversations with the patient, focus on the patient's strengths and what the patient can do; emphasize the positive aspects of aging *to increase the patient's self-esteem.*

■ Encourage the patient to engage in social activities with people from all age-groups *to increase opportunities for human interaction, positive feedback, and development of new interests.*

Suggested NIC interventions

Active Listening; Body Image Enhancement; Counseling; Grief Work Facilitation; Self-Esteem Enhancement

Evaluations for expected outcomes

■ Patient has clean, well-cared-for skin and uses cosmetics appropriately.

■ Patient identifies age-related physical changes and comments on them positively.

■ Patient identifies at least one personal advantage to growing older and one aspect of his life or personality that's better than it was 10 years ago.

■ Patient uses vision and hearing aids comfortably.

■ Patient dresses appropriately.

■ Patient's hair appears clean and well groomed.

- Patient demonstrates increased flexibility and willingness to consider lifestyle changes.
- Patient participates in at least one social activity or group regularly.
- Patient engages in regular, appropriate exercise or activity.

Documentation
- Patient's statements about appearance, ability, and age
- Mental status assessment (baseline and ongoing)
- Physical assessment
- Interventions directed toward improving patient's body image
- Patient's response to nursing interventions
- Evaluations for expected outcomes

Reference
Barba, B.E., and Coleman, P. "What are Old People For?" *Journal of Gerontological Nursing* 32(8):7-8, August 2006.

Risk for imbalanced
BODY TEMPERATURE
related to decreased sensitivity of thermoreceptors

Definition
State of being at risk for failure to maintain body temperature within normal range

Assessment
- Age
- History of present illness
- Medical history, especially endocrine or nervous system illness
- Environmental temperature
- Medication history
- Neurologic status, including level of consciousness, knowledge level, and sensory, motor, and mental status
- Cardiovascular status, including heart rate and rhythm, blood pressure, pulses, capillary refill time, and electrocardiogram results
- Respiratory status, including breath sounds, arterial blood gas results, and respiratory rate, depth, and character
- Integumentary status, including temperature, color, and turgor
- GI status, including evidence of enema or laxative abuse, inspection of abdomen, and auscultation of bowel sounds
- Support systems, including family, friends, volunteer organizations, and clergy

Risk factors
- Advanced age
- Altered metabolic rate
- Dehydration

- Exposure to cold or hot environment
- Extremes of weight (overweight or underweight)
- Illness or trauma that affects temperature regulation
- Inactivity or vigorous activity
- Inappropriate clothing for temperature
- Sedation
- Use of medication that causes vasoconstriction or vasodilation

Expected outcomes
- Patient's body temperature will remain normal.
- Patient's skin will remain warm and dry.
- Patient will state feelings of comfort.
- Patient won't exhibit signs of hypothermia or hyperthermia.
- Patient or family member will identify warning signs of hypothermia and hyperthermia.
- Patient or family member will express understanding of factors that cause hypothermia and hyperthermia.
- Patient or family member will describe ways to prevent imbalanced body temperature.

Suggested NOC outcomes
Risk Control; Risk Detection; Thermoregulation

Interventions and rationales
- Monitor the patient's body temperature every 8 hours or more frequently, as indicated, *to ensure the temperature doesn't vary more than 1° F from average normal (98.6° F [37° C] oral).* If it does, monitor it more frequently.
- Assess the patient's knowledge and lifestyle before teaching about hypothermia and hyperthermia *to gear the teaching plan to the patient's needs.*
- Using large black type, provide the patient with a list of the signs and symptoms of imbalanced body temperature:
– *Hypothermia:* shallow respirations; slow, weak pulse; decreased body temperature; low blood pressure; and pallor
– *Hyperthermia:* shivering, shaking chill; feeling hot; extreme thirst; elevated body temperature; and high blood pressure.
Listing the signs and symptoms helps the patient learn and identify warning signals of imbalanced body temperature. Large black type is easier for the older patient to read.
- Encourage the patient to remain active when in a cool environment *to keep warm and maintain normal metabolism.*
- Explain to the patient or family member why the patient needs warm clothing in cool climates, even indoors. Suggest socks, nonslip house shoes, and leg warmers *to provide warmth to vulnerable lower extremities, where vascular changes may cause decreased temperature sensation.*
- Instruct the patient or family member to label home thermostats with large numbers and to use black or bright contrasting colors to indicate appropriate temperature settings. *Easy-to-read labels will help the patient maintain room temperature.*

■ Teach the patient or family member about the dangers of too much direct sunlight on warm days *to prevent overheating in an older patient with faulty thermoreceptors.*

■ Discuss appropriate clothing for warm and cool climates. Suggest wearing clothes in layers, which can be removed or added, as needed, *to accommodate an increased susceptibility to temperature variations caused by aging vasculature.*

■ Suggest that a friend, family member, or volunteer from a local community organization visit the patient daily *to help ensure the patient's safety.*

Suggested NIC interventions

Environmental Management; Temperature Regulation; Vital Signs Monitoring

Evaluations for expected outcomes
■ Patient's body temperature remains within normal limits.
■ Patient's skin remains warm and dry.
■ Patient reports absence of pain.
■ Patient doesn't exhibit or report signs or symptoms of hypothermia or hyperthermia.
■ Patient or family member identifies warning signs of hypothermia and hyperthermia.
■ Patient or family member correctly identifies factors that may cause hypothermia or hyperthermia.
■ Patient or family member describes changes to lifestyle that will prevent recurrence of imbalanced body temperature.

Documentation
■ Patient's or family member's perception of problem, including reports of excessive cold or heat
■ Patient's temperature
■ Observations of risk factors for imbalanced body temperature
■ Instructions regarding preventive measures
■ Patient's or family member's statements of understanding of instructions
■ Evaluations for expected outcomes

Reference
Day, M.P. "Hypothermia: A Hazard for All Seasons," *Nursing* 36(12 Pt. 1):44-47, December 2006.

Decreased
CARDIAC OUTPUT

related to reduced myocardial perfusion

Definition
Inadequate blood pumped by the heart to meet the metabolic demands of the body

Assessment

- Mental status, especially sudden mental deterioration accompanied by confusion, agitation, and restlessness
- Cardiovascular status, including history of arrhythmias and syncope; skin color, temperature, and turgor; jugular vein distention; hepatojugular reflux; heart rate and rhythm; heart sounds; blood pressure; peripheral pulses; electrocardiogram (ECG), echocardiogram, and phonocardiogram results; serum digoxin level; and aspartate aminotransferase, lactate dehydrogenase, and creatine kinase isoenzyme levels
- Respiratory status, including respiratory rate and depth, breath sounds, chest X-ray, and arterial blood gas results
- Renal status, including weight, intake and output, urine specific gravity, and serum electrolyte levels

Defining characteristics

- Abnormal chest X-ray and cardiac enzyme levels
- Accessory muscle use
- Altered mental state
- Arrhythmias, ECG changes, and increased heart rate
- Audible S_3 or S_4 heart sounds
- Chest pain, coughing and wheezing, fatigue, restlessness, and cold, clammy skin
- Crackles
- Decreased cardiac output and peripheral pulses
- Dyspnea, increased respiratory rate, orthopnea, and paroxysmal nocturnal dyspnea
- Edema
- Ejection fraction less than 40%
- Elevated pulmonary artery pressure
- Jugular vein distention
- Mixed venous oxygen
- Oliguria
- Skin color changes
- Variations in blood pressure readings
- Weight gain

Expected outcomes

- Patient won't experience tachypnea, restlessness, anxiety, dyspnea, confusion, fainting, dizzy spells, light-headedness, nausea, fatigue, or weakness.
- Patient will tolerate exercise and activities at usual level, taking into account any cardiac damage.
- Patient will maintain respiratory status within established parameters.
- Patient's cardiac status will stabilize, with no evidence of arrhythmias.
- Patient and family members will understand and comply with prescribed therapeutic regimen.

Suggested NOC outcomes

Cardiac Disease Self-Management; Cardiac Pump Effectiveness; Circulation Status; Vital Signs

Interventions and rationales

■ Administer medications, as ordered; monitor intake and output; and observe for adverse reactions. *In older patients, decreased renal and liver function may lead to rapid development of toxicity.*

■ Monitor for dyspnea or breathlessness every 2 to 4 hours, and report changes from baseline. *Older patients with silent or painless myocardial infarction frequently develop dyspnea related to left-sided heart failure.*

■ Monitor mental status every 2 to 4 hours and report deviations from baseline. *Dizziness, confusion, light-headedness, and restlessness may indicate decreased cerebral blood flow caused by slow carotid sinus reflex.*

■ Administer diuretics cautiously to the patient. Monitor closely for cardiac overload by taking frequent vital signs and documenting intake and output accurately. Report signs and symptoms of cardiac overload, such as elevated central venous pressure, fluid intake above output, and increased pulmonary artery pressure. *When fluid in the lungs and lower extremities is mobilized and returns to circulation, it may overtax the patient's weakened myocardium.*

■ Assess apical and radial pulses every 2 to 4 hours and report deviations from the baseline *to monitor for arrhythmias, impending cardiac arrest, hypertension, or shock.*

■ Administer oxygen to the patient, as ordered, especially after the patient eats or during increased activity, *to increase oxygenation of the brain and heart.*

■ Make sure the patient gets adequate rest and doesn't exceed his activity tolerance level *to ease dyspnea, decrease oxygen demand on myocardium, and prevent hydrostatic pneumonia, venous thrombosis, and cardiovascular deconditioning.*

■ Teach the patient or family member the symptoms of possible cardiac problems:
– dizziness
– indigestion
– nausea
– retrosternal pain
– shortness of breath
– unusual fatigue and weakness.
Knowing the symptoms of decreased cardiac functioning gives the patient a sense of greater control over the situation and encourages compliance with the treatment plan.

■ Reduce stressful elements, such as excessive noise or light in the patient's environment, *to help decrease anxiety and restlessness, which may lead to arrhythmias.*

■ Encourage the patient to increase fluid intake and dietary fiber and to take natural stool softeners *to avoid Valsalva's maneuver during defecation, which can increase heart rate and blood pressure, cause reflex bradycardia, and decrease cardiac output.*

Suggested NIC interventions

Cardiac Care; Cardiac Precautions; Hemodynamic Regulation; Vital Signs Monitoring

Evaluations for expected outcomes

■ Patient experiences fewer dyspneic episodes, with no syncope or dizzy spells.

■ Patient returns to normal activity and exercise levels, taking into account extent of cardiac damage.

■ Patient maintains normal respiratory status.

■ Physical examination reveals no evidence of arrhythmias.

■ Patient and family members understand and comply with prescribed therapeutic regimen.

Documentation

■ Patient's chief complaint

■ Signs or symptoms of decreased cardiac output

■ Therapeutic interventions and patient's response

■ Activity and exercise tolerance

■ Diet and sleep patterns

■ Teaching provided to patient and family member

■ Evaluations for expected outcomes

Reference

Masse, L., and Antonacci, M. "Low Cardiac Output Syndrome: Identification and Management," *Critical Care Nursing Clinics of North America* 17(4):375-83, December 2005.

Impaired verbal
COMMUNICATION

related to physiologic or psychosocial changes

Definition

Decreased ability to appropriately speak, understand, or use words that's caused by organic and environmental factors

Assessment

■ History of neurologic disease

■ Speech characteristics, including pattern (rate of speech, phrase length, effort, fluency, prosody, repetition, and information content), vocabulary, level of comprehension, and presence of aphasia (Broca's, Wernicke's, transcortical, receptive, or global) or dysarthria

■ Ability to use alternative forms of communication (eye blinks, gestures, pictures, nods, or written notes)

■ Auditory status, including use of hearing aid, history of hearing deficits, and presence of cerumen

■ Vision status, including use of eyeglasses, history of vision deficits, visual acuity (near and distant), and visual fields

■ Neurologic status, including level of consciousness, orientation, cognition, memory (recent and remote), insight, judgment, cranial nerves (IX, X, XII), primitive reflexes (snout, suck, and palm-chin), and results of diagnostic studies (arteriogram, EEG, and computed tomography and magnetic resonance imaging scans)

■ Psychosocial status, including family, friends, other support system; recent relocation; recent losses; and efforts to express sadness, frustration, anxiety, or other emotions associated with verbal communication impairment

■ Medication status, including use of prescription and over-the-counter medications

Defining characteristics
■ Difficulty comprehending and maintaining usual communication pattern
■ Difficulty expressing thoughts verbally (aphasia, dysphasia, apraxia, dyslexia)
■ Difficulty forming words or sentences (aphonia, dyslalia, dysarthria)
■ Difficulty using or inability to use facial expressions or body language
■ Disorientation
■ Dyspnea
■ Impaired articulation
■ Inability or lack of desire to speak
■ Inability to speak dominant language
■ Inappropriate verbalizations
■ Lack of eye contact or poor selective attention
■ Stuttering or slurring
■ Vision deficit (partial or total)

Expected outcomes
■ Patient will improve communication skills to extent possible.
■ Patient will attend sessions with speech therapist.
■ Visitors and staff members will demonstrate appropriate respect when speaking with patient.
■ Patient will communicate needs without excessive frustration.
■ Patient will take steps to decrease isolation from friends and family members.
■ Patient or family member will identify and contact appropriate support services.
■ Patient will indicate through gestures, behavior, writing, or speaking that he's coming to terms with his impaired ability to communicate.

Suggested NOC outcomes
Communication; Communication: Expressive; Communication: Receptive

Interventions and rationales
■ When initiating communication, face the patient, maintain eye contact, speak slowly, and enunciate clearly *to make it easier for the patient to receive and process your message.*

■ Take steps to enhance communication while providing care:
– Communicate one idea at a time.
– Use "yes" and "no" questions.
– Avoid abstract thoughts and controversial topics.
– Use plain, everyday vocabulary.
– Allow longer response time.
– Guess at the meaning of incorrect words.
– Reduce distractions.
– Eliminate unnecessary noise.
– Encourage the patient to use gestures or other alternative means of communication.
Facilitating communication efforts will help decrease the patient's frustration.
■ If the patient's communication problems are exacerbated by hearing deficits, use appropriate techniques to overcome hearing problems:
– Minimize glare in the patient's room *to make it easier for the patient to read your lips.*
– Check for the proper use of adaptive hearing devices. If the patient wears a hearing aid, make sure the battery is working and the hearing aid is placed correctly *to enhance hearing ability.*
– Use paper and a pencil if hearing is severely impaired *to provide alternative means of communication.*
■ If the patient doesn't follow your conversation, rephrase ideas using simpler wording *to overcome differences in language or culture that may block communication.*
■ Don't rush the patient when he's struggling to express his thoughts. Demonstrate tact and willingness to listen. Even if you can't understand the patient, let him know you accept his efforts to communicate and you empathize with his frustration. *A patient with impaired verbal communication experiences isolation, despair, and frustration. Demonstrating compassion and fostering a therapeutic relationship is the most important step for improving communication.*
■ Avoid conversing with the patient when he's tired. *The patient's attention span may deteriorate when he's fatigued, thereby making efforts to communicate even more frustrating.*
■ Encourage the patient to engage in social activities, such as attending therapy sessions and eating with other patients at group tables, *to reduce feelings of isolation.*
■ If appropriate, help the patient reintegrate into family life. *Impaired speech may affect the patient's role in the family. Providing an opportunity to reintegrate the patient into family life, through family gatherings, may diminish loneliness and anxiety.*
■ Encourage the patient to reminisce. Use photographs, gestures, and visits from family members and friends to stimulate the patient's desire to express himself. *Recalling meaningful experiences may motivate the patient to try to communicate and may enhance feelings of self-worth.*
■ Encourage family members and colleagues to use speech appropriate for adults when talking to the patient and not to talk about him within his range of hearing *to convey respect.*

■ Obtain a referral to a speech therapist. Educate family members and colleagues about the methods prescribed by the therapist to enhance communication *to ensure continuity of care.*

■ Refer the patient and family members to appropriate community resources, such as a club for stroke survivors or support group for relatives of Alzheimer's patients, *to help them cope with communication impairment after discharge.*

Suggested NIC interventions

Active Listening; Communication Enhancement: Speech Deficit; Presence; Touch

Evaluations for expected outcomes

■ Patient improves communication skills to extent possible.

■ Patient attends sessions with speech therapist ___ times per week.

■ Visitors and staff demonstrate appropriate respect when speaking with patient by using adult speech and not talking about him within his hearing range.

■ Patient communicates needs, using gestures, behavior, writing, or speech, without excessive frustration.

■ Patient takes steps to decrease isolation from friends and family members.

■ Patient or family member identifies and contacts appropriate support services.

■ Patient indicates that he's coming to terms with his impaired ability to communicate.

Documentation

■ Observations of impaired speaking ability, use of communication aids, and expressions of frustration

■ Interventions implemented to decrease barriers to effective communication

■ Patient's efforts to communicate using gestures, behavior, writing, and speech

■ Patient teaching and patient's response

■ Referrals to speech therapist and other support services

■ Evaluations for expected outcomes

Reference

Liechty, J.A. "The Sounds of Silence: Relating to People with Aphasia," *Journal of Psychosocial Nursing and Mental Health Services* 44(8):53-55, August 2006.

CONSTIPATION

related to diet, fluid intake, activity level, and personal bowel habits

Definition

Decrease in normal frequency of defecation accompanied by difficult or incomplete passage of stool and/or passage of excessively hard, dry stool

Assessment

■ History of bowel disorder or surgery

■ GI status, including nausea and vomiting, usual bowel habits, tenesmus, distention, flatulence, laxative or enema use, and medications

■ Oral status, including inspection of oral cavity (gums, tongue, and dentition), pain or discomfort, and salivation

■ Activity status, including type, duration, and frequency of exercise; lifestyle; and access to toilet facilities during work and recreation

■ Nutritional status, including appetite, dietary intake, amount and type of dietary fiber, fluid intake, food likes and dislikes, meal pattern, access to food supply and storage facilities, access to shopping and transportation, and financial resources available for food

■ Drug history, including use of constipating agents (such as aluminum-based antacids, anticholinergics, antidepressants, iron supplements, laxatives, and opioids) and history of laxative abuse

Defining characteristics

■ Abdominal tenderness or pain and feeling of rectal fullness or pressure

■ Borborygmi, hypoactive or hyperactive bowel sounds, or abdominal dullness on percussion

■ Bright red blood with stools; bark-colored or black, tarry stools; or hard, dry stools

■ Change in bowel pattern

■ Changes in mental status, urinary incontinence, unexplained falls, or elevated body temperature

■ Decreased frequency and stool volume

■ Distended abdomen and increased abdominal pressure

■ General fatigue, anorexia, headache, indigestion, nausea, or vomiting

■ Inability to pass stools

■ Oozing liquid stools

■ Palpable rectal or abdominal mass

■ Severe flatus

■ Soft, pastelike stools in rectum

■ Straining and possibly pain during defecation

Expected outcomes

■ Patient will participate in development of bowel program.

■ Patient will report urge to defecate, as appropriate.

■ Patient will increase fluid and fiber intake.

■ Patient will report easy and complete evacuation of stools.

■ Patient will increase activity level.

■ Patient will have elimination pattern within normal limits.

■ Patient will describe changes in personal habits that will help maintain normal elimination.

Suggested NOC outcomes

Bowel Elimination; Hydration; Symptom Control

Interventions and rationales

■ Monitor the frequency and characteristics of the patient's stools. *Careful monitoring forms the basis of an effective treatment plan.*

■ Monitor and record the patient's fluid intake and output. *Inadequate fluid intake contributes to dry feces and constipation. Monitoring fluid balance ensures adequate fluid intake and promotes elimination.*

■ Provide privacy for elimination *to promote physiologic functioning.*

■ Encourage the patient to use a bedside commode or walk to toilet facilities. Avoid the use of a bedpan *because such use may inhibit normal positioning for evacuation, thereby exacerbating constipation.*

■ Work with the patient to plan and implement an individualized bowel regimen *to establish a regular elimination schedule.*

■ Emphasize to the patient the importance of responding to the urge to defecate. Be alert for any mental status changes that may impair the patient's ability to recognize or attend to the need to defecate or to report the need to the caregiver. *A timely response to the urge to defecate is necessary to maintain normal physiologic functioning and to avoid pressure and discomfort in the lower GI tract.*

■ Teach the patient to locate public restrooms and to wear easily removable clothing on outings *to promote normal bowel functioning.*

■ Teach the patient to massage his abdomen once per day. Show him how to locate and gently massage along the transverse and descending colon. *In the older patient, the neural centers in the lower intestinal wall may be impaired, making it more difficult for the body to evacuate feces. Massage may help stimulate peristalsis and the urge to defecate.*

■ If abdominal pressure is inadequate to complete defecation, encourage the patient to perform a rocking motion of his upper body *to aid in elimination.*

■ Plan and implement an exercise routine, such as walking, leg raising, abdominal muscle strengthening, and Kegel exercises. *Exercise promotes the abdominal and pelvic muscle tone necessary for normal elimination.*

■ Encourage the intake of high-fiber foods. *Many older patients have reduced intestinal muscle tone and decreased strength in abdominal muscles, resulting in slower peristalsis, dry feces, and decreased ability to exert pressure for evacuation. High-fiber foods supply bulk for normal elimination and improve intestinal muscle tone.*

■ Unless contraindicated, encourage fluid intake of 6 to 8 glasses (1,420 to 1,900 ml) daily *to maintain normal metabolic processes and prevent excessive reabsorption of fluid from GI contents.*

■ Teach the patient sensible use of laxatives and enemas *to avoid laxative dependency. Overuse of laxatives and enemas may cause fluid and electrolyte loss and damage to intestinal mucosa.*

■ Help the patient understand his diet modification plan. If appropriate, have the patient consult with a dietitian *to encourage compliance with the prescribed diet.*

Suggested NIC interventions

Bowel Management; Constipation/Impaction Management; Exercise Promotion; Fluid Management; Nutrition Management

Evaluations for expected outcomes

■ Patient participates in planning and implementing bowel program.

- Patient reports urge to defecate, as appropriate.
- Patient's daily diet includes high-fiber foods and adequate fluids.
- Patient reports easy and complete evacuation of stools.
- Patient increases activity level.
- Patient achieves routine bowel function without excessive use of laxatives, enemas, straining, or discomfort.
- Patient makes adaptations to lifestyle to ensure maintenance of bowel function.

Documentation
- Patient's expressions of concern regarding constipation, dietary changes, laxative use, and bowel pattern
- Physical findings
- Intake and output
- Observations of diet, characteristics of stool, and activity level
- Teaching provided and patient's response
- Patient's expressions indicating understanding of bowel program
- Evaluations for expected outcomes

References
Wilson, L.A. "Understanding Bowel Problems in Older People: Part 1," *Nursing Older People* 17(8):25-29, November 2005.

Wilson, L.A. "Understanding Bowel Problems in Older People: Part 2," *Nursing Older People* 17(9):24-29, December 2005.

Compromised family
COPING

related to caring for dependent, aging family member

Definition
Usually supportive primary person (family member or close friend) provides insufficient, ineffective, or compromised support, comfort, assistance, or encouragement that may be needed by the client to manage or master adaptive tasks related to his/her health challenge

Assessment
- Patient status, including age, medical history, self-concept, physical disabilities or limitations, present living arrangements, and role in family
- Family assessment, including communication style, family coping style, perceptions of the aging process (myths versus realities), health problems of other members, financial status, support systems, and additional stressors
- Patient's current health crisis (emotional or physical)

Defining characteristics
- Attempts to assist or support patient with unsatisfactory results (family member)

■ Displays of protective behavior disproportionate to patient's abilities or need for autonomy (family member)
■ Expressed concern about family's response to health problem (patient)
■ Expressed inadequate understanding or knowledge base that interferes with effective assistive or supportive behaviors (family member)
■ Reported preoccupation with personal reaction to patient's health problem (family member)
■ Withdrawal from or limited communication with patient at time of need (family member)

Expected outcomes

■ Family members will assume responsibilities formerly held by patient, as appropriate.
■ Family members will express feelings about responsibilities in caring for an older relative.
■ Patient and family members will express understanding of maturational and developmental issues that contributed to crisis.
■ Patient and family members will identify and make use of appropriate community services.
■ Family members will demonstrate improved capacity to plan care for older relative.
■ Patient and family members will express satisfaction with their improved ability to cope with current crisis.

Suggested NOC outcomes

Caregiver Emotional Health; Caregiver-Patient Relationship; Caregiver Stressors; Family Coping; Family Normalization

Interventions and rationales

■ Identify the primary caregiver in the family and assess the roles of other family members *to establish family hierarchy and plan interventions.*
■ Educate the patient and family members about the aging process. Discuss how changes in the patient have affected the family *to assess the needs of the patient and family members.*
■ Avoid becoming involved in a power struggle among family members. *The patient may no longer be able to fulfill his family role, and the sudden shift in roles may lead to a power struggle among family members. The patient or family members may try to manipulate you as part of this power struggle. Maintaining a neutral, objective approach will help family members adjust to role changes.*
■ As appropriate, arrange and conduct a conference for family members; include the patient when possible. *Long-established communication patterns may interfere with family members' ability to resolve conflicts and make decisions. Your presence may help family members express feelings, identify needs and resources, and develop healthier ways of interacting.*
■ Encourage family members to express their feelings about caring for the older family member. *A nonjudgmental attitude promotes effective communication.*
■ Encourage family members to identify strengths and weaknesses in the family system. Help them explore values, beliefs, perceived changes, and actual role

changes related to the older patient's altered physical or emotional condition *to enhance insight.*

■ Assist the patient and family members in developing short-term and long-term goals and contingency plans *to increase a sense of control and direction for the future.*

■ Help the patient and family members identify appropriate community services, such as adult day care, respite care, and geriatric outreach services, *to provide access to additional sources of support.*

■ Suggest using a care manager to help with the ongoing coordination of the patient's needs. Help the family identify a care manager they can relate to. *A care manager may help simplify decision making and limit family conflict.*

■ Help family members explore coping strategies used effectively during past crises and discuss how to apply these strategies to the present situation *to make family members aware of their demonstrated ability to adapt to change.*

■ Provide emotional support for the primary caregiver. *The family member who takes on the most responsibility for the patient has the double burden of caring for an older adult and adjusting to a new role in the family.*

■ Maintain a nonjudgmental attitude while working with family members. Some families may hesitate to accept outside help. Other families may be unwilling to make even small sacrifices to care for an older relative. Remember that if family members haven't been supportive or close to the patient before, you're unlikely to change their attitudes. *A nonjudgmental outlook benefits the patient and family members. Learning to accept your limitations will help you avoid burnout.*

■ Remain supportive and understanding if the patient or family members are reluctant to use needed community resources, such as adult day care, respite care, and home health care services. *An older patient may feel that using outside resources means sacrificing independence; family members may feel that asking for help indicates lack of caring.*

Suggested NIC interventions

Caregiver Support; Coping Enhancement; Family Involvement Promotion; Respite Care

Evaluations for expected outcomes

■ Family members assume responsibilities formerly held by patient, as appropriate.

■ Patient and family members share feelings about current crisis.

■ Patient and family members express understanding of maturational and developmental issues that led to crisis.

■ Patient and family members acknowledge need for outside help to cope with crisis and identify and contact community resources.

■ Family members demonstrate improved capacity for short-term and long-term planning.

■ Patient and family members express satisfaction with their improved ability to cope with current crisis.

Documentation
■ Patient's and family members' understanding of aging process and current health crisis
■ Observations of patient's and family members' reactions to crisis
■ Family members' willingness to become involved in patient care
■ Nursing interventions
■ Teaching provided
■ Patient's and family members' response to interventions and instructions
■ Referrals to community agencies
■ Evaluations for expected outcomes

Reference
Garity, J. "Caring for a Family Member with Alzheimer's Disease: Coping with Caregiver Burden Post-nursing Home Placement," *Journal of Gerontological Nursing* 32(6):39-48, June 2006.

Ineffective
COPING

related to inability to solve problems or adapt to demands of daily living

---

Definition
Inability to form a valid appraisal of the stressors, inadequate choices of practiced responses, and/or inability to use available resources

Assessment
■ Age
■ Lifestyle changes necessitated by disease or illness
■ Role changes caused by retirement, relocation, or death of spouse, family members, or friends
■ Changes associated with normal aging, such as decreased vision, hearing, and physical endurance
■ Perceived coping ability
■ Usual coping mechanisms
■ Support systems, including family, friends, and religious and community organizations

Defining characteristics
■ Change in communication patterns
■ Decreased use of social support
■ Destructive behavior toward self or others
■ Difficulty asking for help
■ Fatigue
■ High illness rate
■ Inability to meet basic needs and role expectations

- Lack of goal-directed behavior, such as inability to attend, difficulty organizing information, poor concentration, and poor problem-solving abilities
- Maladaptive coping behaviors
- Risk-taking behaviors
- Sleep disturbance
- Statements indicating inability to cope
- Substance abuse

Expected outcomes
- Patient will verbalize increased ability to cope.
- Patient will expand support network to meet social and emotional needs.
- Patient will locate and use appropriate resources for help in problem solving.
- Patient will report increased ability to meet demands of daily living.
- Patient will make changes to environment to ensure enhanced coping or move into long-term care facility, as needed.

Suggested NOC outcomes

Coping; Decision-Making; Impulse Self-Control; Information Processing; Social Interaction Skills

Interventions and rationales
- Refer the patient to social service agencies, such as geriatric assessment centers, adult day-care programs, and home health care agencies, as appropriate, *to expand his support network and help him cope with physical, psychosocial, and economic stressors.*
- Assist the patient in becoming involved with informal community programs, such as volunteer, foster grandparent, or religious groups, *to provide peer and social contact and decrease the patient's loneliness and isolation.*
- Encourage the patient to reminisce about the past *to help him recall past challenges and successful coping strategies.*
- Provide the patient with information about the aging process, methods of coping with stress, and techniques used by other older adults to meet the demands of daily living *to assist the patient in implementing coping strategies.*
- If the patient must enter a long-term care facility or undergo lengthy home-based convalescence, help him put the situation in perspective. Explain to the patient that extreme stress can overwhelm anyone, even well-adapted individuals with strong support systems. When stress becomes overwhelming, rehabilitation in a secure environment may be the best option. Entering a long-term care facility isn't "the beginning of the end," as many people think, but rather an additional mechanism for ensuring optimal recovery. *Taking time to provide a carefully worded explanation may help the patient come to terms with his situation.*
- If the patient requires treatment in a long-term care facility, provide the least restrictive environment possible *to reduce the patient's fear and anxiety, help him retain a sense of control, and encourage him to use his abilities to the maximum.*
- Discuss with the patient the possibility of making lifestyle changes, such as moving closer to relatives, moving to a retirement community, or hiring someone to help with housework, *to improve his ability to cope.*

Suggested NIC interventions

Coping Enhancement; Decision-Making Support; Emotional Support; Environmental Management; Impulse Control Training; Support System Enhancement

Evaluations for expected outcomes

- Patient verbalizes an increased ability to cope.
- Patient reports success in developing support network to meet social and emotional needs.
- Patient contacts resources to help with problem solving.
- Patient reports increased ability to meet demands of daily living.
- Patient identifies lifestyle changes that will improve his ability to cope or states that he understands and accepts need to move to long-term care facility or retirement community.

Documentation

- Patient's expression of feelings about present life situation and difficulty coping
- Formal and informal sources of support identified by patient or family members
- Observations of patient's behavior in response to stressful situations
- Teaching provided and patient's response
- Use of outside support services
- Evaluations for expected outcomes

Reference

Popejoy, L. "Health-related Decision-making by Older Adults and Their Families: How Clinicians Can Help," *Journal of Gerontological Nursing* 31(9):12-18, September 2005.

Ineffective

DENIAL

related to fear or anxiety about aging

Definition

Conscious or unconscious attempt to disavow knowledge or meaning of an event to reduce fear of growing older

Assessment

- Age
- Appearance
- Activity patterns, including sudden interest or participation in activities that may be dangerous
- Self-concept, including self-esteem, body image, and perception of self in life continuum
- Coping behaviors

■ Mental status, including affect, communication, memory, mood, orientation, perception, abstract thinking, judgment, and insight

Defining characteristics
■ Delay in seeking medical attention or refusal of medical attention to detriment of health
■ Inability to admit impact of aging on life pattern
■ Inappropriate affect
■ Minimization of signs and symptoms of aging
■ Refusal to admit fear of death or invalidism
■ Use of dismissive gestures or comments when speaking of distressing events
■ Use of self-treatment to relieve symptoms

Expected outcomes
■ Patient will discuss aging process and impact on ability to participate in hobbies and other activities.
■ Patient will express interest in age-appropriate community activities.
■ Patient will set aside time for reminiscing as part of daily routine.
■ Patient will express more positive view of growing older.
■ Patient will adapt activities to avoid unnecessary physical stress on body.

Suggested NOC outcomes
Acceptance: Health Status; Anxiety Self-Control; Fear Self-Control

Interventions and rationales
■ Discuss the challenge of being an older adult in today's youth-oriented society *to encourage the patient to express his feelings and help him recognize that he doesn't have to accept society's prejudices about aging.*
■ Discuss with the patient and family members the changes that normally occur as part of the aging process *to correct misconceptions.*
■ Discuss how to adapt activities and hobbies to accommodate the physical changes that occur with aging *to avoid excess physical stress.*
■ Discuss the advantages of growing older, such as having more time to pursue hobbies and other interests, *to help the patient develop a positive view of aging.*
■ Emphasize various activities that the patient can continue to do well *to enhance self-esteem.*
■ Encourage the patient to set aside time for reminiscing as part of his daily routine. *Reminiscing helps the patient to affirm the past and promotes self-esteem.*
■ Provide information about senior volunteer groups and part-time work or volunteer opportunities *to help the patient maintain physical and mental functioning and promote social interaction.*
■ Invite an active member of a senior citizens club, social group, senior sports league, or advocacy group to visit the patient *to provide a positive role model.*

Suggested NIC interventions
Coping Enhancement; Health Education; Self-Awareness Enhancement

Evaluations for expected outcomes
■ Patient expresses positive and negative feelings about aging.
■ Patient states intention to engage in age-appropriate community activity.
■ Patient expresses willingness to set aside time for reminiscing.
■ Patient expresses more positive view of growing older.
■ Patient adapts activities to avoid unnecessary physical stress on body.

Documentation
■ Evidence of patient's difficulty adjusting to the aging process
■ Nursing interventions
■ Referrals provided
■ Patient's response to nursing interventions
■ Patient's statements that indicate more positive attitude toward growing older
■ Evaluations for expected outcomes

References
Chao, S.Y., et al. "The Effects of Group Reminiscence Therapy on Depression, Self-esteem, and Life Satisfaction on Elderly Nursing Home Residents," *The Journal of Nursing Research* 14(1):36-45, March 2006.

Moore, S.L., et al. "The Quest for Meaning in Aging," *Geriatric Nursing* 27(5):293-99, September-October 2006.

Adult
FAILURE TO THRIVE
related to illness, disability, or environmental deprivation

Definition
Progressive functional deterioration of a physical and cognitive nature; individual's ability to live with multisystem diseases, cope with ensuing problems, and manage his/her care are remarkably diminished

Assessment
■ Age
■ Weight and fluctuations in weight
■ Condition of hair, skin, and nails
■ Nutritional status, including daily food intake, meal preparation, and use of supplements or vitamins
■ Sleep patterns
■ Mobility status
■ Socioeconomic status, including ethnic background, education, financial resources, family support system, religious affiliation, activity and exercise patterns, involvement in social activities, and access to transportation
■ Health habits and beliefs, including participation in fad diets, excessive concern with preventing obesity, and recent immigration to United States with little experience in selecting appropriate foods in American markets

■ Mental status, including orientation to time, place, and person; insight regarding current situation; judgment; abstract thinking; mood; affect; recent and remote memory; thought processes; and thought content

Defining characteristics
■ Cognitive decline, as evidenced by problems with responding appropriately to environmental stimuli and decreased perception
■ Consumption of minimal to no food at most meals (i.e., consumes less than 75% of normal requirements)
■ Decreased participation in activities of daily living that were once enjoyed
■ Decreased social skills or social withdrawal
■ Difficulty performing simple self-care tasks
■ Doesn't eat meals when offered
■ Frequent exacerbations of chronic health problems, such as pneumonia or urinary tract infections
■ Neglect of home environment or financial responsibilities
■ No longer looks after or takes charge of physical cleanliness or appearance
■ Physical decline, as evidenced by fatigue, dehydration, and incontinence of bowel and bladder
■ Reports of not having an appetite, not feeling hungry, or not wanting to eat
■ Weight loss (decreased from baseline weight):
– 5% unintentional weight loss in 1 month
– 10% unintentional weight loss in 6 months

Related factors
■ Apathy
■ Depression
■ Fatigue

Expected outcomes
■ Patient will express understanding of causes underlying failure to thrive.
■ Patient will express realization that he's depressed.
■ Patient will consume sufficient amounts of food and nutrients.
■ Patient will sleep for ___ hours without interruption.
■ Family members will demonstrate understanding of measures necessary to meet patient's needs.
■ Patient will gain weight.
■ Patient will report feeling safe.
■ Patient will follow up on referrals for social service assistance.
■ Patient will follow up on referrals for psychiatric evaluation.
■ Patient and family members will use community resources to enhance patient's health.

Suggested NOC outcomes
Nutritional Status; Physical Aging Status; Psychosocial Adjustment: Life Change; Will to Live

Interventions and rationales

■ Spend uninterrupted time with the patient *to learn his perception of problems related to failure to thrive; for example, difficulty maintaining independence in activities.*

■ Encourage the patient and family members to establish a plan for addressing the patient's failure to thrive *to encourage the patient and family members to assume responsibility for meeting the patient's needs to the extent that they're physically, mentally, and emotionally able.*

■ Create a pleasant mealtime environment for the patient. Provide unlimited access to nourishing foods and nutritional supplements. Attempt to accommodate ethnic food preferences. *These measures help promote weight gain.*

■ Measure and record the patient's weight at the same time every day *to ensure accuracy and monitor the patient's progress.*

■ Monitor fluid intake and output. *A decrease in body weight may result from fluid loss.*

■ Monitor electrolyte levels and report abnormal values. *Poor nutritional status can cause electrolyte imbalance.*

■ Urge participation in exercise and activities consistent with capabilities. *Mild exercise and socialization may improve self-esteem.*

■ Teach the patient, family members, or caregiver how to maintain progress in reversing failure to thrive without direct supervision by a nurse. *Education helps prepare the patient to live as independently as possible and helps the family to understand how best to support the patient.*

■ Refer the patient and family members to appropriate agencies in the community, such as Meals On Wheels, that can help meet the patient's needs *to ensure continuity of care.*

■ Refer the patient and family members to appropriate resources if the patient has additional needs, such as the need for financial assistance, psychiatric help, or more in-depth nutritional counseling. *This will help ensure adherence to a comprehensive care plan.*

Suggested NIC interventions

Coping Enhancement; Home Maintenance Assistance; Nutritional Monitoring; Spiritual Support

Evaluations for expected outcomes

■ Patient expresses understanding of causes underlying failure to thrive.
■ Patient expresses realization that he's depressed.
■ Patient consumes sufficient amounts of food and nutrients.
■ Patient sleeps for ___ hours without interruption.
■ Family members demonstrate understanding of measures necessary to meet patient's needs.
■ Patient gains weight.
■ Patient reports feeling safe.
■ Patient follows up on referrals for social service assistance.
■ Patient follows up on referrals for psychiatric evaluation.
■ Patient and family members use community resources to enhance patient's health.

Documentation

■ Description of patient's physical condition
■ Daily weight
■ Fluid intake and output
■ Patient's mental and emotional status
■ Teaching provided to patient and family
■ Patient's and family members' expressions indicating understanding of patient's problem
■ Referrals to community agencies and response from these agencies
■ Patient's response to nursing interventions
■ Evaluations for expected outcomes

References

Lennie, T.A., et al. "Factors Influencing Food Intake in Patients with Heart Failure: A Comparison with Healthy Elders," *The Journal of Cardiovascular Nursing* 21(2):123-29, March-April 2006.

Zulkowski, K. "Nutrition and Aging: A Transdisciplinary Approach," *Ostomy/Wound Management* 52(10):53-57, October 2006.

Impaired
GAS EXCHANGE

related to carbon dioxide retention or excess mucus production

Definition

Excess or deficit in oxygenation and/or carbon dioxide elimination at the alveolar/capillary membranes

Assessment

■ Age
■ Gender
■ Smoking history
■ Occupational or environmental risk factors, such as exposure to asbestos, smog, and pollutants
■ Respiratory status, including history of respiratory disorders, breath sounds, sputum characteristics, accessory muscle use, cyanosis, and arterial blood gas (ABG) levels
■ Cardiovascular status, including skin color and temperature, heart rate and rhythm, heart sounds, blood pressure, hemoglobin levels, hematocrit, red and white blood cell and platelet counts, prothrombin and partial thromboplastin times, and serum iron concentrations
■ Psychosocial status, including mental status, knowledge level, lifestyle, and support systems
■ Activity status, including ability to perform activities of daily living (ADLs)

Defining characteristics

- Abnormal arterial pH and ABG levels
- Abnormal respiratory rate, rhythm, and depth
- Confusion
- Diaphoresis
- Dyspnea
- Headache on awakening
- Hypoxia and hypoxemia
- Irritability
- Nasal flaring
- Pale, dusky skin
- Restlessness or somnolence
- Tachycardia
- Vision disturbances

Expected outcomes

- Patient will exercise and perform ADLs without experiencing dyspnea or excessive fatigue.
- Patient will maintain adequate fluid intake.
- Patient will maintain adequate ventilation and have clear breath sounds on auscultation.
- Patient or family members will state understanding of causes for impaired gas exchange and behaviors to prevent it.

Suggested NOC outcomes

Fluid and Electrolyte Balance; Respiratory Status: Gas Exchange; Tissue Perfusion: Pulmonary; Vital Signs

Interventions and rationales

- Establish baseline values for respiratory assessment *to distinguish age-related changes that may mimic disease states from disease. Older adults take shorter breaths. This decreases maximum breathing capacity, vital capacity, residual volume, and functional capacity.*
- Auscultate lungs every 4 hours, taking into account anatomic changes that may occur in older patients, such as kyphosis, deviated trachea, and dowager's hump, *to detect abnormal breath sounds.* Report abnormalities.
- Administer and monitor oxygen therapy, as ordered, *to enhance oxygenation and detect signs of decompensation. Older patients have a high incidence of chronic cardiac and chronic pulmonary disorders. Detecting early changes in condition allows for early intervention.*
- Teach the patient relaxation techniques and ask for a return demonstration. *Using relaxation techniques may help reduce tissue oxygen demand.*
- Incorporate the patient's past experiences into the teaching plan when conveying information about disease, medications, and lifestyle changes. *Information becomes more meaningful when related to previous experiences.*
- Help the patient schedule ADLs to allow for rest periods. *The older patient has more fibrous, less elastic alveoli that contain fewer functional capillaries, which de-*

creases exertional capacity. The patient needs rest periods to conserve respiratory effort.

■ Help the patient identify positions that maximize ventilatory capacity, such as leaning over the bedside table when sitting or using a large wedge pillow under the shoulders. *In an older patient, accessory muscles of the pharynx and larynx may atrophy, making it necessary for the patient to assume breathing positions that maximize ventilation, perfusion, and thoracic expansion.*

■ Encourage adequate fluid intake. *Older adults may have a diminished sense of thirst, which may lead to dry mucous membranes. Dry mucous membranes, in turn, may impede removal of secretions and promote respiratory infection. Consuming adequate fluids helps to liquefy secretions, reducing the energy required to mobilize them.* Record intake and output *to monitor fluid status.*

■ Perform bronchial hygiene, such as positioning, coughing, deep breathing, percussion, postural drainage, and suctioning, *to promote and maintain a patent airway.*

■ Evaluate the home environment and recommend changes, such as moving the patient's bedroom to the first floor, *to reduce exertion.*

Suggested NIC interventions

Acid-Base Management; Hemodynamic Regulation; Oxygen Therapy; Vital Signs Monitoring

Evaluations for expected outcomes

■ Patient performs exercise and ADLs with minimum fatigue and increased endurance.

■ Patient maintains adequate fluid intake.

■ Patient maintains adequate ventilation and has clear breath sounds on auscultation.

■ Patient or family members state understanding of causes for impaired gas exchange and behaviors to prevent it.

Documentation

■ Patient's complaints of dyspnea or fatigue

■ Observations of patient's condition

■ Patient's response to nursing interventions

■ Teaching provided and patient's response

■ Patient's expressions indicating understanding of care plan

■ Evaluations for expected outcomes

Reference

Dahlin, C. "It Takes my Breath Away End-stage COPD. Part 2: Pharmacologic and Nonpharmacologic Management of Dyspnea and Other Symptoms," *Home Healthcare Nurse* 24(4):218-24, April 2006.

GRIEVING

related to perceived potential loss of life

Definition
Intellectual and emotional responses through which an individual attempts to adjust self-concept based on a perceived personal loss; concept of anticipatory grieving can be applied to families and communities as well

Assessment
- Age
- Developmental stage
- Presence of living will, durable power of attorney for health care, and other advance directives
- History of chronic illness or terminal diagnosis
- Mental status, including level of consciousness and orientation
- Emotional status, including evidence of anger, apathy, depression, or hostility
- Support systems, including family members, significant other, friends, and clergy
- Spiritual practices, including religious affiliation and use of spiritual support systems
- Customs and beliefs related to illness, death, and suffering

Defining characteristics
- Altered communication patterns
- Change in eating habits, sleep and dream patterns, activity level, or libido
- Denial of potential loss of life
- Difficulty taking on different roles
- Expressed guilt, anger, sorrow, and bargaining
- Expressions of distress over potential loss of life
- Resolution of grief before loss of life

Expected outcomes
- Patient will express and accept feelings about anticipated death.
- Patient will progress through stages of grieving process in his own way.
- Patient will practice religious rituals and use other coping mechanisms appropriate to end of life.
- Family members or significant other will participate in providing supportive care and comfort to patient.

Suggested NOC outcomes
Coping; Family Coping; Grief Resolution; Psychosocial Adjustment: Life Change

Interventions and rationales
- Provide time for the patient to express his feelings about death or terminal illness. *Active listening helps the patient lessen feelings of loneliness and isolation.*

Don't approach the patient with a busy, hurried attitude, *which can block communication.*

■ Establish a relationship that encourages the patient to express concerns about death. *Basic nursing care combined with genuine interest in the patient fosters trust and understanding.*

■ Guide the patient in life review. Encourage him to write or tape record his life history as a lasting gift to family members. *Life review allows the patient to survey events from his past and give them meaningful interpretation.*

■ Involve an interdisciplinary team (including a psychologist, nurse, the patient, a nutritionist, physician, physical therapist, and chaplain) in providing care for a dying patient. *Each team member offers unique expertise for meeting the dying patient's needs.*

■ Encourage family members to become involved in the care of the dying patient. Communicate with the patient and family members honestly and compassionately. *Giving family members a role in patient care helps relieve anxiety and lessen feelings of regret and guilt. Honest communication is important because family members need an opportunity to acknowledge their loss and say farewell.*

■ Demonstrate acceptance of the patient's response to his anticipated death, whatever that response may be: crying, sadness, anger, fear, or denial. *Each patient responds to dying in his own way. Helping him express his feelings freely will enhance his ability to cope.*

■ Help the patient progress through the psychological stages associated with anticipated death, including shock and denial, anger, bargaining, depression, and acceptance, *to help you anticipate the dying patient's psychological needs. Keep in mind, however, that not all dying patients go through each stage.*

■ Support the patient's spiritual coping behaviors. For example, arrange for the patient to have objects that provide spiritual comfort (such as a Bible, prayer shawl, pictures, statues, or rosary beads) at the bedside. *Even patients for whom religious practice hasn't been a dominant part of life usually turn to religion when confronted by death or serious illness.*

■ Inform the patient about hospice services. Hospice services emphasize symptomatic relief and caring, with the aim of improving patient and family comfort until death occurs, instead of prolonging life for its own sake. *Hospice care is an appropriate alternative for a patient with an incurable illness.*

■ Provide referrals for home health care assistance if the patient will be cared for at home *to support the patient's decision to remain at home.*

Suggested NIC interventions

Anticipatory Guidance; Coping Enhancement; Family Support; Grief Work Facilitation

Evaluations for expected outcomes

■ Patient expresses and accepts feelings brought about by anticipated death.
■ Patient progresses through stages of grieving in his own way.
■ Patient participates in religious rituals and uses other appropriate coping mechanisms.
■ Patient receives adequate support during end of life from family members, friends, and members of health care team.

Documentation
- Patient's verbal expressions indicating feelings about anticipated death
- Observations of emotional responses, such as crying, anger, and withdrawal
- Interventions to help patient cope with anticipated death
- Patient's requests for assistance in achieving spiritual comfort (spiritual objects and visits from minister, priest, or rabbi)
- Patient's responses to interventions
- Evaluations for expected outcomes

Reference
Zimmerman, C., and Wennberg, R. "Integrating Palliative Care: A Postmodern Perspective," *The American Journal of Hospice and Palliative Care* 23(4):255-58, August-September 2006.

Impaired
HOME MAINTENANCE
related to impaired cognitive, emotional, or psychomotor functioning

Definition
Inability to independently maintain a safe, growth-promoting immediate environment

Assessment
- Age
- Gender
- Home environment
- Financial resources
- Patient's psychosocial status, including perception of reality, communication patterns, role responsibilities, degree of awareness and concern, history of psychiatric-related illness, support systems, and cognitive, memory, and motor abilities
- Caregiver's psychosocial status, including stressors, support systems, and understanding of patient's care requirements

Defining characteristics
- Description of outstanding debts or financial crisis
- Expressed difficulty in maintaining comfortable home
- Expressed sense of being overtaxed, marked by exhaustion and anxiety
- Household in disrepair, marked by excessive clutter, unwashed clothing and cooking equipment, offensive odors, presence of rodents and insects, accumulation of dirt and food wastes, and inappropriate temperature
- Lack of necessary equipment or aids
- Requests for assistance with home maintenance

Expected outcomes

■ Patient and caregiver will express concern about poor home maintenance and verbalize plans to correct health and safety hazards in the home.

■ Patient and caregiver will identify community organizations that can help ease transition from hospital to home or long-term care facility.

■ Patient and caregiver will develop schedule for doing household tasks.

Suggested NOC outcomes

Family Functioning; Role Performance; Self-Care: Instrumental Activities of Daily Living (IADL)

Interventions and rationales

■ Help the patient and caregiver identify the strengths and weaknesses in current home maintenance practices *to provide a focus for interventions.*

■ Discuss with the patient and caregiver obstacles to meeting home maintenance needs *to provide the basis for a program to meet health and safety requirements.*

■ Determine the patient's ability and motivation to achieve a higher level of home maintenance. *Self-motivation is necessary to ensure change.*

■ Help the patient and caregiver explore community resources, such as Meals On Wheels, senior centers, home health care agencies, homemaker services, cleaning services, self-help groups, religious programs, and retired senior volunteer programs, *to ease the transition from hospital to home.*

■ Allow the caregiver to express his feelings about having responsibility for the patient's health care regimen and household upkeep. When appropriate, discuss opportunities for the caregiver to assign responsibility to other family members or make use of community resources. Encourage the caregiver to ask questions, seek help, and make decisions *to enhance communication and help the caregiver and family members form realistic expectations.*

■ Conduct a home visit or evaluate the patient's description of his home *to assess safety needs and make recommendations for structural alterations. For example, the patient may benefit from installing ramps, enlarging doorways, or moving a second-floor bedroom to the first-floor family room.*

■ Discuss alternative housing opportunities with the patient and caregiver, such as moving the patient to a life-care community, *to provide necessary information to make appropriate decisions regarding the patient's future.*

■ Based on assessment of the patient's health and home environment, determine the need for assistive devices, including:

– hearing aids
– handheld or table-stand magnifying glasses
– hospital bed
– large-print items
– telephones for hearing impaired
– telephone dial covers with large numbers
– telephones with programmed dialing
– wheelchair
– amplifiers for phone receivers
– clocks that chime or recite time
– canes

– walkers
– handrails
– safety bars for toilet and bath
– automatic chair lifts
– commode chairs
– shower chairs
– orthotics.
Using assistive devices helps the patient remain independent and improves self-confidence and self-esteem.

▪ Help the patient develop written daily and weekly schedules for performing household tasks *to provide structure and consistency and set standards for measuring progress.*

▪ Involve the patient in the decision-making process by providing a choice of where, when, and how to carry out appropriate home maintenance activities *to increase the patient's feelings of independence and self-esteem.*

▪ If the patient can't perform certain tasks without assistance, teach the caregiver or others how to provide help *to ensure the patient's needs are met.*

Suggested NIC interventions

Environmental Management; Family Integrity Promotion; Home Maintenance Assistance; Role Enhancement

Evaluations for expected outcomes

▪ Patient and caregiver express understanding of changes needed to promote maximum health and safety in home.

▪ Patient and caregiver list community resources to assist with home maintenance deficits.

▪ Patient and caregiver establish and follow daily and weekly schedules for home maintenance activities.

Documentation

▪ Patient's perception of problems in home maintenance
▪ Observations regarding magnitude of home maintenance deficits
▪ Interventions to alleviate home maintenance deficits
▪ Responses of caregiver and others asked to assist patient with home maintenance
▪ Evaluations for expected outcomes

Reference

Leff, E.W., and Sonstegard-Gamm, J. "The Home Care Team Approach to Self-neglecting Elders," *Home Healthcare Nurse* 24(4):249-57, April 2006.

Risk for urge urinary
INCONTINENCE

Definition
Potential for involuntary passage of urine occurring shortly after a strong sense of urgency to void

Assessment
- Age and gender
- Vital signs
- Drug history
- History of illness that may cause neuromuscular dysfunction, including stroke, spinal cord injury, head injury, urinary tract disease, and infection
- Genitourinary status, including pain or discomfort, urinalysis, urine specific gravity, use of urinary assistive devices, voiding pattern, and cystometrogram results
- Fluid and electrolyte status, including intake and output, mucous membranes, postvoiding residual volume, skin turgor, and serum electrolyte, blood urea nitrogen, and creatinine levels
- Neuromuscular status, including ambulation ability, cognitive status, sensory ability, and degree of neuromuscular function
- Sexuality status, including patient's or partner's expressions of concern
- Psychosocial status, including coping skills, self-concept, stressors (finances, family, job), patient's and family members' perceptions of health problem, and patient's motivation to meet self-care needs

Risk factors
- Effects of medication, caffeine, or alcohol
- Detrusor hyperreflexia from cystitis, urethritis, tumors, renal calculi, central nervous system disorders above pontine micturation center
- Detrusor muscle instability with impaired contractility
- Ineffective toileting habits
- Involuntary sphincter relaxation
- Small bladder capacity

Expected outcomes
- Patient will state if he can anticipate when episodes of incontinence are likely to occur.
- Patient will state understanding of potential causes of urge incontinence and its treatment.
- Patient will avoid complications of urge incontinence or such complications will be minimized.
- Patient will discuss potential effects of urologic dysfunction on self and family members.
- Patient or family members will demonstrate skill in managing incontinence.

■ Patient and family members will identify community resources to help them cope with alterations in urinary status.

Suggested NOC outcomes

Knowledge: Treatment Regimen; Urinary Continence; Urinary Elimination

Interventions and rationales

■ Observe the patient's voiding pattern, and document intake and output *to ensure correct fluid replacement therapy and provide information about the patient's ability to void adequately.*

■ Determine the patient's premorbid elimination status *to ensure that interventions are realistic and based on the patient's health status and goals.*

■ Use an interdisciplinary approach to caring for incontinence. Incorporate recommendations from a urologist, urology nurse specialist, other health care providers, and the patient. Monitor progress and report the patient's response to interventions. *An interdisciplinary approach helps to ensure that the patient receives adequate care. Encouraging patient participation on the team will help foster motivation.*

■ Assess the patient's ability to sense and communicate elimination needs *to maximize self-care.*

■ Make sure the patient's toilet environment is warm, clean, and free from odor *to promote continence.*

■ Place a commode beside the bed. *A bedside commode requires less energy expenditure than using a bedpan or ambulating to a bathroom.*

■ Keep the bed and commode at same level *to facilitate easy access.*

■ Provide good lighting from bed to bathroom *to reduce confusion and risk of falls.*

■ Remove all obstacles between bed and bathroom *to reduce risk of falls.*

■ Provide a clock *to promote the patient's orientation to time.*

■ Unless contraindicated, provide 2½ to 3 qt (2.5 to 3L) of fluid daily *to moisten mucous membranes and ensure adequate hydration.* Space out fluid intake through the day and limit it to 150 ml after supper *to reduce the need to void at night.*

■ Have the patient wear easily removed articles of clothing (a gown instead of pajamas, Velcro fasteners instead of buttons or zippers) *to facilitate the removal of clothing and foster independence.*

■ Instruct the patient to stop and take a deep breath if he experiences an intense urge to urinate before he can reach a bathroom. *Anxiety and rushing may increase bladder contraction.*

■ Have the patient keep a diary recording episodes of incontinence. Use the information from the diary as a basis for planning interventions. Possible bladder training interventions may include voiding every 2 hours, avoiding high fluid intake, maintaining proper hygiene, or notifying a health care professional if urge incontinence occurs frequently. *Individualized interventions help promote self-care, foster motivation, and avoid incontinence.*

■ Incorporate the patient's suggestions for managing incontinent episodes into a care plan *to foster motivation.*

■ Encourage the patient to express his feelings regarding incontinence *to provide emotional support and identify areas for further patient teaching.*

■ Explain urge incontinence to the patient and family members, especially preventive measures and potential underlying causes, *to foster compliance.*

■ Note if the patient expresses concern about the effect of incontinence on sexuality. If appropriate, refer him to a sex therapist *to promote sexual health.*

■ Refer the patient and family members to community resources such as support groups, as appropriate, *to help ensure continuity of care.*

Suggested NIC interventions

Fluid Monitoring; Urinary Elimination Management; Urinary Habit Training; Urinary Incontinence Care

Evaluations for expected outcomes

■ Patient states if he can anticipate when episodes of incontinence are likely to occur.

■ Patient states understanding of potential causes of urge incontinence and its treatment.

■ Patient avoids complications of urge incontinence or complications are minimized.

■ Patient discusses potential effects of urologic dysfunction on self and family members.

■ Patient or family members demonstrate skill in managing incontinence.

■ Patient and family members identify community resources to help them cope with alterations in urinary status.

Documentation

■ Patient's urologic status

■ Episodes of urge incontinence

■ Nursing interventions and patient's response

■ Instruction given to patient and family and their response

■ Demonstrated ability to meet self-care needs

■ Patient's expression of concern about potential changes in urologic status and its impact on body image and lifestyle

■ Patient's statements indicating motivation to meet self-care needs

■ Evaluations for expected outcomes

Reference

Dingwall, L., and McLafferty, E. "Do Nurses Promote Urinary Continence in Hospitalized Older People? An Exploratory Study," *Journal of Clinical Nursing* 15(10):1276-86, October 2006.

Stress urinary
INCONTINENCE

Definition

Loss of less than 50 ml of urine occurring with increased abdominal pressure

Assessment

■ History of incontinence symptoms, including onset and pattern
■ Physical observations, including personal and perineal hygiene and complete bladder assessment
■ Mental status, including cognition and affect
■ Mobility status
■ Emotional status, including evidence of social withdrawal
■ Current medication regimen

Defining characteristics

■ Dribbling with increased abdominal pressure
■ Frequency
■ Urgency

Expected outcomes

■ Patient will understand causes of stress incontinence.
■ Patient will establish plan compatible with lifestyle to manage symptoms.
■ Patient will resume normal social activities.
■ Patient will maintain continence with the aid of incontinence pads or frequent toileting.
■ Patient will perform Kegel exercises.

Suggested NOC outcomes

Knowledge: Treatment Regimen; Tissue Integrity: Skin/Mucous Membranes; Urinary Continence; Urinary Elimination

Interventions and rationales

■ Discuss stress incontinence and associated social stigma with the patient in a nonjudgmental manner. Tell the patient many people experience incontinence. *The patient may be reluctant to discuss incontinence, which can have a negative effect on self-image. A nonjudgmental approach may help ease embarrassment and encourage open discussion of the problem.*
■ Assist the patient in obtaining appropriate evaluation and care for the underlying causes of stress incontinence *to ensure prompt diagnosis and treatment.*
■ Review the current medication regimen for drugs that can contribute to stress incontinence, including diuretics, central nervous system depressants, and anticholinergics. Discuss with the physician the possibility of changing medications or the medication schedule *to relieve symptoms.*

■ Develop an individualized toileting schedule, increasing intervals by 30 minutes until the patient achieves a 2- to 3 hour pattern. *Bladder retraining may help alleviate symptoms.*

■ Teach the patient to do Kegel exercises to strengthen pelvic floor muscles. Instruct the patient to tighten the muscles of the pelvic floor to stop the flow of urine while urinating and then to release the muscles to restart the flow *to strengthen the urinary sphincter muscle and restore control.*

■ Discuss the benefits and costs of adult incontinence pads with the patient. *Pads, although costly, are nonintrusive, easy to manage, and easily removed.*

■ Encourage the patient to take short trips outside the home when his symptoms are under control *to enhance the patient's confidence and reduce social embarrassment.*

■ When mobility is a problem, help the patient obtain a bedside commode *to reduce the need for adult incontinence pads, which can adversely affect the patient's self-image.*

Suggested NIC interventions

Pelvic Muscle Exercise; Urinary Elimination Management; Urinary Incontinence Care

Evaluations for expected outcomes

■ Patient expresses, without embarrassment, understanding of causes of stress incontinence.

■ Patient manages symptoms successfully.

■ Patient begins to resume social activity.

■ Patient maintains continence with aid of incontinence pads or frequent toileting.

■ Patient performs Kegel exercises.

Documentation

■ Patient's symptoms of stress incontinence, including onset and pattern

■ Patient teaching, including Kegel exercises, use of incontinence pads, and other control strategies

■ Patient's response to nursing interventions

■ Evaluations for expected outcomes

Reference

Zurakowski, T., et al. "Effective Teaching Strategies for the Older Adult with Urologic Concerns," *Urologic Nursing* 26(5):355-60, October 2006.

Risk for
INJURY

related to elder abuse

Definition
At risk of injury as a result of environmental conditions interacting with the individual's adaptive and defensive resources

Assessment
- Age
- Gender
- Patient's health status, including presence of acute or chronic illness and changes or deterioration in mental or physical functioning
- Family status, including communication patterns and presence or absence of extended family
- Family members' willingness and ability to provide physical and emotional support to patient
- Evidence of physical abuse, including malnutrition, imprint of hand or fingers, marks from restraints, and unexplained bruises, burns, welts, cuts, dislocations, or abrasions
- Evidence of emotional abuse, including observation or reports of insults, ridicule, or humiliation
- Evidence of financial abuse, including unexplained changes in bank accounts and transfer of funds to caregivers
- Evidence of neglect, including inappropriate clothing, unsanitary living conditions, inadequate food supplies, lack of medication, and absence of needed eyeglasses, hearing aids, cane, or walker

Risk factors
- Dependence on family members for daily care (patient)
- Deteriorating health, frailty, or impaired mobility (patient)
- Expressed frustration over responsibilities of caring for older family member (caregiver)
- Isolation from community, without relatives living nearby (caregiver)
- Limited education or inadequate financial resources (caregiver)
- Reported lack of social contacts outside family (patient)

Expected outcomes
- Patient will remain free from injury and will state that incidents of abuse no longer occur.
- Patient will express understanding of right to be free from abuse.
- Patient will report increased social contact outside family.
- Patient will establish "buddy system," whereby he and friend visit or telephone each other at regularly scheduled intervals.
- Patient will maintain control over mail, telephone, and other personal effects.

■ Caregiver will state intention to contact respite care services, support groups, and other community resources.

■ Caregiver will report increased ability to cope with responsibilities of caring for older family member.

■ Patient and caregiver will report improved communication patterns.

Suggested NOC outcomes

Risk Control; Safe Home Environment

Interventions and rationales

■ Monitor the patient closely at each visit for evidence of physical or mental abuse or neglect. Observe for bruises or abrasions, body odor, or a dirty, unkempt appearance *to ensure his safety and well-being.* Question him privately about findings *to encourage trust and promote open communication.*

■ Encourage the patient to discuss incidents of abuse or threats of abuse. Be willing to listen and be careful to convey a nonjudgmental attitude. *Older patients may be reluctant to discuss abuse or threats of abuse because of the fear of retaliation, embarrassment, or a reluctance to report family members to authorities. By communicating that you care and are willing to listen, you may help the patient overcome these barriers.*

■ Teach the patient about his right to be free from abuse. Discuss the responsibility of law enforcement agencies to investigate incidents of abuse. Provide a list of social service agencies that can provide counseling *to empower the patient to resist or prevent episodes of abuse.*

■ Encourage the patient to maintain the use of a personal telephone and open his own mail *to promote a sense of control and self-worth and maintain contact with people outside the home.*

■ Encourage the patient to participate in community activities, such as religious groups and senior volunteer organizations, *to establish social contacts and develop a strong support network.*

■ Suggest the use of Meals On Wheels or a community geriatric outreach for the homebound patient *to prevent isolation and provide respite for the family caregiver.*

■ Encourage friends to visit the patient at home. Suggest that the patient and a friend develop a "buddy system," whereby each takes turns telephoning or visiting the other at regular intervals *to provide social contact, respite for the caregiver, and an additional safeguard against abuse.*

■ If appropriate, encourage the patient and family members to periodically hold conferences. Help the patient and family members identify productive topics for discussion, such as strategies for dealing with the patient's self-care deficits or scheduling respite care, *to foster open communication, defuse tension, and develop solutions to practical problems of caring for an older family member.*

■ Inform the caregiver about state and county services for the elderly, respite services, adult day care, support groups for children of aging parents, and other community resources *to enhance the caregiver's ability to cope and thereby diminish the likelihood of abuse.*

■ Report actual or suspected elder abuse to local authorities and provide follow-up or emergency care, if needed. *Nearly every state has laws mandating that suspected elder abuse be reported to authorities.*

Suggested NIC interventions

Abuse Protection Support; Environmental Management: Violence Prevention; Family Mobilization; Risk Identification; Surveillance: Safety

Evaluations for expected outcomes

- Patient doesn't exhibit injuries and states that incidents of abuse have stopped.
- Patient expresses understanding of right to be protected from abuse.
- Patient reports satisfaction with ability to maintain or increase social contacts outside family.
- Patient establishes "buddy system" with friend outside home.
- Patient maintains control over mail, telephone, and other personal effects.
- Caregiver regularly attends community support group and contacts appropriate social service agencies and other sources of support.
- Caregiver reports increased ability to cope with responsibilities of caring for older family member.
- Patient and caregiver report improved communication.

Documentation

- Evidence of emotional, physical, or financial neglect or abuse
- Patient's statements that indicate risk of abuse
- Caregiver's statements indicating feelings about caring for older family member
- Caregiver's statements indicating willingness to attend support groups or use community resources
- Patient's and caregiver's expressed understanding of teaching provided by nurse
- Patient's response to nursing interventions
- Evaluations for expected outcomes

Reference

Muehlbauer, M., and Crane, P.A. "Elder Abuse and Neglect," *Journal of Psychosocial Nursing and Mental Health Services* 44(11):43-48, November 2006.

Deficient
KNOWLEDGE
related to difficulty understanding disease process and its effect on self-care

Definition

Absence or deficiency of cognitive information related to a specific topic

Assessment

- Current knowledge level
- Interest and motivation to learn
- Preferred learning style
- Comprehension ability and reading level

■ Other factors that may affect learning, such as cultural influences; religious practices and beliefs; sensory, cognitive, or physical impairment; support systems; economic status; and feelings of anger, depression, or hopelessness

Defining characteristics
■ Inability to follow through with instruction
■ Inappropriate or exaggerated behaviors (hysteria, hostility, agitation, apathy)
■ Poor performance on test of knowledge
■ Verbalization of problem

Expected outcomes
■ Patient will express understanding of disease process, medication regimen, and treatment plan.
■ Patient will make informed choices when addressing health care problems and self-care deficits.
■ Patient will demonstrate ability to effectively implement chosen health care strategy.

Suggested NOC outcomes

Knowledge: Disease Process; Knowledge: Medication; Knowledge: Treatment Procedure(s)

Interventions and rationales
■ Consider the older patient's life experiences when developing a teaching plan. *New information is easier to assimilate if it's built on existing knowledge.*
■ Provide a quiet, calm environment for learning *to enable the patient to process information without distraction from background noise or stress.*
■ Limit the length of each teaching session *to avoid information overload.*
■ Ask the patient if he wants to learn new or additional information. If not, discuss why. *Open discussion helps identify barriers to learning and determines if these barriers may be eliminated. Discussion also promotes acceptance of the patient's right to choose his own level of participation.*
■ Encourage the patient to use memory aids, such as preset alarms on a watch, a calendar for noting scheduled appointments, and a small notepad for recording questions or symptoms, *to help compensate for memory lapses.*
■ Write instructions in large letters, using black ink or contrasting colors. *Older patients see black best and may have difficulty distinguishing pastels or monochromatic color schemes.*
■ Modify your teaching style to accommodate normal aging changes:
– Face the patient when speaking.
– Use a well-modulated voice.
– Allow ample time for teaching sessions.
Understanding normal age-related changes enhances teaching effectiveness.
■ Set aside time during each session for answering questions and clarifying information. *An older patient may need affirmation that the knowledge he possesses is current and correct. Discussion may also stimulate an exchange of ideas and further learning.*

■ Encourage the patient to join a support group, such as a club for stroke survivors or a support group for cancer patients, *to reinforce education and promote contact with others in the same situation.*

■ Involve the caregiver in teaching sessions, when appropriate, *to reinforce information and ensure continuity of care at home.*

Suggested NIC interventions

Family Support; Health System Guidance; Support Group; Teaching: Disease Process; Teaching: Prescribed Medication; Teaching: Procedure/ Treatment

Evaluations for expected outcomes

■ Patient expresses increased understanding of disease process, medication regimen, and treatment plan, describing at least three basic concepts relevant to disease process and its impact on activities of daily living (ADLs).

■ Patient states at least four strategies to improve self-care and expresses understanding of how chosen strategies will provide relief from disease process and improve his ability to perform ADLs.

■ Patient demonstrates ongoing ability to implement chosen health care strategies.

Documentation

■ Patient's verbal statements and behavior that indicate deficient knowledge

■ Teaching provided and patient's or caregiver's response, including questions and comments made during teaching sessions

■ Patient's description of chosen intervention strategies

■ Patient's statements and behaviors that indicate implementation of strategies

■ Evaluations for expected outcomes

Reference

Stotts, N.A., and Hopf, H.W. "Facilitating Positive Outcomes in Older Adults with Wounds," *The Nursing Clinics of North America* 40(2):267-79, June 2005.

Impaired bed
MOBILITY
related to neuromuscular dysfunction

Definition

Limitation of ability to move about in bed

Assessment

■ Age and gender

■ Vital signs

■ History of neuromuscular disorder or dysfunction

■ Drug history

■ Musculoskeletal status, including coordination, muscle size and strength, muscle tone, range of motion (ROM), and functional mobility as follows:

0 = completely independent

1 = requires use of equipment or device

2 = requires help, supervision, or teaching from another person

3 = requires help from another person and equipment or device

4 = dependent; doesn't participate in activity

■ Neurologic status, including level of consciousness, motor ability, and sensory ability

Defining characteristics

■ Impaired ability to:

– move from supine to long sitting or long sitting to supine

– move from supine to prone or prone to supine

– move from supine to sitting or sitting to supine

– "scoot" or reposition self in bed

– turn side to side

Expected outcomes

■ Patient won't exhibit complications associated with impaired bed mobility, such as altered skin integrity, contractures, venous stasis, thrombus formation, depression, altered health maintenance, and falls.

■ Patient will maintain or improve muscle strength and joint ROM.

■ Patient will achieve highest level of bed mobility possible (independence, independence with device, verbalization of needs for assistance with bed mobility, requires assistance of one person, requires assistance of two people).

■ Patient will maintain safety while in bed.

■ Patient will demonstrate ability to use equipment or devices to assist with moving about in bed safely.

■ Patient will adapt to alteration in ability to move about in bed.

■ Patient will participate in social, physical, and occupational activities to the extent possible.

Suggested NOC outcomes

Body Positioning: Self-Initiated; Immobility Consequences: Physiological; Immobility Consequences: Psycho-Cognitive; Mobility

Interventions and rationales

■ Perform ROM exercises to affected joints, unless contraindicated, at least once per shift. Progress from passive to active ROM, as tolerated, *to prevent joint contractures and muscle atrophy.*

■ Assist the patient in maintaining anatomically correct and functional body positioning. Encourage repositioning every 2 hours while in bed. Establish a turning schedule for immobile patients. *Proper positioning relieves pressure, thereby preventing skin breakdown, and helps prevent fluid accumulation in dependent extremities.*

■ Identify the patient's level of independence using the functional mobility scale. Communicate your findings to staff *to provide continuity of care and preserve the documented level of independence.*

■ Monitor and record daily evidence of complications related to impaired bed mobility (contractures, venous stasis, skin breakdown, thrombus formation, depression, altered health maintenance or self-care skills, falls). *Patients with neuromuscular dysfunction are at risk for complications.*

■ Perform a medical regimen to manage or prevent complications (for example, administer prophylactic heparin for venous stasis) *to promote the patient's health and well-being.*

■ Assess the patient's skin every 2 hours *to maintain skin integrity.*

■ Help the patient move about in bed. Encourage progressive mobility up to the limits imposed by the patient's condition *to maintain muscle tone, prevent complications associated with immobility, and promote self-care.*

■ Refer the patient to a physical therapist for development of a program to improve bed mobility *to assist with rehabilitation of musculoskeletal deficits.*

■ Refer the patient to an occupational therapist for development of a program to maximize self-care *to promote restoration of self-care skills.*

■ Encourage the patient to participate in physical and occupational therapy sessions. Incorporate equipment, devices, and techniques used by therapists into your care. Request written instructions from the patient's therapists to use as a reference *to help ensure continuity of care and reinforce learned skills.*

■ If you're uncertain about your ability to move the patient, request help from colleagues *to maintain safety.*

■ Instruct the patient and family members in techniques to improve bed mobility and ways to prevent complications *to help prepare the patient and family members for discharge.*

■ Demonstrate the patient's bed mobility regimen and note the date. Have the patient and family members perform a return demonstration *to ensure continuity of care and use of proper technique.*

■ Assist the patient in identifying and contacting resources for social and spiritual support *to promote the patient's reintegration into the community and help him maintain psychosocial health.*

Suggested NIC interventions

Bed Rest Care; Body Mechanics Promotion; Circulatory Precautions; Exercise Promotion: Strength Training; Exercise Therapy: Joint Mobility; Fall Prevention; Positioning; Skin Surveillance

Evaluations for expected outcomes

■ Patient doesn't exhibit complications associated with impaired bed mobility, such as altered skin integrity, contractures, venous stasis, thrombus formation, depression, altered health maintenance, and falls.

■ Patient maintains or improves muscle strength and joint ROM.

■ Patient achieves highest level of bed mobility possible (independence, independence with device, verbalization of needs for assistance with bed mobility, requires assistance of one person, requires assistance of two people).

■ Patient maintains safety while in bed.

■ Patient demonstrates ability to use equipment or devices to assist with moving about in bed safely.

■ Patient adapts to alteration in ability to move about in bed.

■ Patient participates in social, physical, and occupational activities to the greatest extent possible.

Documentation

■ Patient's bed mobility status

■ Presence of complications

■ Referrals for physical or occupational therapy

■ Response to program to improve or restore bed mobility

■ Patient's statements regarding the loss of bed mobility skills and his goals for improving bed mobility

■ Teaching provided to patient and family members

■ Patient's and family members' demonstrated skill in carrying out bed mobility program

■ Evaluations for expected outcomes

References

de Laat, E.H., et al. "Epidemiology, Risk and Prevention of Pressure Ulcers in Critically Ill Patients: A Literature Review," *Journal of Wound Care* 15(6):269-75, June 2006.

Lyder, C.H. "Assessing Risk and Preventing Pressure Ulcers in Patients with Cancer," *Seminars in Oncology Nursing* 22(3):178-84, August 2006.

Impaired wheelchair
MOBILITY
related to neuromuscular disorder or dysfunction

Definition
Limitation in independent, purposeful physical movement of the body or one or more extremities

Assessment
■ Age and gender

■ Vital signs

■ History of neuromuscular disorder or dysfunction

■ Drug history

■ Musculoskeletal status, including coordination, gait, muscle size and strength, muscle tone, range of motion (ROM), and functional mobility as follows:

0 = completely independent

1 = requires use of equipment or device

2 = requires help, supervision, or teaching from another person

3 = requires help from another person and equipment or device

4 = dependent; doesn't participate in activity

■ Neurologic status, including level of consciousness, motor ability, and sensory ability

■ Characteristics of patient's wheelchair (for example, whether standard or motorized) and adequacy of wheelchair for meeting patient's needs (right size, appropriate safety features, and easy for patient to operate)

■ Endurance (length of time patient can operate wheelchair before becoming fatigued)

Defining characteristics

■ Postural instability during routine activities of daily living
■ Decreased reaction time
■ Difficulty turning
■ Engages in substitutions for movement
■ Gait changes
■ Limited ability to perform gross motor skills
■ Limited ROM
■ Movement-induced shortness of breath
■ Movement-induced tremor
■ Slowed movement
■ Uncoordinated or jerky movements

Expected outcomes

■ Patient won't exhibit complications associated with impaired wheelchair mobility, such as skin breakdown, contractures, venous stasis, thrombus formation, depression, alteration in health maintenance, and falls.
■ Patient will maintain or improve muscle strength and joint ROM.
■ Patient will achieve highest level of independence possible with regard to wheelchair use.
■ Patient will express feelings regarding alteration in ability to use wheelchair.
■ Patient will maintain safety when using wheelchair.
■ Patient will adapt to alteration in ability.
■ Patient will participate in social and occupational activities to the greatest extent possible.
■ Patient will demonstrate understanding of techniques to improve wheelchair mobility.

Suggested NOC outcomes

Ambulation: Wheelchair; Balance; Immobility Consequences: Physiological; Immobility Consequences: Psycho-Cognitive; Mobility

Interventions and rationales

■ Perform ROM exercises for affected joints, unless contraindicated, at least once per shift. Progress from passive to active ROM, as tolerated, *to prevent joint contractures and muscle atrophy.*

■ Make sure the patient maintains anatomically correct and functional body positioning while in the wheelchair *to promote comfort.* Explain to the patient where vulnerable pressure points are and teach him to shift and reposition his weight *to prevent skin breakdown.*

■ Assess whether the patient's wheelchair is adequate to meet his needs *to help maintain mobility and independence.* Consider the following:

– Is the seat the right size? It should be wide and deep enough to support the patient's thighs and allow him to sit comfortably. It should be low enough so that the patient's feet touch the floor but high enough to allow easy transfer from bed to chair. The chair's back should be tall enough to support the patient's upper body.

– Is the chair easy for the patient to operate when weak? If the patient has little or no arm strength, he may need a motorized wheelchair.

– Is the chair safe? All wheelchairs have safety features, such as brakes that lock the wheels, but some safety features can be modified to meet the patient's needs. For example, seat belts can be attached at the waist, hips, or chest.

■ Identify the patient's level of independence using the functional mobility scale. Communicate findings to staff *to promote continuity of care and preserve the documented level of independence.*

■ Monitor and record daily evidence of complications related to impaired wheelchair mobility (contractures, venous stasis, skin breakdown, thrombus formation, depression, and alteration in health maintenance or self-care skills). *Patients with neuromuscular dysfunction are at risk for complications.*

■ Encourage the patient to operate his wheelchair independently to the limits imposed by his condition *to maintain muscle tone, prevent complications of immobility, and promote independence in self-care and health maintenance skills.*

■ Refer the patient to a physical therapist for development of a program to enhance wheelchair mobility *to assist with rehabilitation of musculoskeletal deficits.*

■ Encourage attendance at physical therapy sessions and reinforce prescribed activities on the unit by using equipment, devices, and techniques used in the therapy session. Request a written copy of the patient's rehabilitation program to use as a reference *to maintain continuity of care and promote patient safety.*

■ Assess the patient's skin on his return to bed and request a wheelchair cushion, if necessary, *to maintain the patient's skin integrity.*

■ Demonstrate techniques to promote wheelchair mobility to the patient and family members, and note the date *to help prepare the patient for discharge and maintain safety.* For example, teach the patient and family members how to perform wheelchair push-ups. If the patient can move his arms, have him grip the arms of the chair and push down hard with his hands and arms to try to raise his body off the seat. Have the patient and family members perform a return demonstration *to ensure continuity of care and use of proper technique.*

■ Assist in identifying resources for helping the patient maintain the highest level of mobility, such as a community stroke program, sports associations for people with disabilities, or the National Multiple Sclerosis Society, *to promote the patient's reintegration into the community.*

Suggested NIC interventions

Exercise Promotion: Strength Training; Exercise Therapy: Balance; Exercise Therapy: Muscle Control; Mutual Goal Setting; Positioning: Wheelchair

Evaluations for expected outcomes
- Patient doesn't exhibit complications associated with impaired wheelchair mobility, such as skin breakdown, contractures, venous stasis, thrombus formation, depression, alteration in health maintenance, and falls.
- Patient maintains or improves muscle strength and joint ROM.
- Patient achieves highest level of independence possible with regard to wheelchair use.
- Patient expresses feelings regarding alteration in ability to use wheelchair.
- Patient maintains safety when using wheelchair.
- Patient adapts to alteration in ability.
- Patient participates in social and occupational activities to the greatest extent possible.
- Patient demonstrates understanding of techniques to improve wheelchair mobility.

Documentation
- Observations of changes in patient's mobility status and related complications
- Patient's expression of concern about loss of wheelchair mobility
- Patient's goals for future regarding mobility status
- Teaching provided to patient
- Patient's return demonstration of skills in carrying out wheelchair mobility program
- Patient's response to nursing interventions
- Evaluations for expected outcomes

Reference
Gavin-Dreschnack, D., et al. "Wheelchair-related Falls: Current Evidence and Directions for Improved Quality Care," *Journal of Nursing Care Quality* 20(2):119-27, April-June 2005.

Imbalanced
NUTRITION: MORE THAN BODY REQUIREMENTS
related to a decline in basal metabolic rate and physical activity

Definition
Intake of nutrients that exceeds metabolic needs

Assessment
- Activity level
- Health history, including evidence of impaired mobility, chronic illness, use of appetite-stimulating medications, lack of exercise, and family history of obesity
- Nutritional status, including height and weight, usual dietary pattern, stated food preferences, and weight fluctuations

■ Psychosocial factors, including lifestyle, ethnic background, socioeconomic status, education level, mode of transportation, internal and external cues that trigger desire to eat, motivation to lose weight, and rate of food consumption
■ Home environment, including presence of family members or significant other, responsibility for grocery shopping and meal preparation, food storage and preparation facilities, and access to transportation

Defining characteristics
■ Body weight 10% or more over ideal weight
■ Dysfunctional eating patterns, such as concentrating food intake at end of day, eating in response to internal cue other than hunger (such as boredom), eating in response to external cues (such as social situations), and pairing food with other activities
■ Sedentary lifestyle
■ Triceps skin-fold measurement greater than 15 mm in men and 25 mm in women

Expected outcomes
■ Patient will express understanding of why obesity is a problem.
■ Patient will develop realistic goals for weight reduction and will plan to achieve these goals.
■ Patient will lose specified amount of weight per week.
■ Patient will carry out exercise and activity plan.

Suggested NOC outcomes
Adherence Behavior; Knowledge: Treatment Regimen; Nutritional Status; Nutritional Status: Nutrient Intake; Weight Control

Interventions and rationales
■ Assess the patient's perception of his weight problem. Determine whether the patient understands that obesity affects his lifestyle and creates health risks *to evaluate the patient's motivation to lose weight and determine an appropriate plan of action.*
■ Encourage the patient to keep a food diary *to track dietary intake accurately.*
■ Teach the patient about changes in nutrient and vitamin needs that occur with aging *to promote well-informed food choices. Dietary requirements diminish with age; the older patient's caloric requirements decrease by 10% to 25%.*
■ If the patient lacks motivation or resources for preparing balanced meals, provide information on appropriate community services, such as Meals On Wheels or federally sponsored nutrition programs, *to help the patient obtain healthier meals.*
■ Encourage the patient to make gradual improvements in eating habits; for example, slowly introduce low-calorie, nutritious foods into the diet. Keep in mind that the older patient has developed his current habits over many years. *Planning for gradual changes increases the chances of success.*
■ Set a realistic goal for weight loss; weekly loss of ½ to 1 lb (0.2 to 0.5 kg) is adequate. *Realistic goals increase motivation and ensure the success of a weight-control program.*

■ If appropriate, have a registered dietitian discuss meal planning and food preparation with the patient, taking into account physical, psychological, socioeconomic, and cultural factors, *to provide appropriate nutritional guidance.*

■ Help the patient develop a modified exercise plan, such as regular walking, *to burn calories, increase endurance, and maintain musculoskeletal strength. Regular exercise enhances the patient's motivation and self-concept.*

■ Provide ongoing support and recognition of the patient's progress *to reinforce changes in eating habits and help the patient assess progress accurately.*

■ Provide the patient with information on social events and artistic, cultural, and educational programs *to stimulate the patient to become more active.*

Suggested NIC interventions

Behavior Modification; Nutrition Management; Nutritional Monitoring; Weight Reduction Assistance

Evaluations for expected outcomes

■ Patient expresses understanding of consequences of continued obesity.
■ Patient actively participates in developing weight-reduction goals.
■ Patient loses specified amount of weight per week.
■ Patient carries out exercise and activity plan.

Documentation

■ Patient's weight
■ Patient's expression of feelings about obesity
■ Observations of patient's eating patterns
■ Weight-reduction plan
■ Teaching provided and patient's response
■ Evaluations for expected outcomes

Reference

Gallagher Camden, S., and Gates, J. "Obesity: Changing Face of Geriatric Care," *Ostomy/Wound Management* 53(10):36-38, 40-44, October 2006.

Readiness for enhanced
NUTRITION

Definition

A pattern of nutrient intake that's sufficient for meeting metabolic needs and can be strengthened

Assessment

■ Biological factors, including age, gender, and height, weight, and body mass index

■ Psychological factors, including self-esteem, history of depression, and attitudes toward food and eating

■ Sociocultural factors, including moral or health concerns about food and eating, financial status, and cultural background and influences of same in food choices

■ Environmental factors, including ability to read and understand food labels, percentage of meals that are take-out, fast food, or eaten in restaurants, and cost of food in a particular geographical area

Defining characteristics
■ Adequate food and fluid consumed
■ Attitude toward eating and drinking congruent with health goals
■ Regular eating
■ Willingness to enhance nutrition

Expected outcomes
■ Patient will articulate present understanding of factors that enable and hinder enhanced nutritional status.
■ Patient will evaluate each of the barriers to enhancing nutritional status.
■ Patient will articulate the personal value of practicing positive behaviors.
■ Patient will plan modifications of environment, which will reinforce change in eating habits.
■ Patient will express positive feelings about self.

Suggested NOC outcomes

Knowledge: Diet; Nutritional Status; Nutritional Status: Biochemical Measures

Interventions and rationales
■ Provide the patient with materials that are intellectually and culturally appropriate for enhancing nutritional knowledge. *It's important to engage the patient in information gathering before beginning to develop a plan to change behavior.*
■ Help the patient list the internal and external barriers to improving nutritional status. *Lack of understanding of the patient's individual barriers, such as unclear goals, lack of skill, or lack of motivation will prevent change from occurring.*
■ Have the patient make a list of the positive outcomes of changing the behaviors, such as wearing smaller size clothing, feeling better about being with others who are health conscious, enjoying feelings of physical and emotional well-being. *Positive reinforcers make the changes more appealing to effect.*
■ Teach the patient to read food labels, to plan meals using a standard method such as the Food Guide Pyramid (American Dietetic Association), and to shop for and stock the refrigerator and pantry with smart food choices. *New behaviors require practice in a practical sense for the kind of reinforcement that will produce the desired change.*
■ Encourage the patient to join or form some type of group *to help maintain the motivation to continue new behaviors.*

Suggested NIC interventions

Nutrition Management; Nutritional Monitoring; Nutritional Counseling; Teaching: Prescribed Diet

Evaluations for expected outcomes

■ Patient articulates present understanding of factors that enable and hinder enhanced nutritional status.

■ Patient evaluates each of the barriers to enhancing nutritional status.

■ Patient articulates the personal value of practicing positive behaviors.

■ Patient plans modifications of environment, which will reinforce change in eating habits.

■ Patient expresses positive feelings about self.

Documentation

■ Weight changes

■ Patient's expressed attitudes toward food and eating

■ Patient's expressed feelings about weight, body image, and emotional status

■ Patient's participation in a group

■ Patient's response to nursing interventions

■ Evaluations for expected outcomes

Reference

Green, S.M., and Watson, R. "Nutritional Screening and Assessment Tools for Older Adults: Literature Review," *Journal of Advanced Nursing* 54(4):477-90, May 2006.

Risk for
POISONING

related to drug toxicity or polypharmacy

Definition

Accentuated risk of ingestion of drugs or dangerous products in doses sufficient to cause poisoning

Assessment

■ Age

■ Gender

■ Drug history, including use of prescription and over-the-counter medications

■ Use of alcoholic beverages

■ Health history, including evidence of hepatic or renal impairment

■ Nutritional status, including weight changes, protein intake, and fluid status

■ Psychosocial history, including activity level, knowledge level, financial status, mental status, and living arrangements

■ Laboratory studies, including toxicology screening; serum digoxin, serum electrolyte, blood urea nitrogen, serum creatinine, and bilirubin levels; liver enzymes, such as aspartate aminotransferase, alanine aminotransferase, and alkaline phosphatase; and total serum protein and albumin to globulin ratio

Risk factors
■ Cognitive or emotional difficulties, including forgetfulness or confusion
■ Drugs stored near bedside
■ History of drug abuse or alcoholism
■ Impaired vision
■ Inability to read medication labels
■ Living alone
■ Multiple health care providers, drug prescriptions, and pharmacies
■ Poor bowel habits, including chronic use of enemas or laxative abuse
■ Poor understanding of drug interactions
■ Poor understanding of drug usage
■ Poor understanding of precautions necessary for safe drug therapy

Expected outcomes
■ Patient will express understanding of medication regimen.
■ Patient won't experience episodes of toxicity.
■ Patient's medical condition will remain under control.
■ Patient will take only prescribed medications in correct quantities at correct times.

Suggested NOC outcomes
Personal Safety Behavior; Safe Home Environment

Interventions and rationales
■ Instruct the patient or family member in the drug regimen, including the reasons for taking drugs, safety precautions, and how to monitor the effectiveness of drugs, *to increase compliance.*
■ Regularly review and document the patient's medication regimen *to monitor medication use, assess whether certain medications should be discontinued, and monitor for drug interactions.*
■ Instruct the patient or family member to store drugs in secure area away from the bedside *to prevent accidental ingestion. Many older patients keep medications at their bedside to decrease the need to arise during the night.*
■ If color-coding medications, use only bright, contrasting colors. *Older patients can't distinguish pastel colors well.*
■ Help the patient or family member identify behaviors that contribute to the risk of toxicity, such as obtaining prescriptions from various health care providers or using different pharmacies, *to raise awareness of potential hazards.*
■ Encourage the patient or family member to retain a primary physician who co-ordinates care. *Older patients with multiple health problems may receive care from various providers who are unaware of each other's treatment plans and medication regimens.*
■ Provide instructions for the use of medications, including quantity, frequency, and number of doses, *to enhance understanding of the medication regimen and in-*

crease compliance. Make sure the instructions are clearly written in black or blue ink. *Older patients can read black or blue ink more easily.*

■ Make sure all medication labels are inscribed in large print and include dosage instructions *to avoid medication errors.*

■ Help the patient maintain an accurate and effective system for following the medication regimen, such as a check-off calendar system or separate pill boxes labeled for each day of the week, *to reduce errors.* Encourage the patient to work with a pharmacist when developing this system.

■ Monitor the patient's urine and serum toxicity levels, when indicated, *to reduce the risk of toxicity. Age-related changes in body function may lead to decreased renal, liver, and GI clearance of drugs, increasing the patient's risk of toxicity. Also, various drugs commonly used by the older patient increases the risk of toxicity from drug interactions.*

■ Discuss with the physician the possibility of using alternative drugs, such as long-acting preparations or drugs that require only one dose per day, *to simplify the drug regimen and thereby decrease the risk of toxicity.*

Suggested NIC interventions

Environmental Management: Safety; Health Education; Risk Identification; Substance Use Prevention

Evaluation for expected outcomes

■ Patient expresses understanding of medication regimen.

■ Patient doesn't experience episodes of toxicity.

■ Patient's existing medical condition remains under control.

■ Patient takes only prescribed drugs in correct quantities at correct times.

Documentation

■ Evidence of patient's or family member's lack of understanding of or poor compliance with medication regimen

■ Additional factors that increase patient's risk of drug toxicity

■ Physical findings

■ Instructions provided about safe drug practices

■ Patient's or family member's response to instructions

■ Patient's response to nursing interventions

■ Evaluations for expected outcomes

Reference

Bergman-Evans, B. "Evidence-based Guideline. Improving Medication Management for Older Adult Clients," *Journal of Gerontological Nursing* 32(7):6-14, July 2006.

POWERLESSNESS

related to perceived loss of control over life situation

Definition
Feeling of helplessness, hopelessness, and lack of control

Assessment
■ Environmental factors, such as institutional setting
■ Impact of therapeutic regimens on lifestyle, including use of cane or walker, changes in diet, and medication regimen
■ Economic status, including retirement income, medical expenses such as ongoing home care or placement in nursing home, and Medicare or other insurance coverage
■ Emotional status, including recent loss of spouse and history of dependence on others
■ Physical impairments, including arthritic conditions, loss of limb use, diminished vision, and lengthy or chronic illness

Defining characteristics
■ Apathy
■ Depression over physical deterioration
■ Expressed dissatisfaction over inability to perform previous tasks
■ Expressed lack of control over self-care, current situation, and outcome
■ Expressed resentment, anger, and guilt
■ Expressed self-doubt
■ Failure to defend self-care practices
■ Failure to monitor progress
■ Failure to seek information about care
■ Irritability because of dependence on others
■ Passivity
■ Reluctance to express true feelings because of fear of alienating caregivers
■ Reluctance to participate in decisions about health
■ Uncertainty about fluctuating energy levels

Expected outcomes
■ Patient will identify aspects of life still under his control.
■ Patient will help develop schedule for self-care activities.
■ Patient will participate in decisions about his care and lifestyle.
■ Patient will express more realistic expectations and increased satisfaction with current situation.

Suggested NOC outcomes

Depression Self-Control; Family Participation in Professional Care; Health Beliefs; Health Beliefs: Perceived Resources

Interventions and rationales

■ Guide the patient through a life review. Encourage the patient to reflect on past achievements *to foster a sense of satisfaction and promote acceptance of his current status.*

■ Help the patient establish realistic expectations and goals. *Having realistic expectations helps prevent failures, which might exacerbate feelings of powerlessness.*

■ Help the patient identify the aspects of his life that are still under his control. For example, offer the patient a chance to request changes to the arrangement of the furniture in his room. Recognize the patient's right to express feelings. *Empowering the older patient in any way possible may prevent feelings of powerlessness from becoming overwhelming.*

■ Encourage the patient to make choices in scheduling his daily routine, including personal hygiene, dressing and grooming, meals, and physical therapy. Emphasize that the patient, not staff members, has the authority to make scheduling decisions. *This helps the patient reassert control.*

■ Ask the patient open-ended questions rather than questions that he can answer with "yes" or "no." *Open-ended questions encourage the patient to assert his opinions and thereby regain a feeling of control.*

■ Encourage staff members to express interest in the patient's progress and set aside time to listen attentively to the patient *to acknowledge and reinforce his efforts to regain control.*

■ Encourage the patient to take an active role in choosing among social and recreational activities *to enhance the patient's lifestyle and further diminish feelings of powerlessness.*

Suggested NIC interventions

Decision-Making Support; Family Involvement Promotion; Financial Resource Assistance; Health System Guidance; Self-Esteem Enhancement; Values Clarification

Evaluations for expected outcomes

■ Patient identifies aspects of life still under his control and describes actions he can take to improve or modify his routine.

■ Patient displays an appropriate sense of responsibility in scheduling self-care activities.

■ Patient takes part in decisions about his care and lifestyle.

■ Patient expresses more realistic expectations and increased satisfaction with current situation.

Documentation

■ Patient's verbal and behavioral expressions of powerlessness
■ Patient's level of involvement in self-care activities
■ Patient's level of participation in therapeutic and social milieu
■ Patient's response to nursing interventions
■ Patient's statements indicating increased feelings of control
■ Evaluations for expected outcomes

Reference

Borg, C., et al. "Life Satisfaction among Older People (65+) with Reduced Self-care Capacity: The Relationship to Social, Health and Financial Aspects," *Journal of Clinical Nursing* 15(5):607-18, May 2006.

Ineffective
ROLE PERFORMANCE

Definition
Disruption in ability to perform social, vocational, and family roles

Assessment
- Age
- Gender
- Patient's perception of social, vocational, and family roles
- Neurologic status, including level of consciousness, memory, mental status, orientation, and cognitive and perceptual functioning
- Physical disabilities or limitations
- Coping behaviors
- Developmental status, including evaluation of age-appropriate task resolution, such as accepting changes in mental and physical capacities, relinquishing past roles, creating new social relationships, substituting new activities and interests for those that can no longer be pursued, and revising goals, values, and self-concept to accommodate lifestyle changes
- Family status, including roles of family members, effect of illness on patient's family, and family members' understanding of patient's illness
- Family members' perceptions of patient's ability to perform social, vocational, and family roles

Defining characteristics
- Altered role perceptions
- Change in ability to perform social, vocational, and family roles
- Changes in mental or physical capacity that affect ability to perform social, vocational, and family roles
- Inadequate role competence
- Role strain

Expected outcomes
- Patient will express feelings about limitations imposed by aging.
- Patient will discuss plans to reevaluate social, family, and vocational roles and adapt them to present physical and mental status.
- Family members will express willingness to take over responsibilities previously performed by patient.

■ Patient will continue to perform usual social, family, and vocational roles to extent possible.

■ Family members will express willingness to provide emotional support as patient adjusts to ineffective role performance.

Suggested NOC outcomes

Caregiver Lifestyle Disruption; Coping; Role Performance

Interventions and rationales

■ Discuss with the patient factors that make it difficult to fulfill his usual vocational role. For example, has the patient recently been forced to retire? How does the patient cope with free time? How does the patient feel about no longer being the family breadwinner? *Discussion helps the patient gain insight and rationally define problems and potential solutions.*

■ Help the patient develop an activity program and explore ways the patient can contribute to society, such as participation in a senior volunteer program, *to help restore the patient's sense of purpose.*

■ Discuss factors that make it difficult for the patient to fulfill his usual social roles. For example, have many of the patient's close friends died? Is it difficult for the patient to obtain transportation to social events? *This will help the patient identify the causes of diminished social interaction.*

■ Investigate support groups, senior citizen centers, and other community resources *to help the patient find new outlets for forming social relationships.*

■ Discuss with family members ways they can help the patient cope with ineffective role performance, such as visiting frequently, providing emotional support, and requesting the patient's input into family decisions, *to help maintain the patient's self-esteem.*

■ Encourage the patient to fulfill life roles within the constraints imposed by aging *to maintain a sense of purpose and preserve a connection with others.*

■ Encourage family members to express feelings about the patient's ineffective role performance. Discuss alternate ways for family members to partially or fully assume roles formerly performed by the patient *to enhance family coping.*

■ Provide the patient and family members with information about developmental tasks that the patient must perform to master the process of aging. These may include accepting changes in mental and physical capacities, relinquishing past roles, creating new social relationships, substituting new activities and interests for those he can no longer pursue, and revising goals, values, and self-concept to accommodate lifestyle changes. *Helping the patient and family members understand that these tasks are a normal part of the aging process may enhance coping.*

Suggested NIC interventions

Anticipatory Guidance; Coping Enhancement; Counseling; Mood Management; Role Enhancement

Evaluations for expected outcomes

■ Patient expresses feelings about limitations imposed by aging.

■ Patient describes plans to adapt to role changes related to aging and chronic illness.

■ Family members express willingness to take on responsibilities formerly held by patient.

■ Patient continues to fulfill family, social, and vocational responsibilities to extent possible.

■ Family members express willingness to provide emotional support for patient as he adjusts to ineffective role performance.

Documentation

■ Patient's expression of feelings and concerns associated with ineffective role performance

■ Nursing interventions to help patient understand and accept changes in role performance

■ Patient's response to nursing interventions

■ Statements by family members indicating their attitude toward patient's ineffective role performance

■ Referrals to support services for patient and family members

■ Evaluations for expected outcomes

Reference

Fakouri, C., and Lyon, B. "Perceived Health and Life Satisfaction among Older Adults: The Effects of Worry and Personal Variables," *Journal of Gerontological Nursing* 31(10):17-24, October 2005.

Situational low
SELF-ESTEEM

related to hospitalization and forced dependence on health care team

Definition
Negative self-image that develops in response to a loss or change in individual who previously had a positive self-image

Assessment

■ Changes in physical appearance, including wrinkles, sagging skin, gray hair, aging spots, scoliosis, dowager's hump, and increased truncal fat

■ Changes in social status, including recent retirement (forced or voluntary)

■ Changes in sleep patterns, including trouble falling asleep, frequent awakenings, and restless sleep

■ Family status, including recent loss of spouse or significant other

■ Reason for current hospitalization

■ Medical history, including chronic illnesses

■ Mental status, including evidence of depression, hopelessness, discouragement, preoccupation with body functions, and unrealistic fear of developing serious disease

Defining characteristics

- Difficulty making decisions
- Evaluation of self as unable to handle life events
- Expressed shame or guilt
- Expression of negative feelings about self (such as helplessness or uselessness)
- Expressions of self-negating thoughts
- Negative self-appraisal in response to life events in a patient who previously exhibited positive self-evaluation

Expected outcomes

- Patient will participate in care.
- Patient will maintain eye contact and initiate conversations.
- Patient will maintain upright and open posture.
- Patient's body language and speech content will be congruent.
- Patient will talk about impact of changes caused by chronic illness or aging on lifestyle.
- Patient will express (verbally or through behavior) increased acceptance of changes caused by chronic illness or aging.
- Patient will express increased self-esteem.

Suggested NOC outcomes

Decision-Making; Grief Resolution; Psychosocial Adjustment: Life Change; Self-Esteem

Interventions and rationales

- Ask permission to enter the patient's personal space, including areas around his bed, bedside tables, and closet. *As the patient's self-esteem decreases, the significance of personal space increases. Asking permission provides the patient with a sense of control and raises self-esteem.*
- Encourage the patient to wear his own pajamas or gowns and robes *to contribute to positive self-identity.*
- Arrange the patient's personal items on the bedside stand so that they're in easy reach *to maintain the patient's independence.*
- Incorporate appropriate exercise activities into the patient's daily care *to enhance strength, endurance, and coordination and improve self-esteem.*
- Encourage the patient to reminisce *to focus the patient's attention on past accomplishments.*
- If the patient has limited mobility, install an over-the-bed trapeze *to promote independence.*
- Incorporate tactile stimulation into daily activities through such techniques as back rubs, foot massages, and touching of the hand or arm. *Frequent touching enhances the patient's sense of self-worth.*
- Encourage the patient to express his feelings about chronic illness or aging and fears about loss of independence and ability to participate in work and leisure activities. *This allows the patient to gain insight and to rationally define problems and possible solutions.*

■ Provide information about appropriate support groups and encourage interacting with individuals who have successfully adapted to illness or limitations *to increase the patient's coping skills.*

Suggested NIC interventions
Coping Enhancement; Decision-Making Support; Grief Work Facilitation; Self-Esteem Enhancement

Evaluations for expected outcomes
■ Patient carries out activities of daily living while in hospital.
■ Patient maintains eye contact and initiates conversations.
■ Patient maintains upright and open posture.
■ Patient's body language and speech are congruent.
■ Patient states at least two ways that chronic illness or aging will affect his lifestyle.
■ Patient discusses feelings about aging, chronic illness, loss of independence, and diminished ability to participate in work and leisure activities.
■ At least once per day, patient makes statements reflecting greater self-esteem.

Documentation
■ Patient's expressions that indicate lowered self-esteem
■ Mental status assessment (baseline and ongoing)
■ Interventions to improve patient's self-esteem
■ Patient's response to nursing interventions
■ Evaluations for expected outcomes

Reference
Jonas-Simpson, C., et al. "The Experience of Being Listened to: A Qualitative Study of Older Adults in Long-term Care Settings," *Journal of Gerontological Nursing* 32(1):46-53, January 2006.

Disturbed
SENSORY PERCEPTION (AUDITORY)
related to illness or the aging process

Definition
Changes in the sense of hearing

Assessment
■ Mental status, including mood, affect, comprehension level, and recent stressors
■ Occupational hazards
■ Auditory status, including physical examination of ears (cerumen buildup, excessive hair in canal), previous ear trauma or surgery, and use of hearing aid

■ Audiometric evaluation, including Rinne, Weber's, Schwabach's, and speech and noise tests

■ Adaptive or maladaptive communication-related behaviors, such as lip reading, gestures, withdrawal, and isolation

■ Medication history, including drugs that may cause hearing loss, such as aspirin, streptomycin, kanamycin, and neomycin

Defining characteristics

■ Altered communication pattern

■ Auditory distortions

■ Change in behavior pattern

■ Change in problem-solving abilities

■ Change in usual response to auditory stimuli

■ Disorientation

■ Hallucinations

■ Irritability

■ Poor concentration

■ Reported or measured change in auditory acuity

■ Restlessness

Expected outcomes

■ Patient will express understanding of normal hearing changes that occur with age.

■ Patient will express feelings about hearing changes and impact on lifestyle.

■ Patient will demonstrate correct use of hearing aids.

■ Patient will incorporate alternative communication techniques, such as lip reading, gestures, and written information, into daily activities.

■ Patient will express interest in attending community support groups.

■ Patient will take steps to enhance communication where possible, such as decreasing background noise and looking at speaker's mouth while listening.

Suggested NOC outcomes

Cognitive Orientation; Hearing Compensation Behavior

Interventions and rationales

■ Provide information about the progressive hearing loss that occurs with age (presbycusis) *to enhance the patient's understanding of hearing deficits.*

■ Support and encourage the patient's expression of feelings about hearing loss *to help overcome self-consciousness. Because of the stigma attached to hearing loss, the older patient may be reluctant to discuss this problem.*

■ Incorporate written (flash cards and word lists) and visual (sign language, gestures, and facial expressions) communication methods into daily care *to provide the patient with alternative means of communication and to enhance his sense of control.*

■ When speaking to the patient, eliminate background noises, such as television, air conditioning, fans, chatter, and radios, *to help the patient concentrate on what you're saying.*

■ Speaking slowly and carefully, orient the patient to the topic of conversation *to reduce feelings of paranoia that may cause the patient to withdraw from social interaction.*

■ Speak to the patient in a moderate, low-pitched voice, maintaining an even volume throughout each sentence, *to maximize the patient's hearing. Speaking louder won't improve the patient's hearing because presbycusis first causes loss in high-pitched sound recognition.*

■ Face the patient when speaking and enunciate words, especially consonant sounds, carefully, *to help the patient read lips.*

■ If the patient has difficulty understanding a sentence, rephrase it *to overcome possible barriers in language comprehension.*

■ Encourage the patient to participate in activities, such as cards or checkers, that don't require a high level of verbal communication *to promote social activity.*

■ Describe types of adaptive hearing devices and their care *to help the patient make informed choices and maintain independence.*

■ Provide information about support groups, such as nationally affiliated hearing-impaired support group Self Help for Hard of Hearing People, *to promote continuity of care through community support.*

■ Make sure other staff members are aware of the patient's hearing deficit, which may be related to the patient's decreased ability to hear high frequencies. Explain that fatigue or environmental distractions may contribute to hearing deficits. *Teaching colleagues about presbycusis will help ensure high-quality care.*

Suggested NIC interventions

Cognitive Stimulation; Communication Enhancement: Hearing Deficit; Emotional Support

Evaluations for expected outcomes

■ Patient expresses understanding of hearing loss that occurs with aging.
■ Patient expresses feelings about hearing deficit and discusses how to modify lifestyle to adapt to deficit.
■ Patient demonstrates correct care and use of adaptive hearing devices.
■ Patient uses alternative communication techniques to express needs or wants.
■ Patient expresses interest in attending appropriate community support groups.
■ Patient takes appropriate steps to enhance communication where possible.

Documentation

■ Patient's statements that indicate feelings about hearing deficits
■ Patient's behavioral response to hearing loss
■ Nursing interventions to help patient cope with hearing deficits
■ Patient teaching, including explanation of hearing loss, instructions on how to care for hearing aids, and instructions on alternative communication techniques
■ Patient's response to nursing interventions
■ Evaluations for expected outcomes

Reference

Wallhagen, M.I., et al. "Sensory Impairment in Older Adults: Part 1: Hearing Loss," *AJN* 106(10):40-48, October 2006.

Disturbed
SENSORY PERCEPTION (VISUAL)
related to illness or the aging process

Definition
Change in the sense of sight

Assessment
- Age
- Vision status, including visual fields, corneal reflexes, extraocular movements, visual acuity, intraocular pressure, accommodation, night blindness, physical examination of eye including ophthalmoscopy, use of glasses, and previous eye trauma, infection, or surgery
- State of other senses
- Patient's lifestyle and physical environment
- Mental status, including behavior, mood, affect, and coping mechanisms
- Family history of vision problems

Defining characteristics
- Altered communication pattern
- Change in behavior pattern
- Change in problem-solving abilities
- Change in usual response to stimuli
- Disorientation
- Hallucinations
- Irritability
- Poor concentration
- Reported or measured change in visual acuity
- Restlessness
- Visual distortions

Expected outcomes
- Patient will discuss impact of vision loss on lifestyle.
- Patient will regain vision to extent possible and begin to come to terms with potentially permanent vision loss.
- Patient will express feelings of safety, comfort, and security.
- Patient will show interest in external environment.
- Patient will use adaptive devices to compensate for vision loss.

Suggested NOC outcomes
Body Image; Cognitive Orientation; Sensory Function: Vision; Vision Compensation Behavior

Interventions and rationales
- Teach the patient about normal age-related eye changes (presbyopia) *to increase the patient's understanding of vision changes.*

■ Encourage the patient to undergo annual eye examinations *to monitor for progressive vision loss. Decreased vision can exacerbate acute confusion.*

■ Install night-lights in the patient's room and strategically arrange lighting *to avoid abrupt changes in light. Aging eyes take longer to accommodate changes in lighting levels.*

■ Provide adequate light for performing activities of daily living (ADLs). *The patient over age 60 needs twice as much illumination for close tasks as a patient age 20.*

■ Adjust lighting to reduce glare from shiny surfaces, such as magazine paper and walls. *Aging eyes are more sensitive to glare.*

■ If color coding medications, use only bright, contrasting colors. *Pastel colors, such as light blues and greens, look alike to aging eyes.*

■ When teaching the patient, use large black print, *which is easier to see and read.*

■ Provide large-print objects, such as clocks, calendars, and telephone dials, *to promote a sense of independence.*

■ Confer with the patient before moving furniture or other items in his room *to help the patient maintain independence in ADLs.*

■ Place a brightly colored strip on the edge of the bedside tray and table *to prevent objects from falling on the bed or floor as a result of depth perception problems.*

■ Touch the patient *to communicate that you're listening.*

■ Provide the patient with low-vision aids, such as large-print books and magnifying glasses, *to help increase the patient's independence.*

Suggested NIC interventions

Communication Enhancement: Visual Deficit; Environmental Management; Self-Esteem Enhancement

Evaluations for expected outcomes

■ Patient describes effects of vision loss on lifestyle.

■ Patient regains vision to extent possible and begins to come to terms with potentially permanent vision loss.

■ Patient expresses feelings of safety, comfort, and security.

■ Patient expresses interest in external environment.

■ Patient uses adaptive devices to compensate for vision loss.

Documentation

■ Patient's expression of feelings about vision loss

■ Patient's behavioral response to vision loss

■ Use of adaptive equipment or devices

■ Teaching provided to patient and patient's response

■ Patient's response to nursing interventions

■ Evaluations for expected outcomes

Reference

Whiteside, M.M., et al. "Sensory Impairment in Older Adults: Part 2: Vision Loss," *AJN* 106(11):52-61, November 2006.

Ineffective
SEXUALITY PATTERNS
related to illness, medical treatment, or age-related changes

Definition
State in which a person expresses concern about personal sexuality

Assessment
- Changes in female reproductive organs related to aging
- History of hormone replacement therapy (postmenopause or postoophorectomy), including estrogen, progesterone, or both
- Relationship with spouse or significant other
- Psychosocial status, including self-perception, ability to cope with aging process, usual sexual activity pattern, and social interaction patterns
- Chronic illnesses
- Impaired mobility
- Perceived changes in sexual activity resulting from surgery or illness

Defining characteristics
- Reported difficulties, limitations, or changes in sexual behavior or activity

Expected outcomes
- Patient will express feelings about sexuality and self-concept.
- Patient will discuss options for maintaining intimacy throughout life span.
- Patient will express understanding of normal physiologic changes in reproductive organs that occur with aging.
- Patient will express understanding of options to relieve discomfort associated with menopause or hysterectomy.

Suggested NOC outcomes
Body Image; Role Performance; Sexual Identity

Interventions and rationales
- Provide information about hysterectomy and menopause. *After menopause or hysterectomy, older women may need reassurance that sexual activity can still be enjoyable.*
- Teach the patient about the impact of normal physiologic changes caused by aging on sexuality. For example, the vagina becomes smaller and less elastic, vaginal walls become thin and smooth, and external genitalia may become softer. Also, vaginal lubrication may take longer. Patient may also have abdominal pain or bladder irritability during intercourse. *Explaining how aging affects sexuality may help the patient accept these physiologic changes.*
- Encourage the patient to express feelings about sexuality *to reassure the patient that you're willing to discuss her concerns.*
- Discuss other options for intimacy, such as hugging, touching, and closeness, *to reaffirm the patient's identity as a sexual being.*

■ Provide information about alternative techniques and adaptations that can assist sexual satisfaction *to encourage the patient to explore and accept her sexuality.* Topics may include the use of lubricants, Kegel exercises (for vaginal muscle tone), self-stimulation, and alternative sexual positions and activities.

■ Discuss the impact that a chronic illness or adverse drug reactions can have on the patient's sexuality *to explore ways of eliminating barriers to sexual enjoyment.* Discuss with the physician the possibility of providing alternative medications.

■ Teach the patient the benefits and risks associated with hormone replacement therapy, including:

− reduced postmenopausal osteoporosis
− increased risk of endometrial cancer (with estrogen therapy alone)
− presence of monthly menses with combined estrogen and progestin therapy
− increased risk of breast cancer.

Education helps the patient make the most informed decision possible.

■ Discuss psychosocial issues that may affect the patient's sexuality, such as financial concerns about remarriage or a family member's objections to her relationship with a male companion, *to help the patient focus on specific concerns and avoid misunderstandings.*

■ If the patient lives in a long-term care facility or life-care community, encourage her to participate in social activities *to enhance opportunities for sexual expression.*

Suggested NIC interventions

Body Image Enhancement; Self-Awareness Enhancement; Self-Esteem Enhancement

Evaluations for expected outcomes

■ Patient discusses feelings related to sexuality and self-concept.
■ Patient discusses options for maintaining intimacy throughout life.
■ Patient describes physiologic changes in reproductive organs that occur with aging.
■ Patient describes options to relieve discomfort associated with menopause or hysterectomy, including risks and benefits of hormone replacement therapy.

Documentation

■ Patient's expression of feelings about sexuality and aging
■ Teaching provided and patient's response
■ Patient's behavioral response to care
■ Patient's expression of improved ability to achieve sexual enjoyment and intimacy
■ Evaluations for expected outcomes

Reference

Sveinsdottir, H., and Olafsson, R.F. "Women's Attitudes to Hormone Replacement Therapy in the Aftermath of the Women's Health Initiative Study," *Journal of Advanced Nursing* 54(5):572-84, June 2006.

| Risk for impaired |
| **SKIN INTEGRITY** |
| related to the aging process and impaired mobility |

Definition
Presence of risk factors for interruption in skin integrity

Assessment
- Age
- Physical examination, including inspection of lower limbs, testing for sensation in lower limbs, palpation of peripheral pulses, and presence of edema
- Integumentary status, including color, elasticity, hygiene, lesions, moisture, quantity and distribution of hair, sensation, temperature and blood pressure, texture, turgor, and condition of nails
- Psychosocial status, including coping patterns, lifestyle, presence of family members or significant other, mental status, self-concept, and body image
- Mobility status, including activity level, joint range of motion, contractures, muscle mass, and tone
- Mental status
- Evidence of incontinence
- Recent changes in medication regimen
- History of skin problems, including pressure ulcers, dermatitis, and trauma
- Ability to perform skin care regimen

Risk factors
- External factors, including pressure, friction and shearing, restraints, physical immobilization, humidity and moisture, chemical substances, radiation, excretions and secretions, hypothermia or hyperthermia, and age
- Internal factors, including effects of medications, skeletal prominences, immunologic responses, altered nutritional status (obesity or emaciation), sensation, pigmentation, metabolic state, circulation, and skin turgor

Expected outcomes
- Patient will maintain intact skin.
- Patient or caregiver will describe normal aging changes in skin and risk factors for disturbance in skin integrity.
- Patient or caregiver will implement strategies to prevent skin breakdown and will carry out skin care regimen.

Suggested NOC outcomes

Immobility Consequences: Physiological; Tissue Integrity: Skin & Mucous Membranes

Interventions and rationales
- Educate the patient or caregiver about changes to skin caused by aging *to motivate the patient or caregiver to implement a skin care regimen. Physiologic changes*

associated with aging increase the risk of skin breakdown. For example, older patients, especially those immobilized with chronic health problems, are at high risk for pressure ulcers. Physiologic changes also leave older patients vulnerable to problems associated with dry skin.

■ Help the patient obtain appropriate evaluation and treatment of the underlying skin condition *to promote healing and minimize complications.*

■ Help the patient or caregiver implement a pressure-relief movement and massage program *to prevent pressure ulcers.* The patient should change position at least every 2 hours. *Frequent turning and massage promotes adequate tissue perfusion and prevents necrosis.*

■ Use preventive skin care devices as needed, such as a foam mattress, alternating pressure mattress, sheepskin, pillows, or padding, *to avoid discomfort and skin breakdown. These measures don't replace the need for turning.*

■ Teach the patient about the need for good nutrition, including the importance of meeting caloric requirements and benefits of adequate vitamin and protein intake. *Good nutrition helps maintain adequate tissue nourishment, perfusion, and oxygenation.*

■ Help the patient or caregiver develop and implement a daily routine of skin inspection and care. Discuss the need to maintain good personal hygiene; use nonirritating (nonalkaline) soap; pat rather than rub skin dry; inspect skin regularly; avoid prolonged exposure to water, sun, cold, and wind; and recognize and report signs of skin breakdown (redness, blisters, and discoloration). *A daily program of skin inspection and maintenance will protect the older patient's skin integrity.*

■ Encourage the patient or caregiver to seek immediate attention if skin injury or trauma occurs *to help prevent further injury and conditions that may require extensive treatment.*

■ Monitor wounds or incisions for infection and follow a prescribed treatment regimen *to prevent infection, which may delay healing.*

Suggested NIC interventions

Bed Rest Care; Circulatory Precautions; Pressure Management; Skin Surveillance

Evaluations for expected outcomes

■ Patient's skin remains intact.

■ Patient or caregiver describes skin changes that result from aging and lists risk factors for impaired skin integrity.

■ Patient or caregiver implements daily program of skin inspection and care, including frequent turning and movement.

Documentation

■ Observations of patient's skin
■ Presence of risk factors for impaired skin integrity
■ Patient teaching provided and patient's response
■ Patient's response to nursing interventions
■ Evaluations for expected outcomes

Reference
Fore, J. "A Review of Skin and the Effects of Aging on Skin Structure and Function." *Ostomy/Wound Management* 52(9):24-35, September 2006.

SOCIAL ISOLATION
related to physiologic, environmental, or emotional barriers

Definition
Self-imposed or environmentally imposed lack of contact with others

Assessment
- Age
- Psychosocial status, including support systems, financial resources, coping and problem-solving ability, cultural background, and activities or hobbies
- Health status, including vision or hearing deficits, chronic illness, incontinence, and pain
- Self-care abilities, including knowledge and use of adaptive equipment and supplies, and technical and mechanical skills
- Living conditions, including home environment, site of activities and resources, and transportation
- Mental status, including behavior, mood, and affect
- Musculoskeletal status, including coordination, functional ability, gait, range of motion, presence of tremor or paralysis, and muscle tone, size, and strength

Defining characteristics
- Culturally unacceptable behavior
- Description of lifestyle as solitary or circumscribed by membership in subculture
- Evidence of physical or mental disability or altered state of wellness
- Expressed feelings of being different from others
- Expressed feelings of rejection or aloneness
- Expressed frustration over inability to meet expectations of others
- Inappropriate interests or activities
- Insecurity in public
- Lack of family, friends, and social groups
- Lack of purpose in life
- Preoccupation with own thoughts
- Projection of hostility in voice and behavior
- Repetitive, meaningless actions
- Sad, dull affect
- Uncommunicative and withdrawn behavior, with poor eye contact

Expected outcomes
- Patient will express feelings associated with social isolation.
- Patient will seek assistance or information from staff to overcome social isolation.

■ Patient will make use of community resources.

■ Patient will describe increased number of social contacts.

■ Patient will express satisfaction with level of social contacts.

Suggested NOC outcomes

Leisure Participation; Loneliness Severity; Mood Equilibrium; Social Interaction Skills

Interventions and rationales

■ Assign a primary nurse or case manager to the patient *to provide consistency and promote trust.*

■ Discuss with the patient causes and contributing factors of social isolation. Find out what factors the patient believes interfere most with his ability to develop relationships with others *to determine the patient's wants and needs.*

■ Determine if the patient is willing to make changes in lifestyle or daily routine to increase contact with others. *The patient needs to have motivation for nursing interventions to succeed.*

■ If appropriate, address physical limitations that interfere with the patient's ability to form social relationships. For example, if the patient has a hearing deficit, make a referral to an audiologist for a hearing aid; if the patient has a mobility impairment, make a referral to a physical therapist for an exercise program or for recommendations for assistive devices. *The patient may need physical limitations addressed before he can overcome social isolation.*

■ Assess the influence of the home environment on the patient's social life. For example, is the patient afraid to go outside because of a high crime rate in the neighborhood? If so, consider investigating options, such as a retirement community or residential care facility, which might offer better social opportunities. *The patient may not be aware of alternative living options.*

■ Investigate activity groups, support groups, senior citizens centers, health education programs, and other community resources *to develop an activity program for the patient.*

■ Investigate the availability and cost of public transportation. Familiarize the patient with the route to planned activities. *The patient must overcome barriers to transportation to gain access to the outside world.*

■ Involve the patient in planning activities that will enhance his social life and assist him in identifying resources *to individualize care planning and reduce feelings of dependency and helplessness.*

Suggested NIC interventions

Behavior Modification: Social Skills; Mood Management; Socialization Enhancement

Evaluations for expected outcomes

■ Patient expresses feelings associated with social isolation.

■ Patient expresses desire to overcome social isolation and seeks help from staff to increase participation in social activities.

■ Patient makes use of resources, such as social services, senior citizens centers, American Association of Retired Persons, and religious organizations.
■ Patient indicates that social contacts have increased and feelings of social isolation have diminished.
■ Patient expresses satisfaction with level of social contacts.

Documentation

■ Factors that have caused or contributed to patient's social isolation
■ Patient's statements indicating dissatisfaction with social situation
■ Community resources identified for patient
■ Planning done by patient, family member, primary nurse, and case manager
■ Patient's use of community resources
■ Evaluations for expected outcomes

References

Arthur, H.M. "Depression, Isolation, Social Support, and Cardiovascular Disease in Older Adults," *The Journal of Cardiovascular Nursing* 21(5 Suppl 1):S2-S7, September-October 2006.

Cheng, C.Y. "Living Alone: The Choice and Health of Older Women," *Journal of Gerontological Nursing* 32(9):16-23, September 2006.

Readiness for enhanced
SPIRITUAL WELL-BEING

Definition

Process of developing inner self by interconnecting physical, psychological, and spiritual strengths

Assessment

■ Spiritual status, including personal religious habits; religious or church affiliation; perceptions of faith, life, death, and suffering; support network; embarrassment at practicing religious rituals; beliefs opposed by family members, peers, and health care providers; conflicts with belief system
■ Health history, including medical conditions that change body image, chronic or terminal illness, debilitating disease
■ Psychological status, including reactions to illness and disability; change in appetite, energy level, motivation, personal hygiene, self-image, sleep, and sex drive; alcohol or drug abuse; moodiness; recent divorce, job loss, losses through separation or death; personality traits, maladaptive behaviors; relationships with peers, group involvement, life events in childhood, family pressure; recreational activities; quality of authority relationships, peer relationships; situational crisis; occupation changes; dating and marital history
■ Brief Psychiatric Rating Scale, Hamilton Depression Rating Scale, and others, as needed

■ Self-care status, including neurologic, musculoskeletal, sensory or psychological impairment, ability to carry out activities and adapt

■ Family status, including marital status; communication, methods of conflict resolution; ability of family to meet physical, social, and emotional needs of its members; socioeconomic factors; family health history; evidence of abuse

■ Nutritional status, including height, weight, and any special dietary habits

■ Sleep pattern status, including hours of sleep, energy level before and after sleep, rest and relaxation patterns; difficulty falling asleep, nocturnal awakening, early morning awakening, hypersomnia, insomnia, sleep pattern reversal; sleep EEG; dyssomnia, parasomnia, unipolar depression, bipolar disorder, sleep apnea

Defining characteristics

■ Harmonious interconnectedness (harmony and connection with self, others, higher power, and environment)

■ Inner strengths, such as inner core, transcendence, self-consciousness, and sense of awareness

■ Sense of unfolding mystery

Expected outcomes

■ Patient will discuss spiritual conflicts.

■ Patient will be provided with opportunity to meet with chosen religious authority.

■ Patient will be supported in his efforts to pursue enhanced spiritual well-being.

■ Patient will pursue religious or spiritual practices to the extent that he feels comfortable.

■ Patient will describe plan to continue to enhance spiritual well-being.

■ Patient will receive referrals for continued support.

Suggested NOC outcomes

Hope; Quality of Life; Spiritual Health

Interventions and rationales

■ Monitor the patient for potential signs of spiritual distress that might harm the patient's well-being (altered self-care, sleep pattern disturbance, and change in exercise and eating habits) *to plan appropriate interventions.*

■ Assess the significance of spirituality in the patient's life and in coping with illness. Note whether the patient participates in religious rituals, observes religious practices (such as prayer, meditation, or dietary restrictions), or wishes to discuss spiritual beliefs. Keep an open view of what constitutes spirituality. *Before the nurse can intervene in spiritual matters, she must determine if spirituality is significant for the patient.*

■ Ask the patient if illness has affected his spiritual outlook and tell him you're willing to help him address spiritual issues, if he wishes, *to reduce isolation and help bring issues related to spiritual distress out into the open.*

■ Ask the patient if he wishes to discuss spiritual concerns with a chosen religious authority *to allow access to expert spiritual care resources.*

■ Encourage the patient to pursue spiritual questions. Reassure him that spiritual concerns are valid and that by strengthening spirituality he can enhance his over-all well-being *to demonstrate acceptance.*

■ Provide the patient with resources for coping with spiritual distress (such as re-ferrals to religious or spiritual organizations or books on prayer and meditation) *to enhance the opportunity to attend to spiritual needs.* Make sure the resources se-lected are appropriate with regard to the patient's religious affiliation and spiritual beliefs *to demonstrate respect for his beliefs and values.* If you lack knowledge about the patient's beliefs and practices, consult his chosen religious authority *to best meet the patient's needs.*

■ Help the patient arrange travel to a place selected for prayer, reflection, or con-templation. Use such resources as church-affiliated vans or volunteer escorts *to enhance the patient's contact with outside sources of support.*

■ Demonstrate to the patient that you're willing to discuss issues related to spiri-tuality, such as the patient's view of God, how illness has affected his religious be-liefs, or how hospital stays affect his spiritual practices, *to bring spiritual issues into the open.* Keep an open mind when listening. Keep the conversation focused on the patient's spiritual values and the role they play in recovering from illness and coping with changes in body image *to ensure that interaction between the nurse and patient remains therapeutic.*

■ Discuss with the patient the importance of maintaining a healthy diet, getting regular exercise and sleep, and maintaining healthy interaction with family mem-bers and friends. *A patient in spiritual distress may neglect day-to-day well-being.*

■ Praise the patient for taking time to attend to spiritual needs and encourage him to continue to develop spirituality after he leaves the health care setting *to provide continued encouragement.*

■ Provide the patient with referrals to appropriate religious groups, spiritually centered organizations, and social service organizations *to help provide additional support and to ensure continuity of care.*

■ Consider such resources as parish nurses, home-visiting services, and computer networks *to help provide continued opportunity for spiritual development and to en-sure continuity of care.*

Suggested NIC interventions
Active Listening; Emotional Support; Hope Instillation; Presence; Spiritual Growth Facilitation; Spiritual Support

Evaluations for expected outcomes
■ Patient becomes comfortable discussing spiritual conflicts.

■ Patient is visited by a religious representative of his choice.

■ Patient is supported in his efforts to pursue enhanced spiritual well-being.

■ Patient takes the initiative to pursue his desire for active religious participation.

■ Patient openly discusses effects of illness on his beliefs and other spiritual is-sues.

■ Patient develops a plan for continued involvement in religious activity.

■ Patient accepts referrals for continued religious growth.

Documentation
- Statements about spiritual conflicts
- Visits with chosen religious authority
- Engagement in religious or spiritual practices
- Suggested religious resources outside of hospital
- Statements about ability to cope with changes in body image as a result of illness, to maintain spiritual values in face of long-term or chronic illness, and to pursue spiritual practices during hospital stays
- Eating patterns, exercise schedules, and sleep patterns
- Stated plans to continue to enhance spiritual well-being
- Evaluations for expected outcomes

References
Callaghan, D.M. "The Influence of Growth on Spiritual Self-care Agency in an Older Adult Population," *Journal of Gerontological Nursing* 32(9):43-51, September 2006.

Gaskamp, C., et al. "Evidence-based Guideline: Promoting Spirituality in the Older Adult," *Journal of Gerontological Nursing* 32(11):8-13, November 2006.

Risk for self-directed
VIOLENCE
related to recurrent losses or changes in physical or mental condition

Definition
Presence of risk factors for attempted suicide

Assessment
- Age
- Gender
- Race
- Religion
- Marital status (widowed, divorced, married, or single)
- Life situation, including isolation (living alone or in urban area) and recent retirement, unemployment, or move to new area
- Mental health history, including coping behaviors, statements of low self-esteem, family dynamics, and communication patterns
- Recent stressors, including divorce, death of spouse, and relocation
- Mental status, including orientation, level of consciousness, and thought processes
- Support systems

Risk factors
- Changes in mood or affect
- Changes in physical or mental status
- Confusion

- Direct or indirect statements of intent to commit suicide
- Evidence of getting affairs in order, such as changing or making will
- Evidence of giving away money or valuables
- Experience of multiple losses, such as loss of spouse, income, and friends
- Expressed feelings of hopelessness, helplessness, or depression
- Frequent medical visits about somatic complaints
- History of attempted suicide
- Hoarding of medications
- Purchasing of gun or other weapon
- Suicidal ideation

Expected outcomes

- Patient won't harm himself and will remain in safe environment.
- Patient will discuss sadness, despair, and other feelings.
- Patient will discuss events that led up to current crisis.
- Patient will acknowledge suicidal thoughts.
- Patient will receive referral to mental health professional.
- Patient will express improved self-concept.
- Patient will report decreased desire to kill himself.
- Patient will discuss appropriate coping skills to avoid future suicidal episodes.

Suggested NOC outcomes

Impulse Self-Control; Self-Mutilation Restraint; Suicide Self-Restraint

Interventions and rationales

- Be aware of key facts about suicide in older patients:
– Suicide among older adults is a serious problem. Those with the highest risk of suicide are at least 85 years old, depressed, with high self-esteem and a need to control life.
– The suicide rate for older adult men is seven times that for older women.
– Most suicides by older patients are planned and aren't just gestures or threats; even frail nursing home residents can find strength to carry out suicide, if sufficiently determined.
Awareness of suicide risks may help prevent attempts.
- Remove items from the patient's surroundings that could be used in a suicide attempt *to ensure the patient's safety.*
- Set aside time for listening to the patient *to communicate that you care.*
- Approach the patient with understanding and concern *to alleviate angry or embarrassed feelings related to emotional breakdown or a previous unsuccessful suicide attempt.*
- Communicate a nonjudgmental attitude *to build trust and rapport.*
- Assess the patient for signs and symptoms of depression, such as a persistent depressed mood, diminished interest in daily activities, sleep disturbances, inappropriate guilt, loss of energy, poor concentration, changes in appetite, psychomotor retardation or agitation, and a passive wish for death. *Elderly patients are at increased risk for depression. Depression increases in frequency and intensity with advancing age. Factors that contribute to an increase in depression include*

changes in neurotransmitter levels, multiple losses, diminished health, and decreased resources. Depression may also occur in the early stages of dementia.

■ Discuss the problems that led the patient to this episode of depression. *Talking about specific events may help the patient achieve catharsis and develop appropriate coping skills.* Events that may contribute to depression in older patients include recent major loss, experience of rejection by or isolation from family or friends, recent disability, loss of partner, loss of sexual function, and loss of social, family, or occupational role.

■ Recognize the patient's feelings of inadequacy and take steps to bolster self-esteem. Encourage the patient to participate in a life review, revisit places where significant past events took place, put together a scrapbook, research family genealogy, or attend family, class, or church reunions. *These activities help the patient experience emotions, which ultimately promotes improved self-esteem.*

■ Avoid comparing the patient with others *to reduce stereotyping and foster individuality.*

■ Support the patient but don't give false reassurances that everything will work out. Let him know that, although no easy answer exists, help is available and you'll help him find alternative solutions *to ease despair.*

■ Supervise the administration of prescribed medications. Be aware of drug actions and adverse effects and make sure that the patient doesn't hoard medications *to ensure he won't harm himself, even inadvertently.*

■ Decrease environmental stimuli, when necessary, and provide a safe outlet that allows patient to release emotions and anger. Review situations that cause stress for the patient and help him develop plans for dealing with them. *These measures will help the patient cope better with depression.*

■ Assess for signs of suicidal thinking that warrant further investigation, such as sudden hoarding of medications, giving away possessions, sudden interest in guns, and despondent remarks, *to determine if the patient is at risk for suicide.*

■ Ask the patient directly, "Have you thought about killing yourself?" If so, ask, "What do you plan to do?" *to assess for suicidal ideation.*

■ If you suspect that the patient is at risk for suicide, refer him to a mental health professional for immediate evaluation *to ensure safety.*

■ Educate the patient or family member in the use of prescribed antidepressants. Explain that geriatric doses differ from those for younger patients. *Knowledge of medications and careful monitoring help guard against adverse effects.*

■ Help the patient identify community resources *to obtain continued therapy and support after hospitalization.*

■ Encourage family members to talk with one another and develop improved coping strategies *to foster enhanced family functioning.*

Suggested NIC interventions

Environmental Management: Violence Prevention; Impulse Control Training; Suicide Prevention

Evaluations for expected outcomes

■ Patient doesn't harm himself and his environment is safe, with items that could be used in suicide attempt removed.

■ Patient expresses feelings and thoughts in way that promotes healing process.

■ Patient discusses events that led up to current crisis.
■ Patient acknowledges suicidal thoughts.
■ Patient receives referral to mental health professional.
■ Patient states that he feels better about himself.
■ Patient states that he experiences fewer suicidal thoughts.
■ Patient expresses understanding of importance of increased social support and improved coping skills in avoiding future suicidal episodes.

Documentation
■ Patient's exact description of suicidal thoughts and recent suicide attempt
■ Observations of patient's behavior
■ Interventions to prevent suicide
■ Patient's response to therapy
■ Evaluations for expected outcomes

Reference
Garand, L., et al. "Suicide in Older Adults: Nursing Assessment of Suicide Risk," *Issues in Mental Health Nursing* 27(4):355-70, May 2006.

VI Psychiatric and mental health

INTRODUCTION

Whether or not you work in mental health nursing, you need to develop skills in dealing with patients who have psychiatric disorders or psychological health problems. As a practitioner, you have a responsibility to respond to the psychological as well as the physical needs of your patients. This section includes care plans for patients with such diverse needs as anxiety, coping, fear, and posttraumatic stress disorder. The establishment and maintenance of a therapeutic relationship is an essential skill in providing mental health care. The nurse should also maintain a nonjudgmental attitude and be open to the prospect of recovery throughout care.

As increased attention is being paid to substance abuse, domestic violence, sexual abuse, and related problems, you'll be called on to provide comprehensive care for these patients in outpatient settings, hospitals, and nontraditional health care settings. Recent improvements in drug therapy allow mental health patients to live in community settings with supervision of their medication regimen.

As more patients cope with the effects of chronic disease, nurses are called on to provide support and instruction for families and friends. Likewise, as more patients are cared for across the managed care spectrum, attention to the mental health aspect of care is crucial in meeting patient outcomes. The care plans in this section will aid you in providing care in the areas of psychological and social health.

ANXIETY

related to environmental conflict (phobia)

Definition
Vague, uneasy feeling of discomfort or dread accompanied by an autonomic response (the source often nonspecific or unknown to the individual); a feeling of apprehension caused by anticipation of danger; an alerting signal that warns of impending danger and enables the individual to take measures to deal with threat

Assessment
- History of panic symptoms (choking feeling in throat, hyperventilation, light-headedness, dizziness, and other physical signs and symptoms of anxiety)
- Psychological status, including patient's explanation of problem, onset, duration, precipitating events, past and present coping (note use of repression and denial and escape-avoidance behaviors), insight (note patient's understanding of irrationality of fears), motivation to change, anxiety level (+1, +2, +3, +4), secondary gains (what kind and from whom), current stressors, results of mental status examination (note expression of anxiety in terms of personal fears, concentration, judgment, affect, and impulse control as well as all other aspects of mental status), and personal abilities, talents, and strengths
- Sociologic status, including support systems, hobbies, interests, work history, family makeup, family roles (evidence of harmony or disharmony), family coping mechanisms, evidence of reinforcement of problem by family, and lifestyle (how this reinforces irrational fears)
- Medication history, including response, effectiveness, and adverse effects

Defining characteristics
Behavioral
- Diminished productivity
- Expressed concerns due to change in life events
- Extraneous movement
- Fidgeting
- Glancing about
- Insomnia
- Poor eye contact
- Restlessness
- Scanning and vigilance

Affective
- Anguish
- Increased wariness
- Irritability
- Jittery
- Overexcited
- Painful and persistent thougths
- Rattled

- Regretful
- Scared
- Uncertain

Physiological
- Facial tension
- Hand tremors
- Increased perspiration
- Increased tension
- Voice quivering
- Shakiness

Cognitive
- Awareness of physiologic symptoms
- Blocking of thoughts
- Confusion
- Decreased perceptual field
- Difficulty concentrating
- Forgetfulness
- Impaired attention
- Preoccupation
- Rumination

Expected outcomes
- Patient will experience reduced anxiety by identifying precipitating situations.
- Patient will connect life events to occurrence of anxiety.
- Patient will identify current stressors.
- Patient will set limits and compromises on behavior when ready.
- Patient will develop effective coping behaviors.
- Patient will maintain autonomy and independence without disabling fears or use of phobic behavior.

Suggested NOC outcomes
Aggression Self-Control; Anxiety Level; Anxiety Self-Control; Concentration; Coping; Impulse Self-Control; Psychosocial Adjustment: Life Change

Interventions and rationales
- Identify your feelings toward the patient *to keep your feelings from interfering with treatment.*
- Accept the patient as he is. *Forcing the patient to change before he's ready causes panic.*
- Explore factors that precipitate phobic reactions and anxiety. *This is important for understanding the patient's behavioral dynamics.*
- Reassure the patient that he's safe. *The patient may perceive that he's at risk, which may increase his level of anxiety.*
- Support the patient with desensitization techniques *to help him overcome his problem.*

■ Give the patient a chance to ventilate his feelings. *This reduces the patient's tendency to suppress or repress his bottled-up feelings, which may continue to affect behavior even though the patient may be unaware of them.*

■ Teach relaxation techniques (breathing exercises, progressive muscle relaxation, guided imagery, meditation) *to counteract the fight-or-flight response.*

■ Help the patient set limits and compromises on behavior when he's ready, and allow the patient to be afraid. *Fear is a feeling, neither right nor wrong.*

■ Give the patient facts about fear and anxiety and their consequences *to reduce anxiety and encourage the patient to help manage his problem.*

■ Encourage the patient not to run away when he's afraid *to help the patient learn that fear can be faced and managed.*

■ Help the patient develop his own techniques for dealing with fears *to establish alternatives to escape or avoidance behaviors.*

Suggested NIC interventions
Anger Control Assistance; Anxiety Reduction; Calming Technique; Coping Enhancement; Impulse Control Training; Presence

Evaluations for expected outcomes
■ Patient identifies precipitating situations and demonstrates fewer physical symptoms of anxiety, improved concentration, and reduced preoccupation with fears.

■ Patient discusses possible relationship between anxiety and past and present experiences.

■ Patient lists stressors.

■ Patient limits phobic behavior when ready.

■ Patient participates in desensitization therapy and learns to better manage stress, health, and responsibilities.

■ Patient makes decisions, shows greater independence, and decreases behaviors that limit spontaneous activity.

Documentation
■ Observation of subjective and objective data

■ Interventions to reduce anxiety and increase coping

■ Patient's response to interventions

■ Evaluations for expected outcomes

Reference
Twiss, E., et al. "The Effect of Music Listening on Older Adults Undergoing Cardiovascular Surgery," *Nursing in Critical Care* 11(5):224-31, September-October 2006.

CAREGIVER ROLE STRAIN
related to unpredictability of the care situation

Definition
A caregiver's felt or exhibited difficulty in performing a family caregiver role

Assessment
■ Caregiver's age, sex, level of education, occupation, and marital status
■ Caregiver's physical and mental status, including chronic health problems, self-care abilities and limitations, and level of cognitive function
■ Patient's physical and mental status, including history of psychiatric illness, self-care limitations, and level of cognitive function
■ Support systems, including financial resources, family members and friends, community services, health-related services such as geriatric or psychiatric day care, and religious affiliation
■ Cultural, ethnic, and religious background of family
■ Family roles, coping patterns, family alliances, goals, and values

Defining characteristics
Caregiving activities
■ Apprehension about possible institutionalization of care receiver
■ Apprehension about the care receiver's care if the caregiver becomes ill or dies
■ Apprehension about the future regarding care receiver's health and the caregiver's ability to provide care
■ Difficulty performing or completing required task; preoccupation with care routine
■ Dysfunctional change in caregiving activities

Caregiver health status
■ Physical
– Diabetes
– Fatigue
– Headaches
– Cardiovascular disease
– GI upset
– Hypertension
– Rash
– Weight change
■ Emotional
– Anger
– Depression
– Disturbed sleep
– Frustration
– Impaired individual coping
– Impatience
– Increased emotional lability

- Increased nervousness
- Lack of time to meet personal needs
- Somatization
- Stress
■ Socioeconomic
- Changes in leisure activities
- Lack of interest in career advancement
- Low work productivity
- Withdrawal from social life

Expected outcomes

■ Family members will discuss how patient's illness has altered established roles and responsibilities within family.

■ Family members will assign responsibilities to prevent too much from falling on one individual's shoulders.

■ Family members will establish limits on patient's behavior and will work together to uphold them.

■ Family members will refrain from using destructive coping mechanisms, such as substance abuse and physical or mental abuse of care recipient.

■ Family members will make use of outside support systems, such as community resources, religious organizations, and day hospitals.

■ Family members will recognize need for professional assistance.

Suggested NOC outcomes

Caregiver Emotional Health; Caregiver Lifestyle Disruption; Caregiver Well-Being; Family Coping; Family Support During Treatment; Role Performance

Interventions and rationales

■ Assist family members to clarify needs, set individual goals, and develop plans to meet them. *This will instill in each person a sense of empowerment and control over his life.*

■ Encourage discussion among family members about role changes and added responsibilities that have occurred as a result of the patient's health status *to establish open and honest communication among family members.*

■ Encourage discussion of the family's past experience with crises, comparing them with the present situation *to help the family see they have survived difficulties together and encourage them to seek viable solutions.*

■ Encourage family members to retain involvement with social and religious networks *to avoid feelings of isolation and abandonment.*

■ Refer the family to appropriate professional services *to ensure their needs are being met. Caregiver support groups may provide the family with helpful strategies that have worked for others facing the same problems.*

Suggested NIC interventions

Caregiver Support; Coping Enhancement; Respite Care; Role Enhancement; Teaching: Individual

Evaluations for expected outcomes
■ Family members adjust to changes in roles and responsibilities.
■ Family members share responsibilities of caregiving equally.
■ Patient behaves within limits set by caregiver.
■ Family members don't exhibit signs of stress.
■ Family members use community resources, as needed.
■ Family members attend support groups or seek other forms of professional assistance.

Documentation
■ Family members' beliefs and attitudes about patient's illness
■ Role adjustment and flexibility of family members
■ Coping patterns
■ Patient's behavior
■ Goals articulated by family members
■ Use of support systems
■ Referrals for professional help
■ Patient's and family members' responses to nursing interventions
■ Evaluations for expected outcomes

Reference
Hansen, L., et al. "Family Caregivers Making Life-Sustaining Treatment Decisions: Factors Associated with Role Strain and Ease," *Journal of Gerontological Nursing* 31(11):28-35, November 2005.

Impaired verbal
COMMUNICATION
related to psychological barriers

Definition
Decreased, delayed, or absent ability to receive, process, transmit, and use a system of symbols

Assessment
■ Neurologic status, including history of neurologic disorders, mental status (orientation, level of consciousness, mood or behavior, knowledge and intelligence, vocabulary, and memory), and speech (pattern, language, level of comprehension and expression, and ability to use other forms of communication, such as gestures, pictures, and drawings)
■ Psychological status, including history of mental or psychiatric disorders, history of alcohol or psychoactive drug use, stressors, phobias, and coping strategies

Defining characteristics
■ Disorientation
■ Difficulty comprehending and maintaining usual communication pattern

- Difficulty expressing thought verbally (aphasia, dysphasia, apraxia, dyslexia)
- Difficulty using or inability to use facial expressions or body language
- Dyspnea
- Inability or lack of desire to speak
- Inappropriate verbalizations
- Stuttering or slurring
- Visual deficit (partial or total)

Expected outcomes

- Patient will communicate needs and desires to staff, family, or friends.
- Staff members will meet patient's needs.
- Patient will incur no injury or harm.
- Patient's communication ability will return to baseline level.
- Patient will explain relationship of causative factors, such as alcohol, to inability to communicate effectively.
- Patient will begin to make plans to use self-help groups and other resources to improve psychological status.

Suggested NOC outcomes

Communication; Communication: Expressive; Communication: Receptive

Interventions and rationales

- Observe the patient closely *to anticipate his needs* (for example, restlessness may indicate a need to urinate).
- Minimize environmental stimuli and maintain a quiet, nonthreatening environment *to reduce anxiety.*
- Introduce yourself, and explain procedures in simple terms. Encourage consistent use of the same terms for common objects. *Treating the patient as normal may enhance responsiveness.*
- Encourage communication attempts and allow the patient time to say or write words in response *to decrease frustration.*
- Assess the patient's communication status daily and record. Match communication needs to interventions: For disorientation, use reality orientation techniques; for a manic state, reduce environmental stimuli and talk softly and calmly; for alcohol withdrawal syndrome, reassure the patient, don't reinforce the presence of hallucinations, and provide a quiet environment; for stuttering, use rhythm or song. *Each patient needs communication status interventions tailored to his situation.*
- Determine the patient's past interests and habits from family members and discuss them with the patient *to stimulate nonthreatening two-way conversation.*
- Maintain a safe environment by using side rails, soft restraints, and other safety measures according to established policies *to protect the patient.*
- Refer the patient to a psychiatric liaison nurse, social services, community agencies, and self-help groups such as Alcoholics Anonymous. *Resolution of communication problems may require long-term follow-up.*

Suggested NIC interventions

Active Listening; Anxiety Reduction; Decision-Making Support; Environmental Management; Presence

Evaluations for expected outcomes

■ Patient consistently communicates needs to staff, family, or friends.

■ Staff members meet patient's basic needs.

■ Patient doesn't show signs of neglect (weight loss, dehydration, constipation) or evidence of falls (bruises, contusions, cuts).

■ Patient demonstrates return to baseline communication level by stating name, place, and time.

■ Patient describes relationship between causative factors and impaired communication.

■ Patient expresses intent to attend self-help groups and identifies resources appropriate to resolving underlying psychological problem.

Documentation

■ Patient's concern with level of communication

■ Observations of patient's needs, communication attempts, orientation, and safety measures

■ Interventions carried out to promote communication

■ Contributing factors to poor communication and plans to improve psychological status

■ Patient's response to nursing interventions

■ Evaluations for expected outcomes

Reference

Liechty, J.A. "The Sounds of Silence: Relating to People with Aphasia," *Journal of Psychosocial Nursing and Mental Health Services* 44(8):53-55, August 2006.

Ineffective
COPING
related to personal vulnerability

Definition

Inability to form a valid appraisal of the stressors, inadequate choices of practiced responses, or inability to use available resources

Assessment

■ Patient's perception of present health problem or crisis

■ Usual problem-solving techniques/behaviors used to cope with life problems

■ Physical or emotional impairment

■ Occupation

■ Diversional activities

■ Financial resources

- Support systems, including family members, friends, and clergy
- Reaction of family members to patient's crisis

Defining characteristics
- Change in communication patterns
- Decreased use of social support
- Destructive behavior toward self or others
- Difficulty asking for help
- Fatigue
- High illness rate
- Inability to meet basic needs and role expectations
- Lack of goal-directed behavior, such as inability to attend, difficulty organizing information, poor concentration, and poor problem-solving abilities
- Maladaptive coping behaviors
- Risk-taking behaviors
- Sleep disturbance
- Statements indicating inability to cope
- Substance abuse

Expected outcomes
- Patient will express understanding of the relationship between emotional state and behavior.
- Patient will become actively involved in planning own care.
- Patient will reduce use of manipulative behavior to gratify needs.
- Patient will accept responsibility for behavior.
- Patient will identify effective and ineffective coping techniques.
- Patient will use available support systems, such as family, friends, and psychotherapist, to develop and maintain effective coping skills.

Suggested NOC outcomes
Aggression Self-Control; Coping; Decision-Making; Impulse Self-Control; Social Interaction Skills

Interventions and rationales
- If possible, assign a primary nurse to the patient *to provide continuity of care and promote development of a therapeutic relationship.*
- Spend consistent, uninterrupted time with the patient. Encourage open expression of feelings. *An open environment will help the patient ventilate intense emotion. Through discussion, you can help the patient understand the personal meaning attached to recent events and foster a realistic assessment of his situation.*
- As the patient becomes able to express feelings more openly, discuss the relationship between feelings and behavior. *To change, the patient must understand this relationship.*
- Discourage dependent behavior by assisting the patient only when necessary. Provide positive reinforcement for independent behavior *to enhance self-esteem, encourage repetition of desired behavior, and promote effective coping.*
- Encourage the patient to make decisions about care *to reduce feelings of helplessness and enhance the patient's sense of mastery over the current situation.*

■ Set limits on manipulative behavior. Provide the patient with clear expectations for behavior, and describe the consequences if limits are violated. *If the patient can't curb inappropriate behavior, consistent limit-setting imposes external controls.*

■ Recognize that manipulative behaviors reduce the patient's sense of insecurity by increasing feelings of power. *Understanding the patient's motivation may help you deal better with manipulative behavior.*

■ Help the patient recognize and accept responsibility for his actions. Discourage the patient from unfairly placing blame on others. *Developing a sense of responsibility is necessary before change can occur.*

■ Help the patient recognize and feel good about his positive personal qualities and accomplishments. Provide rewards to reinforce acceptable coping behaviors. *As self-esteem increases, the patient will feel less need to manipulate others.*

■ Help the patient analyze the current situation and evaluate the effectiveness of coping strategies *to foster an objective outlook.*

■ Praise the patient for identifying and using effective coping techniques *to reinforce appropriate behavior.*

■ Suggest alternatives to ineffective behaviors identified by the patient. Encourage the patient to determine what new behaviors can be effectively incorporated into his lifestyle. *Fostering patient participation in care promotes feelings of independence.*

■ Encourage the patient to use support systems, such as a psychotherapist, family, and friends, *to maintain effective coping skills.*

Suggested NIC interventions
Anger Control Assistance; Coping Enhancement; Decision-Making Support; Environmental Management: Violence Prevention; Impulse Control Training; Support System Enhancement

Evaluations for expected outcomes
■ Patient describes emotions triggered by illness or personal crisis and usual coping behaviors.

■ Patient works with primary nurses to plan care.

■ Patient describes two instances in which needs were met through direct communication.

■ Patient describes one difficult interpersonal situation that was solved by identifying the problem, choosing alternative ways to communicate, and taking action.

■ Patient identifies two effective and two ineffective coping behaviors.

■ Patient enlists support and assistance from family and friends.

Documentation
■ Patient's perception of present situation
■ Emotions expressed by patient
■ Observations of patient's behaviors
■ Interventions performed to help patient develop coping skills
■ Patient's response to nursing interventions
■ Evaluations for expected outcomes

Reference

Vatne, S., and Fagermoen, M.S. "To Correct and to Acknowledge: Two Simultaneous and Conflicting Perspectives of Limit-Setting in Mental Health Nursing," *Journal of Psychiatric and Mental Health Nursing* 14(1):41-48, February 2007.

Dysfunctional
FAMILY PROCESSES: ALCOHOLISM
related to biochemical influences

Definition

Psychosocial, spiritual, and physiological functions of the family unit that are chronically disorganized, which leads to conflict, denial of problems, resistance to change, ineffective problem solving, and a series of self-perpetuating crises

Assessment

■ Family status, including alcoholic family member's ability to function in occupational and family roles, ability of other family members to function in their roles, family conflicts, financial status, and rituals during holidays and family celebrations

■ Coping patterns, including type and number of changes family has recently experienced, usual response to stress, ability to adapt to change, and use of support systems

■ Family health history, including medication use, mental illness, stress-related illnesses, history of alcohol or drug abuse, and evidence of emotional, physical, or sexual abuse of spouse or children

■ Parental status, including age, marital status, number and ages of dependent children, and knowledge of normal child behavior

■ Drinking pattern, including continuous or binge drinking, periods of abstinence and relapse, use of other substances, symptoms of withdrawal, and past drinking patterns and treatment

■ Psychological status, including self-image and self-esteem, functional ability, independence level, and problem-solving and decision-making skills

■ Spiritual status, including affiliation with a religious group and religious practices

Defining characteristics

■ Roles and relationships
- Deterioration in family relationships or disturbed family dynamics
- Inconsistent parenting or low perception of parental support
- Altered role function or disruption of family roles
- Chronic family problems
- Closed communication systems
- Disrupted family rituals
- Economic problems
- Family denial

- Inability to demonstrate respect for individuality and autonomy of its members
- Ineffective spouse communication or marital problems
- Intimacy dysfunction
- Lack of cohesiveness
- Lack of skills necessary for relationships
- Neglected obligations
- Pattern of rejection
- Reduced ability to relate to each other for mutual growth and maturation
- Triangulating family relationships
- Unable to meet security needs of its members
- Behavioral
- Agitation
- Alcohol abuse or other substance abuse such as nicotine
- Blaming, criticizing
- Broken promises
- Chaos
- Contradictory, paradoxical communication
- Controlling communication or power struggles
- Dependency
- Difficulty with intimate relationships
- Diminished physical contact
- Disturbances in academic performance in children
- Disturbances in concentration
- Escalating conflict
- Failure to accomplish current or past developmental tasks or difficulty with life-cycle transitions
- Family special occasions that are alcohol centered
- Harsh self-judgment and self-blame
- Immaturity
- Impaired communication
- Inability to adapt to change
- Inability to deal constructively with traumatic experiences
- Inability to express or accept wide range of feelings
- Inability to meet spiritual needs of its members
- Inability to meet emotional needs of its members
- Inadequate understanding or knowledge of alcoholism
- Inappropriate expressions of anger
- Ineffective problem-solving skills
- Isolation
- Lack of dealing with conflict
- Lack of reliability
- Lying
- Manipulation
- Orientation toward tension relief rather than achievement of goals
- Rationalization or denial of problems
- Refusal to get help or inability to accept and receive help appropriately
- Seeking approval and affirmation
- Stress-related physical illnesses

– Unresolved grief
– Use of enabling to maintain alcoholic drinking patterns
– Verbal abuse of spouse or parent
■ Feelings
– Abandonment
– Anger or suppressed rage
– Anxiety, tension, or distress
– Being "different" from other people
– Being unloved
– Confusing love and pity
– Confusion
– Decreased self-esteem or worthlessness
– Depression
– Dissatisfaction
– Emotional control by others
– Emotional isolation or loneliness
– Failure
– Fear
– Frustration
– Guilt
– Hopelessness
– Hostility
– Hurt
– Insecurity
– Lack of identity
– Lingering resentment
– Loss
– Mistrust
– Misunderstood
– Moodiness
– Powerlessness
– Rejection
– Repressed emotions
– Responsibility for alcoholic's behavior
– Shame/embarrassment
– Unhappiness
– Vulnerability

Expected outcomes

■ Family members will acknowledge there's a problem with alcoholism within the family.

■ Alcoholic family member will sign a contract stating that he agrees to abstain from alcohol.

■ Family members will sign contracts stating that they won't engage in abusive behavior.

■ Family members will communicate their needs using "I" statements.

■ Parents will take steps to reassert appropriate boundaries with children and resume parental responsibilities.

■ Family members will discuss problems in an open, safe environment.

■ Family members will acknowledge their strengths and their progress in resolving problems.

■ Number and intensity of family crises will diminish.

■ Family members will state their plans to continue to seek counseling and attend appropriate support group meetings.

Suggested NOC outcomes

Family Coping; Family Functioning; Family Normalization; Role Performance; Substance Addiction Consequences

Interventions and rationales

■ Encourage family members to acknowledge that alcoholism is a problem within the family *to break through family denial.* Encourage individual family members to take responsibility for their problems. *Problems can't be addressed until family members take responsibility for them.*

■ Inform the alcoholic family member that he'll have to address his alcoholism before progress can be made in rebuilding family relations. Tell him that abstinence with the help of a support group such as Alcoholics Anonymous is the only proven effective treatment for alcoholism *to establish abstinence as basis for treatment.*

■ Ask the alcoholic family member to sign a contract stating he'll abstain from alcohol *to help him take responsibility for his behavior.*

■ Help family members evaluate the consequences of abusive and violent behavior. Inform them that any suspected abuse will be reported. Ask family members to sign contracts stating they won't abuse each other *to help ensure the safety of family members.*

■ Teach family members to communicate their needs assertively. Encourage family members to use "I" statements to express feelings, for example, "I'm mad because you didn't show up for the school play like you promised," *to help family members get in touch with and talk about their feelings.*

■ Discuss with the parents their ideas and beliefs regarding parental authority. Ask if they feel they have abdicated authority. Work with the parents to develop steps to reassert parental authority *to reestablish appropriate boundaries and relieve children of the need to assume parental roles.*

■ Provide an opportunity for family members to discuss conflicts in an open, safe atmosphere *to decrease anxiety and help family members develop confidence in their ability to resolve problems.*

■ Assist family members in identifying their strengths and their progress in addressing problems *to build self-esteem.*

■ Encourage family members to continue to seek counseling *to enhance interpersonal skills and strengthen the family unit.*

■ Encourage family members to participate in Al-Anon or Alateen *to foster recovery.*

Suggested NIC interventions

Coping Enhancement; Family Process Maintenance; Family Support; Substance Use Prevention; Substance Use Treatment

Evaluations for expected outcomes

■ Family members acknowledge that alcoholism is a problem in the family.
■ Alcoholic family member signs a contract stating that he agrees to abstain from alcohol.
■ Family members sign contracts stating that they won't engage in abusive behavior.
■ Family members communicate their needs using "I" statements.
■ Parents take steps to reassert appropriate boundaries with children and to resume parental responsibilities.
■ Family members discuss problems in an open, safe environment.
■ Family members acknowledge their strengths and the progress they have made in resolving problems.
■ Number and intensity of family crises diminish.
■ Family members state their plans to continue to seek counseling and attend appropriate support groups.

Documentation

■ Family's reactions to and experience with alcoholism
■ Interventions to assist family and family's response to them
■ Referrals to community agencies
■ Evaluations for expected outcomes

Reference

Fowler, T.L. "Alcohol Dependence and Depression: Advance Practice Nurse Interventions," *Journal of the American Academy of Nurse Practitioners* 18(7):303-308, July 2006.

Interrupted
FAMILY PROCESSES

related to dysfunctional behavior

Definition

A change in family relationship or functioning

Assessment

■ Family status, including marital status, family's developmental stage, family roles, family rules, communication patterns, family goals, and socioeconomic status
■ Family health history, including history of mental illness, stress-related illnesses, history of substance abuse, and sexual abuse of spouse or children

■ Parental status, including ages of dependent children and knowledge of normal child behavior

■ Psychological status, including self-image and self-esteem, functional ability, independence level, and problem-solving and decision-making skills

Defining characteristics

■ Changes in:

– Availability for emotional support

– Communication patterns

– Expressions of conflict with or isolation from community resources

– Expressions of conflict within family

– Mutual support

– Participation in problem solving

– Patterns and rituals

– Somatic complaints

– Stress-reduction behaviors

Expected outcomes

■ Family members won't experience verbal, physical, emotional, or sexual abuse.

■ Family members will communicate clearly, honestly, consistently, and directly.

■ Family members will establish clearly defined roles and equitable responsibilities.

■ Family members will express understanding of rules and expectations.

■ Family members will report that methods of solving problems and resolving conflicts have improved.

■ Family members will report a decrease in the number and intensity of family crises.

■ Family members will seek ongoing treatment.

Suggested NOC outcomes

Family Coping; Family Functioning; Family Normalization; Social Interaction Skills; Substance Addiction Consequences

Interventions and rationales

■ Meet with family members *to establish levels of authority and responsibility in the family.*

■ In family meeting, arrange seating so adults present unified front *to reinforce their function as a decision-making unit.*

■ Hold adults accountable for their alcohol or substance abuse and have them sign a "Use Contract" *to decrease denial, increase trust, and promote change.*

■ Assist family to set limits on abusive behaviors and have them sign "Abuse Contracts" *to foster feelings of safety and trust.*

■ Teach family to communicate clearly and honestly *to increase their ability to express thoughts and feelings in a positive way.*

■ Encourage family members to evaluate communication patterns periodically *to reinforce benefits of effective communication skills.*

■ Refer to outside agencies, if needed, *to ensure continuing support.*

Suggested NIC interventions

Coping Enhancement; Family Integrity Promotion; Family Process Maintenance; Family Support; Normalization Promotion; Substance Use Prevention; Substance Use Treatment

Evaluations for expected outcomes

- Family members don't experience any type of abuse.
- Family members report that family communication is clear, honest, and respectful.
- Family members describe clearly defined roles and responsibilities.
- Family members demonstrate understanding of roles and responsibilities.
- Family members identify problems and work together to solve them.
- Family members report fewer family crises.
- Family members recognize the need for professional assistance.

Documentation

- Problems and conflicts described by family members
- Behavioral contracts signed by family members
- Changes in roles and responsibilities and information about how these changes were negotiated
- Evidence of changes in family communication patterns
- Family's response to nursing interventions
- Evaluations for expected outcomes

Reference

Yonaka, L., et al. "Barriers to Screening for Domestic Violence in the Emergency Department," *Journal of Continuing Education in Nursing* 38(1):37-45, January-February 2007.

HOPELESSNESS

related to child's mood disturbance

Definition

A subjective feeling in which a child sees limited or no alternatives or personal choices available and can't mobilize energy on own behalf

Assessment

- Family status, including family composition, level of education of family members, parents' occupation, child's grade level, ability of family to meet child's physical and emotional needs, coping patterns, and evidence of abuse
- Psychological status, including changes in appetite, energy level, motivation, and personal hygiene
- Sleep pattern
- Social status, including quality of relationships, degree of trust in others, level of self-esteem, and ability to function in social or academic roles

Defining characteristics

- Closing eyes
- Decreased affect
- Decreased appetite
- Decreased or increased sleep
- Decreased response to stimuli
- Decreased verbalization
- Lack of initiative
- Passivity
- Turning away from speaker

Expected outcomes

- Child won't harm himself while in hospital.
- Child will complete activities of daily living (ADLs) with assistance.
- Child will identify feelings and seek help when they're overwhelming.
- Child will identify ways to deal with stress at home and school.
- Child will begin making positive statements about himself and others.

Suggested NOC outcomes

Decision-Making; Depression Self-Control; Hope; Mood Equilibrium; Psychomotor Energy; Quality of Life

Interventions and rationales

- Assign a small, consistent number of caregivers *to allow for the development of a trusting relationship between the child and the caregiver.*
- Provide a safe environment *to maintain the child's safety.*
- Spend time each shift with the child. Allow the child to play in lieu of talking. *Playing is a form of communication for children.*
- Encourage the child to perform self-care activities to the extent possible and praise the smallest efforts *to enhance self-esteem and reduce feelings of hopelessness.*
- Help the child make contact with other children *to reduce feelings of hopelessness.*
- Have family members bring toys, pictures, and other personal belongings *to reduce the child's stress.*
- Teach the child, parents, and teachers about interventions that increase self-esteem *so that the child continues to receive support after discharge.*

Suggested NIC interventions

Energy Management; Family Support; Hope Instillation; Mood Management

Evaluations for expected outcomes

- Child remains safe and unharmed.
- Child completes ADLs.
- Child asks for help when unable to cope with feelings.
- Child demonstrates positive methods of dealing with stress.
- Child attempts to make positive statements about himself and others.

Documentation

- Observations of child's behavior
- Child's participation in self-care activities
- Child's expressions during play therapy
- Nursing interventions that stabilize mood and maintain safety
- Child's response to nursing interventions
- Evaluations for expected outcomes

Reference

Ott, M.J. "I Want to do it Myself! Interferon Self-injection for Children with Chronic Viral Hepatitis," *Gastroenterology Nursing* 28(5):406-409, September-October 2005.

Disturbed personal
IDENTITY
related to lowered self-esteem

Definition
Inability to distinguish between self and nonself

Assessment

- Choices of vocation, sexual orientation, religious orientation, and friendships
- Ability to defend choices regarding long-range goals, to recognize alternatives, and to appreciate consequences
- Comfort level with decisions made about long-range goals
- Degree of anxiety or depression about long-range goals
- Loss of interest or social isolation from usual activities or friends
- Level of irritability about long-range goals
- Sleep difficulties
- Changes in eating habits
- Family status, including method of dealing with general conflicts, level of patient's communication with parents, handling of negotiations regarding restriction of freedom, degree of patient's separation from family, tolerance of patient's expressed opinions, reaction of parents to patient's long-range goals, and age-appropriateness of dating, curfew regulation, and money responsibilities
- Family and cultural standards related to separation issues

Defining characteristics

- Inadequate sense of self
- Relationship problems
- Social, emotional, or psychological immaturity

Expected outcomes

- Patient will establish trusting relationship with caregiver.
- Patient's issues will be discussed.

- Family's issues will be discussed.
- Patient will establish a firm, positive sense of self and personal identity.
- Patient will choose long-range goals using problem-solving techniques and will be comfortable with choices.
- Family will accept patient's choices of long-range goals.

Suggested NOC outcomes

Distorted Thought Self-Control; Identity; Self-Mutilation Restraint

Interventions and rationales

- Assess the patient alone, without his family, *to gather baseline data and begin a therapeutic relationship.*
- Explain your role as a patient advocate; negotiate rules of interaction, including confidentiality and depth and breadth of discussion *to establish your role as a resource for the patient rather than as the family's agent.*
- Explore personal identity issues distressing to the patient *to isolate issues into smaller, more solvable units.*
- Help the patient identify his values, beliefs, hopes, dreams, skills, and interests. *The patient's deficits may lie in a lack of self-exploration, problem-solving methods used, or separation issues with his parents.*
- Integrate personal identity issues into decisions and choices *to help the patient develop skill in problem-solving methods.*
- Help the patient identify the likely consequences of each choice. *Discussion and explanation aid problem-solving skills.*
- Promote choices with the most likelihood of success. *Specific instructions can help the patient gain problem-solving ability and maturity.*
- Encourage family conferences to explore potential reactions to the patient's choices, and promote support for the patient's independent decision making. *Meetings can help the patient and family members identify problems and find better ways to interact. Meetings also allow the patient and family members to ventilate true feelings in a safe environment.*
- Encourage peer support groups *to explore and share personal identity experiences. Adolescents and young adults commonly accept support from peers more readily than from older adults.*
- Promote outpatient counseling and family meetings, as appropriate, to reinforce progress. *Establishing outpatient support systems can reduce regression.*
- Listen to the patient's personal values and beliefs, but remain nonjudgmental, even if his values and beliefs differ from your own. *Remaining nonjudgmental, but attentive, shows your support.*

Suggested NIC interventions

Delusion Management; Environmental Management: Violence Prevention; Hallucination Management; Reality Orientation

Evaluations for expected outcomes

- Patient openly discusses concerns with caregiver.
- Patient describes personal identity struggles.

- Family members discuss their reactions to patient's personal identity choices.
- Patient describes values, beliefs, skills, and interests in positive way.
- Patient identifies choices and possible alternatives, postulates consequences, and makes decisions about long-range goals.
- Family members accept patient's choices of long-range goals.

Documentation

- Assessment of patient's initial issues and problem-solving ability, including family's reactions, as well as assessment of level of separation achieved by patient
- Patient's level of emotional distress and changes in sleep and eating, initially and as hospitalization continues
- Patient's progress in problem solving and making choices
- Patient-family interactions and content of family meetings
- Patient's interaction in peer-group meetings
- Outpatient resources identified and suggested to patient and family members
- Evaluations for expected outcomes

Reference

Barber, S., et al. "Self-perception in Children with Attention Deficit/Hyperactivity Disorder," *Journal of Pediatric Nursing* 20(4):235-45, August 2005.

Risk for
INJURY
related to elder abuse

Definition

A state in which an individual is at risk for injury as a result of environmental conditions interacting with the individual's adaptive and defensive resources

Assessment

- Age
- Health history, including accidents, falls, exposure to environmental hazards, marks from restraints, and unexplained bruising
- Evidence of neglect, including inappropriate clothing, unsanitary living conditions, inadequate food supplies, lack of medication, and absence of needed eyeglasses, hearing aid, cane, or walker
- Family status, including caregiver relationship to patient; time and resources available for caregiving; willingness and ability to meet patient's physical, social, and psychological needs; feelings of frustration; and history of abuse of any family member

Risk factors

- Affective orientation
- Design, structure, and arrangement of community, building, and equipment
- Developmental age

■ Mode of transportation
■ People or provider (nosocomial agents and staffing patterns)
■ Pollutants, drugs, alcohol, caffeine, nicotine, and preservatives

Expected outcomes

■ Patient will remain free from injury.
■ Patient will state that no incidents of abuse occur.
■ Patient will maintain control of mail, telephone, and other personal effects.
■ Caregiver will state intention to contact respite care services and support groups.
■ Patient and caregiver will report improved communication patterns.

Suggested NOC outcomes

Abuse Protection; Falls Occurrence; Personal Safety Behavior; Risk Control; Safe Home Environment

Interventions and rationales

■ Monitor the patient closely for signs of physical or mental abuse or neglect (bruises, abrasions, body odor, and unkempt appearance) *to ensure the patient's safety and well-being.*
■ Encourage the patient to discuss abuse or threats of abuse. Be willing to listen, and be careful to convey a nonjudgmental attitude. *The patient may hesitate to talk openly for fear of retaliation.*
■ Report actual or suspected abuse to local authorities. *Every state has an agency that investigates and makes decisions about how a patient can best be protected from further abuse. Nurses are mandatory reporters of suspected abuse.*
■ Encourage the patient to answer his own telephone and open his own mail. *This gives the patient a sense of control and self-worth.*
■ Inform the patient and caregiver about state and county services for elderly people, respite services, adult day care, and support groups for children of aging parents *to enhance the caregiver's ability to cope.*

Suggested NIC interventions

Environmental Management: Safety; Incident Reporting; Risk Identification; Surveillance: Safety

Evaluations for expected outcomes

■ Patient shows no physical or mental signs of abuse.
■ Patient reaffirms there has been no abuse.
■ Patient can manage his own mail and telephone messages.
■ Caregiver contacts community agencies that offer assistance.
■ Patient and family demonstrate improved communication.

Documentation

■ Evidence of abuse
■ Comments by patient that indicate abuse
■ Reports made to state agencies

- Changes in caregiver-patient relationship
- Outside agencies contacted by caregiver
- Changes occurring as a result of using outside resources
- Evaluations for expected outcomes

Reference

Muehlbauer, M., and Crane, P.A. "Elder Abuse and Neglect," *Journal of Psychosocial Nursing and Mental Health Services* 44(11):43-48, November 2006.

Deficient
KNOWLEDGE
related to informed consent

Definition

Absence or deficiency of cognitive information related to a specific topic

Assessment

- Age
- Developmental stage
- Educational level
- Ethnic group
- Religion
- Beliefs, values, and attitudes about health and illness
- Family status, including marital status, family roles, and family communication patterns
- Mental status, including level of consciousness, thought and speech, mood and affect, orientation, memory, capacity to read and write, and judgment
- Legal status, including patient's authority to give consent, presence of a legal guardian, and nature of treatment

Defining characteristics

- Inability to understand prescribed treatment
- Inaccurate performance of test
- Inaccurate follow-through of instruction
- Inappropriate or exaggerated behavior

Expected outcomes

- Patient will describe treatment and name person who will perform it.
- Patient will express awareness of right to refuse treatment.

Suggested NOC outcomes

Knowledge: Health Resources; Knowledge: Illness Care

Interventions and rationales

■ Ask the patient to describe his understanding of the procedure to be performed *to determine how much the patient can assimilate.*

■ Answer questions in terms the patient can understand. If the patient can't understand, refer him to the physician *to ensure the patient's right to informed consent is protected.*

■ If the patient can't understand, make sure the patient's legal guardian understands the procedure and the reason for doing it. *The nurse can be held liable if informed consent isn't obtained.*

■ If treatment is ongoing, continue to educate the patient about his care and legal rights *to ensure continuity of care.*

Suggested NIC interventions

Health Care Information Exchange; Health System Guidance; Teaching: Individual

Evaluations for expected outcomes

■ Patient explains treatment accurately.

■ Patient states understanding of legitimate right to refuse treatment.

Documentation

■ Patient's or guardian's understanding of treatment

■ Actions taken to ensure informed consent

■ Signed consent (or refusal to sign)

■ Evaluations for expected outcomes

Reference

Steevenson, G. "Informed Consent," *Journal of Perioperative Practice* 16(8):384-88, August 2006.

POSTTRAUMA SYNDROME

related to assault

Definition

Sustained painful response to an unexpected life event

Assessment

■ History and circumstances of assault

■ Patient's perception of event

■ Physical injuries sustained, including cardiopulmonary, genitourinary, integumentary, and musculoskeletal

■ Neurologic status

■ Emotional reactions, including grief reaction and changes in self-concept and sleep pattern

■ Cognitive reactions, including concentration, memory, and orientation

■ Behavioral reactions, including coping patterns and social interactions
■ Available support systems

Defining characteristics

■ Avoidance, alienation, and altered moods
■ Denial, grief, fear, and depression
■ Detachment
■ Exaggerated startle response and flashbacks
■ Guilt
■ Hypervigilance
■ Intrusive dreams, nightmares, or thoughts and difficulty concentrating
■ Irritability
■ Panic attacks
■ Repression
■ Shame

Expected outcomes

■ Patient will recover from physical injuries to extent possible.
■ Patient will express feelings of anger, blame, fear, and guilt. Patient will spend less time recriminating himself.
■ Patient will express feelings of physical safety.
■ Patient will use effective coping mechanisms to reduce fear.
■ Patient will mobilize support systems and professional resources, as needed.
■ Patient will reestablish and maintain adaptive interpersonal relationships.

Suggested NOC outcomes

Abuse Recovery: Emotional; Abuse Recovery: Sexual; Coping; Fear Self-Control

Interventions and rationales

■ Follow the medical regimen to manage physical injuries. *This reduces anxiety as the patient perceives the body's ability to recover from injury.*
■ Provide the patient with psychological support:
– Visit frequently *to decrease the patient's fear of being left alone and to encourage a trusting relationship.*
– Be available to listen *to express empathy with the patient's feelings.*
– Accept the patient's feelings and behaviors *to reassure the patient that they're appropriate and valid.*
– Reassure the patient of his safety, and take appropriate measures to ensure it. *The patient's feelings of safety are compromised by fear of repeated assaults.*
■ Avoid care-related activities and environmental stimuli (loud noises, bright lights, abrupt entrances to room, painful procedures or treatments) that may intensify symptoms. *The patient's traumatic experience may be intensified by misinterpreting procedures or environmental factors as repeated assaults.*
■ Monitor mental status, reorienting the patient to his surroundings and interpreting reality as often as necessary, *to alleviate psychic numbing, a characteristic symptom of assault.*

- Instruct the patient in at least one fear-reducing behavior, such as seeking support from others when frightened, *to help the patient gain a sense of mastery over the current situation.*
- Support family members:
- Provide time for them to express their feelings.
- Help them understand the phases of crisis and the patient's reactions to them. *These measures help reduce anxiety.*
- Offer referrals to community or professional resources, including clergy, mental health professionals, social services, and support groups, *to help the patient regain a sense of universality, decrease isolation, share fears, and deal constructively with feelings.*
- Recognize that the patient's culture may affect his response to assault; remain supportive and nonjudgmental *to show the patient you support and accept his response.*

Suggested NIC interventions

Coping Enhancement; Counseling; Rape-Trauma Treatment; Security Enhancement; Support System Enhancement

Evaluations for expected outcomes

- Patient recovers from injuries to extent possible and resumes normal or near-normal activities of daily living.
- Patient expresses feelings of anger, blame, fear, and guilt. Patient spends less time recriminating himself.
- Patient reports feeling safe.
- Patient demonstrates at least one fear-reducing behavior during times of panic (specify).
- Patient uses available support groups or mental health crisis center.
- Patient interacts socially with others.

Documentation

- Patient's perception of event
- Observations of patient's verbal and nonverbal behaviors
- Observations of patient's interaction with others
- Patient's response to nursing interventions
- Referrals to other support systems
- Evaluations for expected outcomes

Reference

Hegadoren, K.M., et al. "Posttraumatic Stress Disorder Part III: Health Effects of Interpersonal Violence among Women," *Perspectives in Psychiatric Care* 42(3):163-73, August 2006.

POSTTRAUMA SYNDROME

related to incest

Definition
A sustained, maladaptive response to a traumatic, overwhelming event

Assessment
- Age
- Gender
- Education level
- Customs and rituals, especially pertaining to sexuality
- Family roles, rules, and subsystems
- Evidence of physical, sexual, or emotional abuse within family
- Ability of family members to protect children and correctly judge situations as being safe or unsafe
- Family history of alcoholism, substance abuse, or incarceration of family members

Defining characteristics
- Detachment
- Difficulty in concentrating
- Expressed feelings of denial or shame
- Fear
- Flashbacks
- Irritability
- Panic attacks
- Repression

Expected outcomes
- Child won't harm himself or others.
- Child will agree to maintain personal safety.
- Child will begin expressing feelings in words.
- Child will describe steps to take to maintain safety.
- Child will express awareness of placement after discharge (home, foster care, group home, day treatment program).

Suggested NOC outcomes
Abuse Cessation; Abuse Recovery: Sexual; Anxiety Level; Coping; Fear Self-Control; Self-Mutilation Restraint

Interventions and rationales
- Inform members of the treatment team and appropriate community agencies that the child may be victim of incest. *You have a responsibility to ensure the child's safety after discharge.*

■ Observe the child for changes in mood or behavior and for statements of intention to harm himself. *Children who have recently disclosed sexual abuse have a high rate of suicide.*

■ Ask the child to agree to verbal and written safety contracts stating he won't harm himself *to provide the child with a tangible reminder of how to cope with crises.*

■ If the child wants to talk about the traumatic event, actively listen *to reassure him that what he tells you is important.*

■ Praise the child for participating in one-on-one therapy sessions *to enhance his participation and sense of self-worth.*

■ Help the child identify adults who can be trusted, such as a school counselor, clergy person, or school nurse, *to help prevent further episodes of incest.*

■ Make appropriate referrals to mental health professionals and social service agencies *to ensure the child's safety in the community.*

Suggested NIC interventions
Behavior Management: Self-Harm; Coping Enhancement; Counseling; Mutual Goal Setting; Patient Contracting; Security Enhancement

Evaluations for expected outcomes
■ Child doesn't harm himself or others.
■ Child enters into a contract to refrain from injuring himself or others.
■ Child finds positive ways of expressing feelings.
■ Child follows steps defined in his plan to maintain safety.
■ Child cooperates in looking at a positive living environment after discharge.

Documentation
■ Written or verbal safety contract
■ Exact quotes of child if any disclosures are made regarding incest
■ Child's behavior with peers, staff, and family during visits
■ Responses to nursing interventions
■ Evaluations for expected outcomes

Reference
Harrison, E. "Disclosing the Details of Child Sexual Abuse: Can Imaginative Literature Help Ease the Suffering?" *Journal of Child and Adolescent Psychiatric Nurses* 18(3):127-34, July-September 2005.

POWERLESSNESS
related to physical, sexual, or emotional abuse by partner

Definition
Perception that one's own action won't significantly affect an outcome; a perceived lack of control over a current situation or happening

Assessment

- Age
- Gender
- Level of education
- Occupation
- Ethnic group
- Family status, including marital status; developmental stage; socioeconomic status; support systems; history of physical, sexual, or emotional support; and family health history
- Beliefs, values, and attitudes about health and illness
- History of substance abuse
- Description of physical, sexual, or emotional abuse

Defining characteristics

- Apathy
- Expressed feelings of anger, guilt, apathy, or depression
- Expressed feelings of doubt regarding role performance
- Fear of alienation from caregivers
- Inability to seek information regarding care
- Nonparticipation in care or decision making when opportunities are provided
- Passivity
- Reluctance to express true feelings
- Verbal expressions of having no control over outcome
- Verbal expressions of having no control over present situation

Expected outcomes

- Patient will identify feelings of powerlessness.
- Patient will identify risks to personal safety.
- Patient will make decisions related to care.
- Patient will identify life situations over which she has no control.
- Patient will develop a plan to take control of her life.

Suggested NOC outcomes

Depression Self-Control; Health Beliefs: Perceived Control; Health Beliefs: Perceived Resources

Interventions and rationales

- Evaluate the patient's potential for harm. *Ensuring the patient's safety is your primary responsibility.*
- Discuss the patient's abusive relationship with her. Help her identify feelings of powerlessness and the circumstances that lead to such situations *to help her recognize things that threaten her loss of control.*
- Contact social services *to ensure the patient receives legal and financial support, as needed.*
- Assist the patient to take responsibility for making decisions about self-care by setting care goals and making an activity schedule *to increase her feelings of control over her life.*

- Help the patient recognize situations in which she exhibited determination and control over her life *to reinforce past successes and develop a foundation for establishing future goals.*
- Refer the patient to a women's shelter *to ensure continued safety after discharge.*

Suggested NIC interventions

Decision-Making Support; Financial Resource Assistance; Patient Rights Protection; Referral; Self-Responsibility Facilitation

Evaluations for expected outcomes

- Patient discusses feelings of powerlessness.
- Patient describes circumstances in which safety is threatened.
- Patient makes decisions in relation to care.
- Patient understands situations in her life over which she has no control.
- Patient develops plan that will help her take control of her life.

Documentation

- Observations of patient's behavior
- Visits and phone calls from abusive spouse
- Patient's plan for her future
- Patient's response to nursing interventions
- Referrals to specialized professionals and support groups
- Evaluations for expected outcomes

Reference

Beaulaurier, R.L., et al. "Internal Barriers to Help Seeking for Middle-aged and Older Women who Experience Intimate Partner Violence," *Journal of Elder Abuse and Neglect* 17(3):53-74, 2005.

RAPE-TRAUMA SYNDROME

Definition

Sustained maladaptive response to a forced, violent sexual penetration against the victim's will and consent

Assessment

- History and circumstances of traumatic event
- Physical injuries sustained, including genitourinary, integumentary, musculoskeletal, and neurologic
- Emotional reactions, including grief reaction, changes in self-concept, and spiritual distress
- Support systems available to patient, including clergy, family members, and friends
- Problem-solving techniques usually employed by patient

Defining characteristics

- Aggression, anger, and depression
- Agitation
- Changes in relationships
- Denial
- Embarrassment or shame
- Fear or paranoia
- Guilt and self-blame
- Loss of self-esteem
- Nightmares, sleep disturbances, and phobias
- Powerlessness
- Revenge
- Sexual dysfunction
- Shock
- Vulnerability

Expected outcomes

- Patient will recover from physical injuries to fullest extent possible.
- Patient will express feelings and fears.
- Patient will use support systems.

Suggested NOC outcomes

Abuse Protection; Abuse Recovery: Emotional; Coping

Interventions and rationales

- Explain the assessment procedures to the patient *to reduce the level of fear associated with data gathering after a rape.*
- Follow the medical regimen to manage physical injuries caused by the traumatic event. *This is the first step in meeting the patient's hierarchy of needs and depends on the extent of the patient's other injuries and the intensity of the psychological response.*
- Follow the facility's protocol regarding legal responsibilities. Be aware of the potential legal issues of rape and of the role nurses may play as witnesses in legal proceedings. *These steps will help protect the patient's legal rights.*
- Provide emotional support:
- Be available to listen. *Active listening allows an empathetic response to the patient's feelings while being aware of one's own thoughts and behaviors.*
- Accept the patient's feelings *to let her know her feelings are valid and acceptable.*
- Approach the patient in a warm, caring manner *to cultivate her trust and cooperation.*
- Provide privacy during the physical examination and interviewing process. *To protect the patient's rights, no information should be released without prior consent.*
- Assure the patient of her safety, and take all necessary measures to ensure it. *This reduces the patient's fears of repeated assault.*
- Support the patient's family members in their reactions to the traumatic event:
- Provide time for them to express their feelings and concerns.
- Help them understand the patient's reactions.

Giving them time to talk and providing accurate information helps them support their loved one.

■ Offer referral to other support persons or groups, such as clergy, a crisis center, mental health professionals, rape counselors, and Women Organized Against Rape. *This will help the patient express her feelings and develop coping skills.*

Suggested NIC interventions

Abuse Protection Support; Anxiety Reduction; Crisis Intervention; Rape-Trauma Treatment; Self-Esteem Enhancement

Evaluations for expected outcomes

■ Patient recovers from physical injuries.
■ Patient expresses feelings common to rape victims, such as anger, blame, humiliation, and fear of disease or pregnancy.
■ Patient contacts local mental health, rape counseling, or crisis center.

Documentation

■ Patient's expressions of feelings about herself and traumatic event
■ Physical findings and treatment
■ Observations of family's interaction with patient
■ Referrals to support persons
■ Patient's response to nursing interventions
■ Evaluations for expected outcomes

Reference

Boykins, A.D. "The Forensic Exam: Assessing Health Characteristics of Adult Female Victims of Recent Sexual Assault," *Journal of Forensic Nursing* 1(4):166-71, Winter 2005.

RAPE-TRAUMA SYNDROME: COMPOUND REACTION

Definition

Trauma syndrome that develops after rape or attempted rape in which patient undergoes an acute phase of disorganization and a long-term reorganization and experiences drastic changes in behavior, psychological equilibrium, and ability to function

Assessment

■ History and circumstances of traumatic event
■ Physical symptoms reported by patient
■ Physical injuries sustained, including genitourinary, integumentary, musculoskeletal, and neurologic
■ Emotional reactions
■ Behavioral and cognitive changes, such as expansive mood and affect, agitation, extreme alertness, and narrowed attention span

■ Symptoms associated with posttrauma response, including hypervigilance and reexperience of assault

■ Past experience with physical or psychological trauma, including coping strategies and problem-solving skills

■ Available support systems, occupation, educational background, and lifestyle

Defining characteristics

■ Changes in lifestyle (change in residence or recurring nightmares)

■ Emotional reaction (anger, embarrassment, and fear)

■ Multiple physical symptoms (GI irritability, muscle tension, and sleep pattern disturbance)

■ Reactivated symptoms of previous physical or psychiatric conditions

■ Reliance on alcohol or drugs

Expected outcomes

■ Patient will recover from physical injuries to fullest extent possible.

■ Patient will express feelings about the rape.

■ Patient will report feeling safe.

■ Patient will contact appropriate support persons or groups.

■ Patient will report desire to reestablish and maintain interpersonal relationships.

Suggested NOC outcomes

Abuse Protection; Abuse Recovery: Emotional; Self-Mutilation Restraint

Interventions and rationales

■ Explain each phase of the assessment procedure to the patient *to reduce the level of fear the patient might experience during the data gathering following a rape.*

■ Follow the medical regimen to manage physical injuries. *This is the first step in meeting the patient's needs.*

■ Document and report the rape or attempted rape to appropriate authorities *to help protect the patient's legal rights.*

■ When interviewing the patient, use open-ended questions and listen intently *to encourage the patient to talk about the trauma and express her feelings, both verbally and through behavior.*

■ Show the patient that you accept her feelings, but set limits on aggressive behavior. *Demonstrating acceptance reassures the patient that her response to the trauma is valid. Setting limits provides the patient with necessary structure.*

■ Take appropriate measures to reassure the patient of her safety:

– Approach the patient carefully with open hands.

– Stay with the patient.

– Have female staff conduct the patient interview and physical examination.

Safety measures help to decrease the patient's anxiety and reduce fears of another assault.

■ Direct the patient to perform purposeful activities, such as taking medications and following the instructions of health care personnel, *to help reduce the patient's anxiety and restore her sense of control.*

■ Educate the patient about various responses to trauma. *The patient with a compound reaction may feel that the extreme emotional turmoil she experiences after rape is abnormal. Learning that others have undergone the same experience may help reassure her and decrease her isolation.*

■ Provide the patient's family members with opportunities to express their reactions to the trauma and the patient's response. Educate family members about compound reaction to rape *to help them support the patient.*

■ Refer the patient to appropriate support persons, such as clergy, mental health professionals, or a rape counselor. Encourage the patient to participate in support groups or therapy groups offered by a rape counseling center. *The patient may need long-term care to cope with the psychological consequences of rape.*

■ Provide ongoing support as the patient struggles to regain psychological equilibrium. Encourage her efforts to renew involvement in usual activities. *To achieve long-term personality reorganization, the patient will require time, consistent support, and ongoing counseling.*

Suggested NIC interventions

Abuse Protection Support; Coping Enhancement; Emotional Support; Environmental Management: Safety; Rape-Trauma Treatment

Evaluations for expected outcomes

■ Patient recovers from physical injuries and resumes normal or near-normal activities of daily living.

■ Patient expresses feelings associated with the rape.

■ Patient reports feeling safe.

■ After discharge, patient participates in ongoing counseling sessions or support group.

■ Patient reports increased ability to cope with psychological consequences of rape and increased social interactions and activities.

Documentation

■ Patient's expressions of feelings related to trauma
■ Observations of patient's behavior and interactions with others
■ Nursing interventions
■ Patient's response to interventions
■ Referrals accepted by patient
■ Evaluations for expected outcomes

References

Clements, P.T., et al. "Issues and Dynamics of Sexually Assaulted Adolescents and their Families," *International Journal of Mental Health Nursing* 13(4):267-74, December 2004.

Littleton, H.L., et al. "Rape Acknowledgment and Postassault Experiences: How Acknowledgment Status Relates to Disclosure, Coping, Worldview, and Reactions Received from Others," *Violence and Victims* 21(6):761-78, December 2006.

RAPE-TRAUMA SYNDROME: SILENT REACTION

Definition
Trauma syndrome that develops after rape, attempted rape, or sexual assault, in which patient undergoes an acute phase of disorganization and a long-term reorganization and doesn't tell anyone about the rape nor does she deal with her feelings about it

Assessment
■ Symptoms associated with posttrauma response
■ Evidence of emotional distress, including shock, fear, anger, and guilt
■ Behavioral and cognitive changes, such as lack of affect, agitation, decreased alertness, and narrowed attention span
■ Evidence of physical injuries
■ Available support systems
■ Past experience with physical or psychological trauma, including coping strategies and problem-solving skills
■ Laboratory studies, including tests for pregnancy and sexually transmitted diseases

Defining characteristics
■ Abrupt changes in relationships with men
■ Increased anxiety during interview (blocking of associations, long periods of silence, and minor stuttering)
■ Increase in nightmares
■ No expression that rape, attempted rape, or sexual assault occurred
■ Pronounced changes in sexual behavior
■ Sudden onset of phobic reactions

Expected outcomes
■ Patient will disclose that rape, attempted rape, or sexual assault occurred.
■ Patient will recover from physical injuries to fullest extent possible.
■ Patient will make contact with appropriate sources of support.
■ Patient will express willingness to address psychosocial problems associated with traumatic experience.

Suggested NOC outcomes
Abuse Protection; Abuse Recovery: Emotional; Abuse Recovery: Sexual

Interventions and rationales
■ Establish an atmosphere of trust *to help the patient overcome her silence about the rape or sexual assault.*
■ Confront the patient directly but gently with the question of whether she's a victim of rape or sexual assault. For example, you might say, "You seem very upset and you've told me about increased nightmares and a sudden loss of interest in

sexual relations. These are common characteristics of victims of sexual assault. If you've been sexually assaulted, you can tell me. I'll help you." *The patient with a silent reaction needs patience and encouragement to overcome anxiety about disclosing the rape or sexual assault.*

■ Clear up misconceptions the patient may have about the nature of rape or sexual assault. *If, for example, intercourse didn't take place or the attacker was a boyfriend, spouse, or family member, the patient may not believe that sexual assault occurred. Tell the patient that sexual assault can take different forms and that all can be equally traumatic.*

■ If the patient remains unwilling to disclose the rape or sexual assault, tell her that you'll continue to be available to help. Encourage her to contact you if she feels the need *to provide a resource for future help and to maintain communication.*

■ If the patient discloses the rape or sexual assault, be careful to respond in a caring, nonjudgmental manner *to cultivate trust and cooperation.* Follow the medical regimen to manage physical injuries (if the rape or sexual assault was recent) and follow facility protocol for documenting the rape or sexual assault and reporting it to authorities *to ensure the patient's physical well-being and protect her legal rights.* Use open-ended questions and listen intently *to encourage the patient to talk about the trauma.* If the patient is withdrawn, be understanding and supportive when gathering information *to allow the patient to proceed at her own pace.*

■ Emphasize to the patient that the attack wasn't her fault. *The patient with a silent reaction may feel intense guilt and shame over the assault.*

■ Educate the patient about various emotional responses to trauma. Rape-trauma syndrome is a variant of posttraumatic stress disorder. Responses such as suicidal ideation, disorientation, confusion, extreme detachment, nightmares, flashbacks, guilt, and depression are common. *The patient may believe that the emotional turmoil she experiences after rape or sexual assault is abnormal. Pointing out that others have undergone the same experience may lessen the patient's isolation, help her talk about her symptoms, and motivate her to seek follow-up care.*

■ Offer a referral to appropriate support persons or groups, such as clergy, mental health professionals, or a rape counselor. Contact a local rape crisis center for information about support groups or therapy groups. Note that, if only a single assault has occurred, short-term counseling may be sufficient. However, if the patient is a survivor of several assaults or repeated incest, she may need long-term psychotherapy. *Appropriate referrals help ensure that the patient gets needed care.*

Suggested NIC interventions

Abuse Protection Support; Anger Control Assistance; Assertiveness Training; Coping Enhancement; Counseling

Evaluations for expected outcomes

■ Patient discloses that rape, attempted rape, or sexual assault occurred.

■ Patient recovers from physical injuries and resumes normal or near-normal activities of daily living.

■ Patient contacts rape counselor and agrees to participate in therapy group.

■ Patient acknowledges that rape or sexual assault wasn't her fault and that she needs to deal with psychological consequences of trauma.

Documentation

- Evidence that patient has been raped or sexually assaulted, including patient's behavior and physical evidence
- Efforts made to help patient discuss rape or sexual assault and patient's response
- Nursing interventions
- Patient's response to interventions
- Referrals accepted by patient
- Evaluations for expected outcomes

Reference

Burgess, A.W., and Clements, P.T. "Information Processing of Sexual Abuse in Elders," *Journal of Forensic Nursing* 2(3):113-20, Fall 2006.

Risk for

SELF-MUTILATION

related to emotional illness

Definition

At risk for deliberate self-injurious behavior causing tissue damage with the intent of causing nonfatal injury to attain tension relief

Assessment

- Age
- Gender
- Developmental history
- Current stress level and coping behaviors
- Mental status, including judgment, thought content, and mood
- Family history, including abusive behavior
- Previous episodes of self-mutilation or suicide attempts
- Substance abuse history
- Social history, including sexual activity and aggression within peer group

Risk factors

- Borderline personality disorder (especially in females ages 16 to 25)
- Childhood sexual abuse
- Command hallucinations
- Dysfunctional family
- Feelings of depression, rejection, self-hatred, guilt, or depersonalization
- History of physical or sexual abuse, emotional abuse or deprivation, or emotional disturbance
- History of self-injury
- Inability to cope with increased physical or emotional tension
- Labile affect
- Loss of control over problem-solving situations

- Mental retardation and autism
- Psychotic state (typically young, adult males)
- Separation anxiety

Expected outcomes
- Patient won't harm himself while in facility.
- Patient will express increased sense of security.
- Patient will report being able to cope better with disorganization, aggressive impulses, anxiety, and hallucinations.
- Patient will experience fewer or no dissociative states.
- Patient will participate in therapeutic milieu.
- Patient will report suicidal thoughts to staff members.

Suggested NOC outcomes
Abuse Recovery Status; Anxiety Level; Impulse Self-Control; Risk Control; Self-Mutilation Restraint

Interventions and rationales
- Limit the number of staff members interacting with the patient *to provide continuity of care and increase the patient's sense of security.*
- Have staff members make frequent, short contacts with the patient *to reassure the patient without stifling independence.*
- Remove all dangerous objects from the patient's environment *to promote safety.*
- Make short-term verbal contracts with the patient in which the patient states he won't harm himself *to make the patient aware he's ultimately responsible for his own safety and that he can guarantee it.*
- Administer psychotropic medications, as ordered, *to reduce tension, impulsive behavior, hallucinations, and panic.*
- If the patient enters a dissociative state or hallucinates, move him to a quiet room with reduced stimuli. If he needs restraints, remain with him and provide reassurance *to calm him and orient him to reality.*
- As ordered, place the patient under observation *to provide protection and increase the patient's sense of security.* If hospitalized, the patient can be "zoned" or asked to remain in areas within sight of staff members.
- If the patient is participating in a therapeutic milieu, discuss the patient's risk of self-harm with community members *to provide enhanced protection and psychological support.*
- If the patient harms himself, care for injuries in a calm, nonjudgmental manner. Encourage the patient to talk about the feelings that prompted self-mutilation. *Discussion may help the patient connect self-destructive behavior to the feelings that preceded it and allow exploration of alternative ways of dealing with negative thoughts and feelings.*
- If self-destructive acts persist, consider developing a behavior modification program, in which the patient is rewarded with benefits (personal attention, material items) for demonstrating self-control *to reinforce self-control.*
- Ask the patient directly whether he's thinking of suicide and, if so, what plan he has. *A self-destructive patient may become suicidal and may require additional precautions.*

■ Hold frequent treatment team meetings *to ensure consistent care that's appropriate to the patient's current behavior.*

Suggested NIC interventions

Area Restriction; Behavior Management: Self-Harm; Environmental Management: Violence Prevention; Impulse Control Training; Limit Setting

Evaluations for expected outcomes
■ Patient keeps terms of verbal contract that he won't harm himself.
■ Patient expresses increased sense of security.
■ Patient describes coping skills that help him deal better with disorganization, aggressive impulses, anxiety, and hallucinations.
■ Patient experiences fewer or no dissociative states.
■ Patient participates in therapeutic milieu.
■ Patient tells staff member about suicidal thoughts.

Documentation
■ Nursing interventions performed and patient's response to them
■ Verbal contracts between patient and nurse
■ Patient's responses to medication and behavior modification program
■ Revisions to treatment plan
■ Drawing of self-inflicted injuries
■ Evidence of suicidal ideation
■ Evaluations for expected outcomes

Reference
McDonald, C. "Self-Mutilation in Adolescents," *The Journal of School Nursing* 22(4):193-200, August 2006.

SEXUAL DYSFUNCTION

related to decreased libido caused by depression

Definition
Change in sexual function that's viewed as unsatisfying, unrewarding, or inadequate

Assessment
■ Comprehensive sexual history, including attitude toward sex, sexual preference, sexual responsiveness of partner, previous sexual response patterns, and sexual desire, enjoyment, and performance
■ Psychological factors, including self-esteem, body image, guilt, symptoms of depression, and suicidal ideation
■ Support systems, including family, friends, and clergy
■ Attitude of spouse or significant other
■ Sociocultural factors, including educational level, socioeconomic status, ethnic group, and religious beliefs and practices

■ Physiologic factors, including medication history (response, effectiveness, and adverse reactions), current medication regimen (including tricyclic antidepressants or monoamine oxidase [MAO] inhibitors), and substance abuse history (type and effect on mental status)
■ Coping and problem-solving ability and ability to concentrate

Defining characteristics
■ Actual or perceived limitation imposed by disease or therapy
■ Change in relationship with spouse or significant other
■ Change of interest in self and others
■ Conflicts involving values
■ Inability or change in ability to achieve sexual satisfaction
■ Need for confirmation of desirability
■ Verbal expression of problem

Expected outcomes
■ Patient will acknowledge depressive episode and problem in sexual function.
■ Patient will voice feelings about decreases in sexual desire.
■ Patient will identify ways to enhance pleasure and improve interpersonal communication with partner.
■ Patient will regain sexual desire with recovery from depression.
■ Patient will accept referral for sex therapy, if necessary.

Suggested NOC outcomes
Body Image; Fear Level; Self-Esteem; Sexual Functioning

Interventions and rationales
■ Initiate a trusting therapeutic relationship with the patient. Make the purpose, nature, and parameters of this relationship clear *to help the patient feel secure and develop trust.*
■ Educate the patient and family members about the nature of depression, its treatment, and its effect on sexual desire. *Understanding the link between depression and sexual desire may diminish feelings of guilt and worthlessness and help raise self-esteem.*
■ Allow the patient to express his feelings openly in a nonthreatening, nonjudgmental atmosphere *to foster communication and help the patient cope with unresolved issues.* Offer feedback *to validate the patient's feelings and promote self-esteem.*
■ Include the patient and partner in planning care and interventions *to enhance a feeling of control for both partners.*
■ Reinforce compliance with the treatment plan for depression. *Even though tricyclic antidepressants and MAO inhibitors may diminish sexual desire, the patient needs to comply to resolve depression.*
■ Discuss with the patient and partner alternative expressions of affection to enhance their relationship during treatment *to help the couple preserve intimacy during a temporary loss of libido.*
■ Refer the patient for sex counseling or therapy if low sexual desire persists after the resolution of depression. *Sexual desire should return to its usual level after suc-*

cessful treatment for depression. If it doesn't, the patient should receive professional therapy.

Suggested NIC interventions

Self-Awareness Enhancement; Self-Responsibility Facilitation; Sexual Counseling; Teaching: Sexuality

Evaluations for expected outcomes

■ Patient describes depressive episode, treatment plan, and effects on sexual desire.
■ Patient expresses concerns to staff and family members.
■ Patient identifies at least three activities to enhance pleasure and communication with partner.
■ Patient reports return of sexual fantasies and desire for sexual activity.
■ Patient communicates willingness to follow through with referral for sex therapy.

Documentation

■ Patient's perceptions and concerns
■ Observation of patient's behavior, depressive symptoms, and suicidal risk
■ Interventions to assist patient and family members
■ Patient's and partner's responses to nursing interventions
■ Evaluations for expected outcomes

Reference

Kingsberg, S.A. "Taking a Sexual History," *Obstetrics and Gynecology Clinics of North America* 33(4):535-47, December 2006.

SEXUAL DYSFUNCTION

related to hypersexuality

Definition

Change in sexual function that's viewed as unsatisfying, unrewarding, or inadequate

Assessment

■ History of behaviors indicating excessive elation, such as hypersexuality, intrusiveness, grandiose thoughts, looseness of association, flight of ideas, extreme levels of energy, lack of sleep, lack of proper nutrition, poor judgment, elevated mood, expansiveness, pressured and rapid speech, and strained interpersonal relationships
■ History of psychiatric illness, including personality disorders exemplified by lack of impulse control
■ Sexual history, including attitude toward sex, previous sexual patterns, sexual preference, sexual response of partners, and appropriateness of sexual behavior

■ Sociocultural factors, including educational level, socioeconomic status, and ethnic group

■ Patient's perception of sexual behaviors and practices

■ Partner's perception of patient's sexual behaviors

■ Coping and problem-solving abilities

■ Health history, including medication history (response, effectiveness, and adverse reactions), use of psychosis-inducing drugs (such as phencyclidine and amphetamines), use of disinhibiting drugs (such as alcohol, amphetamines, and cocaine), and other substance abuse (type and effect on mental status)

Defining characteristics

■ Disturbances in interpersonal relationships caused by inappropriate sexual behavior

■ Excessive motor activity

■ Excessive sexual activity

■ Frustration and anger if sexual behavior is thwarted

■ General lack of impulse control

■ Impulsive acting out of sexual urges

■ Inability to conform sexual behavior to social norms

■ Inability to control outcome of sexual encounters

■ Inappropriate and provocative verbalizations that are sexual in content

■ Intrusiveness with peers, including excessive physical closeness and inappropriate touching

■ Periods of excessive elation or cycles of elation and depression

■ Poor perception of reality caused by psychosis or organic mental disorders

■ Sexual encounters that appear self-destructive; inability to maintain lasting relationships because of sexual behavior

Expected outcomes

■ Patient will meet sexual needs in socially appropriate manner.

■ Patient will reduce or eliminate sexual behaviors that may harm self or others.

■ Patient will learn how to recognize indicators of impending episodes of hypersexuality and how to prevent such episodes from occurring.

■ Patient will state plan to participate in recommended therapy.

Suggested NOC outcomes

Anxiety Level; Self-Esteem; Sexual Functioning; Sexual Identity

Interventions and rationales

■ Help the patient recognize potentially harmful sexual behavior. Set limits on high-risk sexual behavior. *Indiscriminate, impulsive sexual behavior can lead to unwanted pregnancy, sexually transmitted diseases, and physical and emotional trauma.*

■ Encourage the patient to express sexual urges in socially acceptable ways (including masturbation in a private setting) *to help the patient discover positive methods of relieving sexual tension.*

■ Discuss with the patient hypersexual behaviors and feelings associated with hypersexuality *to promote insight into behavior.*

■ Refer the patient to a medical and psychiatric specialist or sex therapist, if needed. *Indiscriminate and impulsive hypersexuality usually indicates a physical or psychiatric illness that requires further evaluation and treatment by an appropriate professional.*

Suggested NIC interventions
Behavior Management: Sexual; Energy Management; Sexual Counseling

Evaluations for expected outcomes
■ Patient states desire to express sexual drive in socially acceptable manner.
■ Patient reports sexual relationships that aren't harmful to self or others.
■ Patient develops increased understanding of hypersexual urges and the ability to cope with intense sexual desire.
■ Patient expresses willingness to participate in psychiatric care or sex therapy, if needed.

Documentation
■ Patient's perception of sexual behaviors and level of sexual activities
■ Patient's statements about sexual behaviors
■ Observations of patient's behavior, including inappropriate sexual expression
■ Interventions to help patient set limits on hypersexuality
■ Patient's response to nursing interventions
■ Evaluations for expected outcomes

References
Higgins, A., et al. "Hypersexuality and Dementia: Dealing with Inappropriate Sexual Expression," *British Journal of Nursing* 13(22):1330-34, December 2004-January 2005.

Mick, T.M., and Hollander, E. "Impulsive-Compulsive Sexual Behavior," *CNS Spectrums* 11(12):944-55, December 2006.

SOCIAL ISOLATION
related to inability to engage in satisfying personal relationships

Definition
Aloneness experienced by an individual and perceived as a negative or threatened state imposed by others

Assessment
■ Age
■ Gender
■ Level of education
■ Ethnic group
■ Family status, including marital status, family roles, ability of family to meet patient's physical and emotional needs, and communication style

- Coping patterns
- Evidence of physical, sexual, or emotional abuse
- Mental status, including motor activity, thought and speech, mood and affect, perceptions, orientation, memory, general information, attention span, abstraction, and judgment

Defining characteristics

- Absence of supportive significant other
- Behavior unacceptable to the dominant cultural group
- Expressed feelings of aloneness imposed by others
- Expressed feelings of difference from others
- No eye contact
- Projection of hostility in voice
- Sad, dull affect
- Uncommunicative behavior
- Withdrawal

Expected outcomes

- Patient will articulate feelings of isolation.
- Patient will agree to spend time daily talking to others.
- Patient will express comfort in talking to others.
- Patient will plan to continue social interactions with family and friends after discharge.

Suggested NOC outcomes

Family Social Climate; Loneliness Severity; Personal Well-Being; Social Interaction Skills; Social Involvement; Social Support

Interventions and rationales

- Spend time with the patient each shift *to establish a trusting relationship.*
- Encourage the patient to articulate his feelings. Listen nonjudgmentally *to let the patient know his ideas are valued.*
- Demonstrate eye contact, appropriate physical boundaries, and other socially appropriate behavior *to provide a model for the patient.*
- Encourage the patient to begin relating to others through participation in unit activities *to help the patient practice newly acquired social skills.*
- Encourage the patient to increase his level of social contact gradually *to avoid becoming overwhelmed.*
- Help the patient locate community resources and support groups *to decrease isolation and provide support.*

Suggested NIC interventions

Caregiver Support; Family Integrity Promotion; Mood Management; Socialization Enhancement

Evaluations for expected outcomes

- Patient discusses his difficulty interacting with others.

- Patient is observed communicating with others.
- Patient appears to communicate with increasing ease.
- Patient has developed a personal plan for continued ease in communicating with others.

Documentation
- Patient's comments about his interpersonal problems
- Patient's expression of loneliness
- Patient's participation in group activities
- Resources provided to patient for ongoing care
- Evaluations for expected outcomes

Reference
Perese, E.F., and Wolf, M. "Combating Loneliness among Persons with Severe Mental Illness: Social Network Interventions' Characteristics, Effectiveness, and Applicability," *Issues in Mental Health Nursing* 26(6):591-609, July 2005.

SOCIAL ISOLATION
related to inadequate personal resources

Definition
Aloneness experienced by the individual and perceived as imposed by others as a negative or threatening state

Assessment
- Reason for hospitalization (physiologic or psychiatric)
- Support systems, including clergy, family members, and friends
- Diversional interests
- Attitudes of family members toward patient in this situation
- Financial resources
- Occupation
- Level of education and intelligence
- Coping and problem-solving ability
- Self-esteem

Defining characteristics
- Description of lifestyle as solitary or circumscribed by membership in subculture
- Evidence of physical or mental disability or altered state of wellness
- Expressed feelings of being different from others
- Expressed feelings of rejection or aloneness
- Expressed frustration over inability to meet expectations of others
- Inappropriate or immature interests or activities
- Insecurity in public
- Lack of family, friends, and social groups
- Lack of purpose in life

■ Uncommunicative and withdrawn behavior, with poor eye contact

Expected outcomes

■ Patient will interact positively with caregivers.

■ Patient will express feelings about lack of supportive relationships.

■ Patient will express desire to be involved with others.

■ Patient will express desire to improve himself and current condition—for example, by obtaining further education or learning how to better manage finances.

■ Patient will use available resources (social services, home health care, psychology services, self-improvement classes) to establish realistic plan for future.

■ Patient will state plan to participate in social activity.

Suggested NOC outcomes

Client Satisfaction: Communication; Mood Equilibrium; Personal Well-Being; Social Involvement; Social Support

Interventions and rationales

■ Assign the same caregivers to the patient *to promote a trusting relationship with staff members. Consistent care promotes the patient's ability to communicate openly.*

■ Assign a primary nurse to coordinate the patient's care. *This reduces the potential for fragmented nursing interventions.*

■ Plan a 15-minute period each shift to sit with the patient. If the patient doesn't wish to talk, remain silent. *Active listening communicates concern, allows time to collect thoughts, and encourages the patient to initiate interaction.*

■ Involve the patient in planning care and have him participate in self-care continuously *to provide structure, reduce feelings of helplessness, and foster independent action.*

■ Discuss the patient's living accommodations and lifestyle outside the facility to *help you understand the patient and facilitate discharge planning.*

■ Refer the patient to social services for follow-up, if necessary, *to ensure a comprehensive approach to care.*

■ Help the patient identify social outlets (peer group, associations, group activity) *to draw the patient's attention to specific data and promote goal-directed interaction.*

Suggested NIC interventions

Coping Enhancement; Family Support; Referral; Socialization Enhancement; Support System Enhancement

Evaluations for expected outcomes

■ Patient seeks information from and expresses feelings to caregivers.

■ Patient acknowledges concern about absence of supportive relationships.

■ Patient expresses desire to develop meaningful relationships.

■ Patient states at least two methods of achieving personal growth and improving current situation.

■ Patient identifies and contacts social service agencies.

■ Patient states plan to participate in social activities.

Documentation
- Patient's perceptions of current situation
- Patient's expressions of plans for future
- Observations of patient's behavior
- Planning done by patient with nurse, physician, social worker, and others
- Patient's response to nursing interventions
- Evaluations for expected outcomes

Reference
Lauder, W., et al. "Social Capital, Age, and Religiosity in People Who are Lonely," *Journal of Clinical Nursing* 15(3):334-40, March 2006.

Chronic
SORROW
related to chronic mental illness

Definition
A cyclical, recurring, and potentially progressive pattern of pervasive sadness that's experienced in response to continual loss throughout the trajectory of an illness or disability

Assessment
- Age and sex
- History of recent loss
- Patient's usual pattern of coping with loss, including cultural, intellectual, and emotional responses
- Expressed feelings of loss of control over current situation
- Behavioral manifestations of grieving, including their intensity
- Somatic problems associated with grieving, including changes in appetite, sleep patterns, activity level, and libido
- Lifestyle changes related to illness (mobility restrictions, risk of complications, and medication regimen)
- Psychosocial status, including religious beliefs and practices, personal philosophy, educational background, and effect of altered health status on social life
- Physical and social environment
- Sources of support, including family members, friends, and clergy

Defining characteristics
- Expressed feelings that vary in intensity, are periodic, may progress and intensify over time, and may interfere with patient's ability to reach highest level of personal and social well-being
- Expressions of one or more of the following: anger, being misunderstood, confusion, depression, disappointment, emptiness, fear, frustration, guilt or self-blame, helplessness, hopelessness, loneliness, low self-esteem, recurring loss, and being overwhelmed

■ Expressions of periodic, recurrent feeling of sadness

Expected outcomes

■ Patient will identify losses associated with changes in health status.
■ Patient will express feelings about changes in health status.
■ Patient will seek assistance in dealing with emotions related to loss.
■ Patient will begin to develop healthy coping mechanisms such as open expression of grief.
■ Patient will seek out support from family, friends, clergy, or others when necessary.
■ Patient will begin to plan for discharge and for future.
■ Patient will express realistic expectations with regard to health status.

Suggested NOC outcomes

Acceptance: Health Status; Depression Self-Control; Hope; Mood Equilibrium

Interventions and rationales

■ Spend at least 15 minutes each shift with the patient to focus on expression of feelings. Encourage the patient to express thoughts and feelings openly. *Dysfunctional grieving may result from the inability to freely express feelings.*
■ Communicate to the patient that feelings of anger are acceptable, but place limits on destructive behavior. *Inability to identify anger as normal response to loss may cause the patient to express aggression inappropriately.*
■ Help the patient focus realistically on changes in health status because of loss *to help the patient plan for the future.*
■ Encourage the patient to reach out to people who can offer support, such as family, friends, and clergy, *to increase emotional strength.*
■ Encourage the patient and family members to reminisce. *Engaging in life review promotes a peaceful atmosphere and helps in understanding the meaning of loss in relation to health and life.*
■ Inform the patient and family members about additional sources of support within the facility or community *to facilitate adaptive responses to loss and encourage community integration.*
■ Encourage the patient to take an active part in setting goals for health care *to facilitate independence and enhance self-esteem.*
■ Help the patient and family set realistic goals for discharge and the future *to help the patient place the loss in perspective and move on to new opportunities and relationships.*
■ Encourage the patient to be as independent as possible in self-care activities *to enhance self-esteem and promote optimal functioning.*
■ Refer the patient to a psychologist, psychiatrist, or social worker as appropriate. *Restoring emotional health may require assistance from a mental health professional.*

Suggested NIC interventions

Coping Enhancement; Decision-Making Support; Emotional Support; Hope Instillation; Mood Management; Spiritual Support; Support Group

Evaluations for expected outcomes
- Patient identifies losses associated with changes in health status.
- Patient expresses feelings about changes in health status.
- Patient seeks assistance in dealing with emotions related to loss.
- Patient begins to develop healthy coping mechanisms such as open expression of grief.
- Patient seeks out support from family, friends, clergy, or others when necessary.
- Patient begins to plan for discharge and for future.
- Patient expresses realistic expectations with regard to health status.

Documentation
- Patient's statements regarding loss
- Patient's behavioral response to loss, including interactions with family members and staff
- Nursing interventions to help patient overcome chronic sorrow
- Patient's response to nursing interventions
- Patient's statements indicating understanding that grief is normal
- Patient's statements regarding goals for discharge and future
- Referrals to a mental health professional
- Evaluations for expected outcomes

Reference
Chao, S.Y., et al. "The Effects of Group Reminiscence Therapy on Depression, Self-esteem, and Life Satisfaction of Elderly Nursing Home Residents," *The Journal of Nursing Research* 14(1):36-45, March 2006.

Risk for other-directed
VIOLENCE
related to excitement or antisocial behavior

Definition
At risk for behaviors in which an individual demonstrates that he or she can be physically, emotionally, and/or sexually harmful to others

Assessment
- Age
- Gender
- Recent stressors and coping strategies
- Patient history, including health history, substance abuse history (type and effects on mental status), and previous episodes of violence (circumstances, behavior, arrests)
- Reactions of family members to episodes of violence
- Mental status examination (with emphasis on insight and judgment)
- Physical findings, including neurologic examination
- Laboratory studies, including EEG, toxicology screening, and blood chemistry

Risk factors
- Body language: rigid, clenching of fists and jaw, hyperactivity, pacing
- Cognitive impairment
- History of childhood abuse
- History of threats of violence against person or personal proterty
- History of violence, including hitting, kicking, scratching, throwing objects at someone, attempting rape, sexual molestation
- History of violent antisocial behavior
- Neurological impairment
- Psychotic symptomatology

Expected outcomes
- Patient will maintain control over anger.
- Patient will successfully rechannel hostility into socially acceptable behaviors.
- Patient will discuss angry feelings and will verbalize ways to tolerate frustration appropriately.
- Patient will express need for long-term treatment by appropriate professional.

Suggested NOC outcomes
Abuse Cessation; Abusive Behavior Self-Restraint; Aggression Self-Control; Impulse Self-Control

Interventions and rationales
- Maintain a low level of stimuli in the patient's environment *to avoid increasing agitation and provoking violent behavior.*
- Remove all objects from the environment that the patient could use to injure others *to provide for the patient's safety and protect potential victims of violence.*
- Instruct staff members to maintain and convey a calm attitude toward the patient. *Anxiety is contagious and can be transferred to the patient. A calm attitude reinforces a feeling of safety.*
- Explain in a firm, calm voice that you'll help the patient remain in control. *Communicating willingness to help the patient maintain self-control encourages the patient to take control of his behavior.*
- Set limits on the patient's behavior *to reinforce the expectation that the patient will act in a responsible, controlled manner.*
- Express understanding of the patient's feelings and encourage open discussion *to provide support, reassurance, and positive reinforcement for desirable behaviors.*
- Administer prescribed medications to help the patient control aggressive behavior and remain calm. Monitor for effectiveness. *When used appropriately, medications commonly remove the need for physical restraint.*
- Explain the medication program to the patient *to promote compliance* and make sure he takes medications, as prescribed, *to help keep him calm.*
- According to facility policy, restrain or seclude the patient, as necessary, *to prevent serious injury to himself or others.* Use seclusion or restraint only after less restrictive measures have failed. Both measures require a physician's order as well as accurate documentation.

■ Establish a daily routine of strenuous exercise, and encourage the patient to adhere to it. *Exercise provides an alternative way to handle frustration.*

■ Encourage the patient to gradually begin discussing hostile feelings *to help him develop more appropriate ways of dealing with hostility.*

■ Refer the patient for appropriate long-term treatment—for example, to a drug or alcohol rehabilitation center, psychiatrist, or psychologist. *The patient may require help from specialized professionals or agencies.*

Suggested NIC interventions

Anger Control Assistance; Behavior Management; Environmental Management: Violence Prevention; Impulse Control Training

Evaluations for expected outcomes

■ Patient behaves in nonaggressive manner.

■ Patient rechannels hostility by participating in strenuous physical exercise on daily basis.

■ Patient states what precipitates anger and describes consequences of failing to control it.

■ Patient expresses need for ongoing treatment.

Documentation

■ Patient behaviors that indicate escalating agitation

■ Other observations about patient's verbal and nonverbal behavior

■ Factors that precipitate acts of violence

■ Nursing interventions performed to reduce or prevent violent behavior

■ Nursing interventions performed to ensure safety of other patients and staff members

■ Patient's response to nursing interventions

■ Referrals to specialized professionals and agencies

■ Evaluations for expected outcomes

Reference

Nelstrop, L., et al. "A Systematic Review of the Safety and Effectiveness of Restraint and Seclusion as Interventions for Short-term Management of Violence in Adult Psychiatric Inpatient Settings and Emergency Departments," *Worldviews on Evidence-based Nursing* 3(1):8-18, 2006.

Risk for self-directed
VIOLENCE
related to suicide attempt

Definition

At risk for behaviors in which an individual demonstrates that he or she can be physically, emotionally, and/or sexually harmful to others

Assessment
- Age
- Gender
- Medical history
- Patient's life situation
- Recent stressors and coping behaviors
- Available support systems
- History of suicide attempts, including aggressiveness of suicide attempts, lethality of suicide attempts, and number of prior suicide attempts
- History of substance abuse (type and effects on mental status)
- Reaction of family members
- Safety hazards
- Mental status, including abstract thinking, affect, content of thought, general information, insight, judgment, mood, orientation, recent and remote memory, and thought processes

Risk factors
- Body language: rigid, clenching of fists and jaw, hyperactivity, pacing
- Cognitive impairment
- History of childhood abuse
- History of threats of violence against person or personal property
- History of violence, including hitting, kicking, scratching, throwing objects at someone, attempting rape, sexual molestation
- History of violent antisocial behavior
- Neurological impairment
- Psychotic symptomatology
- Suicidal behavior

Expected outcomes
- Patient's environment will be free from potential suicide weapons.
- Patient will recover from suicidal episode.
- Patient will discuss feelings that precipitated suicide attempt.
- Patient will consult mental health professional.
- Patient will describe available resources for crisis prevention and management.
- Patient will voice improvement in self-worth.

Suggested NOC outcomes
Impulse Self-Control; Self-Mutilation Restraint; Suicide Self-Restraint

Interventions and rationales
- Ask the patient directly, "Have you thought about killing yourself?" If so, ask, "What do you plan to do?" *Suicide risk increases if the patient has a definite plan.*
- Initiate appropriate safety protocols by removing from the patient's environment anything that could be used to inflict further self-injury (razor blades, belts, glass objects, pills) *to help ensure the patient's safety.*
- Make a short-term contract with the patient that he won't harm himself during a specific period. Continue negotiating until no evidence of suicidal ideation ex-

ists. *A contract gets the subject of suicide out in the open, places some responsibility for safety on the patient, and conveys acceptance of the patient as a worthwhile person.*

■ Supervise the administration of prescribed medications. *Medications may be appropriate alternative to verbal interventions.* Be aware of drug actions and adverse effects. Make sure that the patient doesn't hoard medications.

■ Provide supervision (one-on-one observation when possible) for the patient based on facility policy *to ensure compliance with legal requirements to protect the patient and to reassure the patient of staff concern.*

■ Use a warm, caring, nonjudgmental manner *to show unconditional positive regard.*

■ Listen carefully to the patient and don't challenge him *to communicate caring and support.*

■ Demonstrate understanding, but don't reinforce denial of the current situation *because denial can mask the roots of suicidal feelings.*

■ Make appropriate referrals to mental health professionals *to help the patient work through suicidal feelings and develop healthier alternatives.*

■ Help the patient set a goal for obtaining long-term psychiatric care. *Ambivalence about psychiatric care or refusal to consult with a therapist marks the suicidal patient's lack of insight and use of denial.*

■ Provide the patient with telephone numbers and other information about crisis centers, hot lines, and counselors. *Alternatives may ease anxiety about the perceived threat of long-term psychotherapy.*

Suggested NIC interventions

Behavior Management: Self-Harm; Environmental Management: Violence Prevention; Impulse Control Training; Suicide Prevention

Evaluations for expected outcomes

■ Patient won't harm self in hospital.
■ In aftermath of initial suicide attempt, patient makes commitment not to act on suicidal thoughts.
■ Patient states reasons for suicide attempt.
■ Patient contacts mental health professional.
■ Patient identifies crisis prevention resources, such as hot line phone number, local crisis center, and name of therapist.
■ Patient expresses positive feelings about self.

Documentation

■ Patient's comments about suicide attempt and current feelings about it
■ Observations of patient's behavior
■ Interventions to reduce or prevent self-destructive behavior
■ Patient's observable response to interventions
■ Evaluations for expected outcomes

Reference

Ortiz, M. "Staying Alive! A Suicide Prevention Overview," *Journal of Psychosocial Nursing and Mental Health Services* 44(12):43-49, December 2006.

VII Community-based health

INTRODUCTION

Today, more and more nurses must provide care in nontraditional settings, including patients' homes, hospices, subacute care facilities, geriatric care centers, ambulatory care centers, schools, homeless shelters, prisons, faith communities, day care centers (child and geriatric), community nursing centers, centers for the disabled, and other community-based facilities. This section on community-based health will help you meet your care-planning needs in nontraditional clinical placements.

One of the most important recent changes in health care delivery is the reduction in hospital care and the subsequent shift toward home care. Nurses provide home care for patients with complex chronic illnesses, acute conditions, and postoperative care needs. In this section, you'll find plans written specifically to help you administer home care safely and effectively, including plans that focus on home infusion therapy and home ventilation therapy.

In all nontraditional settings, a key nursing role is fostering patient and family participation. Both patient and family must be knowledgeable about care and motivated to take responsibility for their health. This section provides care plans that will help you manage the therapeutic relationship when working in the community. Several scenarios are depicted: helping an overburdened caregiver cope with a family member who has Alzheimer's disease, helping a patient understand the intricacies of managed care, helping a hospice patient adjust to the course of terminal illness, and more.

In the community setting, teaching patients effectively may demand a creative approach. In addition to educating patients about their health condition, your role may include helping patients access health information. What's more, patients may need help sorting through the vast amount of information available to them. Several care plans directly address the opportunities and challenges of teaching patients in the community, including a plan about health care resources on the Internet.

Through teaching efforts, you may have the opportunity not only to improve the lives of individual patients but also to enhance the well-being of an entire community. Therefore, this section also includes care plans that address community-wide health issues, such as high levels of teenage pregnancy, drug and alcohol abuse, and timely immunizations for children. These plans can help you meet your documentation needs when working in community-based health — and they can also give you a taste of the expanding horizons of contemporary nursing.

Risk for
CAREGIVER ROLE STRAIN
related to caring for family member with Alzheimer's disease

Definition
Feelings of vulnerability or difficulty in performing the family caregiver role

Assessment
- Caregiver's age, gender, and general health
- Cultural status, including level of education, occupation, nationality, area of residence (rural, suburban, or urban), beliefs and attitudes about Alzheimer's disease, and race, ethnicity, and religion
- Family status, including caregiver's relationship to patient, roles, rules, communication skills, family subsystems, support network, ability of family members to meet caregiver's and patient's physical and emotional needs, social and economic factors, coping patterns, and evidence of abuse
- Caregiver's psychological status, including quality of relationship with patient, sense of self-worth, hobbies, recreational activities, and recent life changes
- Patient's self-care status, including functional ability and ability to perform activities of daily living
- Caregiver's spiritual status, including religious affiliation, religious practices, and attitudes about life, death, suffering, and faith

Risk factors
- Codependency (between caregiver and patient)
- Competing role commitments (caregiver)
- Developmental delay or disability (caregiver or patient)
- Deviant, bizarre behavior (patient)
- Discharge of family member with significant home care needs
- Drug or alcohol addiction (caregiver or patient)
- Female gender (caregiver)
- History of poor relationship (between caregiver and patient)
- Impaired health (caregiver)
- Inadequate housing, transportation, community services, or equipment for providing care
- Isolation (caregiver)
- Lack of developmental readiness for caregiver role
- Lack of experience (caregiver)
- Lack of respite or recreation (caregiver)
- Numerous, complex caregiving tasks (caregiver)
- Poor coping ability (caregiver)
- Preexisting dysfunctional family coping patterns
- Preexisting role as spouse (caregiver)
- Presence of abuse or violence
- Presence of other stressors, such as significant personal loss, natural disaster, economic hardship, and major life events

- Probability of long duration of caregiving
- Psychological or cognitive problems (patient)
- Unpredictable course or severity of illness or instability of health (patient)

Expected outcomes

- Caregiver will realistically describe current obligations and challenges that lie ahead.
- Caregiver will distinguish obligations she must fulfill from those that she can control or limit.
- In conjunction with nurse, caregiver will develop care plan for patient and demonstrate ability to follow care plan.
- Caregiver will exhibit positive sense of self-worth.
- Caregiver will describe emotional response to caring for patient.
- Caregiver will express less role strain.
- Caregiver will describe help available from informal and formal support systems in community and will take steps to obtain help.

Suggested NOC outcomes

Caregiver Emotional Health; Caregiver Home Care Readiness; Caregiver Physical Health; Caregiving Endurance Potential

Interventions and rationales

- Assess the caregiver's stress level. Several tools allow such assessment, including one in the book *Alzheimer's: A Caregiver's Guide and Sourcebook* by Howard Gruetzner. *Pinpointing specific areas of stress will enable the nurse to assist the caregiver more precisely in developing a "stress relief" plan.*
- Describe the five stages of Alzheimer's disease to the caregiver (early and late confusional states and early, middle, and late dementia). Discuss the characteristics of each stage and ways to respond to the behavioral problems of each stage. *Understanding the progressive nature of the disease will help the caregiver cope and adapt to each new stage.*
- Help the caregiver develop a realistic care plan that considers the patient's abilities and limitations. The plan will require modification as the patient decompensates. *A plan provides consistency for both the caregiver and the patient.*
- Instruct the caregiver to encourage the patient to participate in social and self-care activities, such as bathing, dressing, dining out with friends, and playing cards, to the greatest extent possible. *Allowing the patient to become dependent too soon increases the caregiver's stress.*
- Facilitate a family meeting to help the primary caregiver seek assistance from other family members. *The caregiver may feel guilty about asking for help. A nurse's presence may lend support and validity to the request for assistance and decrease the caregiver's feelings of guilt and embarrassment.*
- Support the caregiver and family members as they adjust to the degenerative nature of the disease. Be aware that over time the stress associated with caring for the patient increases. *Providing ongoing support will help family members avoid physical and emotional problems associated with stress.*
- Identify community resources that may offer the caregiver relief from constant supervision of the patient. Examples of resources include home health nursing as-

sistants, respite care, and adult day care. *Caregivers can use outside resources to provide care for the patient while the caregiver tends to her own needs.*

■ Help the caregiver contact informal sources of support, such as religious groups, extended family, and community volunteers, *for support and relief.*

■ If the patient is taking drug therapy for Alzheimer's disease, ensure that the caregiver understands dosages, adverse effects, and signs and symptoms to report to the physician. *Patients receiving drug therapy for Alzheimer's disease require careful monitoring.*

■ Encourage the caregiver to accept help from a care manager, *who can coordinate the patient's care.*

■ Encourage the caregiver to attend an Alzheimer's support group *for an opportunity to interact with people who share similar experiences.*

■ Refer the caregiver to the Alzheimer's Association *so the caregiver can be aware of current advances in treatment.*

Suggested NIC interventions

Caregiver Support; Coping Enhancement; Decision-Making Support; Family Involvement Promotion; Respite Care

Evaluations for expected outcomes

■ Caregiver develops realistic assessment of situation.

■ Caregiver distinguishes obligations she must fulfill from those she can control or limit.

■ Caregiver develops care plan for patient and demonstrates ability to carry out the plan.

■ Caregiver exhibits positive sense of self-worth.

■ Caregiver describes emotional response to caring for patient.

■ Caregiver expresses less role strain.

■ Caregiver describes and accepts help from informal and formal support systems and resources.

Documentation

■ Caregiver's comments related to:
– Fatigue
– Family members' reactions to caregiver's experience
– Feelings about patient's behavior
– Financial concerns
– Contact with friends or feelings of isolation
– Attendance at support group meetings
– Feelings of self-worth
■ Contacts made in community on behalf of caregiver
■ Evaluations for expected outcomes

References

Gruffydd, E., and Randle, J. "Alzheimer's Disease and the Psychosocial Burden for Caregivers," *Community Practitioner* 79(1):15-18, January 2006.

Spurlock, W.R. "Spiritual Well-being and Caregiver Burden in Alzheimer's Caregivers," *Geriatric Nursing* 26(3):154-61, May-June 2005.

Ineffective
COMMUNITY COPING

related to increased levels of teen pregnancy and deficits of social support services and resources

Definition
Pattern of community activities (for adaptation and problem solving) that's unsatisfactory for meeting the demands or needs of the community

Assessment
■ Community demographics, including age and sex distribution, education and income levels, and ethnic, racial, and religious groups
■ Family status, including family composition (percentage of single-parent families in community), responsibilities assumed by teenagers in caring for siblings, and ability of families to meet their physical, social, emotional, and economic needs
■ Community health status, including prevalence of health problems in community, attitudes toward sex and sexuality, availability of health care services, community members' use of health care services, and beliefs, values, and attitudes about health and illness
■ Prevalence of teen pregnancies, attitudes toward teen mothers and their infants, and incidence of sexually transmitted diseases, low-birth-weight neonates, and congenital abnormalities
■ Education system, including availability of sex education in schools, availability of programs to help pregnant teens complete their education, and willingness of parents to allow children to participate
■ Teenagers' knowledge about sex and sexuality
■ Political system, including government officials' support for or opposition to sex education
■ Attitude of religious groups toward sex and sexuality and religious groups' influence on educators
■ Transportation availability to clinics and other social services and recreation opportunities for adolescents
■ Welfare and health care system and reliance of teen mothers on welfare for support

Defining characteristics
■ Deficits in participation
■ Excessive conflicts
■ Expressed powerlessness and vulnerability
■ Failure of community to meet its own expectations
■ High illness rate
■ Increased social problems (abuse, divorce, and unemployment)

■ Perception of stressors as excessive

Expected outcomes

■ Community members will express awareness of seriousness of high adolescent pregnancy rate in their community.
■ Community members will express need for plan to reduce prevalence of teen pregnancies.
■ Community members will develop and implement plans to reduce teen pregnancy.
■ Community members will evaluate success of plan in meeting goals and objectives and will continue to revise it, as necessary.
■ Community members will report reduction in rate of teen pregnancy.

Suggested NOC outcomes

Community Competence; Community Health Status

Interventions and rationales

■ Assess teenagers' knowledge about sex and sexuality *to determine their educational needs.*
■ Work with schools to develop pregnancy prevention programs *to provide adolescents with information about risks, problems, and complications of early pregnancy.*
■ Work closely with individual pregnant adolescents *to assess their needs and provide care.*
■ Implement an outreach and health promotion program *to raise community members' awareness of the need to approach teen pregnancy as a community problem.* Consider these steps:
– Work with teachers, school psychologists, counselors, school nurses, students, and the parent-teacher association *to determine the extent of the teen pregnancy problem among the adolescent population.*
– Encourage local youth groups and religious and social service organizations to feature guest speakers on pregnancy prevention at their meetings. *Speakers with expertise in the area of teen pregnancy are able to provide information that may help teens make better choices in sexual behaviors.*
– Contact representatives of local corporations *to ask for funding for educational programs.*
– Help community members (school nurses, counselors, and teachers) recognize adolescent girls who need counseling about such issues as peer pressure to be sexually active and long-term consequences of pregnancy. Remind community members of the importance of listening attentively and remaining nonjudgmental. *Adults who take a nonjudgmental approach will have more success in effectively communicating advice to adolescents.*
– Provide education on birth-control measures (including abstinence from sex) and have this information available at school. *Access to information at school provides adolescents with a safe environment in which to seek help.*
■ Establish clubs for adolescent girls in the community. During club meetings, members should have the opportunity to discuss difficult questions openly, such as why girls consider babies as status symbols and how to respond to peer pres-

sure to be sexually active. *Such clubs foster self-esteem, and improved self-esteem is the most effective way to reduce teen pregnancies.*

■ Encourage adolescents to participate in peer-support networks that allow them to discuss social and dating pressure and other issues related to teen pregnancy *to give adolescents a chance to express their feelings openly and obtain support from peers.*

■ Encourage community members to establish school-based clinics that allow teens access to reproductive-system models, pregnancy tests, and nonprescription birth-control measures *to support teenagers who make the decision to protect themselves from unwanted pregnancies.*

■ Develop a referral list for teenagers that includes such resources as hospitals with human sexuality courses, charities that provide prenatal care and childbirth services, women's clinics, and Planned Parenthood *to compensate for restricted access to information in the adolescent's home or school.*

■ Encourage community members to implement an information campaign to educate adolescents, parents, and community members about problems associated with teen pregnancy. *To effectively reduce pregnancy rates, the education program must involve the entire community.*

■ Work with community members to evaluate the effectiveness of the teen pregnancy prevention program and assist with modifying the program, as needed, *to ensure the program's effectiveness and promote use of the program as a model for preventive health.*

■ Collect statistical data from schools to analyze teen pregnancy rates *to help evaluate the effectiveness of the prevention program.*

Suggested NIC interventions

Community Health Development; Health Education; Health Screening; Program Development

Evaluations for expected outcomes

■ Community members express awareness of seriousness of teen pregnancy problem.

■ Community members express need for plan to reduce teen pregnancy.

■ Community members develop and implement plan to reduce incidence of teen pregnancies, including outreach and health promotion and school-based sex education and self-esteem programs.

■ Community members evaluate success of plan and revise it, as needed.

■ Community members report reduction in rate of teen pregnancy.

Documentation

■ Community perception of problem
■ Statistics that support existence of problem
■ Community resources that already exist to alleviate problem
■ Future plans to deal with problem
■ Evaluations for expected outcomes

Reference

Brindis, C.D. "A Public Health Success: Understanding Policy Changes Related to Teen Sexual Activity and Pregnancy," *Annual Review of Public Health* 27:277-95, 2006.

FEAR

related to physical, emotional, or sexual abuse

Definition

Response to perceived threat that's consciously recognized as a danger

Assessment

■ Patient's age and sex
■ Developmental status, including cognitive, psychosexual, and psychosocial stages; cognitive and motor capabilities; and communication and socialization skills
■ Temperature, pulse rate, blood pressure, respiratory rate, and skin color and temperature
■ Health history, especially past or present bruises, burns, fractures, dislocations, and other injuries
■ Changes in behavior, eating or sleeping habits, and ability to concentrate
■ Parental status, including parents' age and maturity level, marital status, stability of parental relationship, educational levels, financial needs and resources, employment status, developmental state of family, parents' knowledge of normal growth and development, relationship with child, understanding of child's fear, past responses to crises, and coping mechanisms

Defining characteristics

■ Aggression
■ Bedwetting
■ Decreased self-assurance
■ Expressed feelings of alarm, apprehension, dread, horror, panic, and terror
■ Identification of and concentration on object of fear
■ Immediate response to object of fear
■ Impulsive behavior
■ Increased alertness
■ Increased heart rate
■ Increased tension, worrying, and wariness
■ Jitteriness
■ Physical arousal
■ Wide-eyed appearance
■ Withdrawal

Expected outcomes

■ Child will identify sources of fear.

■ Child will exhibit marked decrease in physiologic and behavioral manifestations of fear and will report feeling safe and comfortable.

■ Child will experience no further injury or abuse.

■ Child will attend school regularly, participate actively in activities, and develop positive relationships with peers, teachers, and school nurse.

■ If removed from home, child will grieve loss of parents.

■ Parents will acknowledge abuse and will do everything possible to protect child.

■ Parents will seek individual and group support.

■ Parents will receive counseling for problems that might lead to abuse, such as dysfunction in family and lack of food, shelter, or medical care.

Suggested NOC outcomes

Anxiety Self-Control; Comfort Level; Coping; Fear Self-Control

Interventions and rationales

■ Observe the child for signs of possible abuse, and elicit as much information from the child about his injuries as possible. *Discrepancies between physical evidence and reported history may be important signs of possible child abuse.* Report the case to a social service agency as soon as possible.

■ Spend as much time as possible establishing rapport with the child. Communicate at the child's eye level. Speak in a soft, reassuring voice. *Establishing rapport encourages the child to express feelings and provides comfort.*

■ Help the child identify sources of fear *to enable the child to put emotions into perspective.*

■ During your discussion with the child, be careful not to condemn the parents in any way for their actions. *Listening nonjudgmentally helps to maintain a therapeutic relationship.*

■ Refrain from asking the child too many questions. *Excessive questioning may upset the child and make it more difficult for professionals who will investigate the incident formally.*

■ Emphasize to the child that he has done nothing wrong *to prevent feelings of guilt that may interfere with the child's ability to communicate about the problem.*

■ Reassure the child that no one is permitted to hurt him. Tell him he has a right to refuse to let anyone touch him in a way that makes him uncomfortable. *Accurate information dispels misconceptions that exacerbate the child's fear.*

■ Report suspected abuse to the appropriate social service agency as soon as the problem is discovered. *In many states, failure to report abuse constitutes a crime.*

■ Evaluate whether to tell the parents that you're reporting suspected abuse. *The child might be in danger if the parents know they're being reported. Protecting the child is the first priority.*

■ Be available to the child if he wishes to talk about interactions with outside social service agencies or ways in which his life has changed. *Having someone he trusts will enhance the child's ability to cope.*

Suggested NIC interventions

Anxiety Reduction; Coping Enhancement; Security Enhancement; Therapeutic Play

Evaluations for expected outcomes
- Child discusses sources of fear.
- Child exhibits marked decrease in physiologic and behavioral manifestations of fear and reports feeling safe and comfortable.
- Child experiences no further injury or abuse.
- Child attends school regularly, participates in school activities and support groups, and reports improved relationships with peers and adults.
- If removed from home, child grieves loss of parents.
- Parents acknowledge abuse and do everything possible to protect child.
- Parents seek individual and group support.
- Parents receive counseling for problems that might lead to abuse.

Documentation
- Child's verbal and behavioral expressions of fear
- Physical manifestations of fear
- Communication with parents
- Details of report to social service agency
- Child's and parents' responses to nursing interventions
- Evaluations for expected outcomes

Reference
Harrison, E. "Disclosing the Details of Child Sexual Abuse: Can Imaginative Literature Help Ease the Suffering?" *Journal of Child and Adolescent Psychiatric Nursing* 18(3):127-34, July-September 2005.

GRIEVING

related to the need for hospice care

Definition
Intellectual and emotional responses and behaviors by which individuals, families, and communities work through the process of modifying self-concept based on the perception of potential loss

Assessment
- Patient's status, including present condition, estimated life expectancy, and recent treatments and interventions
- Pain control and management, including patient's wishes and the family's expectations
- Patient's and family's status, including events leading to decision to use hospice services, family's cultural and religious beliefs, family members' understanding of hospice care, and family support, including family dynamics, family's special needs, and family member in charge
- Concepts of death, dying, and loss, including willingness of patient and family to discuss terminal illness, willingness to make plans, anger expressed by family members, communication patterns among family members and with health care professionals, awareness of processes and events leading up to death, understand-

ing of what occurs at moment of death, and ethical, financial, and social decisions faced by family members
- Advance directives, including presence of living will
- Involvement with community resources such as religious or support group

Defining characteristics
- Altered activity level
- Altered communication pattern
- Altered libido
- Bargaining with higher power
- Changes in eating habits
- Changes in sleep or dream patterns
- Denial of impending death
- Difficulty taking on new or different roles
- Expressed anger
- Expressed distress at impending death
- Expressed guilt
- Resolution of grief before death
- Sorrow

Expected outcomes
- Patient will report no pain, show no sign of infection, and be as comfortable as possible.
- Patient will express his needs.
- Patient will grieve his loss of life.
- Patient will communicate with family and other members of support network.
- Patient will receive care from family or friends.
- Patient will remain as independent as possible for as long as possible.
- Patient will talk openly about illness and impending death.
- Patient will receive support through stages of dying.
- Patient will die with dignity.

Suggested NOC outcomes
Coping; Dignified Life Closure; Family Coping; Family Social Climate; Grief Resolution

Interventions and rationales
- On each hospice visit, conduct a thorough physical assessment, monitor the patient's vital signs, and note signs of complications or impending death. *Assessment provides information needed to modify the care plan.*
- Assess the patient's and family members' psychosocial status *to determine the need for continued support.*
- Answer all questions honestly *to support the patient's and family members' right to know.*
- Help the patient understand the grieving process and accept the feelings he experiences as normal. Discuss and help the patient progress through the psychological stages of anticipated death: shock and denial, anger, bargaining, depres-

sion, and acceptance. *Knowing these stages will help you and family members antic-ipate the patient's needs. Remember that not all patients go through each stage.*

■ Guide the patient in reviewing his life. Encourage him to write or tape his life history as a lasting gift to family members *to help the patient give events from his past meaningful interpretation.*

■ Encourage the patient to make simple decisions related to his care *to give the patient a sense of functional ability and control.*

■ Express acceptance of the patient's response to his anticipated death, whatever that response: crying, sadness, anger, fear, or denial. *Each patient responds to dying in his own way. Helping the patient express feelings freely enhances coping.*

■ Teach the patient and family members about pain control, comfort measures, diet, medications, hydration, palliative care, skin care, and how to respond to complications or a serious change in the patient's condition. *Knowledge of how to meet the basic needs of the terminally ill enhances the patient's and family members' feeling of control.*

■ Perform skilled care related to indwelling urinary catheters, I.V. therapy, med-ications, supplemental oxygen, and other treatments prescribed by the physician *to fulfill professional nursing responsibilities.*

■ Evaluate the needs of the patient and caregiver for additional resources that hospice can provide. *Commonly, the family may be able to use social, financial, reli-gious, or volunteer services.* Be aware that they may hesitate to ask about such serv-ices.

■ Support the patient's spiritual coping behaviors. For example, arrange for the patient to have at the bedside objects that provide spiritual comfort, such as a bible, prayer shawl, pictures, statues, rosary beads, or other items. *Even nonobser-vant individuals commonly turn to religion when confronted by death.*

■ Recommend that the family call the American Cancer Society at 1-800-ACS-2345 and request publication *Caring for the Patient with Cancer at Home. This guide for patients and families is a good quick reference for caring for terminally ill patients. The information is also appropriate for patients with terminal illnesses oth-er than cancer.*

■ If grief counseling is available, refer family members to this service. Also, pro-vide support to family members after the patient's death *to prevent feelings of be-ing abandoned by the hospice staff.*

Suggested NIC interventions

Anticipatory Guidance; Coping Enhancement; Family Support; Grief Work Facilitation

Evaluations for expected outcomes

■ Patient reports no pain, shows no signs of infection, and indicates state of rela-tive comfort.

■ Patient expresses his needs.

■ Patient grieves his loss of life.

■ Patient communicates with family members and other members of support network.

■ Patient receives care from family or friends.

■ Patient remains as independent as possible for as long as possible.

■ Patient talks openly about impending death and accepts death peacefully.
■ Patient receives support through stages of dying.
■ Patient dies with dignity.

Documentation
■ Assessment of patient's physical and emotional status
■ Patient's and family members' adaptation to situation
■ Interventions to meet patient's needs
■ Patient's response to nursing interventions
■ Referrals to community agencies
■ Evaluations for expected outcomes

Reference
Hindelang, M. "To Help You Live Until You Die: Patient Education in Hospice, Palliative, and Cancer Care," *Home Healthcare Nurse* 24(3):142-44, March 2006.

Delayed
GROWTH AND DEVELOPMENT
related to environmental and stimulation deficiencies

Definition
State in which child demonstrates deviations in norms for age-group

Assessment
■ Psychosocial status, including age, sex, developmental stage, special education status, school attendance record, classroom difficulties or course failures, suspensions or expulsions, physical and mental health (diagnosed medical conditions, *Diagnostic and Statistical Manual of Mental Disorders,* Fourth Edition diagnoses, and medication use), child welfare (including guardianship), alcohol and drug abuse, and history of delinquency
■ Family status, including parents' marital status; family configuration; level of education; employment, socioeconomic status, and public assistance eligibility; familial history of mental illness, substance abuse, criminal activity, or family violence; and types of agencies, placements, and services family members have contacted
■ Cultural influences, including nationality, ethnicity, religious affiliation, and health beliefs and practices
■ Parenting skills, including time spent daily with child by each parent, quality of parent-child interactions, disciplinary history and style of parenting, physical interaction with child, and support from other care providers
■ Social skills and peer interactions, including amount, type, and frequency of interaction with peers and adults; ability to be understood by peers and adults; ability to maintain satisfactory relationships with peers and adults; and ability to maintain self-control, understand directions, and demonstrate appropriate behaviors and feelings

■ Developmental assessment, including motor skills (gross and fine) and language acquisition and use (expressive and receptive ability)

Defining characteristics
■ Altered physical growth
■ Delay or difficulty in performing motor, social, or expressive skills typical of age-group
■ Flat affect
■ Inability to perform self-care activities or maintain self-control at age-appropriate level
■ Listlessness and decreased responses

Expected outcomes
■ Teachers, staff members, administrators, and parents will identify children who exhibit delayed growth and development and will target these children for intervention.
■ Teachers, staff, and administrators will identify children who may be at risk for abuse or neglect and will contact child protective services, as necessary.
■ Children will demonstrate improved motor skills, language acquisition and use, and personal social adaptive skills.
■ Parents will report feeling more comfortable about their parenting skills.
■ Parents will learn basic skills and how to initiate activities that help stimulate children.
■ Children will participate in group activities and will show developmental progress.

Suggested NOC outcomes

Child Development: 4 years; Child Development: Preschool; Growth; Knowledge: Parenting; Parenting Performance

Interventions and rationales
■ Conduct team meetings to identify students with special needs *to initiate needed interventions for children in the community.*
■ Help teachers, staff members, and administrators identify students who may be at risk for child abuse or neglect. Contact child protective services, as necessary, *to initiate investigation and help ensure the child's safety.*
■ Educate teachers about each student's condition and about adaptations that may be needed in the classroom *to promote independence and participation in activity for students with special needs.*
■ Encourage parents, teachers, and staff members to identify socially skilled children and to encourage these children to participate in group activities with peers who exhibit delayed growth and development *to promote interaction for developmentally delayed students.*
■ Discuss with parents and teachers the value of appropriate toys for promoting group activity, including cars, games, and gross motor equipment as well as puppets, dolls, costumes, and other items that encourage emotional and creative expression. *Introducing toys may encourage children to play together. A limited number of materials available promotes sharing and positive peer interaction.*

■ Work with parents and teachers to initiate activities among children that encourage interaction in small groups. *Groups of two or three children are most conducive for peer interaction.*

■ Conduct special activities for children with delayed growth and development, or encourage parents and teachers to conduct such activities. Appropriate activities might include reading to children, showing educational movies and television shows, and taking students on field trips *to provide stimulating experiences.*

■ Work with the school counselor and other school staff members to develop a parenting skills class and make this class available to community members *to improve parents' self-esteem, help them create a more stimulating home environment, and foster realistic expectations about their children's behavior.*

■ Work with parents and teachers to maintain a structured program for children throughout the school year *to ensure consistent intervention.*

■ Continue to work with parents by following up with telephone calls or home visits, conducting conferences, and providing referrals *to monitor the child's development and progress at home and to allow parents to express their needs and concerns about the health of their child and family.*

Suggested NIC interventions

Activity Therapy; Developmental Enhancement: Child; Health Screening; Learning Facilitation; Socialization Enhancement

Evaluations for expected outcomes

■ Children who exhibit signs of delayed growth and development receive appropriate interventions, such as participation in group activities (including small groups) and appropriate stimulation with books, toys, and activities.

■ Children at risk for abuse or neglect receive help from child protective services as needed.

■ Children demonstrate improved skills and language.

■ Parents report feeling more comfortable about their parenting skills.

■ Parents provide more stimulating activities and experiences for children.

■ Children participate in group activities and show ongoing developmental progress.

Documentation

■ Student visits to school nurse, including reason for visit, assessment findings, interventions performed, whether parent was contacted, and whether child was picked up at school or returned to class

■ Information revealed during team meetings with school nurse, staff members, faculty, administrators, and parents, such as child's behavior, developmental progress, test results, planned course of action, and outside agency referrals

■ Instances of suspected child abuse or neglect and date they were reported

■ Evaluations for expected outcomes

Reference

Adams, B.L. "Assessment of Child Abuse Risk Factors by Advanced Practice Nurses," *Pediatric Nursing* 31(6):498-502, November-December 2005.

Ineffective
HEALTH MAINTENANCE

related to lack of familiarity with neighborhood resources

Definition

Inability of community members to meet their needs due to a lack of awareness of community resources, such as social agencies, businesses, and service organizations

Assessment

▪ Community demographics, including age and sex distribution, ethnic and racial groups, education, and income levels
▪ Prevalence of health problems in community, availability of health care services, and use of health care services
▪ Psychosocial status of community members, including cognitive abilities, access to transportation, physical disabilities, communication problems, environmental factors, financial resources, support systems, and beliefs and practices regarding health

Defining characteristics

▪ History of lack of health-seeking behaviors
▪ Impaired personal support systems
▪ Inability to take responsibility for meeting basic health needs
▪ Interest in improving health behaviors
▪ Lack of adaptive behaviors to environmental changes
▪ Lack of knowledge regarding basic health practices
▪ Lack of necessary equipment or financial and other resources

Expected outcomes

▪ Community members will express desire to learn about available resources.
▪ Community members will identify local resources and how to access them.
▪ Community members will contact community agencies.
▪ Community organizations will develop resource information guides for their members and will promote increased access to needed resources.

Suggested NOC outcomes

Health Promoting Behavior; Health Seeking Behavior; Knowledge: Health Behavior; Knowledge: Health Resources

Interventions and rationales

▪ Assess factors that hinder community members learning about neighborhood resources *to identify areas where education may bring about change.*
▪ Assist members in learning about community and resources available to them, such as the American Heart Association, Agency on Aging, American Cancer Society, Meals On Wheels, and Alzheimer's support group, *to help empower community members.*

■ Plan specific programs to familiarize members of community organizations with neighborhood resources, such as having an agency spokesperson attend senior citizen lunch meetings to distribute program materials, *to enhance acceptance and reach more people.*

■ Help community members identify specific neighborhood resources they need. For example, a senior citizen group may need nutrition support services, whereas young families may need information about immunizations and child safety. *Targeting resources that meet specific health needs increases chances that they'll be used.*

■ Assist community organizations—such as neighborhood civic associations, religious groups, or social clubs—develop a manual describing health care resources available to group members *to provide an ongoing resource and help community members become self-sufficient.*

■ Ask members of community organizations to evaluate community resources. Discuss ways in which organizations may become politically active in requesting needed services. *When members are aware of resources, evaluation may help point out the need for changes.*

Suggested NIC interventions

Health Education; Health System Guidance; Self-Responsibility Facilitation; Support System Enhancement

Evaluations for expected outcomes

■ Community members express lack of familiarity with neighborhood resources and desire to learn about them.

■ Community members seek out and obtain information about neighborhood resources.

■ Community members contact appropriate neighborhood resources.

■ Community organizations develop resource information guides for their members and promote increased access to needed resources.

Documentation

■ Perception of problem as expressed by community members

■ Response of community members to presentations by agency spokespeople

■ Evaluation of neighborhood resources

■ Evaluations for expected outcomes

Reference

Downs, M.H., et al. "Open the Door Whenever Opportunity Knocks," *Public Health Nursing* 23(5):433-41, September-October 2006.

Risk for
INFECTION
related to home infusion therapy

Definition
Presence of risk factors associated with home infusion therapy that increase the possibility of bacterial, viral, or fungal infection

Assessment
■ Patient's health status, including age, weight, reason for home infusion therapy, vital signs, nutritional status, and motor skills
■ Health history, including drug allergies, substance abuse, chronic metabolic or systemic disease, and recent or present respiratory, urinary, or oral infection
■ Current medical treatments, including radiation therapy, chemotherapy, antibiotic or antifungal therapy, steroid treatment, and anticoagulant, thrombolytic, or immunosuppressive therapy
■ Mental status, including level of consciousness, orientation, judgment, and affect
■ Caregiver's physical and mental status, including chronic health problems, self-care abilities, mobility limitations, and level of cognitive function
■ Home environment, including structural barriers, availability of soap and water for hand washing, clean preparation area, access to telephone, and need for special equipment
■ Financial status, including insurance coverage and understanding of co-payments and out-of-pocket expenses

Risk factors
■ Absence or incompetence of caregiver in home
■ Impaired cognitive or motor skills of patient or caregiver
■ Implanted vascular access device
■ Inadequate insurance coverage or financial resources
■ Therapy that continues for more than 1 week
■ Unsanitary household conditions

Expected outcomes
■ Patient or caregiver will demonstrate ability to administer drugs and fluids, as prescribed.
■ Patient or caregiver will demonstrate ability to prevent infection from home infusion therapy.
■ Patient or caregiver will monitor site and general condition of patient for complications (redness or tenderness at insertion site, swelling, burning, cool skin, decreased flow rate, blood backup in line, pain along vein, general discomfort, fever, chills, malaise, and respiratory distress) and will report complications immediately.
■ Patient or caregiver will exhibit capability and comfort in carrying out all necessary procedures.

Suggested NOC outcomes

Risk Control; Risk Detection; Safe Home Environment

Interventions and rationales

■ During the initial visit, approach care in a systematic and organized fashion. Have available written materials, checklists, supplies, equipment, and other items. Conduct teaching sessions in a quiet place where you, the patient, and the caregiver will be undisturbed. *An organized approach may reduce anxiety and help the patient and caregiver perceive the responsibility as series of well-defined tasks.*

■ Use verbal and written instructions, demonstrate each step, and have the patient and caregiver perform return demonstrations. *Some patients and caregivers may have difficulty learning new skills and require repeated reinforcement.*

■ Make sure that the patient and caregiver understand the purpose of treatment, and enlist their participation throughout the course of therapy. *Understanding the treatment and its goals helps the home care patient assume a greater role in administering, monitoring, and maintaining therapy.*

■ Provide emotional support and encouragement *to decrease the patient's and caregiver's anxiety regarding home infusion therapy.*

■ Provide all necessary supplies, including solution, sterile I.V. tubing, pole and infusion pump, intake and output record, and dressings. Explain how to get additional supplies and help the patient and caregiver make these arrangements *to promote independence.*

■ Stress the need to use sterile technique *to reduce the risk of infection at the access site.*

■ Emphasize the importance of following safety precautions when disposing of used supplies *to protect caregivers and the patient from injury.*

■ Tell the patient to protect the catheter from coming into contact with granular or lint-producing surfaces. *Airborne particles and surface contaminants can cause localized infection.*

■ Teach the patient to change the site dressing, as ordered (usually every 2 or 3 days), or whenever it becomes wet, soiled, or nonocclusive *to reduce the risk of infection.*

■ Teach the patient and family members drug names, treatment protocols, administration procedures, potential adverse affects and drug toxicity, and signs indicating the need to call a physician or nurse immediately *to reinforce the need to be precise in drug administration.*

■ Teach the patient and caregiver how to manage complications related to improper catheter placement and fluid administration. These may include redness, tenderness, swelling, heat, or fluid leakage at site; streaking or pain along the vein; a decreased flow rate or blood backflow in tubing; and fever, chills, malaise, or shortness of breath. *Detecting complications as early as possible may prevent more serious consequences.*

Suggested NIC interventions

Environmental Management; Health System Guidance; Infection Protection; Venous Access Device (VAD) Maintenance

Evaluations for expected outcomes

■ Patient receives drugs and fluids, as prescribed.

■ Patient remains free from infection associated with home infusion therapy.

■ Patient or caregiver detects and immediately reports complications associated with home infusion therapy.

■ Patient or caregiver exhibits capability and comfort in carrying out all necessary procedures.

Documentation

■ Explanation and demonstration of each procedure and return demonstration by patient (documented on comprehensive teaching checklist)

■ Times of care measures, especially dressing, tubing, and solution changes

■ Observations of patient's condition, complications, and subsequent treatments

■ Evidence of patient's and caregiver's learning

■ Evaluations for expected outcomes

Reference

Polzien, G. "Home Infusion Therapy. First Things First: The Patient and the Prevention of Central Catheter Infections," *Home Healthcare Nurse* 24(10):681-84, November-December 2006.

Risk for
INFECTION
related to increased incidence of tuberculosis

Definition

At increased risk for invasion by pathogenic organisms

Assessment

■ Age, sex, and national origin

■ Health history, including illnesses, treatment, drug therapy, recent hospitalization, history of substance abuse, and time of last chest X-ray

■ Current health beliefs and practices

■ History of exposure to tuberculosis (TB)

■ Living conditions, including number of occupants, sanitation, and ventilation

■ Occupation and work history

■ Sexual activity pattern

■ Support systems, including family members and their willingness to provide support, friends, and community organizations

■ Education level

■ Nutritional status, including height, weight, daily food consumption, and sources of food

■ Financial resources

Risk factors

- Crowded living conditions
- History of TB
- Human immunodeficiency virus infection
- Homelessness
- Incarceration
- Multiple sex partners
- Recent emigration from Africa, Asia, Mexico, or South America
- Recent exposure to TB
- Treatment with immunosuppressants or corticosteroids
- Unsanitary living conditions
- Weak immune system or disease that affects immune system, especially acquired immunodeficiency syndrome (AIDS)

Expected outcomes

- Infection won't be transmitted to other people with whom patient has contact.
- Patient's contacts will receive appropriate screening, monitoring, and education.
- Patient and contacts will comply with anti-infective regimen.
- Patient and contacts will learn about and demonstrate safety precautions, such as washing hands, covering nose and mouth when coughing, and properly disposing of used tissues.
- Patient will demonstrate normal respiratory pattern and absence of dyspnea, cough, and pain.
- Patient will remain free from infection and complications of TB.
- Patient will keep appointments for follow-up care.

Suggested NOC outcomes

Community Risk Control: Communicable Disease; Immune Status; Infection Severity; Knowledge: Infection Control; Risk Control

Interventions and rationales

- Assess for a history of exposure to TB or physical evidence of exposure. *Nurses in community settings contribute significantly to detection of patients with TB. Nurses working in heavily populated cities, especially with large numbers of disenfranchised individuals or immigrants, see a higher incidence of exposure and active disease. Also, nurses who work with patients with AIDS need to be alert for cases of active TB.*
- Perform a purified protein derivative (PPD) test and read it in 48 hours *to provide an initial screening test.*
- If the PPD site shows a positive reaction (measured by induration), refer the patient to a physician *for further evaluation, chest X-ray, and drug prescriptions, if indicated.*
- Emphasize the need to take drugs exactly as prescribed. *Skipping doses and other self-administration errors prolong the length of treatment.*
- Teach the patient about the potential adverse effects of medications *to encourage the patient to recognize and report adverse effects promptly.*

■ Warn patients who are taking rifampin that it will turn their body secretions red-orange. Soft contact lenses worn by the patient may become permanently discolored. *Preparation will help reduce the patient's anxiety about adverse effects.*

■ Teach the patient and contacts about the signs and symptoms of disease that require medical treatment: increased cough, hemoptysis, unexpected weight loss, fever, and night sweats. *Early detection and treatment helps control the spread of disease.*

■ Teach the patient and contacts specific precautions:

– Wash hands in hot, soapy water.

– Cough and sneeze into tissues, and dispose of them properly.

– Wash eating utensils separately in hot, soapy water.

Such measures reduce the spread of TB.

■ Stress the importance of a high-protein, well-balanced diet. When recommending specific foods, take into account the patient's socioeconomic status. *The patient may require assistance in obtaining foods beneficial to his health.*

■ Emphasize the importance of scheduling and keeping follow-up appointments *to promote compliance with treatment. Sputum is cultured monthly during therapy until cultures are negative, and then every 3 months for the duration of therapy.*

■ Refer the patient to a support group or other community resources, as appropriate, *to foster independence and use of available resources.*

Suggested NIC interventions

Environmental Management; Health Screening; Infection Control; Infection Protection

Evaluations for expected outcomes

■ Patient doesn't pass infection to others.

■ Contacts receive appropriate screening, monitoring, and education.

■ Patient and contacts comply with medication regimen.

■ Patient and contacts practice safety measures, such as hand washing and proper disposal of tissues.

■ Patient remains free from cough, hemoptysis, dyspnea, and pain.

■ Patient has negative cultures and remains afebrile.

■ Patient keeps appointments for follow-up care.

Documentation

■ Observations of patient's general condition

■ Detailed assessment of patient's respiratory status

■ Observations about patient's living environment that either support or interfere with recovery

■ Referrals to support groups or other community agencies

■ Evaluations for expected outcomes

Reference

Mishra, P., et al. "Adherence is Associated with the Quality of Professional-Patient Interaction in Directly Observe Treatment Short-course, DOTS," *Patient Education and Counseling* 63(1-2):29-37, October 2006.

Deficient
KNOWLEDGE
related to Americans with Disabilities Act

Definition
Absence or deficiency of cognitive information related to specific topics

Assessment
- Psychosocial status, including age, learning ability (affective, cognitive, and psychomotor domains), decision-making ability, developmental stage, financial resources, health beliefs and attitudes, interest in learning, knowledge and skill regarding current health problem, obstacles to learning, support systems, and usual coping pattern
- Neurologic status, including level of consciousness, memory, mental status, and orientation
- Musculoskeletal status, including coordination, gait, muscle size and strength, muscle tone, range of motion, and functional mobility as follows:
0 = completely independent
1 = requires use of equipment or device
2 = requires help, supervision, or teaching from another person
3 = requires help from another person and equipment or device
4 = dependent; doesn't participate in activity

Defining characteristics
- Difficulty gaining access to public places
- Expressed concern about possible discrimination because of disability
- Lack of familiarity with information about rights of disabled
- Requests for information about rights of individuals with disabilities

Expected outcomes
- Patient will express need for information about rights of individuals with disabilities.
- Patient will state understanding of rights as disabled person under Americans with Disabilities Act (ADA).
- Patient will state intention to seek adaptations to work environment or other accommodations as consequence of learning about ADA.

Suggested NOC outcomes
Knowledge: Health Behavior; Knowledge: Health Resources

Interventions and rationales
- Establish an environment of mutual trust and respect *to enhance learning.*
- Listen to the patient's concerns about coping with a disability in society. *As a community health nurse, you should be concerned not only with the patient's physiologic well-being but also with his ability to function to his maximum potential in the community.*

■ Discuss with the patient whether he feels fully informed about his rights under law. Ask whether he's aware of laws that protect the rights of disabled people. *Open, direct discussion will establish the need for information.*

■ Inform the patient about ADA *to enhance his understanding of his legal rights.* Tell him Congress passed this law in 1990. Explain that many important rights of disabled people, defined as anyone "with a physical or mental impairment that substantially limits one or more major life activities," are set out in the law.

■ Teach the patient about his rights under ADA. Explain that ADA:

– provides for equal employment opportunities for people with disabilities. Explain that the law doesn't mandate for quotas, affirmative action, preferential treatment, or guarantee of job.

– states that employers must make work-related accommodation for a qualified person with a disability.

– prohibits discrimination against a qualified person with a disability by a department or agency of any state or local government.

– requires that programs and services of all state and local governments be readily accessible to and usable by individuals with disabilities.

– provides for access to public accommodations and services; for example, widening or enlarging doors, removing architectural and communication barriers, or providing alternative arrangements if accommodation isn't possible. This provision affects hotels, theaters, shopping centers, professional offices, pharmacies, banks, schools, health centers, and other establishments.

– provides for access to telecommunications for people with hearing and speech impairments.

Discussion of specific provisions of law may help patient to reevaluate past experiences and alert him to possibility of taking appropriate action to assert his rights.

■ If the patient requests more information, refer him to resources available from the library or Internet *to help him increase his knowledge about issues related to disability.* For example, tell him to read *Complying with the Americans with Disabilities Act: A Guidebook for Management and People with Disabilities* by Don Fersh and Peter W. Thomas, Esq., published by Greenwood Publishing Group; or to contact *Americans with Disabilities Act Document Center* Web site (*www.jan.wvu.edu/media/index.htm*).

Suggested NIC interventions

Health Care Information Exchange; Health Education; Health System Guidance

Evaluations for expected outcomes

■ Patient expresses desire to obtain information about ADA.

■ Patient demonstrates initiative in searching for information about ADA and develops realistic understanding of rights under ADA.

■ Patient identifies specific changes he'll seek in response to information about ADA, such as accommodation to disabilities by employer.

Documentation

■ Patient's statements of desire for information related to disability

■ Patient's stated goals of learning more about rights of disabled under law

- Methods used to teach patient
- Patient's statements indicating enhanced understanding of ADA
- Evaluations for expected outcomes

Reference

Ingram, D. "Antidiscrimination, Welfare, and Democracy: Toward a Discourse-ethical Understanding of Disability Law," *Social Theory and Practice* 32(2):213-48, April 2006.

Deficient
KNOWLEDGE
related to lack of familiarity with managed care

Definition
Absence or deficiency of cognitive information related to specific topics

Assessment
- Psychosocial status, including age, developmental stage, learning ability, decision-making ability, health beliefs and attitudes, interest in learning, knowledge and skills regarding current health problem, obstacles to learning, financial resources, support systems, and usual coping pattern
- Neurologic status, including level of consciousness, memory, mental status, and orientation

Defining characteristics
- Expressed lack of understanding of managed care system
- Lack of familiarity with available resources for information
- Requests for information about procedures for obtaining care

Expected outcomes
- Patient will keep insurance card, written material about plan requirements, and name and phone numbers of primary care physician and managed care plan readily available.
- Patient will express understanding of how to use managed care plan, discuss benefits of managed care, and describe role of primary care physician.
- Patient will demonstrate understanding of co-payments, deductibles, and other financial issues and will explain how to get additional information, when needed.
- Patient will schedule preventive screening appointments to which he's entitled.

Suggested NOC outcomes
Knowledge: Health Behavior; Knowledge: Health Resources; Knowledge: Illness Care

Interventions and rationales

■ Allow the patient time to identify his frustrations about managed care. *Managed care concepts are complex and difficult to understand. Providing the patient with an opportunity to express his current understanding of managed care may allow you to identify misperceptions. The patient may view managed care as a mechanism for denying the patient's choice of physicians, hospitals, and other health care options.*

■ Provide a simple explanation of managed care and its benefits. Point out the advantages and disadvantages of managed care to the health consumer. Explain the difference between an HMO and a PPO in simple terms:

– HMO stands for Health Maintenance Organization. There are four different HMO models. A staff-model HMO employs physicians who care for enrollees. In network, group practice, and individual practice association models, the HMO contracts directly with physicians, either individually or in groups, to provide care to their enrollees.

– PPO stands for Preferred Provider Organization. This is a slightly more flexible type of plan. It's less restrictive than an HMO but has many built-in safeguards. In this case, the managed care organization contracts with a group of selected or preferred providers for its members. These physicians then agree to accept whatever reimbursement the PPO determines is fair.

Understanding the structure of managed care may help patients who are accustomed to fee-for-service plans adjust to a new system.

■ Review the highlights of the patient's plan. Explain the importance of keeping the insurance card and phone numbers for the plan handy at all times. *A better understanding of how to use the plan will enhance the patient's opportunity to obtain needed health care.*

■ Explore the patient's understanding of the primary care physician's role. Stress the importance of always going through a primary care physician to meet health care needs. *Understanding the primary care physician's role is the key to using a managed care plan successfully.*

■ Determine what screening examinations are covered under the plan and how often they're allowed. Screening examinations may include routine physical examinations, mammograms, prostate-specific antigen screening, eye examinations, and other procedures. *Accessing these benefits may allow for the diagnosis of major illnesses at an earlier stage.*

■ Have the patient incorporate learned material into a plan that defines how to use a managed care plan for specific medical problems, how and when to obtain referrals, and whom to contact for billing problems. *Developing a plan allows the patient to use new information and receive feedback.*

■ Urge the patient to ask questions *to clarify the need for further information and allow you to evaluate the patient's understanding.*

Suggested NIC interventions

Health Education; Health System Guidance; Learning Facilitation; Teaching: Disease Process

Evaluations for expected outcomes

■ Patient carries his insurance card and keeps essential phone numbers readily available for himself or caregivers.

■ Patient expresses understanding of how to use managed care plan, discusses benefits of plan, and describes role of primary care physician.

■ Patient demonstrates understanding of co-payments, deductibles, and other financial issues, and explains how to get additional information, when needed.

■ Patient schedules preventive screening appointments to which he's entitled.

Documentation
■ Information provided to patient
■ Patient's response to teaching
■ Appointments made by patient as result of teaching
■ Evaluations for expected outcomes

Reference
Siegrist, R. "Helping Patients Become More Educated about Provider Quality," *The Case Manager* 17(2):63-66, March-April 2006.

Imbalanced
NUTRITION: LESS THAN BODY REQUIREMENTS
related to lack of resources or knowledge

Definition
Insufficient intake or absorption of nutrients that results in changed body weight and inability to meet metabolic needs

Assessment
Adult
■ Age, sex, height, and weight
■ Nutritional history, hereditary influences, usual daily intake, meal preparation habits, and use of alcohol or drugs
■ Cultural influences, including education level, occupation, nationality or ethnic group; beliefs, values, and attitudes about health and illness; and health practices and customs

Child
■ Parents' educational level and knowledge of child development
■ Home environment and financial resources
■ Child's capabilities, including communication skills, motor skills, cognitive abilities, and socialization skills

Defining characteristics
■ Abdominal pain or cramping, with or without disorder
■ Altered taste sensation
■ Aversion to or lack of interest in eating
■ Body weight 20% or more under ideal weight
■ Diarrhea and steatorrhea
■ Evidence of lack of food

■ Excessive hair loss
■ Fragile capillaries
■ Hyperactive bowel sounds
■ Inadequate food intake (less than recommended daily allowances)
■ Lack of information or misinformation about nutrition
■ Loss of body weight despite adequate food intake
■ Pale conjunctivae and mucous membranes
■ Perceived inability to ingest food
■ Poor muscle tone
■ Satiety immediately upon eating
■ Sore, inflamed buccal cavity
■ Weakness of muscles required for chewing or swallowing

Expected outcomes
■ Patient will describe reasons for not obtaining adequate nutrition.
■ Patient will state food preferences.
■ Patient will consume adequate calories daily.
■ Patient will gain specified amount of weight weekly.
■ Patient will eat independently without constant encouragement.
■ Patient will use community resources to improve nutritional status as needed.

Suggested NOC outcomes
Nutritional Status; Nutritional Status: Nutrient Intake; Weight Control

Interventions and rationales
Adult
■ Identify patients who don't have resources to eat properly or who neglect nutritional needs. *Nurses working in community settings frequently encounter patients whose nutritional needs aren't met. Nursing responsibilities include identifying these individuals and intervening on their behalf.*
■ Encourage the patient to discuss his reasons for not eating *to assess the cause of the problem and develop a care plan.*
■ Determine the patient's food preferences, and attempt to obtain preferred foods. Offer foods that appeal to the senses *to enhance the patient's appetite.*
■ Suggest the patient eat high-protein, high-calorie foods *to prevent body protein breakdown and provide caloric energy.*
■ If the patient is eligible for food stamps, help him obtain them and teach him how to use them *to buy foods that provide well-balanced meals.*
■ Depending on the patient's resources, help locate soup kitchens for the homeless, senior centers that serve meals for a nominal fee, Meals On Wheels, or similar programs *to promote access to appropriate community resources.*

Child
■ Assess the child for evidence of balanced nutrition patterns. Stress to the parents the importance of good nutrition *to reinforce to the child and parents the value of good nutrition in relation to growth and development.*
■ Encourage the child to take advantage of a school breakfast program *to begin the school day with adequate nutrients.*

■ Determine the child's food preferences *to use as a basis for teaching the child and parents.*

■ Teach the child and parents about required daily nutrients. Stress the need for the parents to supervise the child's meals. *Parental support helps the child develop good eating habits.*

■ If you work in a school, confer with teachers to develop stimulating lessons on nutrition. *Working together, teachers and school nurses can reinforce lessons about nutrition.*

■ Document cases of undernourished children and noncompliant parents. If necessary, refer the family to an appropriate social service agency. *Cases in which parents can't or won't cooperate on the child's behalf may require further intervention.*

Suggested NIC interventions

Eating Disorders Management; Nutrition Management; Nutritional Counseling; Weight Gain Assistance

Evaluations for expected outcomes
■ Patient describes reasons for not obtaining adequate nutrition.
■ Patient states food preferences.
■ Patient consumes adequate calories daily.
■ Patient gains specified amount of weight weekly.
■ Patient eats independently without constant encouragement.
■ Patient uses community resources as needed.

Documentation
■ Patient's weight
■ Daily intake
■ Teaching provided
■ Referrals
■ Patient's response to nursing interventions
■ Evaluations for expected outcomes

Reference
Furman, E.F. "Undernutrition in Older Adults Across the Continuum of Care: Nutritional Assessment, Barriers, and Interventions," *Journal of Gerontological Nursing* 32(1):22-27, January 2006.

Risk for
POISONING

related to ingestion of lead

Definition
Risk of accidental exposure to or ingestion of dangerous products (or some folk remedies) in doses sufficient to cause lead poisoning

Assessment
- Age and gender
- Results of test for blood lead concentration
- Sources of lead in child's environment, such as living in or frequently visiting older building, living in area with heavy traffic, or living near lead smelter
- Occupations and hobbies of family members that include use of lead
- Cultural use of folk remedies that contain lead
- History of pica, such as biting nails or sucking on pencils or other items
- Nutritional deficiencies, such as inadequate amounts of protein, iron, calcium, and zinc
- Mental status, including ability to concentrate and mental acuity
- History of developmental delays
- Behavior such as irritability, restlessness, and hyperactivity

Risk factors
- Chemical contamination of food and water
- History of lead poisoning among siblings or peers
- Home located near lead-related industries
- Household members who have lead-related occupations or hobbies
- Lack of safety or drug education
- Old or deteriorated home or remodeled home in restored urban area
- Pica
- Poor nutrition
- Poverty
- Toys or toy jewelry that contain lead
- Use of certain folk remedies

Expected outcomes
- Laboratory tests will indicate blood lead concentration less than 9 mcg/dl.
- Patient will have no signs or symptoms of elevated blood lead levels.
- Environmental factors for lead poisoning in home will be eliminated as much as possible.
- Parents and teachers will demonstrate understanding of safety guidelines and will promote them at home and in school.
- Children will practice safety measures to prevent lead poisoning.

Suggested NOC outcomes
Personal Safety Behavior; Physical Injury Severity; Safe Home Environment

Interventions and rationales
- Assess the patient for anemia, distractibility, hearing impairment, hyperactivity, impulsivity, and mild intellectual deficit *to detect low-dose lead poisoning. Blindness, coma, seizures, mental retardation, or paralysis may indicate high-dose poisoning.*
- If there's any indication that a child needs his blood level tested, request an order to have a test performed. *Early intervention reduces levels and prevents more se-*

rious complications. When children are registered for preschool, kindergarten, or first grade, their blood should be tested for elevated lead levels. All children under age 6, or as state regulations dictate, should be tested for elevated blood lead levels.

■ In cases of elevated blood levels, communicate with the child's primary physician to determine what actions must be taken. *Nursing responsibilities include following up when the child's health may be jeopardized.*

■ Set up educational programs for children, parents, and teachers about the dangers of lead poisoning. Tailor the sessions to the appropriate educational level. *Education is the first defense against lead poisoning.* Make sure parents understand these critical concepts:

– Before eating, carefully wash hands with hot soapy water. *Dirt and dust on hands may contain lead that may be ingested while eating.*

– Teach children to keep hands, toys, and all other objects out of their mouth *because they contain dirt.* Wash pacifiers and other items meant to be put into the mouth (especially if the item falls on the floor or other dirty surface).

– Provide children with a healthful, balanced diet to ensure that they receive adequate amounts of iron, protein, calcium, and zinc. Be sure to provide fresh fruits, vegetables, whole grains, and meat. *Eating regularly is important because lead is absorbed more quickly on an empty stomach.*

– Allow water to run for 2 minutes before using for drinking, cooking, or making formula *to decrease amount of lead in water.* This is especially important in areas where lead content of water is high.

– Don't store food in open cans, and be cautious about using cookware and ceramic dishes that may contain lead or may have been fired incorrectly. *These can be insidious sources of lead.*

■ Assess whether the child or family members use folk remedies. *Various cultures use folk remedies that contain large quantities of lead. For example, Mexican* azacron *and* greta *(both nearly 100% lead) and Asian* paylooah *are used as remedies for diarrhea and vomiting.* Suggest alternative remedies to these highly toxic compounds.

■ Teach parents to be alert for stomachaches, irritability, and headaches. *These may be early signs of higher-than-normal lead levels.*

Suggested NIC interventions

Environmental Management: Safety; Health Education; Home Maintenance Assistance; Surveillance: Safety

Evaluations for expected outcomes

■ Screening results show normal blood lead levels.
■ Patient doesn't have signs and symptoms of elevated blood lead levels.
■ Environmental factors for lead poisoning in home are eliminated.
■ Parents and teachers promote safety guidelines at home and in school.
■ Children practice safety measures to prevent lead poisoning.

Documentation

■ Blood lead levels
■ Physical and behavioral manifestations of elevated blood lead levels
■ Referrals to physician for treatment and follow-up visits

- Teaching provided
- Response to nursing interventions
- Evaluations for expected outcomes

Reference

Polivka, B.J. "Needs Assessment and Intervention Strategies to Reduce Lead-poisoning Risk among Low-income Ohio Toddlers," *Public Health Nursing* 23(1):52-58, January-February 2006.

Readiness for enhanced
SPIRITUAL WELL-BEING
related to parish nursing

Definition

Ability to experience and integrate meaning and purpose in life through connectedness with self, others, art, music, literature, nature, or a power greater than oneself

Assessment

- Spiritual status, including personal religious habits; religious or church affiliation; perceptions of life, faith, death, and suffering; support network; embarrassment at practicing religious rituals; opposition to beliefs by family, peers, or health care providers; and conflicts with belief system
- Health history, including medical conditions that change body image, chronic or terminal illness, and debilitating disease
- Psychological status, including reactions to illness and disability, job loss, loss through separation or death, relationships with peers, and change in appetite, energy level, motivation, personal hygiene, self-image, and sleep habits
- Self-care status, including neurologic, musculoskeletal, sensory, or psychological impairment and ability to carry out activities and adapt
- Family status, including marital status, communication skills and methods of conflict resolution, cultural factors that affect health practices, socioeconomic factors, family goals, family health history, ability of family to meet physical, social, and emotional needs

Defining characteristics

- Displays creative energy, sings/listens to music, reads spiritual literature, spends time outdoors, prays, and participates in religious activities
- Expresses desire for enhanced hope, meaning, and purpose in life, peace, acceptance, surrender, love, forgiveness of self, satisfying philosophy of life, joy, and courage
- Expresses reverence and awe
- Provides service to others
- Requests forgiveness of others
- Requests interactions with spiritual leaders

Expected outcomes
- Patient will discuss spiritual concerns.
- Patient will meet with appropriate religious figure.
- Patient will openly discuss effect of illness on beliefs and other spiritual issues.
- Patient will receive referrals for continued support.
- Patient will receive support in effort to pursue enhanced spiritual well-being.

Suggested NOC outcomes
Dignified Life Closure; Hope; Quality of Life; Spiritual Health

Interventions and rationales
- Assess the patient's desire for spiritual intervention as part of his care *to promote physical, emotional, and spiritual health.*
- Listen attentively to the patient's concerns *to ascertain the impact of spirituality in the patient's life.*
- Ask the patient if health concerns or other circumstances have affected his spiritual outlook, and tell him you're willing to help him address spiritual issues if he wishes to do so. *This reduces the patient's feeling of isolation and allows for open discussion of spiritual distress.*
- Discuss ways in which the patient believes the community can provide support. *Learning how the patient defines his expectations will help you assess the feasibility of meeting expectations.*
- Help the patient determine a mechanism for soliciting support from the community, such as placing a request for assistance in a parish bulletin or requesting a visit from a member of the clergy. *The patient may know the type of support he needs but may not know how to go about getting it.*
- Demonstrate to the patient that you're willing to discuss issues related to spirituality or to pray with the patient if he wishes. Keep an open mind. Keep the conversation focused on the patient's spiritual values *to maintain the therapeutic value of interaction between patient and nurse.*
- Provide information about other community resources that might benefit the patient and family members *to help provide continuity of care.*

Suggested NIC interventions
Spiritual Growth Facilitation; Spiritual Support; Values Clarification

Evaluations for expected outcomes
- Patient discusses spiritual concerns.
- Patient receives opportunity to meet with clergy member.
- Patient openly discusses effects of illness on beliefs and other spiritual issues.
- Patient receives referrals for continued support.
- Patient recognizes and verbalizes support given to his efforts to pursue enhanced spiritual well-being.

Documentation
- Spiritual needs as defined by patient and nurse
- Interventions initiated by nurse

- Referrals to outside agencies
- Patient's statements about spiritual well-being
- Evaluations for expected outcomes

Reference

Weis, D., et al. "The Process of Empowerment: A Parish Nurse Perspective," *Journal of Holistic Nursing* 24(1):17-24, March 2006.

Ineffective community
THERAPEUTIC REGIMEN MANAGEMENT
related to drug and alcohol abuse among teenagers

Definition

An unsatisfactory pattern of integrating programs for preventing and treating health problems in the community

Assessment

- Community demographics, including age and sex distribution, ethnic groups, and education and income levels
- Prevalence of health problems in community, availability of health care services, and community use of health care services
- Drug and alcohol use among teenagers, including reports of episodes of blackouts, injuries, accidents, and mental health problems; reports from teachers about changes in student behaviors and attitudes and failing grades; increased incidence of school absenteeism, dropouts, and encounters with police and legal system; and reports from school psychologist and counselors
- Problems that may be associated with drug and alcohol abuse in teenagers, such as school violence, automobile accidents, homicides, suicides, domestic violence, burglaries, and increased teenage pregnancy, sexually transmitted diseases, low-birth-weight neonates, and congenital abnormalities

Defining characteristics

- Deficient community activities for secondary and tertiary prevention
- Higher-than-normal drug and alcohol abuse rate among teenagers
- Insufficient advocates for teenagers
- Insufficient number or unavailable health care resources for teenage drug and alcohol abuse
- Insufficient people and programs to be accountable for care of teenage drug and alcohol abusers
- Unexpected acceleration of teenage drug and alcohol abuse rate

Expected outcomes

- Community members will express need for and develop plan to reduce prevalence of drug and alcohol abuse.

■ Community members will demonstrate commitment to maintaining drug education and outreach programs for local teenagers.

■ Teenagers will report understanding of negative effects of drug and alcohol abuse on their health, families, and community.

Suggested NOC outcomes

Community Competence; Community Health Status

Interventions and rationales

■ Implement an outreach and health promotion program *to raise community members' awareness of the need to approach drug and alcohol abuse as a community problem.* Consider these steps:

– Work with teachers, school psychologists, counselors, students, and the parent-teacher association *to educate parents and teenagers about risk factors and signs and symptoms of drug abuse.*

– Place drug education posters in schools and local teenage hangouts *in order to provide useful information to teens in places where they are most comfortable.*

– Encourage local youth groups and religious and social service organizations to feature guest speakers on teen drug and alcohol abuse at their meetings *to foster awareness.*

– Contact representatives of local corporations *to develop partnerships and sources of funding for educational and recreational programs.*

■ Encourage community members to establish a drug and alcohol counseling program *to provide early identification of teenagers at high risk for drug and alcohol abuse.* Educate people who will be working with teenagers about the importance of remaining nonjudgmental and open-minded and of maintaining confidentiality *to foster trust.*

■ Counsel teenagers to participate in outreach and health promotion programs *to allow for early identification, intervention, treatment, and anticipatory guidance.*

■ Establish a school-based drug and alcohol education program *to teach about the risks of drug and alcohol abuse.* A drug and alcohol education program should include teaching about self-esteem issues, assertiveness skills, stress management, coping with peer pressure, and factual information about drugs and alcohol. Participation in recreational activities should also be part of the program. *To be effective, a drug and alcohol education program should use a holistic approach that supports teenagers' emotional needs and encourages them to make informed choices.*

■ Develop a learning packet for community residents *to increase the community's understanding of drug and alcohol abuse. With this knowledge, parents and others can act as advocates for teenagers.*

■ Conduct a follow-up survey on drug and alcohol use *to measure the effectiveness of screening, education, and treatment programs.*

Suggested NIC interventions

Community Health Development; Health Policy Monitoring; Program Development; Risk Identification

Evaluations for expected outcomes

■ Community members express need for and develop plan to reduce incidence (new cases) and prevalence (current number of people with problem) of drug and alcohol abuse.

■ Community members establish outreach and health-promotion programs and school-based drug and alcohol abuse programs.

■ Teenagers report increased understanding of negative effects of drug and alcohol use on their health, families, and community.

Documentation

■ Description of outreach and health-promotion programs developed in community

■ Evidence of participation

■ Results of follow-up survey on drug and alcohol abuse

■ Evaluations for expected outcomes

Reference

VanderWaal, C.J., et al. "Community and School Drug Prevention Strategy Prevalence: Differential Effects by Setting and Substance," *The Journal of Primary Prevention* 26(4):299-320, July 2005.

Impaired spontaneous
VENTILATION
related to home ventilation therapy

Definition

Decreased energy reserves that result in an individual's inability to maintain breathing adequate to support life

Assessment

■ Age and sex

■ Health history, including previous respiratory problems, neurologic or neuromuscular disease, and recent hospitalization

■ Respiratory status, including rate and depth of respiration, chest excursion and symmetry, presence of cyanosis, use of accessory muscles for respiration, effectiveness of cough, suctioning demands, and sputum characteristics

■ Neuromuscular strength and endurance

■ Mental and emotional status, including cognitive state and ability to follow directions

■ Functional status, including ability to perform activities of daily living (ADLs)

■ Family status, including usual coping patterns, family roles, communication patterns, financial resources, effect of patient's illness on family, and beliefs and attitudes about health, illness, death, and other issues

■ Home environment, including electrical safety, availability of hot water, house layout, lighting, and fire hazards

■ Knowledge of safety precautions

Defining characteristics
■ Apprehension
■ Decreased arterial oxygen saturation
■ Decreased cooperation
■ Decreased partial pressure of oxygen
■ Decreased tidal volume
■ Dyspnea
■ Increased metabolic rate
■ Increased partial pressure of arterial carbon dioxide
■ Increased restlessness
■ Increased use of accessory muscles of respiration
■ Tachycardia

Expected outcomes
■ Patient will exhibit clear breath sounds.
■ Patient won't exhibit signs of respiratory distress or infection.
■ Patient will incorporate mechanical ventilation into ADLs and family life.
■ Patient will demonstrate adequate use of communication aids.
■ Patient will remain free from complications.
■ Caregiver will demonstrate ease in using equipment and procedures to keep patient comfortable and free from infection.
■ Caregiver will implement and maintain safety measures for using oxygen in home.

Suggested NOC outcomes

Respiratory Status: Gas Exchange; Respiratory Status: Ventilation; Vital Signs

Interventions and rationales
■ Ascertain what the patient and family members know about home ventilation therapy *to determine what the patient needs to learn. Building on current knowledge enhances learning.*
■ Teach the patient and family members the setup, use, and care of all parts of the equipment *to promote independence and decrease anxiety.*
■ Explain the meanings of ventilator alarms and what to do if alarms sound *to help reduce anxiety and minimize complications.*
■ Explain how to get help in case of emergency *to decrease the potential for injury.*
■ Emphasize the importance of the patient's involvement in family activities, even though he's on mechanical ventilation, *to increase the patient's sense of well-being.*
■ Emphasize to family members that the patient needs to be attended to at all times *to ensure ongoing care.*
■ Demonstrate to family members how to clean and disinfect equipment *to ensure that the patient doesn't develop an infection.*
■ Teach home oxygen safety *to avoid fire or injury to the patient and family members.*

■ Inform the patient and family members about signs and symptoms of complications, such as atelectasis, fluid overload, respiratory infection, and tension pneumothorax. Encourage immediate reporting of complications *to ensure early intervention for respiratory distress.*

Suggested NIC interventions

Airway Management; Mechanical Ventilation; Respiratory Monitoring; Vital Signs Monitoring

Evaluations for expected outcomes

■ Patient has clear breath sounds.

■ Patient doesn't exhibit respiratory distress or infection.

■ Patient incorporates mechanical ventilation into daily life.

■ Patient demonstrates use of communication aids.

■ Patient remains free from complications.

■ Caregiver demonstrates ease in using equipment and procedures to keep patient comfortable and free from infection.

■ Caregiver implements and maintains safety measures for using oxygen in home.

Documentation

■ Assessment results, such as vital signs and breath sounds

■ Checks of ventilator settings, alarms, and backup equipment

■ Arterial blood gas analysis results

■ Patient's response to respiratory treatment

■ Patient's response to nursing interventions

■ Patient teaching and patient's and family members' responses to teaching

■ Evaluations for expected outcomes

Reference

Warren, M.L., et al. "An Interdisciplinary Approach to Transitioning Ventilator-dependent Patients to Home," *Journal of Nursing Care Quality* 19(1):67-73, January-March 2004.

VIII Wellness

INTRODUCTION

This new wellness section focuses on assisting individuals, families, and communities to optimize health and wellness by developing plans that promote healthier lifestyles. These plans emphasize the interconnectedness of body, mind, and spirit by enhancing the existing strengths of an individual, family, or community. The assumption is that by attending to the well-being of one's whole person, a higher level of functioning can be achieved.

In his book *Timeless Healing,* Dr. Herbert Benson describes medicine as a three-legged stool. Well-being or wellness is the seat of the stool, and the three legs are pharmaceuticals, surgery and treatments, and self-care. All three legs are needed proportionately to keep the stool in balance. As a society, we tend to overlook the power of self-care to heal our bodies, minds, and spirit. Instead, we look for answers to our problems in traditional medical solutions.

For decades, nurses have striven to promote health in an illness-oriented model of health care. Now, the opportunity to work actively in a more holistic model is not only accepted but encouraged. This is especially true because of the number of nurses who provide care in nontraditional settings. Such settings include health clubs, health-related spas, weight-control programs, and stress-reduction programs. In addition, the public has been overwhelmed with books, articles, lectures, and Web sites that provide information about the best ways to eat, exercise, reduce stress, and create healthier lifestyles. You, as a nurse, can help your patients navigate through this vast sea of information and design plans with goals that are achievable and interventions that are practical and reasonable.

Ever since the first National Conference on Holistic Health, held in California in June 1975, considerable attention has been given by health care professionals to applying a holistic philosophy to care. In both literature and practice, we see efforts to understand the benefits of and incorporate alternative methods of healing into our care of self and others. The focus on holism, wellness, and the specific alternatives to health has sparked a great deal of interest on the part of health consumers. Many of these methods represent a resurgence of ancient remedies for healing or promoting health. You will be asked about the safety of some of these alternatives. This will involve care on your part not to encourage or include therapies in your plan that fall outside the domain of nursing. If your patient asks about alternative therapies, encourage him to discuss these with his physician.

The wellness plan begins with your assessment. You will want to know about the individual's current health status. Also, include in your assessment all past health problems the patient has had. From your first conversation with the individual, try to determine what areas of wellness the patient is most motivated to improve. Your assessment can then focus on that area so that your plan is individualized when it is completed.

When preforming the assessment, consider the patient's age, gender, ethnicity and culture, education and profession, psychosocial status, self-care status, level of activity, nutritional status, motivation and coping skills, knowledge of health and wellness, and knowledge and experience of alternative therapies. Determine strengths and weaknesses as the patient perceives them. At this point, you may begin to identify your patient's areas of readiness for enhanced wellness. Ascertain what outcomes the patient expects to attain. Because achieving wellness is a process, break the process into outcomes that the individual, family, or community can achieve and measure.

Help your patient look at a variety of activities and or programs that might motivate him to work toward meeting his chosen goals. Help the patient be practical in developing a plan. Stick with goals that can be achieved.

Wellness plans can benefit a large cross section of your patients. There are those individuals or groups who are healthy but who desire to enhance their levels of wellness. You will also find that developing wellness plans for patients with chronic diseases may keep them functioning well without frequent hospitalizations. Seniors who are interested in maintaining good health can modify controllable risk factors for problems such as the prevention of falls.

Also keep in mind that people with physical or mental disabilities, such as limitations in sight, hearing, mobility, intellect, or emotion, will still search for ways to optimize the capabilities they possess.

For each patient in your care, try to identify at least one area in which you can work together to develop a plan that will move the patient toward a higher state of wellness. Refer back to the three-legged stool, and look for self-care activities that will bring the patient's stool into better balance. When caring for patients who have leaned heavily on drugs and other forms of medical treatment with little effort to formulate their own plans for self-care, your challenge as a nurse will be great, but not insurmountable.

Readiness for enhanced
COMFORT

Definition
A pattern of ease, relief, and transcendence in physical, psychospiritual, environmental, and/or social dimensions that can be strengthened

Assessment
- Patient's perception of current state of comfort
- Patient's responsibility for actions taken to maintain a state of comfort
- Support systems, including family members, friends, and clergy
- Attitude of contentment
- Reliance on health care system to resolve complaints

Defining characteristics
- Expresses desire to enhance comfort
- Expresses desire to enhance feeling of contentment
- Expresses desire to enhance relaxation
- Expresses desire to enhance resolution of complaints

Expected outcomes
- Patient will express positive perception of nursing assistance to perform activities that promote comfort.
- Patient will experience physical and psychological ease.
- Patient will develop plans to optimize level of comfort.
- Patient will report an increase in relaxation.

Suggested NOC outcomes
Client Satisfaction; Comfort Level; Comfortable Death

Interventions and rationales
- Assess patient's satisfaction with the amount of assistance the nurse is currently offering *to determine whether patient perceives himself as performing his physical, psychosocial, and spiritual activities at a level that's comfortable for self.*
- Assist patient in developing plan for increasing comfort *to maximize patient's level of contentment and rest.*
- Implement a program to promote resolution of complaints *to prevent or alleviate patient's stress or discomfort.*
- Involve staff, family, and community in promoting patient's comfort *to include all resources that can contribute to patient's comfort and well-being.*

Suggested NIC Interventions
Coping Enhancement; Emotional Support; Environmental Management: Comfort; Touch

Evaluation for expected outcomes
■ Patient expresses positive perception of nursing assistance with activities that promote comfort.
■ Patient reports feelings of encouragement, acceptance, and reassurance during times of stress.
■ Patient develops plan to adapt to perceived stressors, changes, and interferences with a state of comfort.
■ Patient expresses increase in relaxation and level of comfort.

Documentation
■ Patient's perception of level of comfort
■ Patient's plan for increasing comfort
■ Community resources that exist to increase patient comfort
■ Future plans to address comfort and contentment
■ Evaluations for expected outcomes

Reference
Kolcaba, K., and DiMarco, M.A. "Comfort Theory and Its Application to Pediatric Nursing," *Pediatric Nursing* 31(3):187-94, May-June 2005.

Readiness for enhanced
COMMUNICATION
related to wellness diagnosis

Definition
A pattern of exchanging information and ideas with others that's sufficient for meeting one's needs and life goals and can be strengthened

Assessment
■ Gender and age as variables in communication patterns
■ Developmental history of communication patterns and practices
■ Effect of stress on communication
■ Family history of communication patterns
■ Cultural and religious communication patterns
■ Knowledge of difference between passive aggressive and assertive patterns of communication

Defining characteristics
■ Expresses willingness to enhance communication ability
■ Can speak or write language clearly
■ Forms words, phrases, and language with articulation
■ Uses and interprets nonverbal cues appropriately
■ Expresses satisfaction with ability to share information and ideas with others
■ Expresses needs in assertive ways

Expected outcomes

■ Patient will express message clearly as evidenced by feedback that receiver understood message.

■ Patient will express increased sense of confidence in communicating thoughts and feelings to nurse, family, health care teams, and any kind of reference groups in which an individual participates (e.g., friends, school groups, community groups, faith groups, etc.) throughout the life span and the continuum of care.

■ Patient will report enhanced ability to respond assertively to individuals who relate with passive or aggressive communication styles.

■ Patient will report feelings of confidence in social encounters because of enhanced communication skills.

■ Patient will gain practice in applying enhanced communication techniques with individuals, family, and groups.

■ Patient communication will be enhanced by nonverbal means, such as use of electronic mail and Internet connections, pictures, and drawings.

■ Patient will use enhanced communication skills to negotiate and advocate for self with health care providers and in conflict situations.

Suggested NOC outcomes

Communication: Expressive; Communication: Receptive

Interventions and rationales

■ Establish clear purpose for interaction. *This provides the patient with goals and a time frame for interaction.*

■ Provide environment that diminishes physical space between nurse and patient to eliminate such barriers to communications as noise and lack of privacy. *Reducing barriers to communication nonverbally communicates to patient that nurse wants to be involved with patient.*

■ Use verbal and nonverbal communication patterns that integrate warmth, genuineness, empathy, and respect to facilitate patient empowerment and relationship building. *Therapeutic nurse-patient relationship building increase patient's feeling of security. The nurse modeling caring behaviors encourages patient to incorporate the same attitudes.*

■ Provide support through active listening, appropriate periods of silence, reflection of feelings, and paraphrasing and summarizing comments. *Active listening techniques encourage increased patient participation in communication.*

■ Incorporate questions that are open-ended, and start with such words as "what," "how," and "could," rather than "why." *Open-ended, nonthreatening questioning encourages patient to discuss issues of concern and improve communication skills.*

■ Refrain from interrupting, changing subject, revealing too much personal information about self, or responding too quickly to questions during interactions. *Skillful role modeling of positive communication skills keeps focus on patient.*

■ Encourage patient verbally and nonverbally to explore strategies to enhance self-advocacy communication skills with health care providers. *Self-advocacy communication skills can guide patient toward autonomy, confidence, and independence.*

■ Avoid critical, overprotective or overcontrolling communication patterns when working with patient. *Positive communication patterns reflect respect and facilitate development of patient trust and relationship building.*

■ Include role playing as a teaching strategy to model methods of enhanced verbal and nonverbal communication skills. *Role playing of verbal and nonverbal communication methods in a nonthreatening, safe environment can enhance communication skills.*

■ Explore and discuss thoughts and feelings regarding any overuse of negative cognitions and expressions on the part of the patient by suggesting strategies such as rubber band on wrist to snap every time negative expressions start. *Exploration and discussion of negative cognitions may provide an opportunity to explore alternative ways of dealing with negative thoughts and feelings.*

■ Teach theory of assertive behavior, and role-play assertive communication approaches. *Assertiveness training can decrease passive or aggressive communication patterns.*

■ Listen for themes presented during nurse-client interactions *because themes can provide areas of focus for patient discussions with caregiver.*

■ Schedule frequent treatment team meetings regarding communication skill development with patient. *Team meetings with patient can ensure continuity of care and the development of communication patterns, facilitating patient's coping with health and illness.*

■ Communicate a plan to patient regarding mutual decision making (partnering) regarding goals and direction of future encounters *to reinforce patient's role within the relationship.*

■ Consider such factors as age, gender, culture, religion, and spirituality in communicating with patient *to facilitate the provision of holistic and individual care.*

■ Communicate use of positive self-talk to patient *to enhance confidence in communication.*

Suggested NIC interventions

Active Listening; Animal-Assisted Therapy; Anticipatory Guidance; Art Therapy; Assertiveness Training; Behavior Modification: Social Skills; Complex Relationship Building; Music Therapy; Socialization Enhancement

Evaluations for expected outcomes

■ Patient expresses message clearly as evidenced by feedback that receiver understood message.

■ Patient expresses satisfaction with feedback received from caregivers and others.

■ Patient reports that nurse and other health care team members provide an increased sense of security through verbal and nonverbal communication.

■ Patient reports less anxiety and guilt and more control in providing assertive responses when relating to individuals with passive or aggressive communication styles.

■ Patient expresses belief that nurse uses interactions that convey respect, warmth, empathy, and genuineness that can result in enhanced communication skill building.

■ Patient discloses feelings of confidence and increased life quality related to enhanced communication skills with family, groups, health care team, and confrontational persons.

■ Patient describes enhanced ability to advocate for self in coping with chronic and acute illness.

■ Patient reports successful negotiations within health care milieu.

Documentation

■ Efforts made by nurse to provide didactic information on communication theory and to role model enhanced communication skills such as assertiveness training

■ Patient's response to didactic discussions and strategies, such as role playing and interactive videos

■ Nursing interventions regarding coaching and supporting patient progress toward enhanced communication patterns

■ Patient's expressed thoughts and feelings about personal progress toward enhanced communication responses

■ Revisions to treatment plan

■ Evaluations for expected outcomes

Reference

Whyte, R.E., et al. "Nurses' Opportunistic Interventions with Patients in Relation to Smoking," *Journal of Advanced Nursing* 55(5):568-77, September 2006.

Readiness for enhanced
COMMUNITY COPING
related to immunization

Definition

A pattern of community activities for adaptation and problem solving that's satisfactory for meeting the demands or needs of the community but can be improved for management of current and/or future problems

Assessment

■ Community demographics, including age and gender distribution, ethnic groups, racial groups, religious groups, and education and income levels

■ Community health status, including availability of health care services, use of health care services, prevalence of childhood illnesses in the community, epidemiologic statistics, and beliefs, values, and attitudes about health and illness

■ Education system, including educational level of adult population and state law or school system's requirements for immunization before school attendance

■ Religious institutions and their support for, or objections to, immunization

■ Social services, including availability of clinics and other social services, access to health care, welfare system, and parents' dependence on welfare for support

Defining characteristics

■ Active planning to handle predicted stressors

■ Active problem solving when faced with issues

- Agreement that community carries responsibility for stress management
- Deficits in one or more effective coping characteristics
- Existing relaxation and recreation programs
- Positive communication among community members and between members and larger community organizations
- Sufficient resources for managing stressors

Expected outcomes

- Community members will express understanding of problems associated with failure to immunize population and will recognize need for plan to reduce number of children and adults who aren't immunized.
- Community members will establish plan to increase rate of immunizations and ensure adequate protection from communicable diseases.
- Community members will work to reduce spread of communicable diseases and increase rate of immunization within community.
- Community members will evaluate established plans for ensuring that all children become immunized and will make changes to plans as needed.

Suggested NOC outcomes

Community Competence; Community Health Status; Community Health Status: Immunity; Community Risk Control: Communicable Disease

Interventions and rationales

- Work with community members to pinpoint potential problems associated with inadequate immunization of the population *to ensure adequate protection against communicable disease.* Consider taking these steps:
– Identify new members of the community, such as immigrants and refugees, *to help reach parents who need information about immunization.*
– Identify parents who don't follow through with the required series of immunizations *to protect children from incomplete immunization.*
- Encourage community members to implement a program to disseminate information about problems associated with inadequate immunization *to educate residents and promote the community's established immunization program.*
- Provide extensive education about communicable diseases and the importance of immunizations *to empower community residents and help decrease the risk of communicable disease.*
- Encourage health departments, clinics, and practitioners' offices to provide information on the recommended childhood immunization schedule to the public *to foster education about immunization.*
- Contact the parents of children who aren't immunized in person or by handwritten note. Make it clear that your purpose in promoting immunization is to protect their child from illness *to build parents' trust in immunization programs.*
- Provide immunization information in the parents' first language *to overcome a lack of understanding caused by language barriers.*
- Develop a list of referrals for the parents of children who aren't immunized. Include information on low-cost health insurance, city health centers, and well-baby clinics *to encourage compliance.*

■ Coordinate with local nursing schools, health department nurses, and other interested nursing groups to provide the necessary number of professionals to deliver adequate immunizations *to reduce the risk of communicable disease.*

■ Conduct a follow-up survey on immunization rates *to measure the effectiveness of educational efforts.*

■ Collect statistical data from community sources, such as health department and schools, *to continue to identify children who haven't been immunized.*

Suggested NIC interventions

Communicable Disease Management; Community Health Development; Health Education; Health Policy Monitoring; Immunization/Vaccination Management

Evaluations for expected outcomes

■ Community members understand risks of failing to immunize population and recognize need for plan.

■ Community members put forth plan to meet community's immunization needs that contains definite actions yet allows for modifications.

■ Community members implement plan to reduce spread of communicable disease and increase rate of immunization.

■ Community members evaluate plan and make changes, as needed, to help solve problems and further goal of meeting community's immunization needs.

Documentation

■ Evidence of need for immunization program
■ Statistical data documenting problem
■ Written plan to resolve problem
■ Efforts made to disseminate written information to community
■ Evaluations for expected outcomes

Reference

Pender, N.J., et al. *Health Promotion in Nursing Practice,* 5th ed. Upper Saddle River, N.J.: Prentice Hall, 2006.

Readiness for enhanced
COPING

Definition

A pattern of cognitive and behavioral efforts to manage demands that's sufficient for well-being and can be strengthened

Assessment

■ Age
■ Usual coping mechanisms

- Perceived coping ability
- Role responsibilities
- Social support
- Spiritual resources

Defining characteristics

- Defines stressors as manageable
- Seeks knowledge of new strategies
- Seeks social support
- Uses broad range of problem-oriented and emotion-oriented strategies
- Uses spiritual resources

Expected outcomes

- Patient will identify major issues that require ongoing enhancement of coping strategies.
- Patient will express feelings associated with present coping strategies.
- Patient will demonstrate readiness to develop enhanced strategies.
- Patient will identify support persons and activities that will assist in goal attainment.

Suggested NOC outcomes

Coping; Quality of Life

Interventions and rationales

- Establish a trusting relationship with patient. *Building trust will allow patient to be more open.*
- Begin discussions at patient's level of comfort. *If patient wants to discuss feelings, it won't benefit patient for nurse to begin presenting strategies that require logical reasoning.*
- Determine from listening to the patient options that might be attractive to patient in reaching new goals for coping, for example, support group, spiritual direction, and journaling. *The patient will strive to enhance coping skills using those opportunities to which he feels best suited.*
- Arrange to meet with patient regularly to assist in helping patient focus on his goals and evaluate his progress. *Recognizing even small attempts at successful coping encourages patient to increase his efforts.*

Suggested NIC interventions

Active Listening; Coping Enhancement

Evaluations for expected outcomes

- Patient has successfully articulated major areas where enhanced coping strategies are needed.
- Patient expresses feelings associated with current coping strategies.
- Patient demonstrates readiness to develop enhanced strategies.
- Patient identifies the person(s) he perceives as being able to support him therapeutically in his efforts.

■ Patient identifies with group support or attends class or session to learn more about coping.

Documentation
■ Patient's assessment of coping skills
■ Patient's goals for enhanced coping
■ Actions taken by patient to cope from situation to situation
■ Patient's response to nursing interventions
■ Evaluations for expected outcomes

Reference
Fiks, A.G., et al. "Identifying Factors Predicting Immunization Delay for Children Followed in an Urban Primary Care Network Using an Electronic Health Record," *Pediatrics* 118(6):1680-686, December 2006.

Readiness for enhanced
DECISION MAKING

Definition
A pattern of choosing courses of action that's sufficient for meeting short- and long-term health-related goals and that can be strengthened

Assessment
■ Patient's perception of his ability to make decisions
■ Patient's expression of desire to align decisions with his personal values and goals
■ Patient's expression of desire to improve congruence between decisions and sociocultural values and goals
■ Patient's desire to evaluate the efficacy of his decisions
■ Patient's need for reliable information on which to base his decisions

Defining characteristics
■ Expresses desire to enhance decision making
■ Expresses desire to enhance congruency of decisions with personal values and goals
■ Expresses desire to enhance congruency of decisions with sociocultural values and goals
■ Expresses desire to enhance risk benefit analysis of decisions
■ Expresses desire to enhance understanding of choices for decision making
■ Expresses desire to enhance understanding of the meaning of choices
■ Expresses desire to enhance use of reliable evidence for decisions

Expected outcomes

■ Patient will express desire to make effective decisions to meet short- and long-term goals.
■ Patient will share decision-making goals and concerns.
■ Patient will discuss measures used to evaluate quality of decisions made.
■ Patient will make decisions that promote maximal physical, mental, social, and psychological well-being.
■ Patient will involve family, community, friends, and clergy in health care decisions.

Suggested NOC Outcomes

Decision-Making; Participation in Health Care Decisions; Self-Care: Instrumental Activities of Daily Living (IADL)

Interventions and rationales

■ Assess patient's ability to make decisions that affect his well-being *to determine his level of ability to participate in health care decisions.*
■ Work with patient to enhance his decision-making capabilities *to promote personal actions of a competent individual to exercise governance in life decisions.*
■ Provide patient with decision-making support *to enhance self-care and well-being of patient and his family.*
■ Assist patient with decisions that involve family, community, friends, and clergy *to provide opportunities for shared decision making and enhanced support for patient.*

Suggested NIC interventions

Decision-Making Support; Health System Guidance; Self-Responsibility Facilitation

Evaluations for expected outcomes

■ Patient expresses desire to make effective decisions to meet short- and long-term goals.
■ Patient shares decision-making goals and concerns.
■ Patient discusses measures used to evaluate the quality of decisions made.
■ Patient makes decisions that promote maximal physical, mental, social, and psychological well-being.
■ Patient involves his family, community, friends, and clergy in health care decisions.

Documentation

■ Patient's perception of decision-making abilities
■ Patient's involvement of family, community, friends, and clergy in decision-making
■ Future plans to make decisions that improve physical, mental, social, and psychological well-being
■ Evaluation for expected outcomes

Reference

Moser, A., et al. "Patient Autonomy in Nurse-Led Shared Care: A Review of Theoretical and Empirical Literature," *Journal of Advanced Nursing* 57(4):357-65, February 2007.

Readiness for enhanced
FAMILY COPING
related to self-actualization needs

Definition

Effective managing of adaptive tasks by family members involved in the patient's health challenge, who now exhibit desire and readiness for enhanced health and growth in regard to self and relation to the patient

Assessment

■ Family process, including normal pattern of interaction among family members, family's understanding and knowledge of patient's present condition, support systems available (financial, social, and spiritual), family's past response to crises (coping patterns), and communication patterns used to express anger, affection, and confrontation

■ Patient's illness, including progression and severity of illness, patient's perception of health problem, and problem-solving techniques used by patient to cope with life problems

Defining characteristics

■ Interest of family member in making contact with others who have gone through similar situations

■ Attempt by family member to describe impact of crisis on personal values, priorities, goals, or relationships

■ Fostering by family member of a health-promoting and enriching lifestyle that supports and monitors maturational processes and audits and negotiates treatment programs

Expected outcomes

■ Family members will discuss impact of patient's illness and feelings about it.

■ Family members will participate in treatment plan.

■ Family members will establish a visiting routine beneficial to patient and themselves.

■ Family members will demonstrate care needed to maintain patient's health status.

■ Family members will identify and use available support systems.

Suggested NOC outcomes

Family Coping; Family Normalization; Family Participation in Professional Care

Interventions and rationales

■ Allow time for family members to discuss impact of patient's illness and their feelings. Encourage expression of feelings *to allow family members to realistically adjust to patient's problems.*

■ Encourage family conferences; help family members identify key issues and select support services, if needed, *to develop sense of shared responsibility and feelings of safety, adequacy, and comfort.*

■ Help patient and family establish a visiting routine that won't tax patient's or family's resources. Use patient's daily routine to aid in planning—for example, no visiting during treatments or during periods of uninterrupted sleep. *Involving family members reassures patient of their care and reduces family's fear and anxiety.*

■ Reinforce family members' efforts to care for patient *to let them know they're doing their best and to ease adaptation and grieving process.*

■ Demonstrate care procedures, and encourage participation in treatment and planning decisions (such as selecting times for pulmonary toilet for patient with cystic fibrosis). *Meeting others' needs promotes self-esteem.*

■ Provide family members with clear, concise information about patient's condition. Be aware of what they have been told, and help them interpret information. *This information will help alleviate their concerns.*

■ Ensure privacy for patient and family during visits *to foster open communication.*

■ Help family support patient's independence. Encourage attendance at therapy sessions, and allow patient to demonstrate new skills and abilities. *Independence helps patient reach maximum functional level.*

■ Provide emotional support to family by being available to answer questions. *Attentive listening conveys empathy, recognition, and respect for a person.*

■ Inform family of community resources and support groups available to assist in managing patient's illness and providing emotional or financial support to caretakers, such as Easter Seals Association, Visiting Nurse Association, and Meals On Wheels. *Community resources may help patient develop potential, independence, and self-reliance.*

Suggested NIC interventions

Caregiver Support; Family Involvement Promotion; Health Education; Self-Modification Assistance

Evaluations for expected outcomes

■ Family members acknowledge their feelings about patient's illness.

■ Family members spend adequate time with patient and seek to participate in care.

■ Family members establish a visiting routine beneficial to patient and themselves.

■ Family members display competence in caring for patient through return demonstration and provide adequate level of care to maintain patient's health.

■ Family members make contact with support resources available in their community.

Documentation
- Family's response to patient's illness
- Family's current understanding of patient's illness
- Observations about family's interaction with patient and acceptance of current situation
- Evaluations for expected outcomes

Reference
Schure, L.M., et al. "Beyond Stroke: Description and Evaluation of an Effective Intervention to Support Family Caregivers of Stroke Patients," *Patient Education and Counseling* 62(1):46-55, July 2006.

Readiness for enhanced
FLUID BALANCE

Definition
A pattern of equilibrium between fluid volume and chemical composition of body fluids that's sufficient for meeting physical needs and can be strengthened

Assessment
- Cardiovascular status, including pulse and blood pressure, capillary filling, and electrocardiogram (ECG) results
- GI status, including types and amounts of fluid and food intake; maintenance of stable weight; and recent episodes of acute, limited GI disturbance with intestinal loss of fluid (vomiting or diarrhea)
- Fluid and electrolyte status, including skin turgor; mucous membranes (lips) for moistness or cracks; temperature and color of skin; absence or presence of diaphoresis; and presence of dependent edema or fingerprint edema
- Renal-urinary status, including normal pattern and amount of voiding and evidence of straw-colored urine
- Respiratory status, including rate and depth of respirations through nasal passages; cough; and auscultation of lungs for fine crackles
- Neurologic status, including level of consciousness and mental status
- Skeletal muscles, including normal tone and strength and absence of cramping
- Laboratory studies, including serum electrolyte, plasma glucose, and blood urea nitrogen (BUN) levels; plasma osmolarity; hemoglobin level and hematocrit; and urine analysis that includes specific gravity and glucose

Defining characteristics
- Expresses willingness to enhance fluid balance
- Stable weight
- Moist mucous membranes
- Food and fluid intake adequate for daily needs
- Straw-colored urine with specific gravity within normal limits

- Good tissue turgor
- No excessive thirst
- Urine output appropriate for intake
- No evidence of edema or dehydration

Expected outcomes

- Patient's vital signs will remain stable and within normal ranges; ECG shows no abnormality in rhythm.
- Patient's skin temperature, moistness, turgor, and color will be normal.
- Patient's mucous membranes will be moist and noncracked.
- Patient's weight will remain stable.
- Patient's fluid volume intake will remain adequate; patient will experience thirst satiety.
- Patient will produce adequate urine volume (approximately equal to fluid intake) of light to straw-colored urine.
- Patient's urine specific gravity will remain between 1.015 and 1.025.
- Patient's plasma and serum values for electrolytes, osmolarity, glucose, BUN, hematocrit, and hemoglobin will be within normal ranges.
- Patient will be alert and responsive to demands of living and react appropriately to reflex needs such as thirst; patient's muscle reflexes, strength, and tone will be normal.
- Patient will express understanding of factors that contribute to normal fluid and electrolyte balance.
- Patient will adhere to prescribed therapies to manage such coexisting disease processes as diabetes mellitus, heart failure, renal insufficiency, and thyroid excess or deficiency, which interfere with electrolyte and osmolar homeostasis.

Suggested NOC outcomes

Fluid Balance; Hydration; Nutritional Status: Food & Fluid Intake; Tissue Integrity: Skin & Mucous Membranes; Tissue Perfusion: Abdominal Organs; Vital Signs

Interventions and rationales

- Explain and reinforce to patient the need to drink 1½ to 2 qt (1.5 to 2 L) fluids daily, divided equally throughout the day. *Although daily intake should be between 2½ and 3½ qt (2.5 and 3.5 L) daily, food liberates about 1 qt (1 L) of fluid and, in the process of food oxidation, cells liberate up to 0.4 qt (0.4 L) of water.*
- Encourage patient to select healthy, appropriate beverages such as drinking plenty of water; other beverages, such as soda, should be consumed in moderation. *Many beverages, including carbonated soft drinks and fruit juices, have a high sugar content and increase the osmolar content of the body, causing greater thirst and increased load on the renal system and diuresis. Beverages with caffeine cause diuresis and may cause an increased fluid loss. Patient should carefully select and judiciously use beverages and sports drinks that claim to replenish electrolytes. Alcoholic beverages are discouraged during hot weather because these can cause fluid and electrolyte disturbances through excess diuresis.*
- Educate patient on how to read and interpret labels on beverage and food containers. For example, humans require 0.5 g (500 mg) of sodium per day; typical

intake is 5 to 6 g daily. *Reducing the amount of sodium reduces the amount of fluid volume in the vascular system, thus controlling thirst and blood pressure. Individuals with treatment plans that include nutritional therapy should be encouraged to adhere to prescribed restrictions.*

■ Teach patient about adequate water intake during demanding daily events, such as increased exercise or high environmental temperatures. *During extreme exercise conditions, unmeasured fluid losses through diaphoresis and lung evaporation can be significant (1,200 to 2,000 ml). Advise patient to hydrate well before (750 ml), during (250 ml every 15 minutes of activity), and after exercise events (500 ml). To prevent dehydration, gauge fluid need on urine color and amount. It should remain light to straw-colored and normal in volume.*

■ Educate patient on signs and symptoms of dehydration (dry mouth and mucous membranes), light-headedness (blood pressure and vital sign changes), and scant urine output (glycosuria and polyuria). *By recognizing onset of dehydration, one can avoid severe complications.*

■ Educate patient on signs and symptoms of overhydration and fluid retention, such as scant urine output, cough, increased weight gain, dependent edema, and jugular vein distention. *By recognizing onset of overhydration or fluid retention, one can avoid severe complications.*

Suggested NIC interventions

Electrolyte Management; Fluid/Electrolyte Management; Fluid Management; Fluid Monitoring

Evaluations for expected outcomes

■ Patient's vital signs, skin temperature and turgor, and ECG are within normal range.

■ Patient maintains fluid volume equilibrium with normal electrolyte and osmolar balance.

■ Patient responds to natural thirst mechanism and drinks 1,400 to 1,800 ml daily.

■ Patient manages nutrient intake to reduce sodium intake toward daily requirement and maintains serum sodium between 135 to 145 mEq/L.

■ Patient manages food and nutrient intake and treatment plan (if applicable) to maintain plasma glucose level below 120 mg/dl.

■ Patient maintains plasma osmolality between 280 to 295 mOsm/kg.

■ Patient doesn't experience weight gain or loss related to fluid gain or loss.

Documentation

■ Patient's weight and weight changes over time
■ Vital signs; capillary filling
■ Daily intake and types of fluids
■ Daily urine output; characteristics of urine (color, concentration, odor)
■ Thirst and patient's ability to satisfy thirst
■ Skin turgor; moist or dry mucous membranes
■ Laboratory electrolyte results, if available
■ Evaluations for expected outcomes

Reference

Mentes, J. "Oral Hydration in Older Adults: Greater Awareness Is Needed in Preventing, Recognizing, and Treating Dehydration," *AJN* 106(6):40-49, June 2006.

HEALTH-SEEKING BEHAVIORS

related to absence of aerobic exercise as a risk factor for coronary artery disease

Definition

Active seeking (by a person in stable health) of ways to alter personal health habits or the environment in order to move toward a higher level of health

Assessment

- Risk factor analysis, including age, gender, cholesterol level, personal or family history of diabetes, ratio of high-density lipoprotein to low-density lipoprotein, blood pressure, weight, level of exercise, history of smoking, and stressors
- Current health status
- Psychosocial status, including lifestyle and motivation
- Recognition and realization of potential growth, health, and autonomy
- Understanding of risk modification

Defining characteristics

- Expressed or observed desire to seek a higher level of wellness
- Demonstrated or observed lack of knowledge about health promotion behaviors
- Reported or observed unfamiliarity with wellness community resources
- Expressed concern about current environmental conditions on health status
- Expressed or observed desire for increased control of health practices

Expected outcomes

- Patient will communicate understanding of benefits of aerobic exercise program.
- Patient will state guidelines for aerobic exercise.
- Patient will develop exercise routine.
- Patient will state proper target heart rate to achieve during exercise (60% to 80% of 220, minus patient's age).
- Patient will demonstrate ability to take pulse accurately.

Suggested NOC outcomes

Adherence Behavior; Health Beliefs; Health Orientation; Health Promoting Behavior

Interventions and rationales

■ Discuss benefits of regular exercise on cardiovascular and respiratory systems and on mental health status *to introduce patient to various benefits of exercise program.*

■ Review basic components of aerobic exercise routine, including:

– frequency (minimum of three times weekly)

– duration (minimum of 20 minutes, not including 5 to 10 minutes of warm-up and cool-down)

– intensity (workload should progress only according to perceived exertion and target heart rate).

This informs patient of minimum requirements needed to get aerobic benefit from exercise program.

■ Discuss aerobic activities, such as walking, jogging, swimming, cycling, and rowing. *Patient must build individualized program around enjoyable activity that meets aerobic criteria.*

■ Recommend that patient consult with physician before starting exercise program *so patient can have exercise stress test, if necessary, and receive medical clearance for exercise program.*

■ Recommend either a supervised or unsupervised exercise program, depending on patient's motivation to continue program. *Supervised program may help less motivated patients.*

■ Review warm-up and cool-down techniques, which prevent abrupt changes in heart rate, and stretching muscles *to avoid injuries and an overworked heart.*

■ Teach patient how to take his own pulse, and monitor accuracy. *Patient must know how to take pulse to maintain correct heart rate range.*

■ Instruct patient to notify physician of any adverse symptoms experienced while exercising *to detect adverse effects early.*

■ Provide patient with literature on exercise guidelines and community exercise programs *to reinforce teaching and provide references following discharge.*

Suggested NIC interventions

Health Education; Mutual Goal Setting; Teaching: Prescribed Activity/Exercise; Values Clarification

Evaluations for expected outcomes

■ Patient lists several benefits of aerobic exercise program.

■ Patient outlines basic aerobic exercise program.

■ Patient provides example of individualized exercise routine.

■ Patient states personal target heart rate range.

■ Patient demonstrates accurate pulse-taking techniques.

Documentation

■ Patient's expression of concern about promoting a higher level of wellness

■ Patient's response to nursing interventions

■ Instructions given and patient's understanding of instructions

■ Patient's plan of exercise after discharge from facility

■ Patient's ability to take and record pulse

■ Literature provided and referrals made to resources in community
■ Evaluations for expected outcomes

Reference
Klieman, L., et al. "Cardiovascular Disease Risk Reduction in Older Adults," *Journal of Cardiovascular Nursing* 21(5 Suppl 1):S27-39, September-October 2006.

HEALTH-SEEKING BEHAVIORS
related to elevated serum cholesterol level as a risk factor for coronary artery disease

Definition
Active seeking (by a person in stable health) of ways to alter personal health habits or the environment in order to move toward a higher level of health

Assessment
■ Risk factor analysis, including age, gender, cholesterol level, personal or family history of diabetes, ratio of high-density lipoprotein (HDL) to low-density lipoprotein (LDL), blood pressure, weight, level of exercise, history of smoking, and stressors
■ Current health status
■ Psychosocial status, including lifestyle and motivation
■ Recognition and realization of potential growth, health, and autonomy
■ Understanding of risk modification

Defining characteristics
■ Expressed or observed desire to seek a higher level of wellness
■ Demonstrated or observed lack of knowledge about health promotion behaviors
■ Reported or observed unfamiliarity with wellness community resources
■ Expressed concern about current environmental conditions on health status
■ Expressed or observed desire for increased control of health practices

Expected outcomes
■ Patient will state personal cholesterol level.
■ Patient will report that elevated cholesterol level is risk factor for coronary artery disease.
■ Patient will state appropriate dietary intake of fat and cholesterol to reduce cholesterol level.
■ Patient will identify ways to decrease cholesterol level.
■ Patient's cholesterol level will decline to desired level.
■ Patient won't develop illness, or signs and symptoms of disease will be controlled.

Suggested NOC outcomes

Adherence Behavior; Coping; Health Beliefs; Health Orientation; Health Promoting Behavior; Knowledge: Health Promotion

Interventions and rationales

■ Discuss patient's cholesterol level and HDL/LDL ratio *to inform patient of desirable results.*

■ Discuss patient's understanding of cholesterol and its sources *to increase understanding of intrinsic and extrinsic sources and connection between high levels and coronary disease.*

■ Discuss ways to lower cholesterol level *to encourage compliance with postdischarge diet plan.*

■ Provide literature on cholesterol *to reinforce teaching after discharge.*

■ Have patient meet with dietitian *to correct any dietary imbalances and reinforce healthy eating habits.*

■ Review outside resources available to patient *to provide follow-up and reinforcement after discharge.*

■ Review patient's dietary habits, foods high in cholesterol and saturated fats, and importance of adhering to a low-cholesterol, low-fat diet *to reinforce dietary teaching and healthy eating habits.*

Suggested NIC interventions

Active Listening; Coping Enhancement; Counseling; Health Education; Learning Facilitation; Risk Identification; Self-Responsibility Facilitation

Evaluations for expected outcomes

■ Patient states cholesterol level.

■ Patient states that elevated cholesterol level is risk factor for coronary artery disease.

■ Patient communicates understanding of how diet affects cholesterol level.

■ Patient describes other factors, such as exercise, that can decrease cholesterol level.

■ Patient's cholesterol level declines to desired level.

■ Patient doesn't exhibit signs or symptoms of disease associated with elevated cholesterol level.

Documentation

■ Patient's expression of concern about promoting a higher level of wellness

■ Patient's response to nursing interventions

■ Instructions provided and patient's understanding of instructions

■ Literature recommended or provided to patient

■ Evaluations for expected outcomes

Reference

Pins, J.J., and Keenan, J.M. "Dietary and Nutraceutical Options for Managing the Hypertriglyceridemic Patient," *Progress in Cardiovascular Nursing* 21(2):89-93, Spring 2006.

HEALTH-SEEKING BEHAVIORS

related to hypertension as a risk factor for coronary artery disease

Definition

Active seeking (by a person in stable health) of ways to alter personal health habits or the environment in order to move toward a higher level of health

Assessment

■ Risk factor analysis, including age, sex, cholesterol level, personal or family history of diabetes, ratio of high-density lipoprotein to low-density lipoprotein, blood pressure, weight, level of exercise, history of smoking, and stressors
■ Current health status
■ Psychosocial status, including lifestyle and motivation
■ Recognition and realization of potential growth, health, and autonomy
■ Understanding of risk modification

Defining characteristics

■ Expressed or observed desire to seek a higher level of wellness
■ Demonstrated or observed lack of knowledge about health promotion behaviors
■ Reported or observed unfamiliarity with wellness community resources
■ Expressed concern about current environmental conditions on health status
■ Expressed or observed desire for increased control of health practices

Expected outcomes

■ Patient will express interest in learning new behaviors to help reduce blood pressure.
■ Patient will state that hypertension is a risk factor for coronary artery disease.
■ Patient will identify and demonstrate appropriate interventions for lowering blood pressure.
■ Patient will state own blood pressure range.
■ Patient will express and demonstrate appropriate dietary measures used to reduce high blood pressure.
■ Patient will maintain blood pressure within desired limits.
■ Patient won't develop illness, or signs and symptoms of disease will be controlled.

Suggested NOC outcomes

Adherence Behavior; Health Beliefs; Health Orientation; Health Promoting Behavior; Knowledge: Health Promotion; Personal Well-Being; Risk Control: Cardiovascular Health

Interventions and rationales

■ Discuss patient's understanding of hypertension and how it affects body. Clarify any misconceptions. *This increases patient's awareness of hypertension's dangers.*
■ Inform patient of blood pressure reading each time it's taken *to reinforce acceptable range and give patient responsibility for maintaining it.*

- Provide patient with pamphlets on hypertension *for reinforcement and easy reference after discharge.*
- Encourage patient to continue prescribed antihypertensives, as ordered, *to control blood pressure.*
- Teach patient how to monitor own blood pressure *to help maintain normal pressure.*
- Instruct patient on methods to lower blood pressure *using simple exercise and dietary guidelines.*
- Have patient meet with dietitian *to discuss low-sodium diet, assess eating habits, and make appropriate modifications.*

Suggested NIC interventions

Active Listening; Health Education; Health System Guidance; Teaching: Procedure/Treatment; Telephone Consultation

Evaluations for expected outcomes

- Patient expresses desire to control blood pressure.
- Patient communicates that hypertension is a risk factor for coronary artery disease.
- Patient reports at least three methods to help control blood pressure.
- Patient states blood pressure range.
- Patient demonstrates use of appropriate dietary measures to reduce high blood pressure.
- Patient's blood pressure remains within desired limits.
- Patient doesn't exhibit signs or symptoms of disease associated with hypertension.

Documentation

- Patient's expression of concern about promoting a higher level of wellness
- Patient's response to nursing interventions
- Instructions provided and patient's understanding of instructions
- Literature recommended or provided to patient
- Referrals made to community resources
- Evaluations for expected outcomes

Reference

Sol, B.G., et al. "Vascular Risk Management Through Nurse-led Self-management Programs," *Journal of Vascular Nursing* 23(1):20-24, March 2005.

HEALTH-SEEKING BEHAVIORS

related to locating health-related information on the Internet

Definition

Active seeking (by a patient in stable health) of ways to alter personal health habits or the environment in order to move toward optimal health

Assessment

- Current health status
- Risk factors, including age, gender, health history, family health history, and smoking history
- Psychosocial status, including lifestyle, motivation to learn about health, and recognition of potential for growth and autonomy
- Cognitive status, including level of consciousness, educational level, abstract thinking ability, and reasoning and problem-solving abilities
- Mobility status, including muscle strength and mass and use of assistive devices
- Internet access, including availability of computer, modem, and software to support Internet research

Defining characteristics

- Desire for increased control of health status
- Desire to seek higher level of wellness
- Expressed concern about effect of environmental conditions on health status
- Lack of knowledge about ways to promote health
- Unfamiliarity with sources for obtaining health-related information

Expected outcomes

- Patient will state desire for additional health care information.
- Patient will identify health-related resources available on Internet.
- Patient will voice understanding of how to evaluate Internet health resources.
- Patient will share relevant information obtained from Internet with health care provider.

Suggested NOC outcomes

Adherence Behavior; Health Beliefs; Health Orientation; Health Promoting Behavior

Interventions and rationales

- Inform patient that he can obtain information on health-related topics on the Internet *to make patient aware of a valuable resource for health information and help patient take an active role in health care decisions.*
- Explain to patient that the Internet is a large interconnected network of computers. No single entity owns it, and no person or organization controls it. The World Wide Web is a multimedia-based portion of the Internet, which offers color, graphics, sound, video, and dynamic navigation systems. *Clear explanation will help patient understand depth and scope of the Internet and World Wide Web.*
- Provide patient with basic information on how to use the Internet. For example, discuss common Internet terms, such as:
- *Universal resource locator (URL).* Each Web site has its own unique address, or URL, a series of words and symbols that help identify the site. When seeking a particular Web site, the patient must enter the URL exactly as indicated.
- *Home page.* When visiting the Web site, the patient may first arrive at an opening page, called the home page.

– *Hypertext links.* Usually underlined and displayed in a different color on the Web document, hypertext links connect the user to other web documents. Hypertext links may be called *hyperlinks* or simply *links.*

– *Search engine.* Type of Web site that lists different categories and allows the user to search for information on chosen topics using key words. Popular search engines include Google, AltaVista, Yahoo, Lycos, and Excite. One search engine dedicated to health-related topics is HealthAtoZ *(www.healthatoz.com).*

The Internet world is filled with jargon. Helping the patient understand this terminology will reduce anxiety about using the Internet.

■ Provide the patient with information about getting on the Internet. Explain that, in addition to a computer, the patient will need a modem, browser, and Internet connection.

– The patient can obtain an Internet connection through an Internet Service Provider (ISP) or commercial on-line service, such as America Online (AOL), Compuserve, or Prodigy.

– Browsers, such as Super Mosaic, Netscape Navigator, or Microsoft Internet Explorer, are software applications that allow the user to navigate and view the Web. *Providing fundamental information will make exploring the Web less intimidating.*

■ Encourage the patient to locate established Internet sites for health information. For more information on specific sites, recommend that the patient read reference books such as *Dr. Tom Linden's Guide to Online Medicine,* published by McGraw-Hill Book Co. *Reference publications will help the patient gain general knowledge about the Web and specific sites and help him find the information he wants.*

■ Help the patient find general health information on the Internet. Recommended sites include:

– Centers for Disease Control and Prevention *(www.cdc.gov)*
– Health and Medicine in the News, which provides information on medical advances reported in media *(www.biomed.lib.umn.edu)*
– Healthfinder, which provides consumer health and human services information *(www.healthfinder.gov)*
– Medical Matrix, which provides general medical information *(www.medmatrix.org)*
– National Institutes of Health (NIH) Information Center, which provides links to NIH Consumer Health Information, a list of online consumer health resources *(www.nih.gov/)*
– Nursing World, sponsored by the American Nurses Association, provides general nursing information *(www.nursingworld.org)*
– United States Department of Health and Human Services *(www.os.dhhs.gov)*
– The Virtual Hospital *(www.vh.org).*

The Internet has a huge volume of information available. Pointing the patient to specific sites will make the experience of using the Web more efficient and productive.

■ Help the patient locate Internet sites appropriate for his specific needs. Examples of useful sites are listed below:

– AIDS information from HIVnet Information Server *(www.ahrq.gov/data/hivnet.htm)*
– Cancer information from National Cancer Institute *(www.cancer.gov)*
– OncoLink *(www.oncolink.upenn.edu)*

– Information from Alcoholics Anonymous *(www.alcoholics-anonymous.org)*
– Information on diabetes mellitus *(www.diabetes.com)*
– Information on multiple sclerosis *(www.nationalmssociety.org)*
– Information on spinal cord injury from Cure Paralysis Now
(www.cureparalysisnow.org)
These Internet sites may provide relevant information and support for patients and families.

■ Help patient evaluate health information obtained from the Internet *to achieve maximum benefit from the Internet and minimize potential harm.* Emphasize that information found on the Internet isn't always reliable. Information may be reported inaccurately, findings may not be based on valid research methods, or information may be out of date. Patient may want to find the original source of information, verify accuracy, or verify credentials of the organization sponsoring the site.

■ If the patient gains new insight on his own condition or treatment, encourage him to share this information with his primary health care practitioner *to foster a sense of responsibility for obtaining health care.* Suggest patient provide practitioner with a summary of his findings in advance of his appointment to allow the practitioner time to evaluate the information *to promote responsiveness to suggestions.*

Suggested NIC interventions
Health Education; Health System Guidance; Self-Awareness Enhancement; Self-Modification Assistance

Evaluations for expected outcomes
■ Patient reports that he can locate sites on the Internet with health care information.
■ Patient identifies Internet sites for information on specific health-related topics.
■ Patient evaluates information obtained from the Internet for reliability and accuracy.
■ Patient shares relevant information with health care practitioner.

Documentation
■ Patient's expression of desire to find more information about health-related issues
■ Instructions provided and patient's understanding of instructions
■ Internet sites located and information obtained
■ Evaluations for expected outcomes

Reference
Chaffin, A. J., and Maddux, C. D. "Accessibility Accommodations for Older Adults Seeking E-Health Information," *Journal of Gerontological Nursing* 33(3):6-12, March 2007.

HEALTH-SEEKING BEHAVIORS

related to smoking as a risk factor for coronary artery disease

Definition
Active seeking (by a person in stable health) of ways to alter personal health habits or the environment in order to move toward a higher level of health

Assessment
- Risk factor analysis, including age, sex, cholesterol level, ratio of high-density lipoprotein to low-density lipoprotein, blood pressure, weight, level of exercise, history of smoking, and stressors
- Current health status
- Psychosocial status, including lifestyle and motivation
- Recognition and realization of potential growth, health, and autonomy
- Understanding of risk modification

Defining characteristics
- Expressed or observed desire to seek a higher level of wellness
- Demonstrated or observed lack of knowledge about health promotion behaviors
- Reported or observed unfamiliarity with wellness community resources
- Expressed concern about current environmental conditions on health status
- Expressed or observed desire for increased control of health practices

Expected outcomes
- Patient will state need to stop or decrease smoking.
- Patient will state hazards of smoking and how it affects body.
- Patient will understand ways to stop or decrease smoking.
- Patient will choose which smoking cessation alternative to implement.
- Patient will stop smoking or enter a program to stop smoking.
- Patient won't develop illness, or signs and symptoms of disease will be controlled.

Suggested NOC outcomes
Adherence Behavior; Health Beliefs; Health Orientation; Health Promoting Behavior; Knowledge: Health Promotion; Quality of Life; Risk Control: Tobacco Use

Interventions and rationales
- Determine patient's ability and motivation to promote a higher level of wellness. *Patient can't be forced to change; he must have inherent desire.*
- Discuss with patient hazards of smoking *to emphasize nicotine's long-term detriment to body.* Support behavior change.
- Assess patient's understanding of how smoking affects body (blood pressure, cholesterol, clotting, and heart rate). Clarify any misconceptions. *This reinforces patient's desire to change behavior.*

- Emphasize benefits of stopping smoking *to reinforce behavior changes.*
- Review with patient past methods used to decrease or stop smoking (successful or not) *to discover most effective methods for patient.*
- Suggest ways for patient to decrease or stop smoking:
– List reasons to stop.
– Set dates to stop.
– Get support.
– Cut down on number smoked.
– Perform alternative activities.
– Ask physician about pharmacologic interventions such as nicotine patch.
These suggestions provide patient with practical measures he can implement.
- Provide literature on smoking cessation *to reinforce teaching and provide easy reference after discharge.*
- Discuss resources *available to support patient's attempts to stop smoking after discharge.*

Suggested NIC interventions

Behavior Modification; Coping Enhancement; Decision-Making Support; Health Education; Health Screening; Self-Responsibility Facilitation; Values Clarification

Evaluations for expected outcomes

- Patient voices desire to stop or decrease smoking.
- Patient lists several hazards associated with smoking.
- Patient lists several options for assistance with efforts to stop smoking (such as self-help group, smoking cessation class, and hypnosis).
- Patient chooses method to stop smoking and signs a self-contract (including rewards for smoking cessation) to commit to program.
- Patient implements chosen option to stop smoking.
- Patient is free from signs and symptoms of disorders associated with smoking.

Documentation

- Patient's expression of concern about promoting a higher level of wellness
- Patient's response to nursing interventions
- Instructions provided and patient's understanding of instructions
- Referrals made to smoking cessation programs available in hospital and community
- Evaluations for expected outcomes

References

Rempher, K.J. "Cardiovascular Sequelae of Tobacco Smoking," *Critical Care Nursing Clinics of North America* 18(1):13-20, March 2006.

Wynd, C.A. "Guided Health Imagery for Smoking Cessation and Long-term Abstinence," *Journal of Nursing Scholarship* 37(3):245-50, 2005.

HEALTH-SEEKING BEHAVIORS

related to stress as a risk factor for coronary artery disease

Definition

Active seeking (by a person in stable health) of ways to alter personal health habits or the environment in order to move toward a higher level of health

Assessment

■ Risk factor analysis, including age, sex, cholesterol level, ratio of high-density lipoprotein to low-density lipoprotein, blood pressure, weight, level of exercise, history of smoking, and stressors
■ Current health status
■ Psychosocial status, including lifestyle and motivation
■ Recognition and realization of potential growth, health, and autonomy
■ Understanding of risk modification

Defining characteristics

■ Expressed or observed desire to seek a higher level of wellness
■ Demonstrated or observed lack of knowledge about health promotion behaviors
■ Reported or observed unfamiliarity with wellness community resources
■ Expressed concern about current environmental conditions on health status
■ Expressed or observed desire for increased control of health practices

Expected outcomes

■ Patient will state that stress is a risk factor for coronary artery disease.
■ Patient will identify and list factors that create stress in life.
■ Patient will voice understanding of how stress affects body.
■ Patient will state ways to maximize positive aspects and minimize negative aspects of stress.

Suggested NOC outcomes

Adherence Behavior; Health Beliefs; Health Orientation; Health Promoting Behavior

Interventions and rationales

■ Inform patient that stress is a risk factor for many major health problems, including coronary artery disease. *Patient may not know that stress can contribute to disease and death.*
■ Review stressors in patient's personal and professional life and mechanisms used to cope with them. *This increases patient's awareness of stressors and provides baseline for stress management tools.*
■ Discuss how stress affects patient's body and how decreasing stress changes these effects. *This encourages patient to manage stress as a way to improve quality of life.*

■ Discuss difference between type A and type B personalities. *Type A and B behaviors define personality type and provide framework for dealing with stress.*
■ Discuss with patient stress management techniques, including:
– perceiving situation differently
– managing time
– taking a mental health day or evening periodically
– practicing relaxation techniques
– being assertive when faced with unreasonable demands
– improving self-image and self-esteem
– exercising
– facing problems and discussing alternatives with family or friends
– setting realistic goals
– relaxing standards of living.
These measures provide tools to manage stress.
■ Review available community resources for stress management and provide literature *to reinforce teaching after discharge.*

Suggested NIC interventions
Coping Enhancement; Counseling; Decision-Making Support; Health Education; Health System Guidance; Referral; Risk Identification; Simple Relaxation Therapy; Socialization Enhancement

Evaluations for expected outcomes
■ Patient states that stress contributes to coronary artery disease.
■ Patient identifies habits and situations that create stress.
■ Patient identifies physiologic responses to stress.
■ Patient states methods to minimize harmful stressors and ways to cope better with daily stress.

Documentation
■ Patient's expression of concern about promoting a higher level of wellness
■ Patient's response to nursing interventions
■ Instructions provided and patient's understanding of instructions
■ Referrals made and literature provided about stress management courses available in community
■ Evaluations for expected outcomes

Reference
Paquet, M., et al. "Re-engineering Cardiac Rehabilitation Programmes: Considering the Patient's Point of View," *Journal of Advanced Nursing* 51(6):567-76, September 2005.

Readiness for enhanced
HOPE

Definition
A pattern of expectations and desires that's sufficient for mobilizing energy on one's own behalf and that can be strengthened

Assessment
- Patient's perception of ability to set personal goals
- Patient's expression of desire to build on possibilities for the future
- Patient's ability to align desires and expectations
- Patient's expression of hope regarding health situation
- Patient's desire to maintain and enhance relationships with others
- Patient's problem-solving approach to health situation
- Patient's expressed need for increased spiritual connection

Defining characteristics
- Expresses desire to enhance ability to set achievable goals
- Expresses desire to enhance belief in possibilities
- Expresses desire to enhance congruency of expectations with desires
- Expresses desire to enhance hope
- Expresses desire to enhance interconnectedness with others
- Expresses desire to enhance problem solving to meet goals
- Expresses desire to enhance sense of meaning to life
- Expresses desire to enhance spirituality

Expected outcomes
- Patient will express desire for positive health outcomes.
- Patient will share personal goals to increase autonomy and personal satisfaction.
- Patient will discuss measures to increase quality of life.
- Patient will develop plan to promote maximal physical, mental, social, and psychological abilities.
- Patient will share strategies to live a meaningful life.
- Patient will express awareness of the need for developing and maintaining a positive attitude of hope.
- Patient will state plan for own role enhancement.
- Patient will share need for emotional support.
- Patient will maintain a sense of humor and positive sense of self.
- Patient will seek spiritual support as needed.

Suggested NOC outcomes
Hope; Personal Well-Being; Quality of Life; Will to Live

Interventions and rationales

- Assist patient in adapting to disability *to promote acceptance and understanding of physical condition, thereby improving management of therapeutic regimen.*
- Assess patient's adaptation to current health status; *baseline assessment is needed to develop care plan.*
- Implement a plan to build on patient's optimal role performance; *establishing a plan with the patient promotes clear mutual expectations.*
- Facilitate opportunities for spiritual nourishment and growth *to address patient's holistic needs for maximal therapeutic environment.*
- Assist patient to build and maintain meaningful interpersonal relationships *to maintain highest level of well-being.*

Suggested NIC interventions

Hope Instillation; Self-Esteem Enhancement; Spiritual Growth Facilitation

Evaluation for expected outcomes

- Patient expresses desire for positive health outcomes.
- Patient shares personal goals to increase autonomy and personal satisfaction.
- Patient discusses measures utilized to increase quality of life.
- Patient develops a plan to promote maximal physical, mental, social, and psychological abilities.
- Patient shares his strategies for living a meaningful life.
- Patient demonstrates awareness of the need for developing and maintaining a positive attitude of hope.
- Patient states plan for own role enhancement.
- Patient shares the need for emotional support.
- Patient maintains a sense of humor and positive sense of self.
- Patient seeks spiritual support as needed.

Documentation

- Patient's assessment of situation and hopeful resolution of problems
- Community resources to support patient's positive outcomes
- Future plans to maximize patient's preferred outcomes
- Evaluation for expected outcomes

References

Davidson, P.M., et al. "Maintaining Hope in Transition: A Theoretical Framework to Guide Interventions for People with Heart Failure," *Journal of Cardiovascular Nursing* 22(1):58-64, January-February 2007.

Evans, W.G., et al. "Communication at Times of Transitions: How to Help Patients Cope with Loss and Redefine Hope," *Cancer Journal* 12(5):417-24, September-October 2006.

Readiness for enhanced
IMMUNIZATION STATUS

Definition

A pattern of conforming to local, national, and/or international standards of immunization to prevent infectious diseases that's sufficient to protect a person, family, or community and that can be strengthened

Assessment

- Patient's perception of the need for the prevention of infectious diseases
- Patient's responsibility for controlling the spread of communicable disease
- Patient's attitude toward health-seeking behavior that leads to immunization
- Patient's knowledge of infection control through immunization for communicable disease

Defining characteristics

- Expresses desire to enhance behavior to prevent infectious disease
- Expresses desire to enhance identification of possible problems associated with immunizations
- Expresses desire to enhance identification of providers of immunizations
- Expresses desire to enhance immunization status
- Expresses desire to enhance knowledge of immunization standards
- Expresses desire to enhance record keeping of immunizations

Expected outcomes

- Patient will express knowledge of health-seeking behavior necessary to participate in immunization.
- Patient will demonstrate adherence behavior to standard recommended immunization protocols.
- Patient will develop an ongoing plan for maintaining records of immunizations.

Suggested NOC outcomes

Community Health Status: Immunity; Community Risk Control: Communicable Disease; Immunization Behavior; Knowledge: Infection Control

Interventions and rationales

- Assess patient's participation in standard immunization protocol *to determine patient protection from communicable disease.*
- Help patient to understand possible risks associated with immunizations *to assist patient to identify reportable risks and complications resulting from immunizations.*
- Implement a mechanism or device for record keeping of immunizations *to prevent gaps and overlaps in patient immunizations.*

Suggested NIC interventions
Communicable Disease Management; Immunization/Vaccination Management; Infection Control

Evaluation for expected outcomes
■ Patient expresses awareness of risk reduction provided by getting immunizations.
■ Patient expresses need for immunization schedule to protect against communicable disease.
■ Patient reports any problems associated with immunizations.
■ Patient maintains up-to-date immunization records.

Documentation
■ Patient's understanding of the need for immunizations
■ Patient's compliance with immunization schedule
■ Community resources for obtaining immunizations
■ Evaluation for expected outcomes

Reference
Wiggs-Stayner, K.S., et al. "The Impact of Mass School Immunization on School Attendance," *Journal of School Nursing* 22(4):219-22, August 2006.

Readiness for enhanced
KNOWLEDGE

Definition
Presence or acquisition of cognitive information related to a specific topic that's sufficient for meeting health-related goals and that can be strengthened

Assessment
■ Age and gender
■ Developmental state
■ Mental status
■ Health problems, restrictions, and limitations
■ Roles in family and community
■ Socioeconomic factors
■ Cultural background

Defining characteristics
■ Expresses an interest in learning
■ Explains knowledge of topic
■ Behaves congruent with expressed knowledge
■ Describes previous experience related to topic

Expected outcomes
■ Patient will identify new sources for enhancing knowledge in the topic of interest.
■ Patient will make use of all relevant resources to enhance knowledge.
■ Patient will ask questions where new information needs clarification.
■ Patient will begin practicing new behaviors gleaned from enhanced knowledge.

Suggested NOC outcomes
Knowledge: Health Promotion

Interventions and rationales
■ Determine exactly what patient knows and to what level he wishes to and can enhance knowledge and understanding. *This information will assist the nurse in planning with patient.*
■ Provide books and videos that will help patient's quest for enhanced knowledge. *Supplying some materials directly may motivate him to want to search further.*
■ Direct patient to use other sources for information, such as libraries, Internet, or professional organizations. *An independent search results in patient developing confidence in his ability to go much deeper into the area of interest.*
■ Be available to answer questions and correct misconceptions for patient *in order to enhance the effectiveness of what he's learning.*
■ Provide feedback to patient for incorporating new knowledge into lifestyle. *This reinforces behaviors resulting from enhanced knowledge.*

Suggested NIC interventions
Learning Facilitation; Learning Readiness Enhancement

Evaluations for expected outcomes
■ Patient expresses motivation for enhanced knowledge.
■ Patient uses various resources to achieve success.
■ Patient questions things that aren't clearly understood.
■ Patient practices skills derived from enhanced knowledge.

Documentation
■ Patient's current level of knowledge and skill
■ Patient's expressions of motivation to enhance knowledge
■ Resources used to enhance knowledge
■ Patient's response to learning resources
■ Evaluations for expected outcomes

Reference
Eldh, A.C., et al. "Conditions for Patient Participation and Non-participation in Health Care," *Nursing Ethics* 13(5):503-14, September 2006.

Readiness for enhanced
POWER

Definition
A pattern of participating knowingly in change that's sufficient for well-being and that can be strengthened.

Assessment
- Patient's perception of present state of power
- Patient's perception of ability to enhance power
- Support systems, including family members, friends, clergy
- Patient's ability to identify choices
- Patient's readiness for change to occur
- Relience on health care system to resolve complaints or assume power

Defining characteristics
- Expresses readiness to enhance awareness of possible changes to be made
- Expresses readiness to enhance freedom to perform actions for change
- Expresses readiness to enhance identification of choices that can be made for change
- Expresses readiness to enhance involvement in creating change
- Expresses readiness to enhance knowledge for participation in change
- Expresses readiness to enhance participation in choices for daily living and health
- Expresses readiness to enhance power

Expected outcomes
- Patient will express perceived control in influencing health outcomes.
- Patient will participate in choices that enhance his care and well-being.
- Patient will develop a plan for adjusting to significant life changes.

Suggested NOC outcomes
Family Resiliency; Health Beliefs: Perceived Control; Personal Autonomy; Psychosocial Adjustment: Life Change

Interventions and rationales
- Assess patient's understanding of need for changes to improve well-being; *knowledge increases power in independent decisions for change.*
- Assess patient's participation in choices to be made *to enhance care and well-being.*
- Assist patient in acquiring knowledge necessary for positive decision making. *Making positive decisions that produce benefits will reinforce health seeking behaviors.*

■ Help patient to involve family, community, clergy, and friends with changes to the care plan *to increase patient's perceived control to affect maximal self-care outcomes.*

Suggested NIC interventions

Assertiveness Training; Coping Enhancement; Self-Modification Assistance; Self-Responsibility Facilitation

Evaluation for expected outcomes

■ Patient expresses understanding of the need for changes to improve well-being.
■ Patient participates in choices that enhance his care and well-being.
■ Patient develops a plan for adjusting to significant life changes.

Documentation

■ Patient's understanding of needed changes for his care and well-being
■ Patient's choices that enhance his care and well-being
■ Patient's knowledge to make ongoing changes to his care and well-being
■ Evaluations for expected outcomes

Reference

Klam, J., et al. "Personal Empowerment Program: Addressing Health Concerns in People with Schizophrenia," *Journal of Psychosocial Nursing and Mental Health Services* 44(8):20-28, August 2006.

Readiness for enhanced
SELF-CARE

Definition

A pattern of performing activities for oneself that helps to meet health-related goals and that can be strengthened

Assessment

■ Patient's perception of adequacy of self-care
■ Family responsibilities assumed in caring for patient
■ Patient's attitude toward use of health care services
■ Patient's use of family, friends, and clergy support systems
■ Health history, including self-care abilities, disabilities, or deformities
■ Patient's reliance on community for health and welfare support

Defining characteristics

■ Expresses desire to enhance independence in maintaining life
■ Expresses desire to enhance independence in maintaining health
■ Expresses desire to enhance independence in maintaining personal development

■ Expresses desire to enhance independence in maintaining well-being
■ Expresses desire to enhance knowledge of responsibility and strategies for self-care

Expected outcomes

■ Patient will demonstrate positive decision making toward maximizing potential for self-care.
■ Patient will express satisfaction with independence in assuming responsibility for planning self-care
■ Patient will involve staff, family, and community in developing strategies for self-care.

Suggested NOC outcomes

Adherence Behavior; Client Satisfaction: Functional Assistance; Discharge Readiness: Independent Living; Health Beliefs: Perceived Ability to Perform

Interventions and rationales

■ Assess patient's satisfaction with level of self-care *in order to support general well-being.*
■ Assist patient to develop plan to promote autonomous decision making *to increase patient's responsibility for facilitating care.*
■ Support patient's implementation of a program to sustain health-seeking behavior *to promote patient autonomy in self-care.*
■ Promote health team, family, and community efforts to participate in patient's self-care initiatives *to promote satisfactory mutual goal setting and group efforts.*
■ Encourage patient and his family to participate in support networks that promote patient independence, where possible, *to promote patient and family resilience.*
■ Develop a referral list for community resources *to promote patient's enhanced self-care.*

Suggested NIC interventions

Mutual Goal Setting; Resiliency Promotion; Self-Responsibility Facilitation

Evaluations for expected outcomes

■ Patient expresses awareness of his need to maintain independence in health management.
■ Patient develops and maintains a plan for enhanced self-care.
■ Patient involves staff, family, and community in developing strategies for self-care.

Documentation

■ Patient's perception of readiness for enhancing self-care
■ Family, friends, community, and clergy resources available to promote patient's independence

■ Future plans to maintain and enhance independence in self-care
■ Evaluations for expected outcomes

Reference

Moser, A., et al. "Patient Autonomy in Nurse-Led Shared Care: A Review of Theoretical and Empirical Literature," *Journal of Advanced Nursing* 57(4):357-65, February 2007.

Readiness for enhanced
SELF-CONCEPT

Definition

A pattern of perceptions or ideas about self that's sufficient for well-being and that can be enhanced

Assessment

■ Age
■ Gender
■ Developmental stage
■ Health problems
■ Past experience with health care system
■ Mental status
■ Belief system (norms, values, religion)
■ Social interaction patterns
■ Family system
■ Perception of self (past and present), including body image, coping mechanisms, problem-solving ability, and self-worth

Defining characteristics

■ Accepts strengths and limitations
■ Actions are congruent with expressed feelings and thoughts
■ Expresses confidence in abilities
■ Expresses satisfaction with thoughts about self, sense of worthiness, role performance, body image, and personal identity
■ Expresses willingness to enhance self-concept

Expected outcomes

■ Patient will articulate long- and short-term goals.
■ Patient will express motivation necessary to achieve goals.
■ Patient will develop realistic plan to achieve stated goals.
■ Patient will practice self-management strategies needed to be successful.
■ Patient will evaluate progress and modify behavior as needed.

Suggested NOC outcomes

Body Image; Neglect Recovery; Personal Autonomy; Self-Esteem

Interventions and rationales

■ Provide patient with materials and resources on health-related issues that affect this individual's attitude. *Knowledge will enhance or inhibit patient's motivation or resolve.*

■ Answer questions related to written material *so patient is adequately prepared to establish realistic goals.*

■ Assist patient in writing long- and short-term goals. *These goals can serve as tools for self-evaluation as new behaviors are being practiced.*

■ Have patient list one or two realistic, practical behaviors that will facilitate achieving goals. *The more positive his behaviors are, the greater the chance patient has of being successful.*

■ Assist patient to determine positive rewards for successful behavior changes. *Reinforcers are needed for new behavior to continue.*

Suggested NIC interventions

Hope Instillation; Self-Awareness Enhancement; Self-Responsibility Facilitation

Evaluations for expected outcomes

■ Patient has realistic goals and workable plan for change.
■ Patient responds positively to changes in self-concept.
■ Patient demonstrates interest in evaluating progress.
■ Patient shows a willingness to modify plan to continue reaching goals.

Documentation

■ Patient's expressions of self-concept
■ Patient's adherence to plan
■ Modifications to plan
■ Patient's response to nursing interventions
■ Evaluations for expected outcomes

Reference

Schulman-Green, D.J., et al. "Goal Setting as a Shared Decision Making Strategy Among Clinicians and Their Older Patients," *Patient Education and Counseling* 63(1-2):145-51, October 2006.

Readiness for enhanced
SLEEP

Definition
A pattern of natural, periodic suspension of consciousness that provides adequate rest, sustains a desired lifestyle, and can be strengthened

Assessment
■ Age
■ Daytime activity and work patterns
■ Cognitive status
■ Possible precipitating factors
■ Daytime consequences of sleeplessness
■ Underlying conditions or medications
■ Situational daily stressors
■ Overall quality and duration of sleep
■ Sleep environment
■ Exposure to bright lights, exercise, and social interaction
■ Recent changes in health status or lifestyle
■ Dietary and drug history, including ingestion of caffeine or other stimulants, nicotine, alcohol, sedatives, hypnotics, and fluid intake

Defining characteristics
■ Amount of sleep and rapid-eye-movement (REM) sleep congruent with developmental needs
■ Feeling of being rested after sleep
■ Occasional or infrequent use of medications to induce sleep
■ Sleep routines that promote sleep habits
■ Use of sleep-disrupting drugs
■ Willingness to enhance sleep

Expected outcomes
■ Patient will identify factors that enhance readiness for sleep.
■ Patient will demonstrate readiness for enhanced sleep through the use of appropriate sleep hygiene measures.
■ Patient's amount of sleep and REM sleep will be congruent with developmental needs.
■ Patient will express feeling rested after sleep.
■ Institutional policies and staff behaviors will reflect measures to enhance readiness for sleep.

Suggested NOC outcomes
Anxiety Level; Rest; Sleep

Interventions and rationales

■ Ask patient to keep a log of sleep and wake times, number of awakenings, total time asleep, quality of sleep, and any precipitating factors that may influence sleep *to determine sleep efficiency.*

■ Educate patient about normal age-related changes to sleep and strategies to improve sleep that are specific to patient's health status, lifestyle, and environment *to decrease anxiety about sleeplessness.*

■ Make a behavior modification plan based upon the assessment of condition, patient history, and precipitating factors *to enhance compliance.*

■ Provide education about sleep *to dispel myths about sleep requirements and faulty strategies.*

■ Increase exposure to light, exercise, and social interaction as synchronizers *to help rematch the circadian rhythms with normal day and night cycles.*

■ Provide an environment conducive to relaxation, including low level of stimuli, dimmed lights, silence, and comfortable furniture, *to maximize sleep response.*

■ Develop interventions within the facility that address quality sleep; for example, scheduling procedures and care activities *to avoid unnecessary awakenings;* modifying environmental factors *to promote a quiet, warm, relaxed sleep setting;* addressing lifestyle changes, such as having a roommate and the unfamiliarity of relocation; and orienting older adults to facility's setting *to enhance the ability to sleep.*

■ Implement environment strategies that cause people to lower their voices and thereby reduce noise; for example, closing patient's door, placing phones on low volume, speaking at lower volumes, and dimming lights *to reduce extraneous sounds.*

■ Instruct the patient to avoid dietary substances and drugs that may influence sleep, including ingestion of caffeine or other stimulants, nicotine, alcohol, sedatives, hypnotics, and fluid intake *to enhance the ability to sleep.*

■ Provide warm, light snacks containing protein at bedtime and small amounts of liquids *to promote a sense of comfort.*

■ Provide a cup of water close to the bed *to avoid a dry mouth and facilitate returning to sleep after awakening.*

■ Advise the patient to avoid strenuous exercise at least 2 hours before bedtime *to enhance the ability to sleep.*

■ Teach the patient to relax before going to bed with reading, music, meditation, or other comforting and soothing activity *to enhance the ability to sleep.*

■ Educate the patient about sleep hygiene measures: to use the bedroom and bed only for sleep (or sexual activity), and to avoid other activities in the bedroom, such as watching television, reading, and eating, *to enhance the ability to sleep.*

Suggested NIC interventions

Environmental Management; Environmental Management: Comfort; Progressive Muscle Relaxation; Sleep Enhancement

Evaluations for expected outcomes

■ Patient identifies factors that enhance readiness for sleep.

■ Patient demonstrates readiness for enhanced sleep through the use of appropriate sleep hygiene measures.

■ Patient's amount of sleep and REM sleep is congruent with developmental needs.
■ Patient expresses feeling rested after sleep.
■ Institutional policies and staff behaviors reflect measures to enhance readiness for sleep.

Documentation
■ Patient's sleep history
■ Patient's plan for behavioral modification
■ Observations of sleep hygiene behaviors
■ Nursing interventions to enhance sleep readiness
■ Patient's response to nursing interventions
■ Evaluations for expected outcomes

Reference
Page, M.S., et al. "Putting Evidence into Practice: Evidence-based Interventions for Sleep-Wake Disturbances," *Clinical Journal of Oncology Nursing* 10(6):753-67, December 2006.

Readiness for enhanced
SPIRITUAL WELL-BEING

Definition
Process of developing the inner self by interconnecting physical, psychological, and spiritual strengths

Assessment
■ Spiritual status, including personal religious habits, religious or church affiliation, embarrassment at practicing religious rituals, and opposition to beliefs by family, peers, and health care providers
■ Health history, including medical conditions that change body image, chronic or terminal illness, and debilitating disease
■ Psychological status, including reactions to illness and disability; change in appetite, energy level, motivation, personal hygiene, self-image, sleep, and sex drive; alcohol or drug abuse; moodiness; recent divorce, job loss, or losses through separation or death; personality traits; and relationships with peers
■ Self-care status, including neurologic, musculoskeletal, sensory, or psychological impairment and ability to carry out activities and adapt
■ Family status, including marital status and communication patterns
■ Nutritional status, including malabsorption or nutritional deficiencies, obesity, anorexia, bulimia, weight loss or gain, nausea, vomiting, fainting, constipation, diarrhea, pallor, irritability, cravings, food hoarding, and alteration in such personal habits as exercise, drug and alcohol use, and use of laxatives

■ Sleep pattern status, including hours of sleep, energy level before and after sleep, difficulty falling asleep, nocturnal awakening, early morning awakening, hypersomnia, insomnia, and sleep pattern reversal

Defining characteristics

■ Harmonious interconnectedness (harmony and connection with self, others, higher power, and environment)
■ Inner strengths, such as inner core, transcendence, self-consciousness, and sense of awareness
■ Sense of unfolding mystery
■ Displays creative energy
■ Sings, listens to music
■ Reads spiritual literature
■ Spends time outdoors
■ Prays
■ Participates in religious activities

Expected outcomes

■ Patient will discuss spiritual conflicts.
■ Patient will have opportunity to meet with chosen religious figure.
■ Patient will receive support in his efforts to pursue enhanced spiritual well-being.
■ Patient will pursue religious or spiritual practices to the extent he feels comfortable.
■ Patient will openly discuss effects of illness on his beliefs and other spiritual issues.
■ Patient will describe plan to continue to enhance spiritual well-being.
■ Patient will receive referrals for continued support.

Suggested NOC outcomes

Hope; Quality of Life; Spiritual Health

Interventions and rationales

■ Monitor for potential signs of spiritual distress that might harm the patient's well-being (altered self-care, sleep pattern disturbance, and change in exercise and eating habits) *to plan appropriate interventions.*
■ Assess the significance of spirituality in the patient's life and his ability to cope with illness. Note whether the patient participates in religious rituals, observes religious practices (prayer, meditation, and dietary restrictions), or wishes to discuss spiritual beliefs. Keep an open view of what constitutes spirituality. *Before you can intervene in spiritual matters, you must determine the significance of spirituality for the patient.*
■ Ask the patient whether his illness has affected his spiritual outlook, and tell him you're willing to help him address spiritual issues if he wishes *to reduce isolation and help bring issues related to spiritual distress out into the open.*
■ Ask the patient whether he wishes to discuss spiritual concerns with a religious figure *to allow access to expert spiritual care resources.*

■ Encourage the patient to pursue spiritual questions. Reassure him that spiritual concerns are valid and that by strengthening his spirituality, he can enhance his overall well-being *to demonstrate acceptance.*

■ Provide the patient with resources for coping with spiritual distress (referrals to religious or spiritual organizations and books on prayer and meditation) *to enhance his opportunity to attend to spiritual needs.* Make sure he receives materials appropriate to his religious affiliation and spiritual beliefs *to demonstrate respect for his beliefs and values.* If you lack knowledge about the patient's beliefs and practices, consult a religious figure *to best meet the patient's needs.*

■ Help the patient arrange travel to a place selected for prayer, reflection, or contemplation. Use such resources as church-affiliated vans or volunteer escorts *to enhance the patient's contact with outside sources of support.*

■ Demonstrate to the patient that you're willing to discuss issues related to spirituality, such as the patient's view of God, how illness has affected his religious beliefs, and how hospital stays affect his spiritual practices *to bring spiritual issues into the open.* Keep an open mind when listening. Keep conversation focused on the patient's spiritual values and the role they play in recovering from illness and coping with changes in body image *to ensure that interaction between you and the patient remains therapeutic.*

■ Discuss with the patient the importance of maintaining a healthful diet, getting regular exercise and sleep, and maintaining healthy interaction with family and friends. *A patient in spiritual distress may neglect his day-to-day well-being.*

■ Praise the patient for taking time to attend to his spiritual needs, and encourage him to continue to develop his spirituality after he leaves the facility *to provide continued encouragement.*

■ Provide the patient with referrals to appropriate religious groups, spiritually centered organizations, and social service organizations. Consider such resources as parish nurses, home-visiting services, and computer networks *to help provide a continued opportunity for spiritual development and to ensure continuity of care.*

Suggested NIC interventions
Coping Enhancement; Self-Awareness Enhancement; Spiritual Growth Facilitation; Spiritual Support; Values Clarification

Evaluations for expected outcomes
■ Patient discusses spiritual conflicts.
■ Patient has opportunity to meet with chosen religious figure.
■ Patient recognizes and expresses support he has received in his efforts to pursue enhanced spiritual well-being.
■ Patient pursues religious or spiritual practices to extent he feels comfortable.
■ Patient discusses effects of illness on his beliefs and other spiritual issues openly.
■ Patient describes plan to continue to enhance spiritual well-being.
■ Patient identifies religious resources offered outside facility or agency.

Documentation
■ Statements about spiritual conflicts
■ Visits with religious representative

- Engagement in religious or spiritual practices
- Religious resources suggested outside facility or agency
- Statements about ability to cope with changes in body image as a result of illness, to maintain spiritual values in the face of long-term or chronic illness, and to pursue spiritual practices during hospital stays
- Eating patterns, exercise schedules, and sleep patterns
- Stated plans to continue to enhance spiritual well-being
- Evaluations for expected outcomes

Reference

Baldacchino, D.R. "Nursing Competencies for Spiritual Care," *Journal of Clinical Nursing* 15(7):885-96, July 2006.

Readiness for enhanced
THERAPEUTIC REGIMEN MANAGEMENT

Definition

A pattern of regulating and integrating into daily living programs for treatment of illness and its sequelae that's sufficient for meeting health-related goals and that can be strengthened

Assessment

- Cultural status, including age, gender, level of education, occupation, race, ethnic group, beliefs, values, and attitudes about health and illness
- Family status, including marital status, family composition and developmental stage, adaptability, family need, and coping patterns
- Psychological status, including changes in appetite, behavior, energy level, mood, motivation, self-image, sleep, alcohol and drug use, life changes, psychiatric history, and blood and urine toxicology
- Self-care status, including ability to carry out voluntary activities, use of adaptive devices, and neurologic, sensory, or psychological impairment
- Social status, including communication skills, size of social network, quality of relationships, degree of trust in others, and ability to function in social and occupational roles
- Spiritual status, including religious or church affiliation; current perception of faith and religious practices; perceptions about life, death, and suffering; and support network (family, clergy, friends)

Defining characteristics

- Appropriate choices of daily living for meeting goals of treatment or prevention
- Expressed desire to manage treatment of illness and prevention of sequelae
- Little to no difficulty expressed with regulation and integration of one or more prescribed regimens for treatment of illness or prevention of complications
- No unexpected acceleration of illness symptoms
- Reduction of risk factors for progression of illness and sequelae

Expected outcomes

- Patient will be able to articulate strengths and competencies in managing therapeutic regimen.
- Patient will set goals related to enhancement of therapeutic regimen.
- Patient will develop plan to maximize behaviors directed at enhancing therapeutic regimen and preventing sequelae.
- Patient will identify types of support needed to enhance health behaviors.

Suggested NOC outcomes

Knowledge: Treatment Regimen; Symptom Control; Treatment Behavior: Illness or Injury

Interventions and rationales

- Review assessment data with the patient in order *to validate understanding of the current regimen.*
- Assist the patient with setting goals and developing a plan *to provide concrete direction to the patient's desire to enhance the therapeutic regimen.*
- Provide suggestions to the patient for sources of support that will help reinforce enhanced behaviors (support group, classes, periodicals) *to broaden ideas the patient may already have in order to reinforce positive behaviors.*
- Provide feedback *to recognize patient's success in meeting new goals.*

Suggested NIC interventions

Decision-Making Support; Support System Enhancement

Evaluations for expected outcomes

- Patient successfully prevents sequelae in managing therapeutic regimen.
- Patient expresses determination to meet the goals.
- Patient adheres (over time) to plan and modifies it as needed.
- Patient uses a variety of support systems available to him.

Documentation

- Patient's description of skills, competencies, and barriers to success in managing therapeutic regimen
- Patient's progress toward meeting stated goals
- Response to nursing interventions
- Evaluations for expected outcomes

Reference

Schulman-Green, et al. "Goal Setting as a Shared Decision Making Strategy Among Clinicians and Their Older Patients," *Patient Education and Counseling* 63(1-2):145-51, October 2006.

Liver Dysfunction

Monitor:
- Liver function tests (ALT/AST/GGT/Bili): increase with impaired liver function
- Platelet count: increase c̄ impaired liver function
- PT/INR: increase c̄ impaired liver function
- albumin: decrease c̄ impaired liver function

Report changes in laboratory data to physician immediately.
Report onset of jaundice to physician immediately
Report changes in patient status as appropriate
  - onset or increase in bleeding gums
  - increased bleeding time c̄ everyday cuts/scrapes
  - increased fatigue

Selected nursing diagnoses by medical diagnosis

Abnormal rupture of membranes
- Deficient fluid volume
- Hyperthermia
- Risk for infection

Abortion
- Complicated grieving
- Ineffective tissue perfusion (specify)
- Moral distress
- Risk for complicated grieving
- Situational low self-esteem

Abruptio placentae
- Acute pain
- Anxiety
- Complicated grieving
- Ineffective tissue perfusion
- Readiness for enhanced hope

Acoustic neuroma
- Chronic pain
- Disturbed sensory perception (auditory)
- Imbalanced nutrition: Less than body requirements
- Impaired skin integrity
- Ineffective breathing pattern
- Ineffective tissue perfusion (cerebral)
- Insomnia
- Risk for deficient fluid volume

Acquired immunodeficiency syndrome
- Caregiver role strain
- Chronic confusion
- Death anxiety
- Defensive coping
- Grieving
- Hopelessness
- Impaired memory
- Ineffective community coping

- Ineffective denial
- Ineffective protection
- Ineffective sexuality patterns
- Ineffective therapeutic regimen management
- Moral distress
- Powerlessness
- Readiness for enhanced communication
- Risk for caregiver role strain
- Risk for complicated grieving
- Risk for compromised human dignity
- Risk for contamination
- Risk for infection
- Risk for loneliness
- Risk-prone health behavior
- Social isolation

Acute pancreatitis
- Acute pain
- Deficient knowledge (specify)
- Insomnia
- Nausea
- Risk for imbalanced nutrition: More than body requirements
- Risk for impaired liver function
- Risk for unstable glucose level
- Risk-prone health behavior

Acute renal failure
- Death anxiety
- Decreased cardiac output
- Deficient fluid volume
- Disturbed thought processes
- Dressing or grooming self-care deficit
- Excess fluid volume
- Fear
- Impaired physical mobility
- Impaired skin integrity
- Ineffective tissue perfusion (renal)
- Interrupted family processes
- Risk for acute confusion
- Risk for complicated grieving
- Risk for infection
- Risk-prone health behavior
- Sexual dysfunction
- Sleep deprivation

Acute respiratory distress syndrome
- Anxiety
- Bathing or hygiene self-care deficit

- Deficient fluid volume
- Denial
- Dysfunctional ventilatory weaning response
- Fear
- Imbalanced nutrition: Less than body requirements
- Impaired gas exchange
- Impaired skin integrity
- Impaired spontaneous ventilation
- Impaired verbal communication
- Ineffective airway clearance
- Ineffective breathing pattern
- Ineffective coping
- Ineffective tissue perfusion (cardiopulmonary)
- Insomnia
- Risk for acute confusion
- Risk for infection

Acute respiratory failure
- Activity intolerance
- Death anxiety
- Decreased cardiac output
- Denial
- Disturbed sensory perception
- Disturbed thought processes
- Fear
- Impaired gas exchange
- Impaired verbal communication
- Ineffective tissue perfusion (cardiopulmonary)
- Insomnia
- Powerlessness
- Readiness for enhanced spiritual well-being
- Risk for acute confusion
- Risk for aspiration
- Risk for infection
- Risk for suffocation
- Spiritual distress

Adrenal insufficiency
- Acute pain
- Chronic low self-esteem
- Compromised family coping
- Disturbed body image
- Hypothermia
- Readiness for enhanced self-care
- Risk for imbalanced body temperature
- Risk for impaired skin integrity
- Risk for infection
- Risk-prone health behavior

- Sexual dysfunction
- Sleep deprivation

Adrenocortical insufficiency
- Risk for disproportionate growth

Affective disorders
- Anxiety
- Disturbed sensory perception (specify)
- Disturbed thought processes
- Hopelessness
- Impaired religiosity
- Ineffective coping
- Ineffective role performance
- Insomnia
- Risk for loneliness
- Risk for other-directed violence
- Risk-prone health behavior
- Sexual dysfunction
- Stress overload

Alcohol addiction and abuse
- Acute confusion
- Bathing or hygiene self-care deficit
- Defensive coping
- Deficient knowledge (specify)
- Dysfunctional family processes: Alcoholism
- Functional urinary incontinence
- Imbalanced nutrition: Less than body requirements
- Impaired physical mobility
- Ineffective community therapeutic regimen management
- Ineffective coping
- Ineffective denial
- Ineffective family therapeutic regimen management
- Insomnia
- Powerlessness
- Readiness for enhanced family processes
- Risk for acute confusion
- Risk for compromised human dignity
- Risk for poisoning
- Risk for self-directed violence
- Risk-prone health behavior
- Sexual dysfunction
- Sleep deprivation
- Social isolation
- Stress overload

Alzheimer's disease

- Adult failure to thrive
- Anxiety
- Bathing or hygiene self-care deficit
- Bowel incontinence
- Caregiver role strain
- Chronic confusion
- Chronic low self-esteem
- Complicated grieving
- Compromised family coping
- Deficient knowledge (specify)
- Disturbed sensory perception
- Disturbed thought processes
- Functional urinary incontinence
- Grieving
- Hopelessness
- Imbalanced nutrition: Less than body requirements
- Impaired environmental interpretation syndrome
- Impaired home maintenance
- Impaired memory
- Impaired verbal communication
- Ineffective coping
- Ineffective health maintenance
- Ineffective role performance
- Ineffective sexuality patterns
- Interrupted family processes
- Moral distress
- Readiness for enhanced knowledge
- Readiness for enhanced self-care
- Relocation stress syndrome
- Risk for caregiver role strain
- Risk for compromised human dignity
- Risk for injury
- Risk for poisoning
- Risk for trauma
- Social isolation
- Stress urinary incontinence

Amniotic fluid embolism

- Ineffective tissue perfusion (cardiopulmonary)
- Risk for injury

Amputation

- Acute pain
- Chronic low self-esteem
- Chronic pain
- Decisional conflict

- Deficient knowledge (specify)
- Delayed surgical recovery
- Denial
- Disturbed body image
- Energy field disturbance
- Grieving
- Readiness for enhanced self-care
- Risk for compromised human dignity
- Risk for injury
- Risk-prone health behavior

Amyotrophic lateral sclerosis
- Bowel incontinence
- Caregiver role strain
- Chronic low self-esteem
- Complicated grieving
- Compromised family coping
- Death anxiety
- Dressing or grooming self-care deficit
- Dysfunctional ventilatory weaning response
- Grieving
- Hopelessness
- Impaired physical mobility
- Impaired skin integrity
- Impaired spontaneous ventilation
- Impaired verbal communication
- Ineffective airway clearance
- Ineffective breathing pattern
- Ineffective coping
- Ineffective health maintenance
- Ineffective sexuality patterns
- Readiness for enhanced knowledge
- Risk for aspiration
- Risk for caregiver role strain
- Risk for infection
- Social isolation

Anaphylactic shock
- Decreased cardiac output
- Ineffective tissue perfusion (cardiopulmonary)
- Ineffective tissue perfusion (renal)

Anemias
- Activity intolerance
- Adult failure to thrive
- Decreased cardiac output
- Fatigue
- Impaired gas exchange

- Impaired skin integrity
- Ineffective breathing patterns
- Ineffective protection
- Ineffective tissue perfusion (cardiopulmonary)
- Risk for infection

Angina pectoris
- Acute pain
- Anxiety
- Deficient knowledge (specify)
- Impaired environmental interpretation syndrome
- Ineffective denial
- Ineffective role performance
- Ineffective sexuality patterns
- Stress overload

Anorexia nervosa
- Anxiety
- Constipation
- Deficient fluid volume
- Disturbed body image
- Hyperthermia
- Imbalanced nutrition: Less than body requirements
- Ineffective denial
- Interrupted family processes
- Readiness for enhanced nutrition
- Risk for constipation
- Risk-prone health behavior
- Sleep deprivation
- Social isolation
- Spiritual distress
- Stress overload

Antisocial personality disorder
- Chronic low self-esteem
- Disturbed sensory perception
- Dysfunctional family processes: Alcoholism
- Impaired home maintenance
- Ineffective coping
- Ineffective role performance
- Risk for other-directed violence
- Risk for self-mutilation
- Risk for suicide
- Sexual dysfunction
- Social isolation

Anxiety disorder

- Anxiety
- Caregiver role strain
- Chronic low self-esteem
- Constipation
- Defensive coping
- Diarrhea
- Disturbed sensory perception
- Disturbed thought processes
- Hopelessness
- Imbalance nutrition: More than body requirements
- Impaired home maintenance
- Ineffective denial
- Interrupted family processes
- Posttrauma syndrome
- Powerlessness
- Readiness for enhanced communication
- Readiness for enhanced coping
- Readiness for enhanced nutrition
- Readiness for enhanced self-concept
- Risk for imbalanced nutrition: More than body requirements
- Risk for impaired religiosity
- Risk for loneliness
- Risk for posttrauma syndrome
- Social isolation
- Stress overload

Aortic aneurysm

- Acute pain
- Excess fluid volume
- Impaired gas exchange
- Ineffective tissue perfusion (cardiopulmonary)
- Ineffective tissue perfusion (peripheral)
- Ineffective tissue perfusion (renal)

Aortic insufficiency

- Activity intolerance
- Decreased cardiac output
- Deficient knowledge (specify)
- Ineffective tissue perfusion (cardiopulmonary)

Aortic stenosis

- Activity intolerance
- Decreased cardiac output
- Deficient knowledge (specify)
- Ineffective tissue perfusion (cardiopulmonary)

Appendicitis
- Acute pain
- Imbalanced nutrition: Less than body requirements
- Risk for infection

Arterial insufficiency
- Impaired tissue integrity

Arterial occlusion
- Acute pain
- Deficient knowledge (specify)
- Disturbed sensory perception (tactile)
- Impaired skin integrity
- Ineffective tissue perfusion (peripheral)
- Risk-prone health behavior

Asphyxia
- Delayed growth and development
- Hypothermia
- Ineffective breathing pattern
- Risk for aspiration
- Risk for suffocation

Asthma
- Activity intolerance
- Anxiety
- Deficient knowledge (specify)
- Dressing or grooming self-care deficit
- Impaired gas exchange
- Impaired oral mucous membrane
- Ineffective airway clearance
- Ineffective breathing pattern
- Ineffective coping
- Ineffective therapeutic regimen management
- Latex allergy response
- Readiness for enhanced family coping
- Readiness for enhanced knowledge
- Readiness for enhanced therapeutic regimen management
- Risk for infection
- Risk for latex allergy response
- Risk-prone health behavior
- Stress overload

Atelectasis
- Anxiety
- Bathing or hygiene self-care deficit
- Impaired gas exchange
- Impaired physical mobility

- Ineffective airway clearance
- Ineffective breathing pattern

Attention deficit hyperactivity disorder

- Interrupted family processes
- Readiness for enhanced family processes
- Risk for delayed development
- Stress overload

Autism

- Delayed growth and development
- Risk for delayed development
- Risk for self-mutilation

Bell's palsy

- Anxiety
- Chronic low self-esteem
- Disturbed body image
- Disturbed sensory perception (gustatory)
- Impaired swallowing
- Impaired verbal communication
- Ineffective sexuality patterns
- Risk for compromised human dignity
- Social isolation
- Stress overload
- Unilateral neglect

Benign prostatic hypertrophy

- Deficient knowledge (specify)
- Impaired urinary elimination
- Ineffective sexuality patterns
- Sexual dysfunction
- Urinary retention

Bipolar disorder: Depressive phase

- Chronic low self-esteem
- Constipation
- Disturbed sensory perception
- Disturbed thought processes
- Feeding self-care deficit
- Hopelessness
- Imbalanced nutrition: Less than body requirements
- Ineffective coping
- Ineffective denial
- Ineffective health maintenance
- Insomnia
- Risk for compromised human dignity
- Risk for injury

- Risk for self-directed violence
- Sexual dysfunction
- Sleep deprivation
- Social isolation
- Spiritual distress
- Stress overload

Bipolar disorder: Manic phase
- Chronic low self-esteem
- Disturbed sensory perception
- Disturbed thought processes
- Feeding self-care deficit
- Impaired home maintenance
- Impaired physical mobility
- Impaired verbal communication
- Ineffective coping
- Ineffective denial
- Insomnia
- Risk for injury
- Risk for other-directed violence
- Risk-prone health behavior
- Sexual dysfunction

Bladder cancer
- Acute pain
- Fear
- Impaired tissue integrity
- Impaired urinary elimination
- Readiness for enhanced self-care
- Risk for compromised human dignity
- Urge urinary incontinence

Blindness
- Deficient diversional activity
- Deficient knowledge (specify)
- Disturbed body image
- Disturbed sensory perception (visual)
- Fear
- Impaired physical mobility
- Powerlessness
- Risk for injury
- Risk for loneliness

Bone marrow transplantation
- Activity intolerance
- Complicated grieving
- Contamination
- Decreased cardiac output

- Deficient diversional activity
- Diarrhea
- Disturbed body image
- Excess fluid volume
- Grieving
- Imbalanced nutrition: Less than body requirements
- Impaired oral mucous membrane
- Impaired skin integrity
- Ineffective protection
- Risk for infection

Bone sarcomas
- Activity intolerance
- Acute pain
- Impaired physical mobility
- Impaired tissue integrity

Borderline personality disorder
- Chronic low self-esteem
- Fear
- Impaired religiosity
- Ineffective coping
- Risk for self-directed violence
- Risk for self-mutilation
- Social isolation

Bowel fistula
- Risk for deficient fluid volume

Bowel resection
- Delayed surgical recovery
- Risk for infection

Brain abscess
- Acute pain
- Decreased intracranial adaptive capacity
- Disturbed body image
- Impaired physical mobility
- Impaired skin integrity
- Ineffective sexuality patterns
- Ineffective tissue perfusion (cerebral)
- Risk for aspiration
- Risk for injury
- Risk for urge urinary incontinence

Brain tumors
- Acute confusion
- Bowel incontinence

- Constipation
- Decreased intracranial adaptive capacity
- Disturbed sensory perception
- Disturbed thought processes
- Fear
- Grieving
- Impaired environmental interpretation syndrome
- Impaired tissue integrity
- Impaired urinary elimination
- Impaired verbal communication
- Ineffective coping
- Ineffective thermoregulation
- Risk for injury
- Total urinary incontinence

Breast cancer

- Acute pain
- Anxiety
- Complicated grieving
- Decisional conflict (specify)
- Deficient knowledge (specify)
- Disturbed body image
- Fear
- Grieving
- Impaired skin integrity
- Ineffective coping
- Risk for compromised human dignity
- Spiritual distress

Breast engorgement

- Acute pain
- Impaired skin integrity
- Ineffective breast-feeding
- Risk for infection

Bronchiectasis

- Compromised family coping
- Deficient knowledge
- Imbalanced nutrition: Less than body requirements
- Impaired gas exchange
- Ineffective airway clearance
- Ineffective breathing pattern
- Risk for infection

Bulimia nervosa

- Anxiety
- Constipation
- Deficient fluid volume

- Disturbed body image
- Hyperthermia
- Imbalanced nutrition: Less than body requirements
- Ineffective denial
- Interrupted family processes
- Risk for constipation
- Sleep deprivation
- Social isolation

Burns

- Acute pain
- Constipation
- Deficient diversional activity
- Deficient fluid volume
- Disabled family coping
- Disturbed body image
- Dysfunctional ventilatory weaning response
- Grieving
- Hyperthermia
- Hypothermia
- Imbalanced nutrition: Less than body requirements
- Impaired physical mobility
- Impaired skin integrity
- Impaired spontaneous ventilation
- Ineffective breathing pattern
- Ineffective tissue perfusion (renal)
- Powerlessness
- Readiness for enhanced hope
- Readiness for enhanced self-care
- Risk for deficient fluid volume
- Risk for imbalanced body temperature
- Risk for infection
- Risk for injury

Cancer

- Adult failure to thrive
- Chronic sorrow
- Death anxiety
- Disabled family coping
- Energy field disturbance
- Grieving
- Ineffective health maintenance
- Readiness for enhanced knowledge
- Readiness for enhanced religiosity
- Readiness for enhanced self-concept
- Readiness for enhanced spiritual well-being
- Risk for infection
- Risk for spiritual distress

Cardiac arrhythmias

- Decreased cardiac output
- Excess fluid volume
- Fear
- Ineffective sexuality patterns
- Ineffective tissue perfusion (cardiopulmonary)
- Risk for sudden infant death syndrome
- Stress overload

Cardiac disease: End-stage

- Activity intolerance
- Adult failure to thrive
- Caregiver role strain
- Death anxiety
- Decisional conflict
- Decreased cardiac output
- Defensive coping
- Excess fluid volume
- Grieving
- Hopelessness
- Ineffective coping
- Risk for caregiver role strain
- Risk for infection
- Risk for injury
- Sedentary lifestyle
- Situational low self-esteem

Cardiogenic shock

- Decreased cardiac output
- Excess fluid volume
- Impaired gas exchange
- Ineffective tissue perfusion

Carpal tunnel syndrome

- Acute pain
- Impaired physical mobility
- Ineffective tissue perfusion (peripheral)
- Risk for peripheral neurovascular dysfunction

Cataracts

- Disturbed body image
- Disturbed sensory perception (visual)
- Impaired physical mobility
- Ineffective coping
- Ineffective health maintenance
- Risk for injury

Cellulitis
- Acute pain
- Anxiety
- Deficient knowledge (specify)
- Impaired physical mobility
- Impaired skin integrity

Cerebral aneurysm
- Decreased intracranial adaptive capacity
- Impaired physical mobility
- Impaired skin integrity
- Ineffective airway clearance
- Ineffective breathing pattern
- Ineffective tissue perfusion
- Risk for injury

Cerebral edema
- Decreased intracranial adaptive capacity
- Ineffective thermoregulation

Cerebral palsy
- Delayed growth and development
- Impaired physical mobility
- Readiness for enhanced self-care
- Risk for caregiver role strain
- Risk for compromised human dignity
- Toileting self-care deficit
- Total urinary incontinence

Cervical cancer
- Acute pain
- Disturbed body image
- Fatigue
- Fear
- Impaired skin integrity
- Risk-prone health behavior

Chemotherapy
- Constipation
- Deficient diversional activity
- Deficient fluid volume
- Diarrhea
- Disturbed sensory perception (auditory)
- Imbalanced nutrition: Less than body requirements
- Impaired gas exchange
- Impaired oral mucous membrane
- Impaired physical mobility
- Ineffective protection

- Ineffective tissue perfusion
- Nausea
- Risk for impaired skin integrity
- Risk for infection
- Sexual dysfunction

Chest trauma
- Dysfunctional ventilatory weaning response
- Impaired spontaneous ventilation
- Ineffective airway clearance
- Ineffective breathing pattern
- Risk for aspiration

Child abuse
- Delayed growth and development
- Impaired parenting
- Readiness for enhanced parenting
- Risk for impaired parenting

Childbirth
- Deficient knowledge (specify)
- Interrupted family processes
- Readiness for enhanced parenting

Chlamydia
- Ineffective sexuality patterns
- Risk for infection

Chloride imbalance
- Imbalanced nutrition: Less than body requirements

Cholecystitis
- Acute pain
- Deficient fluid volume
- Imbalanced nutrition: Less than body requirements
- Risk for impaired liver function
- Risk for infection

Chronic bronchitis
- Activity intolerance
- Deficient knowledge (specify)
- Fatigue
- Fear
- Hopelessness
- Impaired gas exchange
- Impaired spontaneous ventilation
- Ineffective airway clearance

- Ineffective breathing pattern
- Risk for infection

Chronic fatigue syndrome

- Acute pain
- Fatigue
- Hopelessness
- Ineffective therapeutic regimen management
- Readiness for enhanced therapeutic regimen management
- Sleep deprivation

Chronic obstructive pulmonary disease

- Activity intolerance
- Adult failure to thrive
- Anxiety
- Caregiver role strain
- Compromised family coping
- Defensive coping
- Deficient fluid volume
- Deficient knowledge (specify)
- Dysfunctional ventilatory weaning response
- Fatigue
- Fear
- Hopelessness
- Imbalance nutrition: More than body requirements
- Imbalanced nutrition: Less than body requirements
- Impaired gas exchange
- Impaired home maintenance
- Impaired oral mucous membrane
- Impaired spontaneous ventilation
- Impaired verbal communication
- Ineffective airway clearance
- Ineffective breathing pattern
- Ineffective denial
- Ineffective health maintenance
- Ineffective tissue perfusion (cardiopulmonary)
- Insomnia
- Powerlessness
- Readiness for enhanced coping
- Risk for infection
- Risk for injury
- Risk for suffocation
- Sleep deprivation

Chronic pain

- Chronic low self-esteem
- Chronic pain
- Defensive coping

- Hopelessness
- Risk-prone health behavior

Chronic renal failure
- Compromised family coping
- Death anxiety
- Deficient knowledge (specify)
- Disturbed body image
- Excess fluid volume
- Ineffective denial
- Ineffective tissue perfusion (renal)
- Interrupted family processes
- Powerlessness
- Risk for impaired skin integrity
- Risk for infection
- Sexual dysfunction

Cirrhosis
- Compromised family coping
- Deficient fluid volume
- Disturbed thought processes
- Imbalanced nutrition: Less than body requirements
- Ineffective breathing pattern
- Interrupted family processes: Alcoholism
- Moral distress
- Risk for impaired liver function
- Risk for impaired skin integrity
- Risk for injury
- Stress urinary incontinence

Cleft lip or palate
- Compromised family coping
- Imbalanced nutrition: Less than body requirements
- Impaired verbal communication
- Ineffective breast-feeding
- Ineffective infant feeding pattern
- Risk for aspiration
- Risk for compromised human dignity

Colic
- Disorganized infant behavior

Colitis
- Acute pain
- Deficient fluid volume
- Diarrhea
- Disturbed body image
- Imbalanced nutrition: Less than body requirements

- Ineffective tissue perfusion (GI)
- Risk for imbalanced body temperature
- Risk-prone health behavior

Colon and rectal cancer
- Acute pain
- Anxiety
- Constipation
- Deficient fluid volume
- Deficient knowledge (specify)
- Diarrhea
- Fear

Colostomy
- Complicated grieving
- Deficient fluid volume
- Disturbed body image
- Imbalanced nutrition: Less than body requirements
- Impaired skin integrity
- Ineffective sexuality patterns
- Ineffective tissue perfusion (GI)
- Readiness for enhanced hope
- Readiness for enhanced self-care
- Risk for compromised human dignity
- Situational low self-esteem
- Spiritual distress

Conduct disorder
- Chronic low self-esteem
- Hopelessness
- Interrupted family processes

Congenital anomalies
- Disabled family coping
- Total urinary incontinence

Congenital heart disease
- Activity intolerance
- Decreased cardiac output
- Ineffective breathing pattern
- Interrupted family processes
- Risk for disproportionate growth
- Risk for infection
- Risk for injury

Coronary artery disease
- Activity intolerance
- Acute pain

- Anxiety
- Decreased cardiac output
- Deficient knowledge (specify)
- Health-seeking behaviors
- Imbalance nutrition: More than body requirements
- Impaired gas exchange
- Impaired home maintenance
- Ineffective sexuality patterns
- Ineffective tissue perfusion (cardiopulmonary)
- Risk for injury
- Risk-prone health behavior
- Sedentary lifestyle
- Stress overload

Cor pulmonale
- Activity intolerance
- Decreased cardiac output
- Excess fluid volume
- Fatigue
- Grieving
- Hopelessness
- Impaired gas exchange
- Ineffective airway clearance
- Ineffective breathing pattern
- Ineffective coping
- Risk for infection

Craniotomy
- Acute pain
- Bathing or hygiene self-care deficit
- Decreased intracranial adaptive capacity
- Delayed surgical recovery
- Disturbed body image
- Disturbed sensory perception
- Impaired physical mobility
- Impaired skin integrity
- Ineffective airway clearance
- Ineffective breathing pattern
- Ineffective tissue perfusion (cerebral)
- Risk for infection
- Sleep deprivation

Crohn's disease
- Acute pain
- Anxiety
- Compromised family coping
- Deficient fluid volume
- Deficient knowledge (specify)

- Diarrhea
- Fear
- Imbalanced nutrition: Less than body requirements
- Impaired skin integrity
- Insomnia
- Nausea
- Readiness for enhanced hope
- Readiness for enhanced self-care
- Risk for imbalanced fluid volume
- Risk for infection
- Stress overload

Cushing's syndrome
- Activity intolerance
- Complicated grieving
- Disturbed body image
- Disturbed thought processes
- Excess fluid volume
- Hopelessness
- Imbalance nutrition: More than body requirements
- Impaired skin integrity
- Ineffective coping
- Risk for acute confusion
- Risk for imbalanced body temperature

Cystic fibrosis
- Activity intolerance
- Compromised family coping
- Deficient diversional activity
- Deficient fluid volume
- Imbalanced nutrition: Less than body requirements
- Impaired gas exchange
- Ineffective airway clearance
- Ineffective breathing pattern
- Parental role conflict
- Risk for delayed development
- Risk for deficient fluid volume
- Risk for imbalanced body temperature
- Risk for imbalanced fluid volume
- Risk for infection

Cystitis
- Acute pain
- Impaired urinary elimination
- Noncompliance
- Overflow urinary incontinence
- Risk for urge urinary incontinence

- Sleep deprivation
- Urge urinary incontinence

Deafness
- Chronic low self-esteem
- Defensive coping
- Disturbed sensory perception (auditory)
- Fear
- Impaired verbal communication
- Ineffective coping
- Readiness for enhanced coping
- Risk for injury

Delusional disorder
- Disturbed thought processes
- Impaired home maintenance

Dementia
- Activity intolerance
- Acute confusion
- Caregiver role strain
- Chronic confusion
- Disturbed thought processes
- Functional urinary incontinence
- Impaired environmental interpretation syndrome
- Impaired memory
- Impaired verbal communication
- Interrupted family processes
- Risk for loneliness
- Powerlessness
- Risk for injury
- Risk for self-directed violence
- Social isolation

Depression
- Adult failure to thrive
- Caregiver role strain
- Chronic low self-esteem
- Constipation
- Deficient diversional activity
- Disturbed body image
- Fatigue
- Functional urinary incontinence
- Hopelessness
- Imbalance nutrition: More than body requirements
- Imbalanced nutrition: Less than body requirements
- Impaired home maintenance
- Ineffective coping

- Ineffective denial
- Posttrauma syndrome
- Powerlessness
- Readiness for enhanced nutrition
- Risk for constipation
- Risk for imbalanced nutrition: More than body requirements
- Risk for injury
- Risk for loneliness
- Risk for poisoning
- Risk for posttrauma syndrome
- Risk for self-directed violence
- Sexual dysfunction
- Sleep deprivation
- Social isolation
- Spiritual distress

Detached retina

- Acute pain
- Anxiety
- Disturbed sensory perception (visual)
- Risk for injury

Developmental disorder

- Disabled family coping
- Risk for impaired parent-infant-child attachment
- Risk for injury
- Risk for self-mutilation

Diabetes insipidus

- Deficient fluid volume
- Impaired oral mucous membrane
- Risk for deficient fluid volume
- Risk for imbalanced body temperature
- Risk for unstable glucose level

Diabetes mellitus

- Chronic low self-esteem
- Compromised family coping
- Constipation
- Decreased cardiac output
- Deficient knowledge (specify)
- Disturbed body image
- Disturbed sensory perception
- Grieving
- Hopelessness
- Hyperthermia
- Imbalance nutrition: More than body requirements
- Impaired oral mucous membrane

- Impaired skin integrity
- Impaired urinary elimination
- Ineffective coping
- Ineffective health maintenance
- Ineffective sexuality patterns
- Ineffective therapeutic regimen management
- Ineffective tissue perfusion (peripheral)
- Ineffective tissue perfusion (renal)
- Noncompliance
- Powerlessness
- Readiness for enhanced fluid balance
- Readiness for enhanced nutrition
- Readiness for enhanced therapeutic regimen management
- Readiness for enhanced urinary elimination
- Risk for deficient fluid volume
- Risk for imbalanced body temperature
- Risk for imbalanced nutrition: More than body requirements
- Risk for impaired skin integrity
- Risk for infection
- Risk for injury
- Risk for unstable glucose level
- Risk-prone health behavior
- Social isolation
- Total urinary incontinence

Diabetic ketoacidosis
- Deficient fluid volume
- Disturbed thought processes
- Risk for acute confusion
- Risk for imbalanced body temperature
- Risk for unstable glucose level

Diarrhea
- Deficient fluid volume
- Diarrhea
- Disturbed body image
- Readiness for enhanced fluid balance
- Risk for deficient fluid volume
- Risk for imbalanced fluid volume

Digoxin toxicity
- Decreased cardiac output
- Deficient knowledge (specify)
- Risk for poisoning

Disseminated intravascular coagulation
- Decreased cardiac output
- Deficient fluid volume

- Fear
- Impaired gas exchange

Disorder, dissociative
- Disturbed thought processes
- Impaired home maintenance
- Interrupted family processes

Diverticulitis
- Acute pain
- Constipation
- Deficient fluid volume
- Diarrhea
- Imbalanced nutrition: Less than body requirements

Down syndrome
- Compromised family coping
- Deficient knowledge (specify)
- Delayed growth and development
- Interrupted family processes
- Readiness for enhanced knowledge
- Readiness for enhanced self-care
- Risk for aspiration
- Risk for delayed development
- Risk for infection
- Risk for injury
- Situational low self-esteem
- Toileting self-care deficit

Drug addiction
- Acute confusion
- Adult failure to thrive
- Decisional conflict
- Defensive coping
- Dysfunctional family processes: Alcoholism
- Ineffective community therapeutic regimen management
- Ineffective coping
- Ineffective denial
- Ineffective family therapeutic regimen management
- Ineffective health maintenance
- Moral distress
- Risk for compromised human dignity
- Risk for impaired liver function
- Risk for poisoning
- Risk for self-directed violence
- Risk for sudden infant death syndrome
- Sexual dysfunction
- Sleep deprivation

Drug overdose
- Disturbed thought processes
- Functional urinary incontinence
- Hyperthermia
- Hypothermia
- Impaired gas exchange
- Ineffective coping
- Ineffective thermoregulation
- Risk for compromised human dignity
- Risk for poisoning
- Risk for suffocation
- Risk for trauma

Drug toxicity
- Functional urinary incontinence
- Hyperthermia
- Hypothermia
- Impaired gas exchange
- Risk for poisoning

Duodenal ulcer
- Acute pain
- Anxiety
- Imbalanced nutrition: Less than body requirements
- Ineffective tissue perfusion (GI)

Eating disorders (anorexia nervosa and bulimia nervosa)
- Decisional conflict
- Disturbed body image
- Imbalanced nutrition: Less than body requirements
- Posttrauma syndrome
- Risk for loneliness

Ectopic pregnancy
- Acute pain
- Deficient fluid volume
- Ineffective tissue perfusion (cardiopulmonary)

Emphysema
- Activity intolerance
- Deficient knowledge (specify)
- Fatigue
- Fear
- Hopelessness
- Imbalanced nutrition: Less than body requirements
- Impaired gas exchange
- Impaired spontaneous ventilation
- Ineffective airway clearance

- Ineffective breathing pattern
- Noncompliance
- Risk for infection

Empyema
- Deficient fluid volume
- Impaired gas exchange
- Ineffective breathing pattern
- Risk for infection

Encephalitis
- Activity intolerance
- Acute pain
- Anxiety
- Constipation
- Deficient fluid volume
- Delayed growth and development
- Disturbed thought processes
- Hyperthermia
- Impaired physical mobility
- Ineffective coping
- Ineffective thermoregulation
- Risk for infection

Endocarditis
- Activity intolerance
- Anxiety
- Contamination
- Decreased cardiac output
- Deficient knowledge (specify)
- Excess fluid volume
- Imbalanced nutrition: Less than body requirements
- Risk for infection

Endometrial cancer
- Acute pain
- Fear
- Grieving
- Impaired tissue integrity

Endometriosis
- Anxiety
- Deficient fluid volume
- Deficient knowledge (specify)
- Grieving
- Risk for infection
- Sexual dysfunction
- Spiritual distress

Esophageal cancer
- Acute pain
- Fatigue
- Fear
- Imbalanced nutrition: Less than body requirements
- Risk for aspiration
- Risk for deficient fluid volume
- Risk for infection

Esophageal fistula
- Imbalanced nutrition: Less than body requirements
- Risk for aspiration
- Risk for deficient fluid volume

Esophageal varices
- Deficient fluid volume
- Dysfunctional family processes: Alcoholism
- Imbalanced nutrition: Less than body requirements
- Readiness for enhanced hope
- Risk for deficient fluid volume
- Risk for impaired skin integrity

Failure to thrive
- Deficient fluid volume
- Delayed growth and development
- Disorganized infant behavior
- Imbalanced nutrition: Less than body requirements
- Impaired parenting
- Ineffective community coping
- Risk for deficient fluid volume
- Risk for disorganized infant behavior
- Risk for impaired parenting

Fetal alcohol syndrome
- Compromised family coping
- Delayed growth and development
- Dysfunctional family processes: Alcoholism
- Ineffective community coping
- Moral distress
- Risk for delayed development
- Risk for disproportionate growth

Food poisoning
- Contamination
- Diarrhea
- Disturbed sensory perception (visual)
- Hyperthermia
- Impaired physical mobility

- Impaired verbal communication
- Ineffective breathing pattern
- Nausea

Fractures
- Activity intolerance
- Acute pain
- Bathing or hygiene self-care deficit
- Compromised family coping
- Deficient diversional activity
- Deficient fluid volume
- Disturbed sensory perception
- Hopelessness
- Impaired parenting
- Impaired physical mobility
- Impaired skin integrity
- Ineffective breathing pattern
- Ineffective denial
- Risk for constipation
- Risk for disuse syndrome
- Risk for falls
- Risk for injury
- Risk for peripheral neurovascular dysfunction
- Risk for trauma

Gallbladder disease
- Acute pain
- Anxiety
- Fear

Gastric cancer
- Imbalanced nutrition: Less than body requirements
- Ineffective tissue perfusion (GI)

Gastric ulcer
- Acute pain
- Anxiety
- Imbalanced nutrition: Less than body requirements
- Ineffective tissue perfusion (GI)
- Risk-prone health behavior
- Stress overload

Gastroenteritis
- Deficient fluid volume
- Diarrhea
- Risk for deficient fluid volume
- Risk for imbalanced body temperature

Genital herpes

- Deficient knowledge (specify)
- Ineffective community coping
- Ineffective sexuality patterns
- Powerlessness
- Risk for infection
- Risk for loneliness
- Risk-prone health behavior
- Social isolation

Gestational diabetes

- Risk for infection
- Risk for unstable glucose level

Gestational hypertension

- Activity intolerance
- Acute pain
- Deficient fluid volume
- Deficient knowledge (specify)
- Disturbed sensory perception (visual)
- Excess fluid volume
- Fear
- Ineffective tissue perfusion (cerebral)
- Urinary retention

Glaucoma

- Acute pain
- Anxiety
- Complicated grieving
- Deficient knowledge (specify)
- Disturbed sensory perception (visual)
- Grieving
- Risk for falls
- Risk for injury

Glomerulonephritis

- Compromised family coping
- Excess fluid volume
- Imbalanced nutrition: Less than body requirements
- Ineffective tissue perfusion (renal)
- Risk for infection

Gonorrhea

- Deficient knowledge (specify)
- Ineffective community coping
- Ineffective sexuality patterns
- Moral distress

- Risk for infection
- Risk-prone health behavior

Gout
- Activity intolerance
- Acute pain
- Deficient knowledge (specify)
- Disturbed body image
- Imbalance nutrition: More than body requirements
- Impaired physical mobility

Guillain-Barré syndrome
- Activity intolerance
- Acute pain
- Anxiety
- Bathing or hygiene self-care deficit
- Bowel incontinence
- Fatigue
- Impaired gas exchange
- Impaired physical mobility
- Impaired spontaneous ventilation
- Ineffective airway clearance
- Ineffective breathing pattern
- Ineffective coping
- Risk for urge urinary incontinence

Headaches
- Acute pain
- Ineffective coping
- Insomnia

Head injury
- Activity intolerance
- Acute confusion
- Bowel incontinence
- Chronic confusion
- Chronic sorrow
- Decreased intracranial adaptive capacity
- Deficient knowledge (specify)
- Delayed growth and development
- Disturbed body image
- Disturbed sensory perception
- Disturbed thought processes
- Dressing or grooming self-care deficit
- Fear
- Imbalanced nutrition: Less than body requirements
- Impaired environmental interpretation syndrome

- Impaired gas exchange
- Impaired memory
- Impaired parenting
- Impaired physical mobility
- Impaired social interaction
- Impaired swallowing
- Impaired verbal communication
- Ineffective thermoregulation
- Ineffective tissue perfusion
- Posttrauma syndrome
- Powerlessness
- Risk for activity intolerance
- Risk for aspiration
- Risk for constipation
- Risk for delayed development
- Risk for disuse syndrome
- Risk for imbalanced body temperature
- Risk for imbalanced fluid volume
- Risk for impaired parenting
- Risk for injury
- Risk for trauma
- Risk for urge urinary incontinence
- Sleep deprivation
- Total urinary incontinence
- Unilateral neglect

Head or neck cancer
- Acute pain
- Anxiety
- Disturbed body image
- Disturbed sensory perception (gustatory)
- Impaired oral mucous membrane
- Impaired tissue integrity
- Impaired verbal communication
- Ineffective airway clearance

Heart failure
- Activity intolerance
- Acute pain
- Caregiver role strain
- Death anxiety
- Decreased cardiac output
- Deficient knowledge (specify)
- Excess fluid volume
- Fatigue
- Hopelessness
- Imbalance nutrition: More than body requirements
- Impaired gas exchange

- Impaired home maintenance
- Ineffective airway clearance
- Ineffective breathing pattern
- Ineffective tissue perfusion
- Powerlessness
- Risk for activity intolerance
- Risk for caregiver role strain
- Risk for imbalanced fluid volume
- Risk for injury

Hemodialysis
- Complicated grieving
- Deficient fluid volume
- Deficient knowledge (specify)
- Disturbed body image
- Disturbed thought processes
- Excess fluid volume
- Interrupted family processes
- Readiness for enhanced hope
- Risk for falls
- Risk for infection
- Spiritual distress

Hemophilia
- Acute pain
- Chronic low self-esteem
- Impaired gas exchange
- Ineffective protection
- Parental role conflict
- Readiness for enhanced coping family
- Risk for falls
- Risk for imbalanced body temperature
- Risk for injury
- Risk for trauma
- Risk-prone health behavior

Hemorrhage
- Deficient fluid volume
- Impaired oral mucous membrane
- Ineffective thermoregulation
- Ineffective tissue perfusion (renal)
- Risk for aspiration

Hemorrhoids
- Acute pain
- Constipation
- Deficient knowledge (specify)

Hemothorax
- Acute pain
- Anxiety
- Deficient fluid volume
- Fear
- Impaired gas exchange
- Impaired spontaneous ventilation
- Ineffective breathing pattern
- Ineffective tissue perfusion

Hepatic coma
- Acute confusion
- Deficient fluid volume
- Disturbed sensory perception
- Disturbed thought processes
- Imbalanced nutrition: Less than body requirements
- Impaired skin integrity
- Moral distress
- Risk for acute confusion
- Risk for infection
- Risk for injury

Hepatitis
- Deficient knowledge (specify)
- Ineffective community coping
- Nausea
- Readiness for enhanced community coping

Hip fracture
- Compromised family coping
- Deficient knowledge (specify)
- Ineffective denial
- Ineffective sexuality patterns
- Powerlessness
- Risk for activity intolerance
- Risk for falls
- Risk for impaired skin integrity
- Risk for injury
- Spiritual distress

Hodgkin's disease
- Grieving
- Imbalanced nutrition: Less than body requirements
- Impaired physical mobility
- Impaired skin integrity
- Impaired tissue integrity
- Ineffective breathing pattern
- Ineffective protection

- Risk for complicated grieving
- Risk for infection

Huntington's disease
- Bathing or hygiene self-care deficit
- Bowel incontinence
- Caregiver role strain
- Compromised family coping
- Deficient knowledge (specify)
- Hopelessness
- Impaired physical mobility
- Impaired verbal communication
- Ineffective health maintenance
- Risk for loneliness
- Moral distress
- Risk for injury
- Social isolation

Hydatidiform mole
- Acute pain
- Deficient fluid volume
- Grieving

Hydrocephalus
- Acute pain
- Anxiety
- Compromised family coping
- Delayed growth and development
- Disturbed body image
- Imbalanced nutrition: Less than body requirements
- Interrupted family processes
- Risk for impaired skin integrity
- Risk for infection

Hyperbilirubinemia
- Interrupted breast-feeding
- Risk for injury

Hyperemesis gravidarum
- Deficient fluid volume
- Imbalanced nutrition: Less than body requirements

Hyperosmolar hyperglycemic nonketotic syndrome
- Deficient fluid volume
- Disturbed thought processes
- Impaired skin integrity
- Ineffective tissue perfusion

- Risk for infection
- Risk for unstable glucose level

Hyperparathyroidism
- Acute pain
- Anxiety
- Hopelessness
- Imbalanced nutrition: Less than body requirements
- Ineffective breathing pattern
- Ineffective coping
- Risk for imbalanced body temperature
- Risk for impaired skin integrity

Hyperpituitarism
- Acute pain
- Disturbed body image
- Ineffective coping
- Risk for compromised human dignity
- Sexual dysfunction

Hypertension
- Decreased cardiac output
- Deficient knowledge (specify)
- Excess fluid volume
- Health-seeking behaviors
- Imbalance nutrition: More than body requirements
- Impaired environmental interpretation syndrome
- Ineffective denial
- Ineffective sexuality patterns
- Ineffective therapeutic regimen management
- Noncompliance (specify)
- Powerlessness
- Readiness for enhanced urinary elimination
- Risk-prone health behavior
- Situational low self-esteem

Hyperthermia
- Deficient knowledge (specify)
- Hyperthermia
- Impaired oral mucous membrane
- Ineffective thermoregulation

Hyperthyroidism
- Activity intolerance
- Decreased cardiac output
- Disturbed body image
- Disturbed thought processes
- Ineffective thermoregulation

- Risk for imbalanced body temperature
- Sleep deprivation

Hypochondriasis
- Disturbed thought processes
- Ineffective coping
- Ineffective health maintenance

Hypoparathyroidism
- Anxiety
- Compromised family coping
- Decreased cardiac output
- Imbalanced nutrition: Less than body requirements
- Ineffective coping
- Ineffective thermoregulation
- Risk for trauma

Hypopituitarism
- Risk for delayed development
- Risk for disproportionate growth

Hypothermia
- Deficient knowledge (specify)
- Hypothermia
- Ineffective thermoregulation

Hypothyroidism
- Activity intolerance
- Compromised family coping
- Constipation
- Decreased cardiac output
- Disturbed body image
- Disturbed thought processes
- Functional urinary incontinence
- Ineffective coping
- Ineffective sexuality patterns
- Ineffective thermoregulation
- Risk for delayed development
- Risk for disproportionate growth
- Risk for imbalanced body temperature

Ileostomy
- Anxiety
- Deficient fluid volume
- Disturbed body image
- Fear
- Imbalanced nutrition: Less than body requirements
- Impaired skin integrity

- Ineffective sexuality patterns
- Ineffective tissue perfusion (GI)
- Risk for infection
- Situational low self-esteem

Impotence
- Deficient knowledge (specify)
- Disturbed body image
- Risk for compromised human dignity
- Sexual dysfunction
- Situational low self-esteem
- Urinary retention

Incest
- Ineffective coping
- Interrupted family processes
- Moral distress
- Posttrauma syndrome
- Rape-trauma syndrome: Compound reaction
- Rape-trauma syndrome: Silent reaction

Infertility
- Complicated grieving
- Deficient knowledge (specify)
- Ineffective coping
- Situational low self-esteem
- Stress overload

Inhalation injuries
- Ineffective thermoregulation
- Risk for injury
- Risk for suffocation

Interstitial pulmonary fibrosis
- Activity intolerance
- Deficient knowledge (specify)
- Grieving
- Impaired gas exchange
- Ineffective breathing pattern
- Ineffective coping
- Spiritual distress

Intestinal obstruction
- Acute pain
- Constipation
- Imbalanced nutrition: Less than body requirements
- Ineffective tissue perfusion (GI)
- Risk for aspiration

- Risk for deficient fluid volume
- Risk for imbalanced fluid volume
- Urinary retention

Intoxication

- Disturbed sensory perception
- Disturbed thought processes
- Hypothermia
- Impaired verbal communication
- Ineffective community therapeutic regimen management
- Moral distress
- Risk for aspiration

Joint replacement

- Acute pain
- Compromised family coping
- Deficient knowledge (specify)
- Disturbed sensory perception (kinesthetic)
- Impaired physical mobility
- Ineffective tissue perfusion
- Risk for contamination
- Risk for infection
- Risk for injury

Juvenile rheumatoid arthritis

- Compromised family coping
- Defensive coping
- Disturbed sensory perception (tactile)
- Grieving
- Impaired physical mobility
- Ineffective health maintenance
- Risk for unstable glucose level

Kidney transplantation

- Deficient fluid volume
- Deficient knowledge (specify)
- Delayed surgical recovery
- Disturbed body image
- Ineffective protection
- Interrupted family processes
- Risk for infection

Labor and delivery

- Acute pain
- Anxiety
- Deficient knowledge (specify)
- Effective breast-feeding

- Impaired skin integrity
- Ineffective coping
- Risk for injury
- Total urinary incontinence
- Urinary retention

Laryngeal cancer
- Grieving

Leukemia
- Acute pain
- Grieving
- Hopelessness
- Imbalanced nutrition: Less than body requirements
- Impaired gas exchange
- Impaired oral mucous membrane
- Impaired tissue integrity
- Ineffective protection
- Ineffective tissue perfusion (cardiopulmonary)
- Ineffective tissue perfusion (renal)
- Risk for falls
- Risk for imbalanced body temperature
- Risk for infection
- Risk for injury

Liver transplantation
- Anxiety
- Compromised family coping
- Deficient knowledge (specify)
- Delayed surgical recovery
- Fear
- Ineffective coping
- Ineffective protection
- Ineffective tissue perfusion (cardiopulmonary)
- Ineffective tissue perfusion (GI)
- Ineffective tissue perfusion (renal)
- Moral distress
- Risk for impaired liver function
- Risk for infection

Lung abscess
- Acute pain
- Anxiety
- Impaired gas exchange
- Ineffective airway clearance
- Ineffective breathing pattern
- Ineffective coping

see page 940 & 813 for

★ liver dysfunction

★ Monitor patient for signs and symptoms of jaundice, dark colored urine, decreased thirst, frequent urination, increase in liver function tests and increase in platelet count. Report changes in condition and lab values to physician immediately to detect risk for impaired liver function.

- Ineffective tissue perfusion (cardiopulmonary)
- Risk for imbalanced body temperature

Lung cancer
- Activity intolerance
- Death anxiety
- Fear
- Hopelessness
- Imbalanced nutrition: Less than body requirements
- Impaired gas exchange
- Impaired tissue integrity
- Impaired verbal communication
- Ineffective airway clearance
- Ineffective breathing pattern
- Powerlessness

Lupus erythematosus
- Decreased cardiac output
- Imbalanced nutrition: Less than body requirements
- Impaired physical mobility
- Ineffective tissue perfusion
- Risk for infection
- Risk-prone health behavior

Lyme disease
- Activity intolerance
- Acute pain
- Fatigue
- Hyperthermia
- Impaired skin integrity

Lymphomas
- Death anxiety
- Grieving
- Hopelessness
- Impaired tissue integrity
- Ineffective protection
- Risk for infection

Macular degeneration
- Activity intolerance
- Disturbed sensory perception (visual)
- Ineffective denial
- Powerlessness
- Readiness for enhanced hope
- Risk for caregiver role strain
- Risk for falls

Malnutrition
- Imbalanced nutrition: Less than body requirements
- Ineffective community coping
- Risk for injury

Maternal psychological stress
- Anxiety
- Ineffective breast-feeding
- Interrupted breast-feeding
- Powerlessness

Meconium aspiration syndrome
- Ineffective breathing pattern
- Risk for injury

Melanoma
- Decisional conflict
- Defensive coping
- Disturbed body image
- Fatigue
- Hopelessness
- Impaired oral mucous membrane
- Powerlessness
- Spiritual distress

Ménière's disease
- Disturbed sensory perception (auditory)
- Impaired physical mobility
- Insomnia
- Nausea
- Risk for falls
- Risk for trauma

Meningitis
- Acute pain
- Bowel incontinence
- Deficient fluid volume
- Disturbed sensory perception (auditory)
- Disturbed sensory perception (visual)
- Excess fluid volume
- Fear
- Hyperthermia
- Ineffective airway clearance
- Ineffective breathing pattern
- Risk for imbalanced fluid volume
- Risk for infection

Menopause

- Ineffective sexuality patterns
- Insomnia
- Sexual dysfunction
- Situational low self-esteem
- Stress overload

Metabolic acidosis

- Deficient knowledge (specify)
- Disturbed thought processes
- Impaired oral mucous membrane
- Ineffective breathing pattern
- Risk for injury

Metabolic alkalosis

- Deficient fluid volume
- Disturbed thought processes
- Impaired oral mucous membrane
- Ineffective breathing pattern
- Risk for injury

Mitral insufficiency

- Activity intolerance
- Decreased cardiac output
- Deficient knowledge (specify)
- Fatigue
- Ineffective tissue perfusion (cardiopulmonary)

Mitral stenosis

- Activity intolerance
- Decreased cardiac output
- Deficient knowledge (specify)
- Fatigue
- Ineffective tissue perfusion (cardiopulmonary)

Mood disorders

- Impaired religiosity
- Ineffective community therapeutic regimen management
- Powerlessness
- Risk for suicide
- Self-mutilation
- Social isolation
- Spiritual distress

Multiple births

- Anxiety
- Deficient knowledge (specify)
- Impaired parenting

- Ineffective coping
- Risk for injury
- Stress urinary incontinence

Multiple myeloma
- Activity intolerance
- Acute pain
- Excess fluid volume
- Fatigue
- Grieving
- Imbalanced nutrition: Less than body requirements
- Ineffective tissue perfusion (cerebral)
- Risk for infection

Multiple sclerosis
- Acute pain
- Bowel incontinence
- Caregiver role strain
- Chronic low self-esteem
- Death anxiety
- Deficient knowledge (specify)
- Disturbed sensory perception
- Dressing or grooming self-care deficit
- Fatigue
- Grieving
- Imbalanced nutrition: Less than body requirements
- Impaired memory
- Impaired physical mobility
- Impaired spontaneous ventilation
- Impaired urinary elimination
- Ineffective airway clearance
- Ineffective health maintenance
- Ineffective sexuality patterns
- Ineffective therapeutic regimen management
- Readiness for enhanced family coping
- Risk for activity intolerance
- Risk for caregiver role strain
- Risk for infection
- Risk for spiritual distress
- Risk for urge urinary incontinence
- Risk-prone health behavior
- Total urinary incontinence

Multisystem trauma
- Anxiety
- Bathing or hygiene self-care deficit
- Deficient fluid volume
- Dysfunctional ventilatory weaning response

- Ineffective tissue perfusion
- Powerlessness
- Risk for infection
- Risk for suffocation
- Risk for trauma

Muscular dystrophy

- Caregiver role strain
- Deficient knowledge (specify)
- Disturbed sensory perception (kinesthetic)
- Feeding self-care deficit
- Hopelessness
- Impaired physical mobility
- Ineffective health maintenance
- Readiness for enhanced family coping
- Risk for caregiver role strain
- Risk for urge urinary incontinence
- Risk-prone health behavior

Myasthenia gravis

- Bowel incontinence
- Chronic low self-esteem
- Dressing or grooming self-care deficit
- Dysfunctional ventilatory weaning response
- Fatigue
- Fear
- Impaired gas exchange
- Impaired physical mobility
- Impaired verbal communication
- Ineffective airway clearance
- Readiness for enhanced self-care
- Risk for urge urinary incontinence

Myocardial infarction

- Activity intolerance
- Acute pain
- Anxiety
- Compromised family coping
- Death anxiety
- Decreased cardiac output
- Health-seeking behaviors
- Ineffective coping
- Ineffective denial
- Ineffective role performance
- Ineffective sexuality patterns
- Ineffective tissue perfusion
- Readiness for enhanced spiritual well-being
- Risk for spiritual distress

- Risk-prone health behavior
- Sedentary lifestyle
- Sexual dysfunction
- Situational low self-esteem
- Sleep deprivation
- Spiritual distress

Narcissistic personality disorder
- Fear
- Ineffective coping

Neonatal asphyxia
- Compromised family coping
- Delayed growth and development
- Hypothermia
- Ineffective breathing pattern
- Risk for aspiration
- Risk for injury

Neonatal hyperbilirubinemia
- Interrupted breast-feeding

Neurologic impairment (neonatal)
- Compromised family coping
- Ineffective infant feeding pattern

Neuromuscular trauma
- Impaired skin integrity
- Overflow urinary incontinence
- Posttrauma syndrome
- Risk for aspiration
- Risk for constipation
- Risk for disuse syndrome
- Total urinary incontinence
- Unilateral neglect

Nutritional deficiencies
- Disturbed thought processes
- Imbalanced nutrition: Less than body requirements
- Impaired skin integrity
- Risk for impaired parenting
- Risk for infection

Obesity
- Imbalance nutrition: More than body requirements
- Readiness for enhanced nutrition
- Readiness for enhanced self-concept
- Risk for constipation

- Risk for impaired skin integrity
- Situational low self-esteem
- Stress urinary incontinence

Obsessive-compulsive disorder
- Anxiety
- Decisional conflict
- Disturbed personal identity
- Impaired home maintenance
- Ineffective coping
- Ineffective denial
- Insomnia
- Risk for impaired religiosity
- Risk for injury
- Risk for suicide
- Self-mutilation
- Sleep deprivation
- Social isolation

Organic brain syndrome
- Adult failure to thrive
- Risk for deficient fluid volume

Osteoarthritis
- Activity intolerance
- Acute pain
- Compromised family coping
- Deficient knowledge (specify)
- Disturbed body image
- Dressing or grooming self-care deficit
- Health-seeking behaviors
- Imbalance nutrition: More than body requirements
- Impaired home maintenance
- Impaired physical mobility
- Ineffective health maintenance
- Risk for falls
- Risk for injury

Osteomyelitis
- Acute pain
- Disturbed body image
- Impaired physical mobility
- Impaired skin integrity
- Ineffective coping
- Ineffective tissue perfusion (specify)
- Risk for infection
- Risk for injury

Osteoporosis

- Deficient knowledge (specify)
- Disturbed body image
- Fear
- Health-seeking behaviors
- Ineffective denial
- Ineffective sexuality patterns
- Loneliness
- Powerlessness
- Risk for falls
- Risk for injury
- Risk for trauma
- Social isolation

Ovarian cancer

- Constipation
- Death anxiety
- Fear
- Grieving
- Imbalanced nutrition: Less than body requirements
- Impaired tissue integrity
- Nausea
- Powerlessness
- Readiness for enhanced hope
- Risk for falls
- Spiritual distress
- Urinary retention

Panic disorder

- Anxiety
- Chronic low self-esteem
- Deficient knowledge (specify)
- Fear
- Ineffective coping
- Insomnia
- Powerlessness
- Risk for posttrauma syndrome
- Sleep deprivation

Paralysis

- Bowel incontinence
- Caregiver role strain
- Complicated grieving
- Compromised family coping
- Hopelessness
- Impaired physical mobility
- Impaired skin integrity

- Ineffective coping
- Ineffective health maintenance
- Ineffective role performance
- Ineffective sexuality patterns
- Powerlessness
- Reflex urinary incontinence
- Risk for caregiver role strain
- Risk for impaired skin integrity

Parkinson's disease
- Activity intolerance
- Bowel incontinence
- Chronic low self-esteem
- Compromised family coping
- Death anxiety
- Deficient knowledge (specify)
- Disturbed body image
- Disturbed sensory perception (tactile)
- Feeding self-care deficit
- Grieving
- Hopelessness
- Imbalanced nutrition: Less than body requirements
- Impaired home maintenance
- Impaired physical mobility
- Ineffective breathing pattern
- Ineffective coping
- Ineffective health maintenance
- Ineffective role performance
- Ineffective sexuality patterns
- Ineffective therapeutic regimen management
- Powerlessness
- Readiness for enhanced therapeutic regimen management
- Risk for aspiration
- Risk for caregiver role strain
- Risk for compromised human dignity
- Risk for injury
- Risk for loneliness
- Risk for urge urinary incontinence
- Social isolation

Passive-aggressive personality disorder
- Anxiety
- Disturbed personal identity
- Fear
- Ineffective coping

Pelvic inflammatory disease
- Acute pain
- Deficient fluid volume
- Sexual dysfunction

Pericarditis
- Activity intolerance
- Acute pain
- Anxiety
- Decreased cardiac output
- Ineffective tissue perfusion (cardiopulmonary)

Perinatal trauma
- Delayed growth and development
- Hypothermia
- Risk for injury

Peripheral vascular disease
- Activity intolerance
- Acute pain
- Deficient diversional activity
- Deficient knowledge (specify)
- Impaired physical mobility
- Impaired skin integrity
- Impaired tissue integrity
- Risk for falls
- Risk for impaired skin integrity
- Risk for infection
- Risk for injury
- Risk for peripheral neurovascular dysfunction

Peritoneal dialysis
- Defensive coping
- Deficient fluid volume
- Deficient knowledge (specify)
- Disturbed body image
- Excess fluid volume
- Imbalanced nutrition: Less than body requirements
- Interrupted family processes
- Risk for infection

Peritonitis
- Acute pain
- Anxiety
- Decreased cardiac output
- Deficient fluid volume
- Nausea
- Risk for infection

Personality disorders
- Decisional conflict
- Interrupted family processes
- Risk for loneliness
- Risk for self-directed violence
- Risk for suicide
- Sexual dysfunction
- Social isolation

Phobic disorder
- Anxiety
- Disturbed personal identity
- Fear
- Ineffective coping
- Powerlessness
- Risk for loneliness
- Social isolation

Placenta previa
- Anxiety
- Fear
- Ineffective denial

Pleural effusion
- Acute pain
- Dysfunctional ventilatory weaning response *
- Hyperthermia
- Ineffective breathing pattern
- Risk for infection

Pleurisy
- Acute pain
- Fatigue
- Impaired gas exchange
- Ineffective breathing pattern

Pneumonia
- Bathing or hygiene self-care deficit
- Deficient fluid volume
- Imbalanced nutrition: Less than body requirements
- Impaired gas exchange
- Impaired physical mobility
- Impaired spontaneous ventilation
- Impaired verbal communication
- Ineffective airway clearance
- Ineffective breathing pattern
- Ineffective tissue perfusion (cardiopulmonary)
- Readiness for enhanced sleep

a state in which an individual cannot adjust to lowered levels of mechanical ventilator support which interrupts & prolongs the weaning process.

- *risk for impaired respiratory function*
- *ineffective airway clearance*
- *ineffective breathing patterns*
- *impaired gas exchange*

- Risk for aspiration
- Risk for infection

Pneumothorax
- Anxiety
- Ineffective breathing pattern
- Fear
- Impaired gas exchange
- Acute pain
- Ineffective tissue perfusion (cardiopulmonary)
- Impaired spontaneous ventilation

Poisoning
- Contamination
- Delayed growth and development
- Disturbed sensory perception (olfactory)
- Disturbed sensory perception (tactile)
- Ineffective tissue perfusion (renal)
- Risk for aspiration
- Risk for injury
- Risk for poisoning

Polycystic kidney disease
- Acute pain
- Defensive coping
- Deficient knowledge (specify)
- Ineffective tissue perfusion (renal)
- Interrupted family processes
- Moral distress
- Risk for infection

Polycythemia vera
- Acute pain
- Disturbed sensory perception (visual)
- Impaired gas exchange
- Impaired skin integrity

Postpartum hemorrhage
- Anxiety
- Deficient fluid volume
- Ineffective tissue perfusion (cardiopulmonary)
- Ineffective tissue perfusion (cerebral)

Posttraumatic stress disorder
- Disturbed sensory perception
- Disturbed thought processes
- Hopelessness
- Posttrauma syndrome

- Powerlessness
- Risk for loneliness
- Risk for posttrauma syndrome
- Situational low self-esteem

Pregnancy
- Anxiety
- Deficient knowledge (specify)
- Impaired tissue integrity
- Ineffective coping
- Ineffective tissue perfusion (peripheral)
- Interrupted family processes
- Readiness for enhanced fluid balance
- Risk for constipation

Premature labor
- Anxiety
- Deficient knowledge (specify)
- Effective breast-feeding
- Impaired parenting
- Ineffective coping
- Risk for infection
- Situational low self-esteem

Premature rupture of membranes
- Deficient fluid volume
- Risk for infection

Prematurity
- Compromised family coping
- Delayed growth and development
- Disorganized infant behavior
- Hypothermia
- Imbalanced nutrition: Less than body requirements
- Impaired verbal communication
- Ineffective breast-feeding
- Ineffective breathing pattern
- Ineffective infant feeding pattern
- Ineffective thermoregulation
- Interrupted breast-feeding
- Readiness for enhanced parenting
- Risk for aspiration
- Risk for delayed development
- Risk for disorganized infant behavior
- Risk for impaired parent-infant-child attachment
- Risk for sudden infant death syndrome

Pressure ulcers
- Imbalanced nutrition: Less than body requirements
- Impaired physical mobility
- Impaired skin integrity
- Impaired tissue integrity
- Ineffective protection
- Risk for deficient fluid volume
- Risk for infection

Prolapsed intervertebral disk
- Acute pain
- Impaired physical mobility
- Reflex urinary incontinence
- Urinary retention

Prostate cancer
- Acute pain
- Chronic sorrow
- Impaired tissue integrity
- Sexual dysfunction
- Urinary retention

Prostatectomy
- Disturbed body image
- Impaired skin integrity
- Risk for infection
- Urinary retention

Pseudomembranous colitis
- Deficient fluid volume
- Diarrhea
- Impaired skin integrity
- Ineffective tissue perfusion (cardiopulmonary)
- Ineffective tissue perfusion (GI)
- Ineffective tissue perfusion (renal)

Psoriasis
- Disturbed body image
- Impaired skin integrity
- Powerlessness
- Risk for imbalanced body temperature
- Social isolation

Pulmonary edema
- Activity intolerance
- Bathing or hygiene self-care deficit
- Decreased cardiac output
- Dysfunctional ventilatory weaning response

- Excess fluid volume
- Fear
- Impaired gas exchange
- Impaired verbal communication
- Ineffective airway clearance
- Ineffective breathing pattern
- Ineffective tissue perfusion (cardiopulmonary)

Pulmonary embolus
- Acute pain
- Anxiety
- Activity intolerance
- Decreased cardiac output
- Deficient fluid volume
- Impaired gas exchange
- Impaired verbal communication
- Ineffective breathing pattern
- Ineffective tissue perfusion (cardiopulmonary)

Pyelonephritis
- Acute pain
- Excess fluid volume
- Impaired physical mobility
- Risk for infection

Pyloric stenosis
- Imbalanced nutrition: Less than body requirements
- Risk for aspiration
- Risk for imbalanced body temperature

Radiation therapy
- Acute pain
- Deficient fluid volume
- Diarrhea
- Imbalanced nutrition: Less than body requirements
- Impaired oral mucous membrane
- Impaired physical mobility
- Impaired tissue integrity
- Nausea
- Sexual dysfunction

Rape
- Anxiety
- Complicated grieving
- Fear
- Posttrauma syndrome
- Rape-trauma syndrome
- Rape-trauma syndrome: Compound reaction

- Rape-trauma syndrome: Silent reaction
- Risk for compromised human dignity
- Situational low self-esteem
- Social isolation

Raynaud's disease
- Deficient knowledge (specify)
- Disturbed sensory perception (tactile)
- Impaired tissue integrity
- Ineffective tissue perfusion (peripheral)
- Risk for impaired skin integrity

Renal calculi
- Acute pain
- Ineffective denial
- Risk for infection
- Urinary retention

Renal cancer
- Acute pain
- Deficient fluid volume

Renal disease: End-stage
- Caregiver role strain
- Chronic low self-esteem
- Decisional conflict
- Defensive coping
- Excess fluid volume
- Grieving
- Hopelessness
- Ineffective coping
- Ineffective denial
- Ineffective role performance
- Ineffective sexuality patterns
- Risk for caregiver role strain
- Risk for disuse syndrome
- Risk for infection
- Risk for poisoning
- Risk for spiritual distress
- Spiritual distress

Respiratory distress syndrome
- Impaired gas exchange
- Ineffective airway clearance
- Ineffective breathing pattern
- Ineffective thermoregulation
- Risk for infection

Reye's syndrome
- Decreased intracranial adaptive capacity
- Delayed growth and development
- Impaired physical mobility
- Ineffective thermoregulation

Rheumatic fever
- Acute pain
- Anxiety
- Decreased cardiac output
- Deficient knowledge (specify)
- Fatigue
- Hyperthermia
- Impaired gas exchange
- Impaired physical mobility
- Ineffective breathing pattern
- Risk for infection

Rheumatoid arthritis
- Activity intolerance
- Acute pain
- Deficient knowledge (specify)
- Disturbed body image
- Dressing or grooming self-care deficit
- Impaired physical mobility
- Ineffective coping
- Ineffective denial
- Ineffective health maintenance
- Ineffective protection
- Ineffective therapeutic regimen management
- Insomnia
- Risk for disuse syndrome
- Risk for falls
- Risk for injury
- Sexual dysfunction

Salmonella
- Constipation
- Diarrhea
- Hyperthermia
- Risk for deficient fluid volume
- Risk for infection
- Urinary retention

Sarcoidosis
- Activity intolerance
- Acute pain
- Decreased cardiac output

- Disturbed body image
- Impaired gas exchange
- Ineffective breathing pattern

Schizophrenia

- Anxiety
- Bathing or hygiene self-care deficit
- Caregiver role strain
- Disturbed sensory perception
- Disturbed thought processes
- Functional urinary incontinence
- Hopelessness
- Impaired home maintenance
- Impaired social interaction
- Ineffective coping
- Ineffective health maintenance
- Ineffective role performance
- Interrupted family processes
- Insomnia
- Risk for caregiver role strain
- Risk for injury
- Risk for poisoning
- Risk for self-directed violence
- Risk for suicide
- Sexual dysfunction
- Social isolation

Seizure disorders

- Anxiety
- Chronic low self-esteem
- Delayed growth and development
- Disturbed sensory perception (tactile)
- Impaired environmental interpretation syndrome
- Impaired memory
- Ineffective airway clearance
- Ineffective breathing pattern
- Ineffective coping
- Risk for delayed development
- Risk for spiritual distress
- Risk for trauma
- Social isolation

Self-destructive behavior

- Anxiety
- Chronic low self-esteem
- Ineffective denial
- Risk for poisoning
- Risk for self-directed violence

■ Risk for self-mutilation

Sepsis
■ Acute confusion
■ Acute pain
■ Diarrhea
■ Dysfunctional ventilatory weaning response
■ Hyperthermia
■ Hypothermia
■ Imbalanced nutrition: Less than body requirements
■ Impaired spontaneous ventilation
■ Ineffective thermoregulation

Sexual assault
■ Posttrauma syndrome
■ Rape-trauma syndrome
■ Rape-trauma syndrome: Compound reaction
■ Rape-trauma syndrome: Silent reaction
■ Risk for self-directed violence

Shaken baby syndrome
■ Impaired parenting
■ Risk for impaired parenting

Shock
■ Decreased cardiac output
■ Deficient fluid volume
■ Impaired gas exchange
■ Impaired oral mucous membrane
■ Impaired spontaneous ventilation
■ Ineffective airway clearance
■ Ineffective tissue perfusion (cardiopulmonary)
■ Ineffective tissue perfusion (cerebral)
■ Ineffective tissue perfusion (renal)
■ Risk for infection

Sickle cell anemia
■ Acute pain
■ Impaired gas exchange
■ Impaired physical mobility
■ Ineffective protection
■ Ineffective tissue perfusion (peripheral)
■ Ineffective tissue perfusion (renal)

Sjögren's syndrome
■ Acute pain
■ Disturbed sensory perception (gustatory)
■ Impaired oral mucous membrane

Somatic disorder
- Caregiver role strain

Spina bifida
- Latex allergy response
- Risk for latex allergy response

Spinal cord defects
- Chronic low self-esteem
- Delayed growth and development
- Impaired urinary elimination
- Overflow urinary incontinence
- Readiness for enhanced coping family
- Risk-prone health behavior
- Total urinary incontinence

Spinal cord injury
- Activity intolerance
- Autonomic dysreflexia
- Bathing or hygiene self-care deficit
- Bowel incontinence
- Chronic pain
- Chronic sorrow
- Complicated grieving
- Constipation
- Deficient diversional activity
- Deficient knowledge (specify)
- Delayed growth and development
- Disturbed body image
- Disturbed sensory perception
- Fear
- Hopelessness
- Impaired physical mobility
- Impaired spontaneous ventilation
- Impaired transfer ability
- Impaired urinary elimination
- Ineffective airway clearance
- Ineffective health maintenance
- Ineffective sexuality patterns
- Ineffective therapeutic regimen management
- Moral distress
- Posttrauma syndrome
- Powerlessness
- Readiness for enhanced communication
- Readiness for enhanced therapeutic regimen management
- Reflex urinary incontinence
- Risk for autonomic dysreflexia
- Risk for constipation

- Risk for delayed development
- Risk for disuse syndrome
- Risk for impaired skin integrity
- Risk for infection
- Risk for trauma
- Risk for urge urinary incontinence
- Risk-prone health behavior
- Sleep deprivation
- Social isolation
- Total urinary incontinence
- Urinary retention

Spinal tumor

- Autonomic dysreflexia
- Bowel incontinence
- Chronic low self-esteem
- Disturbed sensory perception (kinesthetic)
- Dressing or grooming self -care deficit
- Impaired physical mobility
- Impaired urinary elimination
- Ineffective breathing pattern
- Reflex urinary incontinence
- Risk for autonomic dysreflexia
- Risk for impaired skin integrity
- Risk for injury
- Risk for urge urinary incontinence
- Sexual dysfunction
- Situational low self-esteem
- Total urinary incontinence

Spouse abuse

- Anxiety
- Defensive coping
- Deficient knowledge (specify)
- Fear
- Posttrauma syndrome
- Rape-trauma syndrome
- Rape-trauma syndrome: Compound reaction
- Rape-trauma syndrome: Silent reaction
- Risk for other-directed violence
- Stress overload

Streptococcal throat

- Acute pain
- Hyperthermia
- Impaired oral mucous membrane
- Risk for infection

Stroke

- Acute confusion
- Bathing or hygiene self-care deficit
- Bowel incontinence
- Caregiver role strain
- Chronic confusion
- Chronic sorrow
- Compromised family coping
- Constipation
- Death anxiety
- Decreased intracranial adaptive capacity
- Deficient knowledge (specify)
- Disturbed body image
- Disturbed sensory perception (tactile)
- Fatigue
- Functional urinary incontinence
- Hopelessness
- Imbalance nutrition: More than body requirements
- Imbalanced nutrition: Less than body requirements
- Impaired environmental interpretation syndrome
- Impaired gas exchange
- Impaired home maintenance
- Impaired memory
- Impaired physical mobility
- Impaired social interaction
- Impaired swallowing
- Impaired urinary elimination
- Impaired verbal communication
- Impaired walking
- Ineffective airway clearance
- Ineffective breathing pattern
- Ineffective health maintenance
- Ineffective sexuality patterns
- Ineffective thermoregulation
- Ineffective tissue perfusion (cerebral)
- Interrupted family processes
- Powerlessness
- Readiness for enhanced family processes
- Risk for activity intolerance
- Risk for aspiration
- Risk for caregiver role strain
- Risk for compromised human dignity
- Risk for disuse syndrome
- Risk for impaired skin integrity
- Risk for injury
- Risk for poisoning
- Situational low self-esteem
- Sleep deprivation

- Social isolation
- Stress urinary incontinence
- Total urinary incontinence
- Unilateral neglect

Suicidal behavior
- Anxiety
- Chronic low self-esteem
- Ineffective denial
- Readiness for enhanced spiritual well-being
- Risk for poisoning
- Risk for self-directed violence
- Risk for self-mutilation

Syphilis
- Deficient knowledge (specify)
- Ineffective community coping
- Ineffective sexuality patterns
- Risk for infection
- Risk for injury

Tendinitis
- Activity intolerance
- Impaired physical mobility
- Ineffective role performance

Testicular cancer
- Acute pain
- Disturbed body image
- Fear
- Sexual dysfunction

Thoracic surgery
- Acute pain
- Deficient fluid volume
- Fatigue
- Fear
- Impaired gas exchange
- Ineffective airway clearance
- Ineffective breathing pattern
- Risk for infection

Thrombophlebitis
- Acute pain
- Impaired gas exchange
- Impaired skin integrity
- Ineffective tissue perfusion (peripheral)

- Risk for impaired skin integrity
- Risk for infection

Tracheoesophageal fistula
- Imbalanced nutrition: Less than body requirements
- Risk for aspiration

Tracheostomy
- Imbalanced nutrition: Less than body requirements
- Impaired skin integrity
- Impaired verbal communication

Transient ischemic attacks
- Acute confusion
- Disturbed sensory perception (tactile)
- Impaired environmental interpretation syndrome
- Impaired memory
- Ineffective tissue perfusion (cerebral)

Trauma
- Death anxiety
- Disabled family coping
- Disturbed sensory perception (auditory)
- Energy field disturbance
- Risk for self-directed violence

Trigeminal neuralgia
- Acute pain
- Anxiety
- Deficient knowledge (specify)
- Imbalanced nutrition: Less than body requirements

Tuberculosis
- Fatigue
- Fear
- Impaired dentition
- Impaired gas exchange
- Ineffective airway clearance
- Ineffective breathing pattern
- Risk for infection
- Risk for loneliness
- Social isolation

Urinary calculi
- Acute pain
- Anxiety

- Impaired urinary elimination
- Ineffective tissue perfusion (renal)
- Readiness for enhanced urinary elimination
- Risk for infection

Urinary diversion
- Acute pain
- Constipation
- Disturbed personal identity
- Grieving
- Impaired skin integrity
- Ineffective breathing pattern
- Ineffective sexuality patterns
- Infection
- Sexual dysfunction

Urinary incontinence
- Anxiety
- Functional urinary incontinence
- Impaired skin integrity
- Overflow urinary incontinence
- Reflex urinary incontinence
- Social isolation
- Stress urinary incontinence
- Total urinary incontinence

Urinary tract infection
- Acute pain
- Impaired urinary elimination
- Readiness for enhanced urinary elimination
- Risk for infection
- Risk for urge urinary incontinence
- Stress urinary incontinence
- Urge urinary incontinence

Uterine prolapse
- Disturbed body image
- Stress urinary incontinence

Uterine rupture
- Acute pain
- Deficient fluid volume
- Ineffective tissue perfusion (cardiopulmonary)
- Ineffective tissue perfusion (cerebral)
- Ineffective tissue perfusion (renal)

Vascular insufficiency
- Impaired tissue integrity
- Risk for peripheral neurovascular dysfunction

Viral hepatitis
- Deficient fluid volume
- Imbalanced nutrition: Less than body requirements
- Impaired skin integrity
- Risk for impaired skin integrity
- Risk for infection
- Social isolation

S+S of liver problems:
- jaundice = skin turns yellow or orange; white portion of eye turns yellow — caused by increased bilirubin in blood

- dark colored urine or tea colored urine
- excessive thirst (polydypsia)
- frequent urination (polyuria)
- enlargement + bloating of abdomen — accompanied by abdominal pain
- lack of color + pigmentation of stool — caused by decrease in the production of bile by the liver
- lack of appetite — leads to anemia + weight loss
- nausea + vomiting

Other signs:
dizziness
headaches
achy eyes
low fever
constipation
fatigue
lethargy

Gordon's functional health patterns

Gordon has described a functional health pattern system to help identify and formulate nursing diagnoses. Based on general categories, this system permits easy organization of basic nursing information obtained during the initial assessment. Flexible and adaptable, these functional health patterns can be used for patients in various states of health and illness, in all age-groups, and in all clinical specialties. Here's a brief outline of Gordon's functional health patterns.

Learning to incorporate Gordon's concepts into your assessment format may require time and practice; however, the rewards of understanding the patient and identifying specific areas where you can intervene are well worth the effort. When using these health pattern categories, obtain the nursing history from the patient's perspective through a series of specific questions designed to elicit information in an organized manner.

1. Health perception and health management pattern
- General health
- Health practices
- Concerns about illness
- Responsibility for health restoration and maintenance

2. Nutritional and metabolic pattern
- Daily food and fluid intake
- Weight loss or gain
- Appetite
- Dietary restrictions
- Healing potential of skin wounds or lesions
- General body status or condition

3. Elimination pattern
- Bowel elimination pattern or problem
- Urinary elimination pattern or problem
- Perspiration pattern or problem

4. Activity and exercise pattern
- Energy level
- Exercise pattern
- Perceived ability for (use Functional level code*, page 947):
_____Bathing
_____Bed mobility
_____Cooking

_____Dressing
_____Feeding
_____General mobility
_____Grooming
_____Home maintenance
_____Shopping
_____Toileting

5. Sleep and rest pattern
- Sleep problems
- Rested or not rested after sleep
- Use of sleep aids

6.Cognitive and perceptual pattern
- Sensory status: Visual, auditory, olfactory, tactile, gustatory
- Memory
- Intelligence
- Pain or discomfort

7. Self-perception and self-concept pattern
- Feelings about self
- Body image
- Self-esteem
- Emotional state

8. Role and relationship pattern
- Living arrangement
- Family or significant others
- Communication
- Role and responsibilities in family
- Socialization
- Finances

9. Sexuality and reproductive pattern
- Sexual relations
- Sexual satisfaction or dissatisfaction
- Contraceptive use and problems
- Reproductive and menstrual history

10. Coping and stress-tolerance pattern
- Stressors
- Coping mechanisms
- Major life changes
- Problem management

11. Value and belief pattern
- Satisfaction with life
- Spirituality and religious beliefs

- Religious practices
- Conflicts

12. Other
- Concerns not already discussed

NURSING DIAGNOSES AND GORDON'S FUNCTIONAL HEALTH PATTERNS

1. Health perception and health management pattern
- Autonomic dysreflexia
- Contamination
- Delayed surgical recovery
- Effective therapeutic regimen management
- Health-seeking behaviors
- Ineffective community therapeutic regimen management
- Ineffective family therapeutic regimen management
- Ineffective health maintenance
- Ineffective protection
- Ineffective therapeutic regimen management
- Latex allergy response
- Noncompliance
- Readiness for enhanced immunization status
- Readiness for enhanced therapeutic regimen management
- Risk for autonomic dysreflexia
- Risk for contamination
- Risk for delayed development
- Risk for disproportionate growth
- Risk for disuse syndrome
- Risk for impaired liver function
- Risk for infection
- Risk for latex allergy response
- Risk for poisoning
- Risk for sudden infant death syndrome
- Risk for suffocation
- Risk for trauma
- Risk for injury

2. Nutritional and metabolic pattern
- Deficient fluid volume
- Effective breast-feeding
- Excess fluid volume
- Hyperthermia
- Hypothermia
- Imbalanced nutrition: Less than body requirements
- Imbalanced nutrition: More than body requirements
- Impaired dentition

- Impaired oral mucous membrane
- Impaired skin integrity
- Impaired swallowing
- Impaired tissue integrity
- Ineffective breast-feeding
- Ineffective infant feeding pattern
- Ineffective thermoregulation
- Interrupted breast-feeding
- Nausea
- Readiness for enhanced fluid volume
- Readiness for enhanced nutrition
- Risk for deficient fluid volume
- Risk for imbalanced body temperature
- Risk for imbalanced fluid volume
- Risk for imbalanced nutrition: More than body requirements
- Risk for impaired skin integrity
- Risk for unstable glucose level

3. Elimination pattern
- Bowel incontinence
- Constipation
- Diarrhea
- Functional urinary incontinence
- Impaired urinary elimination
- Overflow urinary incontinence
- Perceived constipation
- Readiness for enhanced urinary elimination
- Reflex urinary incontinence
- Risk for constipation
- Risk for urge urinary incontinence
- Stress urinary incontinence
- Total urinary incontinence
- Urge urinary incontinence
- Urinary retention

4. Activity and exercise pattern
- Activity intolerance
- Bathing or hygiene self-care deficit
- Decreased cardiac output
- Decreased intracranial adaptive capacity
- Deficient diversional activity
- Dressing or grooming self-care deficit
- Dysfunctional ventilatory weaning response
- Energy field disturbance
- Feeding self-care deficit
- Impaired bed mobility
- Impaired gas exchange
- Impaired home maintenance

- Impaired physical mobility
- Impaired spontaneous ventilation
- Impaired transfer ability
- Impaired walking
- Impaired wheelchair mobility
- Ineffective airway clearance
- Ineffective breathing pattern
- Ineffective tissue perfusion
- Readiness for enhanced self-care
- Risk for activity intolerance
- Risk for aspiration
- Risk for falls
- Risk for perioperative-positioning injury
- Risk for peripheral neurovascular dysfunction
- Sedentary lifestyle
- Toileting self-care deficit
- Unilateral neglect

5. Sleep and rest pattern

- Fatigue
- Insomnia
- Readiness for enhanced sleep
- Sleep deprivation

6. Cognitive and perceptual pattern

- Acute confusion
- Acute pain
- Chronic confusion
- Chronic pain
- Deficient knowledge (specify)
- Disorganized infant behavior
- Disturbed sensory perception (specify)
- Disturbed thought processes
- Impaired environmental interpretation syndrome
- Impaired memory
- Readiness for enhanced comfort
- Readiness for enhanced decision-making
- Readiness for enhanced knowledge
- Readiness for enhanced organized infant behavior
- Risk for acute confusion
- Risk for disorganized infant behavior
- Wandering

7. Self-perception and self-concept pattern

- Anxiety
- Chronic low self-esteem
- Complicated grieving
- Death anxiety

- Disturbed body image
- Disturbed personal identity
- Fear
- Hopelessness
- Powerlessness
- Readiness for enhanced hope
- Readiness for enhanced power
- Readiness for enhanced self-concept
- Risk for complicated grieving
- Risk for other-directed violence
- Risk for powerlessness
- Risk for self-directed violence
- Risk for self-mutilation
- Risk for situational low self-esteem
- Risk for suicide
- Risk-prone health behavior
- Self-mutilation
- Situational low self-esteem

8. Role and relationship pattern
- Complicated grieving
- Dysfunctional family processes: Alcoholism
- Grieving
- Impaired parenting
- Impaired social interaction
- Impaired verbal communication
- Ineffective role performance
- Interrupted family processes
- Parental role conflict
- Readiness for enhanced communication
- Readiness for enhanced parenting
- Readiness for enhanced family processes
- Risk for impaired parent-infant-child attachment
- Risk for impaired parenting
- Risk for loneliness
- Social isolation

9. Sexuality and reproductive pattern
- Ineffective sexuality patterns
- Rape-trauma syndrome
- Rape-trauma syndrome: Compound reaction
- Rape-trauma syndrome: Silent reaction
- Sexual dysfunction

10. Coping and stress-tolerance pattern
- Adult failure to thrive
- Caregiver role strain
- Chronic sorrow

- Complicated grieving
- Compromised family coping
- Decisional conflict
- Defensive coping
- Delayed growth and development
- Disabled family coping
- Ineffective community coping
- Ineffective coping
- Ineffective denial
- Posttrauma syndrome
- Readiness for enhanced community coping
- Readiness for enhanced coping
- Readiness for enhanced family coping
- Relocation stress syndrome
- Risk for caregiver role strain
- Risk for posttrauma syndrome
- Risk for relocation stress syndrome
- Stress overload

11. Value and belief pattern
- Impaired religiosity
- Moral distress
- Readiness for enhanced religiosity
- Readiness for enhanced spiritual well-being
- Risk for compromised human dignity
- Risk for impaired religiosity
- Risk for spiritual distress
- Spiritual distress

Functional level code
0 = Completely independent
1 = Requires use of equipment or device
2 = Requires help, supervision, or teaching from another person
3 = Requires help from another person and equipment or device
4 = Dependent; doesn't participate in activity

Taxonomy II domains, classes, and diagnoses

DOMAIN 1 HEALTH PROMOTION

The awareness of well-being or normality of function and the strategies used to maintain control of and enhance that well-being or normality of function

Class 1 Health Awareness Recognition of normal function and well-being

Class 2 Health Management Identifying, controlling, performing, and integrating activities to maintain health and well-being

Approved diagnoses

00082	*Effective therapeutic regimen management*
00078	*Ineffective therapeutic regimen management*
00080	*Ineffective family therapeutic regimen management*
00081	*Ineffective community therapeutic regimen management*
00084	*Health-seeking behaviors (specify)*
00099	*Ineffective health maintenance*
00098	*Impaired home maintenance*
00162	*Readiness for enhanced therapeutic regimen management*
00163	*Readiness for enhanced nutrition*
00186	*Readiness for enhanced immunization status*

DOMAIN 2 NUTRITION

The activities of taking in, assimilating, and using nutrients for the purposes of tissue maintenance, tissue repair, and the production of energy

Class 1 Ingestion Taking food or nutrients into the body

Approved diagnoses

00107	*Ineffective infant feeding pattern*
00103	*Impaired swallowing*
00002	*Imbalanced nutrition: Less than body requirements*
00001	*Imbalanced nutrition: More than body requirements*
00003	*Risk for imbalanced nutrition: More than body requirements*

Class 2 Digestion The physical and chemical activities that convert foodstuffs into substances suitable for absorption and assimilation

Class 3 Absorption The act of taking up nutrients through body tissues

Class 4 Metabolism The chemical and physical processes occurring in living organisms and cells for the development and use of protoplasm, production of waste and energy, with the release of energy for all vital processes

Approved diagnoses

00178	*Risk for impaired liver function*
00179	*Risk for unstable glucose level*

Class 5 *Hydration* The taking in and absorption of fluids and electrolytes

Approved diagnoses

00027	*Deficient fluid volume*
00028	*Risk for deficient fluid volume*
00026	*Excess fluid volume*
00025	*Risk for imbalanced fluid volume*
00160	*Readiness for enhanced fluid balance*

DOMAIN 3 ELIMINATION/EXCHANGE

Secretion and excretion of waste products from the body

Class 1 *Urinary Function* The process of secretion, reabsorption, and excretion of urine

Approved diagnoses

00016	*Impaired urinary elimination*
00023	*Urinary retention*
00021	*Total urinary incontinence*
00020	*Functional urinary incontinence*
00017	*Stress urinary incontinence*
00019	*Urge urinary incontinence*
00018	*Reflex urinary incontinence*
00022	*Risk for urge urinary incontinence*
00166	*Readiness for enhanced urinary elimination*
00176	*Overflow urinary incontinence*

Class 2 *Gastrointestinal Function* The process of absorption and secretion of the end products of digestion

Approved diagnoses

00014	*Bowel incontinence*
00013	*Diarrhea*
00011	*Constipation*
00015	*Risk for constipation*
00012	*Perceived constipation*

Class 3 *Integumentary Function* The process of secretion and excretion through the skin

Class 4 *Respiratory Function* The process of exchange of gases and removal of the end products of metabolism

Approved diagnosis

00030	*Impaired gas exchange*

DOMAIN 4 ACTIVITY/REST

The production, conservation, expenditure, or balance of energy resources

Class 1 Sleep/Rest Slumber, repose, ease, relaxation, or inactivity

Approved diagnoses

00096	*Sleep deprivation*
00165	*Readiness for enhanced sleep*
00095	*Insomnia*

Class 2 Activity/Exercise Moving parts of the body (mobility), doing work, or performing actions often (but not always) against resistance

Approved diagnoses

00040	*Risk for disuse syndrome*
00085	*Impaired physical mobility*
00091	*Impaired bed mobility*
00089	*Impaired wheelchair mobility*
00090	*Impaired transfer ability*
00088	*Impaired walking*
00097	*Deficient diversional activity*
00100	*Delayed surgical recovery*
00168	*Sedentary lifestyle*

Class 3 Energy Balance A dynamic state of harmony between intake and expenditure of resources

Approved diagnoses

00050 *Energy field disturbance*
00093 *Fatigue*

Class 4 Cardiovascular/Pulmonary Responses Cardiopulmonary mechanisms that support activity/rest

Approved diagnoses

00029	*Decreased cardiac output*
00033	*Impaired spontaneous ventilation*
00032	*Ineffective breathing pattern*
00092	*Activity intolerance*
00094	*Risk for activity intolerance*
00034	*Dysfunctional ventilatory weaning response*
00024	*Ineffective tissue perfusion (specify type: renal, cerebral, cardiopulmonary, gastrointestinal, peripheral)*

Class 5 Self-Care Ability to perform activities to care for one's body and bodily functions

Approved diagnoses

00109	*Dressing/grooming self-care deficit*
00108	*Bathing/hygiene self-care deficit*
00102	*Feeding self-care deficit*

00110   *Toileting self-care deficit*
00182   *Readiness for enhanced self-care*

DOMAIN 5 PERCEPTION/COGNITION

The human information processing system including attention, orientation, sensation, perception, cognition, and communication

Class 1 Attention Mental readiness to notice or observe

Approved diagnosis
00123   *Unilateral neglect*

Class 2 Orientation Awareness of time, place, and person

Approved diagnoses
00127   *Impaired environmental interpretation syndrome*
00154   *Wandering*

Class 3 Sensation/Perception Receiving information through the senses of touch, taste, smell, vision, hearing, and kinesthesia and the comprehension of sense data resulting in naming, associating, and/or pattern recognition

Approved diagnosis
00122   *Disturbed sensory perception (specify: visual, auditory, kinesthetic, gustatory, tactile)*

Class 4 Cognition Use of memory, learning, thinking, problem solving, abstraction, judgment, insight, intellectual capacity, calculation, and language

Approved diagnoses
00126   *Deficient knowledge (specify)*
00161   *Readiness for enhanced knowledge (specify)*
00128   *Acute confusion*
00129   *Chronic confusion*
00131   *Impaired memory*
00130   *Disturbed thought processes*
00184   *Readiness for enhanced decision making*
00173   *Risk for acute confusion*

Class 5 Communication Sending and receiving verbal and nonverbal information

Approved diagnoses
00051   *Impaired verbal communication*
00157   *Readiness for enhanced communication*

DOMAIN 6 SELF-PERCEPTION

Awareness about the self

Class 1 Self-Concept The perception(s) about the total self

Approved diagnoses

00121	*Disturbed personal identity*
00125	*Powerlessness*
00152	*Risk for powerlessness*
00124	*Hopelessness*
00054	*Risk for loneliness*
00167	*Readiness for enhanced self-concept*
00187	*Readiness for enhanced power*
00174	*Risk for compromised human dignity*
00185	*Readiness for enhanced hope*

Class 2 Self-Esteem Assessment of one's own worth, capability, significance, and success

Approved diagnoses

00119	*Chronic low self-esteem*
00120	*Situational low self-esteem*
00153	*Risk for situational low self-esteem*

Class 3 Body Image A mental image of one's own body

Approved diagnosis

00118	*Disturbed body image*

DOMAIN 7 ROLE RELATIONSHIPS

The positive and negative connections or associations between people or groups of people and the means by which those connections are demonstrated

Class 1 Caregiving Roles Socially expected behavior patterns by people providing care who aren't health care professionals

Approved diagnoses

00061	*Caregiver role strain*
00062	*Risk for caregiver role strain*
00056	*Impaired parenting*
00057	*Risk for impaired parenting*
00164	*Readiness for enhanced parenting*

Class 2 Family Relationships Associations of people who are biologically related or related by choice

Approved diagnoses

00060	*Interrupted family processes*
00159	*Readiness for enhanced family processes*
00063	*Dysfunctional family processes: Alcoholism*
00058	*Risk for impaired parent/infant/child attachment*

Class 3 Role Performance Quality of functioning in socially expected behavior patterns

Approved diagnoses

00106	*Effective breast-feeding*
00104	*Ineffective breast-feeding*
00105	*Interrupted breast-feeding*
00055	*Ineffective role performance*
00064	*Parental role conflict*
00052	*Impaired social interaction*

DOMAIN 8 SEXUALITY

Sexual identity, sexual function, and reproduction

Class 1 Sexual Identity The state of being a specific person in regard to sexuality and/or gender

Class 2 Sexual Function The capacity or ability to participate in sexual activities

Approved diagnoses

00059	*Sexual dysfunction*
00065	*Ineffective sexuality pattern*

Class 3 Reproduction Any process by which human beings are produced

DOMAIN 9 COPING/STRESS TOLERANCE

Contending with life events/life processes

Class 1 Post-Trauma Responses Reactions occurring after physical or psychological trauma

Approved diagnoses

00114	*Relocation stress syndrome*
00149	*Risk for relocation stress syndrome*
00142	*Rape-trauma syndrome*
00144	*Rape-trauma syndrome: Silent reaction*
00143	*Rape-trauma syndrome: Compound reaction*
00141	*Posttrauma syndrome*
00145	*Risk for posttrauma syndrome*

Class 2 Coping Responses The process of managing environmental stress

Approved diagnoses

00148	*Fear*
00146	*Anxiety*
00147	*Death anxiety*
00137	*Chronic sorrow*
00072	*Ineffective denial*
00136	*Grieving*
00135	*Complicated grieving*
00069	*Ineffective coping*

00073	Disabled family coping
00074	Compromised family coping
00071	Defensive coping
00077	Ineffective community coping
00158	Readiness for enhanced coping (individual)
00075	Readiness for enhanced family coping
00076	Readiness for enhanced community coping
00172	Risk for complicated grieving
00177	Stress overload
00188	Risk-prone health behavior

Class 3 Neurobehavioral Stress Behavioral responses reflecting nerve and brain function

Approved diagnoses

00009	Autonomic dysreflexia
00010	Risk for autonomic dysreflexia
00116	Disorganized infant behavior
00115	Risk for disorganized infant behavior
00117	Readiness for enhanced organized infant behavior
00049	Decreased intracranial adaptive capacity

DOMAIN 10 LIFE PRINCIPLES

Principles underlying conduct, thought, and behavior about acts, customs, or institutions viewed as being true or having intrinsic worth

Class 1 Values The identification and ranking of preferred modes of conduct or end states

Approved diagnosis

00185	Readiness for enhanced hope

Class 2 Beliefs Opinions, expectations, or judgments about acts, customs, or institutions viewed as being true or having intrinsic worth

Approved diagnoses

00068	Readiness for enhanced spiritual well-being
00185	Readiness for enhanced hope

Class 3 Value/Belief/Action Congruence The correspondence or balance achieved between values, beliefs, and actions

Approved diagnoses

00066	Spiritual distress
00067	Risk for spiritual distress
00083	Decisional conflict (specify)
00079	Noncompliance (specify)
00170	Risk for impaired religiosity
00169	Impaired religiosity

00171   *Readiness for enhanced religiosity*
00175   *Moral distress*
00184   *Readiness for enhanced decision making*

DOMAIN 11 SAFETY/PROTECTION

Freedom from danger, physical injury, or immune system damage; preservation from loss; and protection of safety and security

Class 1 Infection Host responses following pathogenic invasion

Approved diagnoses
00004   *Risk for infection*
00186   *Readiness for enhanced immunization status*

Class 2 Physical Injury Bodily harm or hurt

Approved diagnoses
00045   *Impaired oral mucous membrane*
00035   *Risk for injury*
00087   *Risk for perioperative positioning injury*
00155   *Risk for falls*
00038   *Risk for trauma*
00046   *Impaired skin integrity*
00047   *Risk for impaired skin integrity*
00044   *Impaired tissue integrity*
00048   *Impaired dentition*
00036   *Risk for suffocation*
00039   *Risk for aspiration*
00031   *Ineffective airway clearance*
00086   *Risk for peripheral neurovascular disfunction*
00043   *Ineffective protection*
00156   *Risk for sudden infant death syndrome*

Class 3 Violence The exertion of excessive force or power so as to cause injury or abuse

Approved diagnoses
00139   *Risk for self-mutilation*
00151   *Self-mutilation*
00138   *Risk for other-directed violence*
00140   *Risk for self-directed violence*
00150   *Risk for suicide*

Class 4 Environmental Hazards Sources of danger in the surroundings

Approved diagnoses
00037   *Risk for poisoning*
00180   *Risk for contamination*
00181   *Contamination*

Class 5 Defensive Processes The process by which the self protects itself from the nonself

Approved diagnoses

00041	*Latex allergy response*
00042	*Risk for latex allergy response*
00186	*Readiness for enhanced immunization status*

Class 6 Thermoregulation The physiologic process of regulating heat and energy within the body for purposes of protecting the organism

Approved diagnoses

00005	*Risk for imbalanced body temperature*
00008	*Ineffective thermoregulation*
00006	*Hypothermia*
00007	*Hyperthermia*

DOMAIN 12 COMFORT

Sense of mental, physical, or social well-being or ease

Class 1 Physical Comfort Sense of well-being or ease and/or freedom from pain

Approved diagnoses

00132	*Acute pain*
00133	*Chronic pain*
00134	*Nausea*
00183	*Readiness for enhanced comfort*

Class 2 Environmental Comfort Sense of well-being or ease in/with one's environment

Approved diagnosis

00183	*Readiness for enhanced comfort*

Class 3 Social Comfort Sense of well-being or ease with one's social situations

Approved diagnosis

00053	*Social isolation*

DOMAIN 13 GROWTH/DEVELOPMENT

Age-appropriate increases in physical dimensions, maturation of organ systems, and/or progression through the developmental milestones

Class 1 Growth Increases in physical dimensions or maturity of organ systems

Approved diagnoses

00111	*Delayed growth and development*
00113	*Risk for disproportionate growth*
00101	*Adult failure to thrive*

Class 2 Development Progression or regression through a sequence of recognized milestones in life

Approved diagnoses
00111   *Delayed growth and development*
00112   *Risk for delayed development*

Reprinted with permission from *NANDA-I, Nursing Diagnoses: Definitions & Classification 2007-2008*. Philadelphia: NANDA International, 2007.

NNN taxonomy of nursing practice: Placement of nursing diagnoses

DOMAINS	CLASSES
I. Functional Includes diagnoses, outcomes, and interventions to promote basic needs	*Activity/Exercise*
	Comfort
	Growth and Development
	Nutrition
	Self-Care

DIAGNOSES, OUTCOMES, AND INTERVENTIONS	NANDA-I NURSING DIAGNOSES
Physical activity, including energy conservation and expenditure	*Activity intolerance* *Risk for activity intolerance* *Risk for disuse syndrome* *Risk for falls* *Fatigue* *Impaired bed mobility* *Impaired physical mobility* *Impaired wheelchair mobility* *Impaired transfer ability* *Impaired walking* *Sedentary lifestyle*
A sense of emotional, physical, and spiritual well-being and relative freedom from distress	*Nausea* *Acute pain* *Chronic pain* *Energy field disturbance* *Readiness for enhanced comfort*
Physical, emotional, and social growth and development milestones	*Risk for delayed development* *Adult failure to thrive* *Delayed growth and development* *Risk for disproportionate growth* *Disorganized infant behavior* *Risk for disorganized infant behavior* *Readiness for enhanced organized infant behavior*
Processes related to taking in, assimilating, and using nutrients	*Effective breast-feeding* *Ineffective breast-feeding* *Interrupted breast-feeding* *Ineffective infant feeding pattern* *Imbalanced nutrition: Less than body requirements* *Imbalanced nutrition: More than body requirements* *Risk for imbalanced nutrition: More than body requirements* *Readiness for enhanced nutrition* *Impaired swallowing*
Ability to accomplish basic and instrumental activities of daily living	*Bathing/hygiene self-care deficit* *Dressing/grooming self-care deficit* *Feeding self-care deficit* *Toileting self-care deficit* *Readiness for enhanced self-care*

(continued)

NNN taxonomy of nursing practice: Placement of nursing diagnoses *(continued)*

DOMAINS	CLASSES
I. Functional *(continued)*	*Sexuality*
	Sleep/Rest
	Values/Beliefs
II. Physiological Includes diagnoses, outcomes, and interventions to promote optimal biophysical health	*Cardiac Function*
	Elimination
	Fluid & Electrolyte

DIAGNOSES, OUTCOMES, AND INTERVENTIONS	NANDA-I NURSING DIAGNOSES
Maintenance or modification of sexual identity and patterns	*Sexual dysfunction* *Ineffective sexuality patterns*
The quantity and quality of sleep, rest and relaxation patterns	*Sleep deprivation* *Insomnia* *Readiness for enhanced sleep*
Ideas, goals, perceptions, spiritual and other beliefs that influence choices or decisions	*Spiritual distress* *Risk for spiritual distress* *Readiness for enhanced spiritual well-being* *Impaired religiosity* *Risk for impaired religiosity* *Readiness for enhanced religiosity* *Moral distress*
Cardiac mechanisms used to maintain tissue profusion	*Decreased cardiac output* *Ineffective tissue perfusion*
Processes related to secretion and excretion of body wastes	*Bowel incontinence* *Constipation* *Perceived constipation* *Risk for constipation* *Diarrhea* *Functional urinary incontinence* *Reflex urinary incontinence* *Stress urinary incontinence* *Total urinary incontinence* *Urge urinary incontinence* *Risk for urge urinary incontinence* *Impaired urinary elimination* *Urinary retention* *Readiness for enhanced urinary elimination* *Overflow incontinence*
Regulation of fluids/electrolytes and acid-base balance	*Deficient fluid volume* *Excess fluid volume* *Risk for deficient fluid volume* *Risk for imbalanced fluid volume* *Readiness for enhanced fluid balance*

(continued)

NNN taxonomy of nursing practice: Placement of nursing diagnoses *(continued)*

DOMAINS	CLASSES
II. Physiological *(continued)*	*Neurocognition*
	Pharmacological Function
	Physical Regulation
	Reproduction
	Respiratory Function
	Sensation/Perception

Diagnoses, outcomes, and interventions	**NANDA-I nursing diagnoses**
Mechanisms related to the nervous system and neurocognitive functioning, including memory, thinking, and judgment	*Autonomic dysreflexia* *Risk for autonomic dysreflexia* *Acute confusion* *Chronic confusion* *Risk for acute confusion* *Impaired environmental interpretation syndrome* *Decreased intracranial adaptive capacity* *Impaired memory* *Unilateral neglect* *Disturbed thought processes* *Wandering*
Effects (therapeutic and adverse) of medications or drugs and other pharmacologically active products	
Body temperature, endocrine, and immune system responses to regulate cellular processes	*Latex allergy response* *Risk for latex allergy response* *Risk for imbalanced body temperature* *Hyperthermia* *Hypothermia* *Ineffective thermoregulation* *Risk for infection* *Risk for peripheral neurovascular dysfunction* *Ineffective protection* *Risk for unstable blood sugar* *Risk for impaired liver function*
Processes related to human procreation and birth	
Ventilation adequate to maintain arterial blood gases within normal limits	*Ineffective airway clearance* *Risk for aspiration* *Ineffective breathing pattern* *Impaired gas exchange* *Risk for suffocation* *Impaired spontaneous ventilation* *Dysfunctional ventilatory weaning response*
Intake and interpretation of information through the senses, including seeing, hearing, touching, tasting, smelling	*Disturbed sensory perception*

(continued)

NNN taxonomy of nursing practice: Placement of nursing diagnoses *(continued)*

DOMAINS	CLASSES
II. Physiological *(continued)*	*Tissue Integrity*
III. Psychosocial Includes diagnoses, outcomes, and interventions to promote optimal mental and emotional health and social functioning	*Behavior*
	Communication
	Coping

DIAGNOSES, OUTCOMES, AND INTERVENTIONS	NANDA-I NURSING DIAGNOSES
Skin and mucous membrane protection to support secretion, excretion, and healing	*Impaired dentition* *Impaired oral mucous membrane* *Impaired skin integrity* *Risk for impaired skin integrity* *Impaired tissue integrity*
Actions that promote, maintain, or restore health	*Ineffective health maintenance* *Health-seeking behaviors* *Noncompliance* *Effective therapeutic regimen management* *Ineffective therapeutic regimen management* *Ineffective community therapeutic regimen management* *Ineffective family therapeutic regimen management* *Readiness for enhanced therapeutic regimen management*
Receiving, interpreting, and expressing spoken, written, and nonverbal messages	*Impaired verbal communication* *Readiness for enhanced communication*
Adjusting or adapting to stressful events	*Risk-prone health behavior* *Decisional conflict* *Ineffective coping* *Ineffective community coping* *Readiness for enhanced community coping* *Defensive coping* *Compromised family coping* *Disabled family coping* *Readiness for enhanced family coping* *Ineffective denial* *Grieving* *Complicated grieving* *Risk for complicated grieving* *Posttrauma syndrome* *Risk for posttrauma syndrome* *Rape-trauma syndrome* *Rape-trauma syndrome: Compound reaction* *Rape-trauma syndrome: Silent reaction* *Relocation stress syndrome* *Risk for relocation stress syndrome* *Self-mutilation*

(continued)

NNN taxonomy of nursing practice: Placement of nursing diagnoses *(continued)*

DOMAINS	CLASSES
III. Psychosocial *(continued)*	*Coping (continued)*
	Emotional
	Knowledge
	Roles/Relationships
	Self-Perception

DIAGNOSES, OUTCOMES, AND INTERVENTIONS	NANDA-I NURSING DIAGNOSES
	Risk for self-mutilation *Risk for suicide* *Risk for self-directed violence* *Readiness for enhanced coping* *Stress overload* *Readiness for enhanced decision making*
A mental state or feeling that may influence perceptions of the world	*Anxiety* *Death anxiety* *Fear* *Hopelessness* *Chronic sorrow* *Readiness for enhanced hope*
Understanding and skill in applying information to promote, maintain, and restore health	*Deficient knowledge (specify)* *Readiness for enhanced knowledge (specify)*
Maintenance and/or modification of expected social behaviors and emotional connectedness with others	*Risk for impaired parent/child attachment* *Caregiver role strain* *Risk for caregiver role strain* *Parental role conflict* *Dysfunctional family processes: Alcoholism* *Interrupted family processes* *Impaired parenting* *Risk for impaired parenting* *Ineffective role performance* *Impaired social interaction* *Social isolation* *Risk for other-directed violence* *Readiness for enhanced family processes* *Readiness for enhanced parenting*
Awareness of one's body and personal identity	*Disturbed body image* *Disturbed personal identity* *Risk for loneliness* *Powerlessness* *Risk for powerlessness* *Chronic low self-esteem* *Situational low self-esteem* *Risk for situational low self-esteem* *Readiness for enhanced self-concept* *Readiness for enhanced power* *Risk for compromised human dignity*

(continued)

NNN taxonomy of nursing practice: Placement of nursing diagnoses *(continued)*

DOMAINS	CLASSES
IV. Environmental Includes diagnoses, outcomes, and interventions to promote and protect the environmental health and safety of individuals, systems, and communities	*Healthcare System*
	Populations
	Risk Management

Reprinted with permission from *NANDA-I, Nursing Diagnoses: Definitions & Classification 2007-2008.* Philadelphia: NANDA International, 2007.

DIAGNOSES, OUTCOMES, AND INTERVENTIONS	NANDA-I NURSING DIAGNOSES
Social, political, and economic structures and processes for the delivery of health-care services	
Aggregates of individuals or communities having characteristics in common	
Avoidance of identifiable health threats	*Impaired home maintenance* *Risk for injury* *Risk for perioperative-positioning injury* *Risk for poisoning* *Risk for trauma* *Risk for sudden infant death syndrome* *Readiness for enhanced immunization* *Contamination* *Risk for contamination* **Unable to place in the structure** *Deficient diversional activity* *Delayed surgical recovery*

Index

A

Abdominal incision, impaired skin integrity related to, 637-639

Abortion, 874

Abruptio placentae, 874

Accidental injury, posttrauma syndrome related to, 258-260

Acoustic neuroma, 874

Acquired immunodeficiency syndrome, 874-875

Activity and exercise pattern, Gordon's, 941-942

nursing diagnoses and, 944-945

Activity intolerance

related to generalized weakness, 648-650

related to imbalance between oxygen supply and demand, 2-4

related to immobility, 4-6

risk for, related to presence of circulatory or respiratory problems, 6-8

Activity level, constipation related to, 661-664

Acute renal failure, 875

Acute respiratory distress syndrome, 875-876

Acute respiratory failure, 876

Admission, relocation stress syndrome related to, 273-275

Adrenal insufficiency, 876-877

Adrenocortical insufficiency, 877

Aerobic exercise, absence of, health-seeking behaviors related to, 842-844

Affective disorders, 877

Age-related changes, ineffective sexuality patterns related to, 715-716

Aging process

disturbed auditory sensory perception related to, 710-712

disturbed visual sensory perception related to, 713-714

risk for impaired skin integrity related to, 717-719

Airway clearance, ineffective, related to retained secretions, 9-11

Alcohol abuse among teenagers, ineffective community therapeutic regimen management related to, 818-820

Alcohol addiction and abuse, 877

Allergy response to latex

related to absent immune system response, 11-14

risk for, 14-16

Alveolar-capillary changes, impaired gas exchange related to, 134-136

Alzheimer's disease, 878

risk for caregiver role strain related to, 786-789

Americans with Disabilities Act, deficient knowledge related to, 807-809

Amniotic fluid embolism, 878

Amputation, 878-879

Amyotrophic lateral sclerosis, 879

Anaphylactic shock, 879

Anemias, 879-880

Angina pectoris, 880

Anorexia nervosa, 880

Antisocial behavior, risk for other-directed violence related to, 778-780

Antisocial personality disorder, 880

Anxiety

about aging, ineffective denial related to, 669-671

diarrhea related to, 96-98

ineffective denial related to, 92-94

insomnia related to, 189-191

predisposition for, complicated grieving related to, 141-143

related to environmental conflict, 730-732

related to hospitalization and birth process, 540-542

related to situational crisis, 16-19

related to terminal illness, 19-22

Anxiety disorder, 881

Aortic aneurysm, 881

Aortic insufficiency, 881

Aortic stenosis, 881

Appendicitis, 882

Arterial blood flow, reduced, ineffective peripheral tissue perfusion related to, 399-402

t refers to a table.

t refers to a table.

---

t refers to a table.

t refers to a table.

t refers to a table.

t refers to a table.

t refers to a table.

t refers to a table.

t refers to a table.

t refers to a table.

t refers to a table.

t refers to a table.

---

t refers to a table.

t refers to a table.

---

t refers to a table.

t refers to a table.

t refers to a table.